Cultures Covered in the Text

People of African American Heritage
The Amish
People of Appalachian Heritage
People of Arab Heritage
People of Chinese Heritage
People of Cuban Heritage
People of Filipino Heritage
People of French Canadian Heritage
People of Iranian Heritage
People of Irish Heritage
People of Italian Heritage
People of Japanese Heritage
People of Jewish Heritage
People of Korean Heritage
People of Mexican Heritage
Navajo Indians
People of Polish Heritage
People of Puerto Rican Heritage
People of Vietnamese Heritage

Cultures Covered on the CD-ROM

People of Baltic Heritage: Estonians, Latvians,
  and Lithuanians
People of Brazilian Heritage
People of Egyptian Heritage
People of German Heritage
People of Greek Heritage
People of Haitian Heritage
People of Hindu Heritage
People of Turkish Heritage

Transcultural Health Care

A Culturally Competent Approach

Second Edition

Larry D. Purnell, PhD, RN, FAAN

Professor
College of Health and Nursing Sciences
University of Delaware
Newark, Delaware

Betty J. Paulanka, EdD, RN

Professor and Dean
College of Health and Nursing Sciences
University of Delaware
Newark, Delaware

F.A. Davis Company • Philadelphia

F. A. Davis Company
1915 Arch Street
Philadelphia, PA 19103
www.fadavis.com

Printed in the United States of America

Last digit indicates print number: 10 9 8 7 6 5 4 3 2

Publisher, Nursing: Robert G. Martone
Developmental Editor: David Carroll
Cover Designer: Louis J. Forgione

As new scientific information becomes available through basic and clinical research, recommended treatments and drug therapies undergo changes. The author(s) and publisher have done everything possible to make this book accurate, up to date, and in accord with accepted standards at the time of publication. The author(s), editors, and publisher are not responsible for errors or omissions or for consequences from application of the book, and make no warranty, expressed or implied, in regard to the contents of the book. Any practice described in this book should be applied by the reader in accordance with professional standards of care used in regard to the unique circumstances that may apply in each situation. The reader is advised always to check product information (package inserts) for changes and new information regarding dose and contraindications before administering any drug. Caution is especially urged when using new or infrequently ordered drugs.

Library of Congress Cataloging-in-Publication Data

Transcultural health care: a culturally competent approach / [edited by] Larry D. Purnell,
Betty J. Paulanka – 2nd ed.
    p. cm.
    Includes bibliographical references and index.
    ISBN 0-8036-1057-2
    1. Transcultural medical care–United States. 2. Transcultural medical care–Canada. 3.
Minorities–Medical care–United States. 4. Minorities–Medical care–Canada. I. Purnell,
Larry D. II. Paulanka, Betty J.

RA418.5.T73T73 2003
362. 1'089–dc21
                                        2003040786

Preface

The Purnell Model for Cultural Competence and its accompanying organizing framework has been used in education, clinical practice, administration, and research, giving credence to its usefulness for health-care providers. The model and framework have been translated into Spanish, French, Flemish, and Korean. The first edition of this book is used in numerous associate degree, baccalaureate, master's, and doctoral nursing programs throughout the United States, Canada, and overseas, as well as in medical schools in the United States and overseas and in many cultural anthropology courses. Health-care organizations have adapted the organizing framework as a cultural assessment tool, and numerous students have used the Purnell Model to guide research for theses and dissertations. The model's usefulness has been established in the global arena, recognizing and including the client's culture in assessment, health-care planning, interventions, and evaluation.

The second edition of *Transcultural Health Care: A Culturally Competent Approach* has been revised based on responses from educators, students, and practicing health-care professionals—nurses, physicians, physical therapists, emergency medical technicians, and nutritionists, to name a few. Critical reviews by users of the first edition, which went through eight printings, have resulted in several changes in this second edition.

Chapter 1 has two important changes: (1) the assumptions upon which the Purnell Model for Cultural Competence is based, and (2) a more extensive description of the primary and secondary characteristics of culture that determine the degree to which people identify with their dominant cultural values, practices, and beliefs. Contributors have made a concerted effort to use nonstereotypical language when describing cultural attributes of specific cultures, recognizing that there are exceptions to every description provided, and that the differences within a cultural group may be greater than the diversity between and among different cultural groups. We have also tried to include both the sociological and anthropological perspectives of culture.

Another major change in the second edition is a greater focus on the dominant American culture, which has been integrated into Chapter 2 along with the description, constructs, and concepts related to the 12 domains of culture as identified in the Purnell Model for Cultural Competence. The impetus for this inclusion came in response to American professionals who felt they needed to have a better understanding of their own culture and to foreign graduates working in the United States who need to understand the dominant American culture and workforce. Another important change is the inclusion of cultural attributes of groups from a global perspective, because culture is not border specific. For example, people emigrating from Korea to the United States, Great Britain, Canada, or Central America bring the cultural values, traditions, and practices of their home country. Likewise, Americans who emigrate to another country continue to hold onto, sometimes tenaciously, their cultural attributes, regardless of where they relocate. Chapter 2 expands the description of the Purnell Model for Cultural Competence to include application of the domains and concepts of culture to the dominant American culture in a cross-cultural fashion. This edition includes an appendix of illnesses and diseases by heritage and country of origin. The glossary remains as it did in the first edition because users felt that it was helpful.

Given the world diversity and the diversity within cultural groups, it is impossible to cover each group more extensively. Space and cost concerns limit the number of chapters that can be included in the book; therefore, a CD-ROM is included which addresses additional cultural groups. In addition, the CD also includes a chapter devoted to teaching cultural diversity and additional case studies. Specific criteria were used for identifying the groups represented in the book and those included in electronic format. Groups included in the book were selected based on any of the six criteria that follow.

- The group has a large population in North America, such as people of Mexican, Irish, German, and African American heritage.

- The group is relatively new in its migration status, such as people of Vietnamese, Cuban, and Arab heritage.
- The group is widely dispersed throughout North America, such as people of Iranian, Italian, and Appalachian heritage.
- There is little written about the group in the health-care literature, such as people of Korean and Haitian heritage.
- The group holds significant disenfranchised status, such as people of Navajo heritage, a large American Indian group.
- The group was of particular interest to readers in the first edition, such as people of Amish heritage.

Many chapter authors come from the culture about which they write; others have extensive research or empirical experience with that particular cultural group. They write from the heart, empirical evidence, ethnographic research, and personal experience. A special thanks is extended to all of the authors, to the content reviewers, and to those who teach cultural content in colleges and health-care organizations.

Again, we have strived to portray each culture positively and without stereotyping. We hope you enjoy our book and are as excited about the content as we are.

LARRY D. PURNELL

BETTY J. PAULANKA

Acknowledgments

The editors would like to thank all those who helped in the preparation of the second edition of this book. We especially thank Robert Martone, publisher of nursing, F. A. Davis, for his enthusiasm and personal support of the project; and David Carroll, developmental editor, for his attention to detail, timeliness, sense of humor, and patience during the editing process. Additionally, we wish to thank all the contributing editors, consultants, and reviewers for their many helpful suggestions on multicultural health promotion and wellness and disease and illness-prevention strategies. We thank the copy editors at F. A. Davis for their assistance in ensuring that our ideas have been presented clearly and accurately. We thank Randee Roberts Tobin, secretary at the University of Delaware, for her assistance in bringing the book to completion. Most importantly, we want to thank the many multicultural populations and health professionals who are the impetus for this book. Finally, we thank our families, friends, and colleagues for their patience and support during the preparation of the book.

About the Contributors

CHAPTER 1   TRANSCULTURAL DIVERSITY AND HEALTH CARE

CHAPTER 2   THE PURNELL MODEL FOR CULTURAL COMPETENCE

Larry D. Purnell, PhD, RN, FAAN, is Professor, College of Health and Nursing Sciences, University of Delaware, in Newark, Delaware. He heads the MS and MSN degree programs in Health Services Administration and teaches courses in transcultural health care. Originally from Appalachia, Dr. Purnell has worked with Mexicans and Mexican Americans in Chicago, Delaware, and Maryland. Dr. Purnell's transcultural health-care experience spans the globe, including Africa, Australia, the Caribbean, Central America, China, Finland, Hong Kong, Korea, Great Britain, Mexico, Spain, Sweden, and South America.

Betty J. Paulanka, EdD, RN, is Professor and Dean, College of Health and Nursing Sciences, University of Delaware, in Newark, Delaware. She has fostered the development of international nursing courses in both the undergraduate and graduate health programs.

CHAPTER 3   PEOPLE OF AFRICAN AMERICAN HERITAGE

Cathryn L. Glanville, EdD, RN, CFLE, is Professor, Department of Nursing, Loyola University, New Orleans, Louisiana. She has completed research and publications on cultural diversity, race, and class conflict in the health-care workplace. Dr. Glanville has done consultation and written on working with undergraduate and graduate minority students in the academic environment.

The author wishes to thank Dr. Josepha Campinha-Bacote, who wrote this chapter in the first edition.

CHAPTER 4   THE AMISH

Anna Frances (Fran) Z. Wenger, PhD, RN, FAAN, is an Affiliate Faculty member at the Nell Hodgson Woodruff School of Nursing and a Senior Scholar at the Rollins School of Public Health, Emory University, Atlanta, Georgia

Marion R. Wenger, PhD, is a language and culture specialist, Stone Mountain, Georgia. Dr. Wenger has taught college German and linguistics in Indiana and Ohio, near two of the three largest Amish settlements. His doctoral dissertation was based on descriptive research into the German dialect stock, which provides the basis for the first language of most Amish. His views on Amish communication are drawn from personal observation and language teaching among the Amish.

CHAPTER 5   PEOPLE OF APPALACHIAN HERITAGE

Larry D. Purnell, PhD, RN, FAAN, is Professor, College of Health and Nursing Sciences, University of Delaware, Newark, Delaware. Dr. Purnell spent his formative years in northern Appalachia, where he lived with several families from differing socioeconomic backgrounds. He later returned to Appalachia, where he held positions in nursing service administration and nursing education.

The author wishes to thank Dr. Mona Counts, who assisted with this chapter in the first edition.

CHAPTER 6   PEOPLE OF ARAB HERITAGE

Anahid Dervartanian Kulwicki, DNS, RN, is Professor at Oakland University School of Nursing in Rochester, Michigan. She was the Research Director of several community-based health promotion and disease prevention programs at the Arab Community Center for Economic and Social Services in Dearborn. She has developed the first community-based Teen Health Center for Arab Americans in Dearborn. Dr. Kulwicki was a Fulbright Scholar in Jordan and a consultant in the area of Arab American health. Her presentations and publications have been in the areas of tobacco prevention and cessation, cardiovascular disease, HIV/AIDS, infant mortality, and domestic violence in the Arab American community. Dr. Kulwicki is fluent in Arabic, Armenian, and English. She emigrated from Lebanon in 1977.

The author wishes to thank Dr. Patricia Abu Gharbieh, who wrote this chapter in the first edition.

PEOPLE OF BALTIC HERITAGE: ESTONIANS, LATVIANS, AND LITHUANIANS (Chapter on CD)

Rauda Gelazis, PhD, RN, CS, CTN, is Associate Professor, Ursuline College, Pepper Pike, Ohio. Dr. Gelazis is a Lithuanian American who has done research on Lithuanian Americans and completed her doctoral dissertation on humor, care, and well-being in Lithuanian Americans. She has taught transcultural nursing and psychiatric mental health nursing for several years. She is an active member of the Lithuanian and Baltic communities in Cleveland, Ohio.

PEOPLE OF BRAZILIAN HERITAGE (Chapter on CD)

Larry D. Purnell

The author wishes to thank Marga Simon Coler, who wrote this chapter in the first edition.

CHAPTER 7   PEOPLE OF CHINESE HERITAGE

Yan Wang, MSN, RN, is Clinical Information Systems Administrator, Duke University Hospital and is an active member of American Nurses Association and Sigma Theta Tau International Honor Society of Nursing.

The author wishes to thank Dr. Linda Matocha, who wrote this chapter in the first edition.

CHAPTER 8   PEOPLE OF CUBAN HERITAGE

Larry D. Purnell

The author wishes to thank Dr. Divina Grossman, who wrote this chapter in the first edition.

PEOPLE OF EGYPTIAN HERITAGE (Chapter on CD)

Larry D. Purnell

The author wishes to thank Afaf I. Meleis and Mahmoud Meleis, who wrote this chapter in the first edition.

CHAPTER 9   PEOPLE OF FILIPINO HERITAGE

Dula F. Pacquiao, EdD, RN, CTN, is Professor of Nursing, Director of the Transcultural Nursing Institute, and Coordinator of the Graduate Nursing Program at Kean University in Union, New Jersey. She is Associate Editor of the *Journal of Transcultural Nursing* and President of the Transcultural Nursing Society. In 2000 she received the Leininger Award in recognition of her leadership in Transcultural Nursing. She is a former President of the Philippine Nurses Association in New Jersey, and a lifetime member of its

advisory board. Dr. Pacquiao is a transcultural nursing consultant and presenter who has published and conducted numerous research studies in cultural and transcultural issues.

The author wishes to thank Beatrice R. Miranda, Magelende R. McBride, and Zen Spangler, who wrote this chapter in the first edition.

CHAPTER 10   PEOPLE OF FRENCH CANADIAN HERITAGE

Ginette Coutu-Wakulczyk, PhD, RN, is Associate Professor, School of Nursing, Faculty of Health Sciences, University of Ottawa, Ontario, Canada. French Canadian, born of parents with a genealogy dating to the early settlers from France, Dr. Coutu-Wakulczyk was raised and educated in the French language from elementary school to the end of her graduate studies. Her cross-cultural experiences include overseas practice in Nigeria.

Denise Moreau, MSc, RN, PhD (candidate), is Assistant Professor Lecturer, School of Nursing, Faculty of Health Sciences, University of Ottawa, Ontario, Canada. A community nurse clinical specialist, she teaches maternity and child-care nursing.

Ann C. Beckingham, PhD, RN, is a retired Professor, School of Nursing, Faculty Health Sciences and Vice-Chair, Continuing Education, McMaster University, Hamilton, Ontario, Canada. With more than 20 years' experience in international health, she has been active with the World Health Organization in the Eastern Mediterranean, Southeast Asian, African, and European regions. In addition to her work with gerontology and community nursing, she has published widely and presented numerous papers, seminars, and workshops on cultural diversity.

PEOPLE OF GERMAN HERITAGE (Chapter on CD)

Jessica A. Steckler, MSN, RN, EdD (candidate), RNC, is Associate Director, Lake Area Health Education Center, Veterans Affairs Medical Center, Erie, Pennsylvania. She was born and raised in York County, Pennsylvania, and is a fifth-generation German American who grew up in a family that valued its German heritage and preserved its traditions. She has taught various levels of nursing and professional continuing education classes in the predominantly German communities of York and Erie, Pennsylvania.

PEOPLE OF GREEK HERITAGE (Chapter on CD)

Irena Papadopoulos, PhD, RN, is Co-coordinator for Nursing and Allied Subjects, Head of Research Center for Transcultural Studies in Health at Middlesex University, School of Health and Social Sciences, Middlesex University, Highgate, London. Dr. Papadopoulos has conducted research in Greek and Greek Cypriot communities in Greece and in Great Britain.

Larry D. Purnell

The authors wish to thank Toni Tripp-Reimer and Bernard Sorofman, who wrote this chapter in the first edition.

PEOPLE OF HAITIAN HERITAGE (Chapter on CD)

Jessie M. Colin, PhD, RN, is an Assistant Professor, Barry University School of Nursing, Miami Shores, Florida.

Ghislaine Paperwalla, BSN, RN, is a Research Nurse in Immunology at the Veterans Administration Medical Center in Miami, Florida. Born in Haiti, she immigrated to the United States in 1960. She received her nursing education at Laval University in Canada and at Florida International University. She is president of the Haitian-American Nurses Association of Florida and Vice President of the Haitian Health Foundation of South Florida.

PEOPLE OF HINDU HERITAGE (Chapter on CD)

Jayalakshmi Jambunathan, PhD, RN, RNC, is Professor, College of Nursing, and Director, CON Research Center, University of Wisconsin, Oshkosh Wisconsin. Born in India, she has resided in the United States for the last 25 years. Frequent visits to her homeland keep her current on Indian health care and health-care practices. Her area of cultural interest is the sociocultural factors affecting depression in Asian women.

CHAPTER 11   PEOPLE OF IRANIAN HERITAGE

Homeyra Hafizi, MS, RN, has 16 years of experience in nursing and has served in multiple capacities while in acute care settings ranging from staff nursing, supervision, and nursing administration. She currently works with Workers Compensation case management on the state and federal levels, occupational and environmental health, OSHA record keeping, performance improvement, health training, and corporate wellness promotion at Kennedy Space Center in Florida.

Juliene G. Lipson, PhD, RN, FAAN, a nurse-anthropologist, is a Professor in the Department of Community Health Systems, School of Nursing, University of California, San Francisco, where she teaches graduate students in community health and cross-cultural nursing. Since 1982, she has done research on the health and adjustment of immigrant and refugees to the United States from several Arab countries, Iran, Afghanistan, Bosnia, and the former Soviet Union. She is active in the Council on Nursing and Anthropology and the Council on Refugees and Immigrants in the American Anthropological Association and the Society for Applied Anthropology.

CHAPTER 12   PEOPLE OF IRISH HERITAGE

Sarah A. Wilson, PhD, RN, Associate Professor, Marquette University, College of Nursing, Milwaukee, Wisconsin is a nurse anthropologist. Her research interests are dying and death, and she is currently funded by National Institute on Aging to study cultural influences on dying and death in the African American community. Dr. Wilson teaches community health nursing and a course on culture and health. She is a first-generation Irish American.

CHAPTER 13   PEOPLE OF ITALIAN HERITAGE

Sandra M. Hillman, PhD, RN, is an Associate Professor of Nursing at Kennesaw State University, Kennesaw, Georgia. A second-generation American of Italian descent, she has taught nursing at the undergraduate and graduate levels since 1978. A nursing health professional for the past 31 years specializing in public and international health, she is also president of her own consulting company, Hillman Consulting International. She has incorporated alternative healing strategies into her nursing practice since the early 1980s and has presented programs on humor and health nationally and internationally. From 1989 to 1991 she worked in Bermuda as a consultant and developed the first comprehensive community-based case management program as well as the first inpatient hospice facility for AIDS and other terminally ill patients. Recently she has been involved in the development and implementation of an interdisciplinary course in Complementary Alternative Medicine at Kennesaw State University College of Health and Human Services.

CHAPTER 14   PEOPLE OF JAPANESE HERITAGE

Nancy C. Sharts-Hopko, PhD, RN, FAAN, is Professor, College of Nursing, Villanova University, Villanova, Pennsylvania. Dr. Sharts-Hopko served as an Overseas Associate, Presbyterian Church (U.S.A.) in Tokyo, Japan, for over two years, from 1984 to 1986. In that capacity, she worked at St. Luke's College of Nursing in Tokyo, where she provided counseling to women in the international community and conducted research on the childbearing experiences of American women in Japan. Dr. Sharts-Hopko continues to serve on the American Council for St. Luke's, Tokyo, a national committee associated with the Episcopal Church.

CHAPTER 15   PEOPLE OF JEWISH HERITAGE

Janice Selekman, DNSc, RN, is a Professor in the Department of Nursing, College of Health and Nursing Sciences, University of Delaware, Newark, Delaware.

CHAPTER 16   PEOPLE OF KOREAN HERITAGE

Larry D. Purnell

Susie Kim, PhD, RN, FAAN, is Professor and Director of the Nursing Research Institute, Ewha Woman's University in Seoul, Korea. A native Korean, she has spent considerable time in the United States.

The authors wish to thank Lauren Regan Sabat, who wrote this chapter in the first edition.

CHAPTER 17   PEOPLE OF MEXICAN HERITAGE

Richard Zoucha, DNSc, RN, APRN, BC, CTN, is an Associate Professor at Duquesne University, Pittsburgh, Pennsylvania. He is a Certified Transcultural Nurse and past president of the Transcultural Nursing Society.

Larry D. Purnell

CHAPTER 18   NAVAJO INDIANS

Olivia Still, PhD, RN, is Staff Development and Clinical Education Department Director, Indian Health Service, Shiprock, New Mexico. A native of the Cherokee Indian tribe, she has lived on both Navajo and Zuni Indian reservations.

David Hodgins, MSN, RN, CEN, is Director of the Emergency Room for the Indian Health Service, Shiprock, New Mexico. He has worked with Navajo and Hopi Indians. Half Navajo, he was raised as a Native American on the Hopi Reservation.

CHAPTER 19   PEOPLE OF POLISH HERITAGE

Martha A. From, EdD, RN, CRNP, is a geriatric nurse practitioner. Dr. From is a first-generation Polish American who grew up in a Polish Catholic farming community; she maintains her ethnic heritage by practicing Polish rituals and customs. Dr. From has spent time with relatives in Poland and is part of the Kosciuszko Founda-tion/UNICEF summer program, teaching English to high school students in Poland.

CHAPTER 20   PEOPLE OF PUERTO RICAN HERITAGE

Teresa C. Juarbe, PhD, RN, is a consultant in issues related to promotion of health among Latina women in the United States. She is a first-generation Puerto Rican, living in San Jose, California. She immigrated to the United States in 1983.

PEOPLE OF TURKISH HERITAGE (Chapter on CD)

Cara B. Towle, RN, MSN, MA, is Coordinator of International Clinical Programs, University of California–San Francisco Medical Center. She holds a master's degree in community health nursing administration, with an emphasis on international and cross-cultural nursing. Before entering the field of nursing, she earned a master's degree in international/intercultural administration and worked for several years as a foreign student advisor. She has lived in Turkey and is actively involved in the Turkish American community in California.

Timur Arslanoglu, BSME, CVT, MSBA (candidate), has worked as a business consultant for the medical community in the United States and in Turkey. He has served as president of the Turkish-American Association of Northern California. Currently, he is collaborating on a cardiovascular research project in Turkey for the Gladstone Institute at the University of California–San Francisco.

CHAPTER 21   PEOPLE OF VIETNAMESE HERITAGE

Thu T. Nowak, BSN, RN, a native of Vietnam, came to the United States in 1970 and pursued her education in nursing at George Mason University. Her career in hospital, community health, and home care has emphasized the application of transcultural health-care principles to minority and refugee populations. She is currently a nurse in the Fairfax County Virginia Health Department. She practices alternative medicine and nursing and teaches meditation principles in both the United States and in Vietnam.

The author wishes to thank Ronald M. Nowak, PhD, who assisted in the preparation of the manuscript for this chapter.

Contributors to the First Edition

Consultants
for the Second
Edition

Caroline Camunas, EdD, RN
Professor
Columbia Teacher's College
New York, New York

Lydia DeSantis, RN, PhD, FAAN
Professor
University of Miami
Coral Gables, Florida

Carol Holtz, PhD, RN
Assistant Professor
Kennesaw State University
Kennesaw, Georgia

Suzan E. Karoong-Edgren, MS, RNC, FACCE
Clinical Instructor
University of Texas at Arlington
Arlington, Texas

Connie Vance, EdD, RN, FAAN
Professor
College of New Rochelle
New Rochelle, New York

Diane Weiland, PhD, RN, CS
Assistant Professor
LaSalle University
Philadelphia, Pennsylvania

Contents

Contents for the CD-ROM

Introduction

Worldwide, health-care providers and organizations have embraced the concepts of culturally specific care. Increasingly, educational and service organizations have seen the need to prepare students and staff to provide culturally sensitive and culturally competent care to individuals, families, and communities—care that reflects the unique understanding of the values of racially and culturally diverse populations and individual acculturation patterns. The Joint Commission on Accreditation of Healthcare Organizations, insurance companies, and the federal government with its Cultural and Linguistic Appropriate Services (CLAS Project) have also helped accelerate the people's recognition of the value of culturally competent health-care services. The National Certification Licensing Examinations (NCLEX) for registered nurses and practical nurses have included questions on culture. This change has stimulated nursing programs to address cultural issues in curricula.

Culture has powerful influences on one's interpretation of, and responses to, health care. Clients and staff have the right to be understood, respected, and treated as individuals regardless of their differences. In addition, they have a right to expect employers and health-care providers to realize that their unique perspectives on, and interpretations of, health are legitimate. Respect for such differences is demonstrated by incorporating traditional cultural practices for staying healthy into professional prescriptions and interventions. If clients and staff are forced to relinquish their personal ideologies and cultural beliefs, resentment, anger, and noncompliance may result. In some instances, if non-Western medicines and complementary therapies such as traditional Chinese and ayurvedic medicine, acupressure, acumassage, acupuncture, reflexology, rolfing, moxibustion, cupping, and herbal therapies are not incorporated into health-care regimens, prescribed interventions may be ignored. In some cultures, lay and traditional healers are preferred over Western professional caregivers. These wishes must be respected and incorporated when feasible.

Valuing diversity in health care enhances the delivery and effectiveness of care, both physically and symbolically. Health-care providers need to address their personal views of traditional values, including biases and prejudices about other cultures and ethnic groups. Teaching diversity increases the students' sophistication and understanding of the world in which they live. Educators can improve instruction related to diversity by first determining students' knowledge and perceptions of their own cultures as well as those of other ethnocultural groups. Correcting misconceptions is essential so that prescriptions do not interfere with learning. Allowing students to see the world differently helps them to develop more creative solutions to simple as well as complex problems. Moreover, multicultural education is an important aspect of personal and professional development.

Cultural general knowledge provides a framework with which providers can assess multicultural populations. Health-care providers who have specific cultural knowledge can maximize therapeutic interventions by becoming co-participants and client advocates in diverse health-care settings. The challenge for health-care providers is to understand clients' perspectives. This approach requires that health-care providers develop an open style of communication, be receptive to learning from multicultural clients, and demonstrate tolerance for ambiguities inherent in cultural norms, which evolve and are, thus, continually changing. Whereas many cultural characteristics are readily apparent, others are less obvious and need conscious exploration.

Although physicians, nurses, social workers, nutritionists, technicians, therapists, home health aides, and other health-care providers need similar culturally specific information, the manner in which the information is used differs according to the caregiver's profession, individual experiences, and specific circumstances.

Leadership is a key factor in promoting effective multicultural relationships. Leaders influence policy and practice, create organizational cultures, and set the tone for cultural competence and sensitivity. Leaders must be role models of holistic health care through their interactions with consumers and staff members. Administrative and managerial staff who receive cultural training should be viewed as educational resources for other staff members.

Cultural diversity permeates most societies throughout the world and has often provided causes for concern. Benjamin Franklin addressed cultural differences and values from North America in his account of a short dialogue (Kronenberger, 1970) that took place over 200 years ago between two distinct cultural groups who failed to understand the other's attitudes, beliefs, values, and lifestyle.

> At the treaty of Lancaster, in Pennsylvania, anno 1744, between the Government of Virginia and the Six Nations, the commissioners from Virginia acquainted the Indians by a speech, that there was at Williamsburg a college with a fund for educating youth, and that if the chiefs of the Six Nations would send down half a dozen of their sons to that college, the government would take care that they be well provided for, and instructed in all the learning of the white people.

The Indians' Spokesman replied:

> . . . We are convinced . . . that you mean to do us good by your proposal and we thank you heartily. But you, who are wise, must know that different nations have different conceptions of things; and you will not therefore take it amiss, if our ideals of this kind of education happen not to be the same as yours. We have some experience of it; several of our young people were formerly brought up at the colleges of northern provinces; they came back to us; they were bad runners, ignorant of every means of living in the woods, unable to bear either cold or hunger, knew neither how to build a cabin, take a deer, nor kill an enemy, spoke our language imperfectly, were therefore neither fit for hunters, warriors, nor counselors; they were totally good for nothing.
>
> We are however not the less obligated by your kind offer, though we decline accepting it; and, to show our grateful sense of it, if the gentlemen of Virginia will send us a dozen of their sons, we will take care of their education, instruct them in all we know, and make men of them. (pp. 5–6)

Similar experiences have occurred over millennia, continue today, and will continue into the future if people are not willing to take the time and communicate their individual belief systems. Without this willingness to communicate and understand one another's culture, mutually satisfying relationships are hindered. Lack of communication can threaten the quality of health care provided in a multicultural setting.

This textbook presents a framework for collecting health data about individuals or groups from diverse cultural backgrounds in a nonjudgmental way; this assists health-care providers in delivering competently conscious, congruent, and relevant care in diverse settings. We have attempted to support information with current research where available. However, there continues to be a paucity of literature on specific ethnocultural groups so chapter authors have supplemented the information on the group with their own empirical evidence of the group.

The book is divided into 21 chapters. Chapter 1 provides an overview of culture and ethnicity and defines terms commonly used in the study of culture. Chapter 2 introduces and explains The Purnell Model for Cultural Competence and its organizing framework. Chapters 3 through 21 describe the health-care needs and practices of specific ethnic and cultural groups. The authors and editors are fully cognizant that there are individual exceptions for every description. Given the diversity within cultural groups, it is impossible to describe the attributes of every individual within his or her cultural group. The descriptions are intended as general attributes, and cannot be uniformly applied to all members of the group being discussed. The primary and secondary characteristics of culture, as described in Chapter 1, are just a few reasons that people vary from their dominant culture.

The chapters are organized alphabetically by cultural group, and the format of each chapter follows The Purnell Model for Cultural Competence. Each chapter has pictures or graphics representative of the culture, a cultural case study, and a reference list. The book concludes with a glossary incorporating key terms that appear in each chapter and on the accompanying CD-ROM. The culturally specific chapters on the CD follow the same format of those in the book. A subject index to this text is provided for easy reference.

Reference

Kronenberger, L. (1970). *The cutting edge*. Garden City, NY: Doubleday & Co.

Chapter 1

Transcultural Diversity and Health Care

LARRY D. PURNELL and BETTY J. PAULANKA*

The Need for Culturally Competent Health Care

Diversity has emerged as a major issue for business, health care, and educational organizations. The world is a sea of people on the move. Visit an international airport any place in the world and you will see a host of people from many ethnic and cultural backgrounds boarding airplanes for a variety of reasons. People from Bangladesh are moving to England, people from Pakistan are moving to Scotland, Chinese and Central Americans are moving to the Untied States, Spanish are moving to Argentina, and Arabs are moving to Canada, to name a few. Others are on their way to visit relatives who have already relocated. However, most are probably on business or vacation, or on temporary educational or work assignments. Unfortunately, a few will need health care while they are away from their home country. Whether they are immigrants or vacationers, they have the right to expect health-care providers to respect their personal beliefs and health-care practices. They will need culturally sensitive and culturally competent health care.

Diversity is not always apparent. People may wear the same brand and style of clothes, drive the same make of automobile, and watch the same television shows but still be worlds apart in cultural and ethnic backgrounds that define their basic heritage and values. The more dissimilar in appearance individuals are, the easier it becomes for others to realize that they may have differing beliefs, attitudes, and ideologies. Unfortunately, this observation does not necessarily enhance better acceptance of individual differences. Increased similarity in the appearance of culturally diverse individuals challenges others to be more consciously aware of differences underlying ethnocultural diversity.

The mass media, professional organizations, the workplace, and educational institutions from elementary schools to colleges and universities have addressed the need for individuals to understand and become sensitive to cultural diversity. Health-care personnel provide care to people of diverse cultures in numerous settings. Long-term-care facilities, acute-care facilities, clinics, communities, and clients' homes are common examples of settings where health-care providers encounter culturally diverse clients and staff. Although physicians, nurses, nutritionists, therapists, technicians, morticians, home health aides, and other caregivers need similar culturally specific information, the manner in which the information is used may differ significantly based on the discipline, individual experiences, and specific circumstances of the client. Each discipline has its own unique knowledge base to support its ways of knowing, techniques, roles, norms, values, ideologies, attitudes, and beliefs, which interlock to make a reinforced and supportive system within its defined practice. Thus, an understanding of ethnocultural diversity is essential for all health-care providers.

Before the 1960s, many health-care facilities and places of business openly discriminated against people of color and selected ethnic backgrounds. Organizational practices of discrimination often segregated these ethnic groups into separate settings or locations. After the civil rights movement of the 1960s, a surge of individual and political support developed for treating all people equally regardless of their color, race, ethnicity, culture, religion,

*The authors would like to acknowledge the contribution of Caroline Camunas to the section on ethics in this chapter.

1

gender, disabilities, and, more recently, sexual orientation. Today, each subgroup has the right to be respected for its unique individuality.

Organizations and individuals who understand their clients' cultural values, beliefs, and practices are in a better position to be coparticipants with their clients and provide culturally acceptable care. Accordingly, there will be improved opportunities for health promotion, illness and disease prevention, and health restoration. To this end, health-care providers need both general and specific cultural knowledge.

Diversity in the World and in the United States

The world's population reached 6.1 billion people in the year 2000 and is expected to approach 7.6 billion by 2020. By the year 2050, the estimated population will be 9.3 billion, an increase of 3.2 billion, or approximately 30 percent from the present day. The percent increase in world population has steadily decreased from 22 percent in 1960 to the present 12.6 percent. This trend is expected to continue to decrease to 5.6 percent by the year 2050. Asia has 3.6 billion people, Africa has 770 million, Europe and Latin America each have 507 million people, and North America has 301 million, with most of these living in the United States. A significant number of immigrants to the United States and Canada come from the world's most populous countries: China, India, Indonesia, Brazil, Russia, Pakistan, Bangladesh, Japan, Nigeria, Mexico, Germany, the Philippines, Vietnam, Egypt, Turkey, Iran, Ethiopia, Thailand, and the United Kingdom. Twenty-one of the world's 50 largest cities are located in Asia (*http://www.infoplease.com*, 2001).

Between 1990 and 2000, the U.S. population increased from 248.7 million to 281.4 million. Population growth varied significantly in the last decade, with higher rates in the West (19.7 percent), and South (17.3 percent) (American Factfinder, 2001). Of the people reporting in this census, 75.1 percent are white, 12.5 percent are Spanish/Hispanic/Latino (of any race), 12.3 percent are black or African American, 0.9 percent are American Indian or Alaskan Native, 3.6 percent are Asian, 0.1 percent are Native Hawaiian or other Pacific Islander, 5.5 percent are some other race, and 2.4 percent are of two or more races. Please note: The figures above total more than 100 percent because the federal government considers race and Hispanic origin to be two separate and distinct categories. Race categories as used in Census 2000 are:

1 *White* refers to people having origins in any of the original peoples of Europe, the Near East, and the Middle East, or North Africa. This category includes Irish, German, Italian, Lebanese, Turkish, Arab, and Polish.

2 *Black* or *African American* refers to people having origins in any of the black racial groups of Africa, and includes Nigerians and Haitians or any person who self-designated this category regardless of origin.

3 *American Indian* and *Alaskan Native* refer to people having origins in any of the original peoples of North, South, or Central America, and who maintain tribal affiliation or community attachment.

4 *Asian* refers to people having origins in any of the original peoples of the Far East, Southeast Asia, or the Indian subcontinent. This category includes the terms Asian Indian, Chinese, Filipino, Korean, Japanese, Vietnamese, Burmese, Hmong, Pakistani, and Thai.

5 *Native Hawaiian* and *other Pacific Islander* refers to people having origins in any of the original peoples of Hawaii, Guam, Samoa, Tahiti, the Mariana Islands, and Chuuk.

6 *"Some other race"* was included for people who are unable to identify with the other categories. Additionally, the respondent could identify, as a write-in, with two races (*http://www.census.gov*, 2001).

Over the last decade, the Spanish/Hispanic/Latino population rose from 22.4 million to 35.3 million, an increase of 57.9 percent. Of these, most are Mexicans, followed by Puerto Ricans, Cubans, Central Americans, South Americans, and lastly Dominicans. Salvadorans are the largest group from Central America. Three-quarters of the Hispanics live in the West or South, with 50 percent of the Hispanics living in just two states, California and Texas. It is interesting to note that the median age for the entire U.S. population is 35.3 years, while the median age for Hispanics is 25.9 years (*http://www.census.gov*, 2001). The young age of Hispanics in the United States makes them ideal candidates for recruitment into the health professions, an area with crisis-level shortages of personnel, especially of minority representation.

Before 1940, most immigrants to the United States came from Europe, especially Germany, the United Kingdom, Ireland, the former Union of Soviet Socialist Republics, Latvia, Austria, and Hungary. Since 1940, immigration patterns to the United States have changed: Most are from Mexico, the Philippines, China, India, Brazil, Russia, Pakistan, Japan, Turkey, Egypt, and Thailand. People from each of these countries bring their own culture with them and increase the cultural mosaic of the United States. Many of these groups have strong ethnic identities and maintain their values, beliefs, practices, and languages long after their arrival. Individuals who speak only their indigenous language are more likely to adhere to traditional practices and live in ethnic enclaves and are less likely to assimilate into their new society. The inability of immigrants to speak the language of their new country creates additional challenges for health-care providers working with these populations.

Native Americans, immigrants, and their descendants have transformed the United States into the world's most powerful nation. North America is increasingly becoming a mosaic of many cultures, reflecting a mixture of ideologies, beliefs, and health-care practices. As society has become more diverse, learning about and developing an awareness of cultural and ethnic differences is more important than ever for health-care providers.

Self-Awareness and Health Professionals

Culture has a powerful unconscious impact on health professionals. Each individual health-care provider adds a new and unique dimension to the complexity of providing culturally competent care. The way health-care providers perceive themselves as competent providers is often reflected in the way they communicate with clients. Thus, it is essential for health professionals to take time to think about themselves, their behaviors, and their communication styles in relation to their perceptions of culture. They should also examine the impact they have on others, including clients, who are culturally diverse (Ens, 1999). Before addressing the multicultural backgrounds and unique individual perspectives of each client, health-care professionals must first address their own personal and professional knowledge, values, beliefs, ethics, and life experiences in a manner that optimizes interactions and assessment of culturally diverse clients (Mattson, 2000).

Many trainers of cultural competence believe that the best way to meet the various needs of individual health-care professionals is to promote a high level of self-awareness, knowledge, skills, and a level of professional maturity that fosters the use of effective communication in diversity situations (Anand, 1997). According to Cook (1999), many of these beliefs are based on the assumption that in order to provide optimal care for others, one must first understand oneself. Self-knowledge and understanding promote strong professional perceptions that free health-care professionals from prejudice and allow them to interact with others in a manner that preserves personal integrity and respects uniqueness and differences among individual clients.

The process of professional development and diversity competence begins with self-awareness, sometimes referred to as self-exploration. While the literature provides numerous definitions of self-awareness, there is minimal discussion of research integrating the concept of self-awareness with multicultural competence. Many theorists and diversity trainers imply that self-examination or awareness of personal prejudices and biases is an important step in the cognitive process of developing cultural competence (Anand, 1997; Andrews & Boyle, 1999; Campinha-Bacote, 1998; Giger & Davidhizar, 1999); however, discussions of emotional feelings elicited by this cognitive awareness are somewhat limited given the potential impact of emotions and conscious feelings on behavioral outcomes.

Self-awareness in cultural competence is defined as a deliberate and conscious cognitive and emotional process of getting to know yourself: your personality, your values, your beliefs, your professional knowledge standards, your ethics, and the impact of these factors on the various roles you play when interacting with individuals who are different from yourself. The ability to understand oneself sets the stage for integrating new knowledge related to cultural differences into the professional's knowledge base and perceptions of health interventions.

Cultural Concepts and Essential Terminology

ATTITUDE, BELIEF, AND IDEOLOGY

The definition of culture includes the terms attitude, belief, and ideology. **Attitude** is a state of mind or feeling about some matter of a culture. Attitudes are learned; for example, some people think that one culture is better than another culture. A **belief** is something that is accepted as true, especially as a tenet or a body of tenets accepted by people in an ethnocultural group. A belief among cultures is that if a pregnant woman craves a particular food substance, strawberries, for example, and does not satisfy the craving, the baby will be born with a birthmark in the shape of the craving. Attitudes and beliefs do not have to be proven; they are unconsciously accepted as truths. **Ideology** consists of the thoughts and beliefs that reflect the social needs and aspirations of an individual or an ethnocultural group. For example, some people believe that health care is a right of all people, while others see health care as a privilege.

Anthropologists and sociologists have proposed many definitions of **culture.** For the purposes of this book, culture is defined as the totality of socially transmitted behavioral patterns, arts, beliefs, values, customs, lifeways, and all other products of human work and thought characteristics of a population of people that guide their worldview and decision making.

These patterns may be explicit or implicit, are primarily learned and transmitted within the family, are shared by most members of the culture, and are emergent phenomena that change in response to global phenomena. Culture is largely unconscious and has powerful influences on health and illness. Health-care providers must recognize, respect, and integrate clients' cultural beliefs and practices into health prescriptions.

When individuals of dissimilar cultural orientations meet in a work or therapeutic environment, the likelihood for developing a mutually satisfying relationship is improved if both parties in the relationship attempt to learn about each other's culture. The literature reports many definitions for the terms **cultural awareness, cultural sensitivity,** and **cultural competence**. Sometimes these definitions are used interchangeably. However, cultural awareness has more to do with an appreciation of the external signs of diversity, such as arts, music, dress, and physical characteristics. Cultural sensitivity has more to do with personal attitudes and not saying things that might be offensive to someone from a cultural or ethnic background different from the health-care provider's. Increasing one's consciousness of cultural diversity improves the possibilities for health-care practitioners to provide culturally competent care. Cultural competence, as used in this book, means:

1 Developing an awareness of one's own existence, sensations, thoughts, and environment without letting it have an undue influence on those from other backgrounds.

2 Demonstrating knowledge and understanding of the client's culture, health-related needs, and meanings of health and illness.

3 Accepting and respecting cultural differences.

4 Not assuming that the health-care provider's beliefs and values are the same as the client's.

5 Resisting judgmental attitudes such as "different is not as good."

6 Being open to cultural encounters.

7 Adapting care to be congruent with the client's culture. Cultural competence is a conscious process and not necessarily linear.

Several things must be in place if an organization is to demonstrate cultural competence. The organization must have a mission statement and policies that address diversity. Additionally, diversity must be addressed as part of new employees' orientation, in-service, and continuing-education programs. All employees must be offered general cultural topics and culturally specific needs of populations for whom they provide care. There must be mechanisms in place for translation of written materials and for interpretation services.

One progresses from unconscious incompetence (not being aware that one is lacking knowledge about another culture), to conscious incompetence (being aware that one is lacking knowledge about another culture), to conscious competence (learning about the client's culture, verifying generalizations about the client's culture, and providing culturally specific interventions), and finally, to unconscious competence (automatically providing culturally congruent care to clients of diverse cultures). Unconscious competence is difficult to accomplish and potentially dangerous because individual differences exist within specific cultural groups. To be even minimally effective, culturally competent care must have the assurance of continuation after the original impetus is withdrawn; it must be integrated into, and valued by, the culture that is to benefit from the interventions.

Developing mutually satisfying relationships with diverse cultural groups involves good interpersonal skills and the application of knowledge and techniques learned from the physical, biologic, and social sciences, as well as the humanities. An understanding of one's own culture and personal values, and the ability to detach oneself from "excess baggage" associated with personal views, are essential to cultural competence. Even then, traces of ethnocentrism may unconsciously pervade one's attitudes and behavior. **Ethnocentrism,** the universal tendency of human beings to think that their ways of thinking, acting, and believing are the only right, proper, and natural ways, can be a major barrier to providing culturally competent care. Ethnocentrism perpetuates an attitude in which beliefs that differ greatly from one's own are strange, bizarre, or unenlightened and, therefore, wrong. **Values** are principles and standards that have meaning and worth to an individual, family, group, or community. The extent to which one's cultural values are internalized influences the tendency toward ethnocentrism. The more one's values are internalized, the more difficult it is to avoid the tendency toward ethnocentrism.

The Human Genome Project provides evidence that all human beings share a genetic code that is over 99 percent identical. However, the controversial term **race** must still be addressed when learning about culture. Race is genetic in origin and includes physical characteristics that are similar among members of the group, such as skin color, blood type, and hair and eye color. Although there is less than 1 percent difference, this difference is significant when conducting physical assessments and prescribing medication, as outlined in culturally specific chapters that follow. People from a given racial group may, but do not necessarily, share a common culture. Culture is learned first in the family, then in school, then in the community and other social organizations.

WORLDVIEW, SUBCULTURES, AND ETHNICITY

Worldview is the way individuals or groups of people look at the universe to form values about their lives and the world around them. Worldview includes cosmology, relationships with nature, moral and ethical reasoning, social relationships, magicoreligious beliefs, and aesthetics.

Any **generalization** made about the behaviors of any individual or large group of people is almost certain to be an oversimplification. When a generalization relates less to the actual observed behavior than to the motives thought to underlie the behavior (that is, the *why* of the behavior), it is likely to be oversimplified. Thus, generalizations can lead to **stereotyping,** an oversimplified conception, opinion, or belief about some aspect of an individual or group of people. However, there is value in being able to make generalizations about cultural groups so that the health-care provider knows what questions to ask. For example, knowing if the person comes from an **individualistic** versus a **collectivistic** culture is important. People identifying with a collectivist culture, such as most Asians, are more likely to place a higher value on the family than on the individual. However, people who identify with an individualistic culture, such as the dominant American culture, are more likely to place a higher value on the individual than on the family or the community.

Within all cultures are subcultures and ethnic groups that may not hold all the values of their dominant culture. **Subcultures, ethnic** groups, or **ethnocultural** populations are groups of people who have experiences different from those of the dominant culture. Some of these differences may include socioeconomic status, ethnic background, residence, religion, education, or other factors that functionally unify the group and act collectively on each member with a conscious awareness of these differences. Subcultures differ from the dominant ethnic group and share beliefs according to the primary and secondary characteristics of culture.

Primary and Secondary Characteristics of Culture

Major influences that shape peoples' worldview and the degree to which they identify with their cultural group of origin are called the primary and secondary characteristics of culture. The **primary characteristics** are nationality, race, color, gender, age, and religious affiliation. For example, take two people: one is a 75-year-old orthodox Jewish woman from Israel; the other is a 19-year-old African American fundamentalist Baptist man from Louisiana. Obviously, the two do not look alike, and they probably have very different worldviews and beliefs.

The **secondary characteristics** include educational status, socioeconomic status, occupation, military experience, political beliefs, urban versus rural residence, enclave identity, marital status, parental status, physical characteristics, sexual orientation, gender issues, reason for migration (sojourner, immigrant, or undocumented status), and length of time away from the country of origin. For example, a single lesbian urban business executive will most likely have a different worldview from a married heterosexual rural waitress who has two teenagers. In another case, a migrant farmworker from the highlands of Guatemala, who has an undocumented status, will have a different perspective than an immigrant from Mexico who has lived in New York City for 10 years. People who live in ethnic enclaves and get their work, shopping, and business needs met without learning the language and customs of their host country may be more traditional than people in their home country. Such was the case for a Japanese man who lived in a Japanese ethnic enclave in San Francisco. When he returned to Japan after 20 years to visit relatives, he was criticized for being too traditional. Japanese society had changed, while he had not.

Immigration status influences a person's worldview. For example, people who voluntarily immigrate generally **acculturate** more willingly; that is, they modify their own culture as a result of contact with another culture. Similarly, they **assimilate,** that is, gradually adopt and incorporate the characteristics of the prevailing culture more easily than people who immigrate unwillingly or as sojourners. **Sojourners,** who immigrate with the intention of remaining in their new homeland only a short time, or **refugees,** who think they may return to their home country, may not need to acculturate or assimilate. Additionally, undocumented individuals (illegal aliens) may have a different worldview from those who have arrived legally with work visas or as "legal immigrants."

Transcultural Health Care

The debate regarding the precise definition of the terms **transcultural, crosscultural,** and **intercultural** continues. Many authors and texts define the terms differently. This book uses the terms interchangeably to mean "crossing," "spanning," or "interacting" with a culture other than one's own. When people interact with individuals whose cultures are different from their own, they are engaged in **cultural diversity.** Awareness of the differences and similarities among ethnocultural groups results in a broadened multicultural worldview.

Ethics across Cultures

As globalization grows and population diversity with nations increases, health-care providers are increasingly confronted with ethical issues related to cultural diversity. These are very different issues. At the extremes stand those who favor multiculturalism and **postmodernism** versus those who favor **humanism.** Within the United States, multiculturalism has the universalistic demand that all groups should be recognized (Glazer, 1997). Internationally, multiculturalism asserts that there are no common moral principles shared by all cultures; postmodernism asserts a similar claim against all universal standards, both moral and nonmoral. Postmodernism holds the stance that everything is social construction, which leads to the contention that context is all-important (Baker, 1998). The concern is that universal standards provide a disguise while dominant cultures destroy or eradicate traditional cultures.

Humanism asserts that all human beings are equal in worth, that they have common resources and problems, and that they are alike in fundamental ways (Macklin, 1999). Humanism does not put aside the many circumstances that make individuals' lives different around the world. Many similarities exist as to what people need to live well. Humanism says that there are human rights that should not be violated. Macklin (1998) asserts that universal applicability of moral principles is required, not universal acceptability. Beaucamp (1998) concurs that fundamental principles of morality and human rights allow for cross-cultural judgments of immoral conduct. Of course, there is a middle ground.

Throughout the world, practices are claimed to be cultural, traditional, and beneficial, even when they are exploitive and harmful. For example, the practice of female circumcision, a traditional cultural practice, is seen by some as exploiting women. In many cases, the practice is harmful and can even lead to death. While empirical anthropologic research has shown that different cultures and historical eras contain different moral beliefs and practices, it is far from certain that what is right or wrong can be determined only by the beliefs and practices within a particular culture or subculture. Slavery and apartheid are examples of civil rights violations.

Accordingly, codes of ethics are open to interpretation and are not value-free. Furthermore, ethics belong to the society, not to professional groups. Ethics and ethical decision making are culturally bound. The Western ethical principles of patient autonomy, self-determination, justice, do no harm, truth telling, and promise keeping are not interpreted or shared by many non-Western societies. For example, advance directives give patients the opportunity to decide about their care, and staff members are required to ask patients about this upon admission to a health-care facility. **Western ethics,** with its stress on individualism, asks this question directly of the patient. However, in collectivist societies, such as among ethnic Chinese and Japanese, the preferred person to ask is a family member. In most collectivist societies, a person does not stand alone, but rather is defined in relation to another unit, such as the family. Additionally, translating these forms into another language can be troublesome because a direct translation can be confusing. For example, "informed consent" may be translated to mean that the person relinquishes his or her right to decision making.

Likewise, truth telling is culture-bound. Even in Western cultures that espouse "complete truth telling," truth telling is sometimes tempered under a disguise of civility, such as when someone asks "How do you like my new hair style?" The socially acceptable answer may be less than truthful. However, in health-care decision making, the provider is expected to be completely truthful. For example, an ethical dilemma occurred with a 64-year-old man of German ancestry, who was diagnosed with terminal cancer. The family and patient agreed to his placement in a "long-term-care facility." When the nurse approached the patient about his diagnoses, a necessary policy dictated by the hospice for placement, he refused to acknowledge his terminal diagnosis. He was aware that there would be no "resuscitation" at the long-term-care facility, but he refused to say the word "hospice." This created an ethical dilemma for the nurse, who wanted to do the best for her patient and still follow agency policy. The nurse completed the paperwork that indicated the patient knew his terminal diagnosis. A similar situation could occur with clients of other heritages as well, such as Asian Indians who believe that if you tell a patient that he or she has a terminal diagnosis, it causes the patient to give up hope.

Other cultural situations occur that raise legal issues. For instance, in Western societies, a competent person (or an alternative such as the spouse, if the person is married) is supposed to sign his or her own consent for medical procedures. However, in some cultures, the eldest son is expected to sign consent forms, not the spouse. In this case, both the organization and the family can be satisfied if both the spouse and the son sign the informed consent.

Instead of Western ethics prevailing, some authorities advocate for **universal ethics**. Each culture has its own definition of what is right or wrong and what is good or bad. Accordingly, some health-care providers encourage international codes of ethics, such as those developed by the International Council of Nurses. These codes are intended to reflect the patient's culture and whether the value is placed on individualism or collectivism. Most Western codes of ethics have interpretative statements based on the Western value of individualism. International codes of ethics do not contain interpretative statements, but rather let each culture interpret them according to their culture. As our multicultural society increases its diversity, health-care providers need to rely upon ethics committees that include members from the cultures they serve.

As the globalization of health-care services increases, providers must also address very crucial issues such as cultural imperialism, cultural relativism, and cultural imposition. **Cultural imperialism** is the practice of extending the policies and practices of one group (usually the dominant one) to disenfranchised and minority groups. An example is the U.S. government's forced migration of Native-American tribes to reservations with individual allotments of lands instead of group ownership, as well as forced attendance of children at white people's boarding schools. Proponents of cultural imperialism appeal to universal human rights values and standards.

Cultural relativism is the belief that the behaviors and practices of people should be judged only from the context of their cultural system. Proponents of cultural relativism argue that issues such as abortion, euthanasia, female circumcision, and physical punishment in child rearing should be accepted as cultural values without judgment from the outside world. Opponents argue that cultural relativism may undermine condemnation of human rights violations, and family violence cannot be justified or excused on a cultural basis.

Cultural imposition is the intrusive application of the majority group's cultural view upon individuals and families (Declaration of Human Rights, 2001). Prescription of special diets without regard to clients' cultures and limiting visitors to immediate family, a practice of many acute-care facilities, border on cultural imposition.

Female genital mutilation (FGM) has been discussed frequently. An estimated 100 to 132 million girls and women have been subjected to FGM worldwide, with an estimate of 2 million more annually (United Nations, 2000). Many die from hemorrhage or infection or suffer lifelong and life-threatening health problems. FGM is illegal in most countries where it is practiced, including the United States. The threat of FGM is sufficient for the U.S. Immigration and Naturalization Service to grant political asylum to girls and women seeking it. Those who argue for the procedure claim that keeping the tradition of FGM is valuable and important. Since FGM is predominantly practiced in certain cultures, and is relatively geographically contained, it should be less difficult to eradicate than women's hunger (Nussbaum, 1999).

Health-care professionals must be cautious about forcefully imposing their values regarding genetic testing and counseling. No group is spared from genetic disease. Ashkenazi Jews have been tested for Tay-Sachs disease for many years. Advances in technology and genetics have found that many diseases such as Huntington's chorea have a genetic basis. Some forms of breast and colon cancers, adult-onset diabetes, Alzheimer's disease, and hypertension are some of the newest additions. Currently, only the well-to-do can afford broad testing. Advances in technology will provide the means for access to screening that will challenge genetic testing and counseling. The relationship of genetics to disability, disabled individuals, and the potentially disabled will create moral dilemmas of new complexity and magnitude.

Many questions surround genetic testing. Should health-care providers encourage genetic testing? What is, or should be, done with the results? How do we approach testing for genes that lead to disease or disability? How do we maximize health and well-being without creating a eugenic devaluation of those who are disabled? Should employers and third-party payers be allowed to discriminate based on genetic potential for illness? What is the purpose of prenatal screening and genetic testing?

What are the assumptions for state-mandated testing programs? Should parents and individuals be allowed to "opt out" of testing? What if the individual does not want to know the results? What if the results could have a deleterious outcome to the infant or mother? What if the results got into the hands of insurance companies that then denied payment or refused to provide coverage? Should public policy support genetic testing, which may improve health and health care for the masses of society? Should multiple births from fertility drugs be restricted because of the burden of cost, education, and health of the family? Should public policy encourage limiting family size in the contexts of the mother's health, religious and personal preferences, and the availability of sufficient natural resources (such as water and food) for future survival? What effect do these issues have on a nation with an aging population, a decrease in family size, and decreases in the numbers and percentages of younger people? What effect will these issues have on the ability of countries to provide health care for its citizens? Health-care providers must understand these three concepts and the ethical issues involved because they will increasingly encounter situations in which they must balance the client's cultural practices and behaviors with health promotion and wellness, as well as illness and disease prevention activities for the good of the client, the family, and society. Other international issues that may be less controversial include latex allergies, needle sticks, sustainable environments, pacification, and poverty (Davis, 2001; Purnell, 2001).

REFERENCES

American Factfinder. (2001). http://www.factfinder.census.gov.
Amnesty International. (2001). http://www.amnesty.org.

Anand, R. (1997). *Cultural competence in health care: A guide for trainers.* Washington, DC: National Multicultural Institute.
Andrews, M., & Boyle, J. (1999). *Transcultural concepts in nursing* (3rd ed.). Philadelphia: Lippincott.
Baker, R. (1998). A theory of international bioethics: Multiculturism, postmodernism, and the bankruptcy of fundamentalism. *Kennedy Institute Ethics Journal, 8*(3), 201–231.
Beaucamp, T. (1998). The mettle of moral fundamentalism: A reply to Robert Baker. *Kennedy Institute of Ethics Journal, 8*(4), 389–401.
Bureau of the Census. (2001). http://www.census.gov.
Campinha-Bacote, J. (1998). *The process of cultural competence in the delivery of health services: A culturally competent approach* (3rd ed.). Cincinnati, OH: Transcultural C.A.R.E. Associates.
Cook, S. (1999). The self in self-awareness. *Archives of Psychiatric Nursing, 12*(6), 1292–1299.
Davis, A. (2001). Ethics in international nursing: Issues and questions. In N. L. Chaska (Ed.), *The nursing profession: Tomorrow and beyond* (pp. 65–75). Thousand Oaks, CA: Sage Publications.
Ens, I. (1999). The lived experience of cultural transference in psychiatric/mental health nurses. *Archives of Psychiatric Nursing, 12*(6), 201–212.
Family Education Network. (2001). http://www.infoplease.com.
Giger, J., & Davidhizar, R. (1999). *Transcultural nursing: Assessment and intervention* (3rd ed.). St. Louis: Mosby.
Glazer, N. (1997). *We are all multiculturists now.* Cambridge, MA: Harvard University Press.
Macklin, R. (1998). A defense of fundamental principles and human rights: A reply to Robert Baker. *Kennedy Institute of Ethics Journal, 8*(4), 389–401.
Macklin, R. (1999). *Against relativism: Cultural diversity and the search for ethical universals in medicine.* New York: Oxford University Press.
Mattson, M. (2000). Ethical decision making: The person in the process. *Social Work, 45,* 321–329.
Nussbaum, M. C. (1999). *Sex and social justice.* New York: Oxford University Press.
Purnell, L. (2001). Cultural competence in a changing health-care environment. In N. L. Chaska (Ed.), *The nursing profession: Tomorrow and beyond* (pp. 451–461). Thousand Oaks, CA: Sage Publications.
United Nations (2000). *The world's women: Trends and statistics.* New York: Author.
Universal Declaration of Human Rights. (2001). Available at www.amnesty.org.

Chapter 2

The Purnell Model for Cultural Competence

LARRY D. PURNELL and BETTY J. PAULANKA

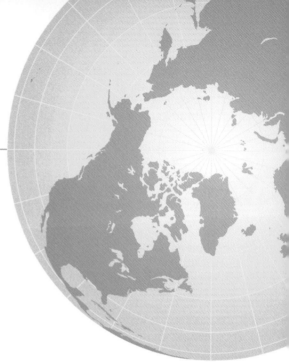

This chapter presents the Purnell Model for Cultural Competence, its organizing framework, and the assumptions upon which the model is based. Additionally, American cultural values, practices, and beliefs are presented to assist nonnative American health-care providers to understand American ways. The American references are meant to describe, not prescribe, behaviors and practices. Although the authors recognize that Canada and Mexico are part of North America, when the words American culture are used in this chapter, they refer to the dominant middle-class values of citizens of the mainland United States. Due to space limitations, this chapter does not deal with the objective culture—arts, literature, humanities, and so on—but rather with the subjective culture. Many Americans are not aware of the subjective culture because they identify differences as individual personality traits and disregard political and social origins of culture. Many view culture as something that belongs only to foreigners or disadvantaged groups. However, when Americans travel abroad, their host country inhabitants many times stereotypically identify them as Americans because of their values, beliefs, attitudes, behaviors, speech patterns, and mannerisms. Some feel that Americans are "fun lovers" and that for some Americans violence is a way of life. However, "the right to bear arms" is guaranteed by the Constitution. Most likely, the United States is not any more violent than, or even as violent as, many other societies, but American media coverage may be better than other countries, thereby giving the impression that the United States is more violent that it actually is. Accordingly, these stereotypes are not always accurate or desirable.

Western academic and health-care organizations stress structure, systematization, and formalization when studying complex phenomena such as culture and ethnicity. Given the complexity of individuals, the Purnell Model for Cultural Competence provides a comprehensive, systematic, and concise framework for learning and understanding culture. The empirical framework of the model can assist health-care providers, managers, and administrators in all health disciplines to provide holistic, culturally competent therapeutic interventions, health promotion, health maintenance, illness and disease prevention, and health teaching across educational and practice settings.

The purposes of this model are to:

1 Provide a framework for all health-care providers to learn concepts and characteristics of culture

2 Define circumstances that affect a person's cultural worldview in the context of historical perspectives

3 Provide a model that links the most central relationships of culture

4 Interrelate characteristics of culture to promote congruence and to facilitate the delivery of consciously sensitive and competent health care

5 Provide a framework that reflects human characteristics such as motivation, intentionality, and meaning

6 Provide a structure for analyzing cultural data

7 View the individual, family, or group within their unique ethnocultural environment

Assumptions upon which the Model Is Based

These are the major explicit assumptions upon which the model is based:

1 All health-care professions need similar information about cultural diversity.

2 All health-care professions share the metaparadigm concepts of global society, family, person, and health.

3 One culture is not better than another culture; they are just different.

4 There are core similarities shared by all cultures.

5 There are differences within, between, and among cultures.

6 Cultures change slowly over time.

7 The primary and secondary characteristics of culture (see Chapter 1) determine the degree to which one varies from the dominant culture.

8 If clients are coparticipants in their care and have a choice in health-related goals, plans, and interventions, their compliance and health outcomes will be improved.

9 Culture has a powerful influence on one's interpretation of and responses to health care.

10 Individuals and families belong to several cultural groups.

11 Each individual has the right to be respected for his or her uniqueness and cultural heritage.

12 Caregivers need both cultural-general and cultural-specific information in order to provide culturally sensitive and culturally competent care.

13 Caregivers who can assess, plan, intervene, and evaluate in a culturally competent manner will improve the care of clients for whom they care.

14 Learning culture is an ongoing process that develops in a variety of ways, but primarily through cultural encounters (Campinha-Bacote, 1999).

15 Prejudices and biases can be minimized with cultural understanding.

16 To be effective, health care must reflect the unique understanding of the values, beliefs, attitudes, lifeways, and worldview of diverse populations and individual acculturation patterns.

17 Differences in race and culture often require adaptations to standard interventions.

18 Cultural awareness improves the caregiver's self-awareness.

19 Professions, organizations, and associations have their own culture, which can be analyzed using a grand theory of culture.

Overview of the Theory, the Model, and Organizing Framework

The Purnell model has been classified as holographic and complexity theory because it includes a model and organizing framework that can be used by all health-care providers in various disciplines and settings. The model is a circle, with an outlying rim representing global society, a second rim representing community, a third rim representing family, and an inner rim representing the person (Fig. 2–1.) The interior of the circle is divided into 12 pie-shaped wedges depicting cultural domains and their concepts. The dark center of the circle represents unknown phenomena. Along the bottom of the model is a jagged line representing the nonlinear concept of cultural consciousness. The 12 cultural domains (constructs) provide the organizing framework of the model. Following the discussion of each of the domains is a box that provides statements that can be adapted as a guide for assessing patients and clients in various settings. Accordingly, health-care providers can use these same questions to better understand their own cultural beliefs, attitudes, values, practices, and behaviors.

MACRO ASPECTS OF THE MODEL

The macro aspects of this interactional model include the metaparadigm concepts of a global society, community, family, person, and conscious competence. The theory and model are conceptualized from biology, anthropology, sociology, economics, geography, history, ecology, physiology, psychology, political science, pharmacology, and nutrition as well as theories from communication, family development, and social support. The model can be used in clinical practice, education, research, and the administration and management of health-care services.

Phenomena related to a **global society** include world communication and politics; conflicts and warfare; natural disasters and famines; international exchanges in education, business, commerce, and information technology; advances in the health sciences; space exploration; and the expanded opportunities for people to travel around the world and interact with diverse societies. Global events that are widely disseminated by television, radio, satellite transmission, newsprint, and information technology affect all societies, either directly or indirectly. Such events create chaos while consciously and unconsciously forcing people to alter their lifeways and worldviews.

In its broadest definition, **community** is a group of people having a common interest or identity and living in a specified locality. Community includes the physical, social, and symbolic characteristics that cause people to connect. Bodies of water, mountains, rural versus urban living, and even railroad tracks help people define their physical concept of community. Today, however, technology and the Internet allow people to expand their community beyond physical boundaries. Economics, religion, politics, age, generation, and marital status delineate the social concepts of community. Sharing a specific language or dialect, lifestyle, history, dress, art, or musical interest are symbolic characteristics of a community. People actively and passively interact with the community, necessitating adaptation and assimilation for equilibrium and homeostasis in their worldview. Individuals may willingly change their physical, social, and symbolic community when it no longer meets their needs.

A **family** is two or more people who are emotionally connected. They may, but do not necessarily, live in close

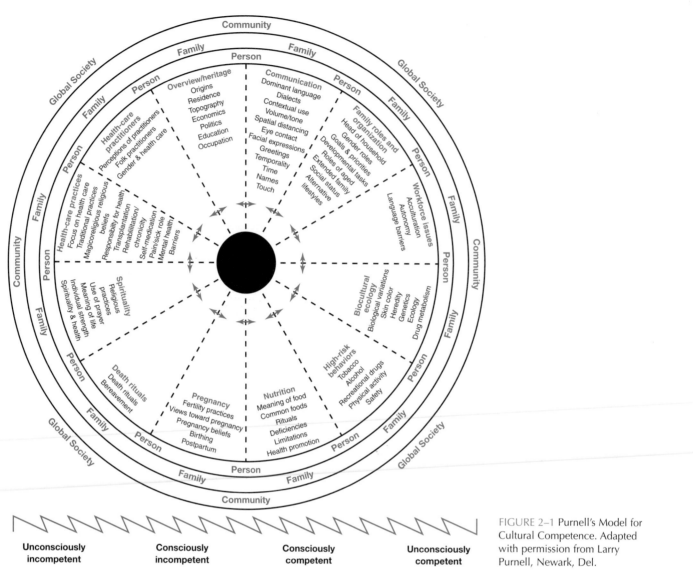

FIGURE 2–1 Purnell's Model for Cultural Competence. Adapted with permission from Larry Purnell, Newark, Del.

proximity to each other. Family may include physically and emotionally close and distant consanguineous relatives as well as physically and emotionally connected and distant non-blood-related significant others. Family structure and roles change according to age, generation, marital status, relocation or immigration, and socioeconomic status, requiring each person to rethink individual beliefs and lifeways.

A **person** is a biopsychosociocultural being who is constantly adapting to his or her community. Human beings adapt biologically and physiologically with the aging process; psychologically in the context of social relationships, stress, and relaxation; socially as they interact with the changing community; and ethnoculturally within the broader global society. In Western cultures, a person is a separate physical and unique psychological being and a singular member of society. The self is separate from others. However, in Asian cultures, the individual is defined in relation to the family, including ancestors or another group rather than a basic unit of nature.

Health, as used in this book, is a state of wellness as defined by people within their ethnocultural group. Health generally includes physical, mental, and spiritual states because group members interact with the family, community, and global society. The concept of health, which permeates all metaparadigm concepts of culture, is defined globally, nationally, regionally, locally, and individually. Thus, people can speak about their personal health status or the health status of the nation or community. Health can also be subjective or objective in nature.

MICRO ASPECTS OF THE MODEL

On a micro level, the model has an organizing framework consisting of 12 domains and their concepts, which are common to all cultures. These 12 domains are interconnected and have implications for health. The utility of this organizing framework comes from its concise structure, which can be used in any setting and applied to a broad range of empirical experiences and can foster inductive and deductive reasoning in the assessment of cultural domains. Once cultural data are analyzed, the practitioner can fully adopt, modify, or reject health-care interventions and treatment regimens in a manner that respects the client's cultural differences. Such adaptations improve the quality of the client's health-care experiences and personal existence.

The 12 Domains of Culture

The 12 domains essential for assessing the ethnocultural attributes of an individual, family, or group are as follows:

1 Overview, inhabited localities, and topography
2 Communication
3 Family roles and organization
4 Workforce issues
5 Biocultural ecology
6 High-risk behaviors
7 Nutrition
8 Pregnancy and childbearing practices
9 Death rituals
10 Spirituality
11 Health-care practices
12 Health-care practitioners

OVERVIEW, INHABITED LOCALITIES, AND TOPOGRAPHY

This domain, *overview, inhabited localities, and topography,* includes concepts related to the country of origin, the current residence, the effects of the topography of the country of origin and current residence on health, economics, politics, reasons for migration, educational status, and occupations. These concepts are interrelated. For example, economic and political conditions may affect one's reason for migration, and educational attainment is usually interrelated with employment choices and opportunities. Sociopolitical and socioeconomic conditions influence individual behavioral responses to health and illness.

Knowing and understanding a different culture includes becoming familiar with the heritage of its people and their part of the world. Salient historical events, such as discrimination in the country of origin, affect culture and influence value systems, beliefs, and explanatory frameworks used in everyday life. Given the primary and secondary characteristics of diversity (see Chapter 1), generalizations and stereotypes may not be part of a specific individual's beliefs or value system.

For most Americans, dominant cultural values and beliefs include individualism, free speech, rights of choice, independence and self-reliance, confidence, "doing" rather than "being," egalitarian relationships,

nonhierarchal status of individuals, achievement status over ascribed status, "volunteerism," friendliness, openness, futuristic temporality, being able to control the environment, and an emphasis on material things and physical comfort. These concepts will be more fully described in other sections of this chapter.

Many Americans are obsessed with self-improvement, youth, beauty, and fear of aging. Advertisements in newspapers, radio and television commercials, and bookstores in major cities and airports have a plethora of self-help and self-improvement books such as *Win Friends and Influence People, Reach the Summit, The Search of the Real Self, Essential Guide to Mental Health, The Age-Defying Diet, Asserting Yourself, The Biology of Success, Sources of Power, The Winning Attitude, Put Your Best Foot Forward,* and *Attracting Terrific People,* to name a few. The media and Americans' conversations are filled with phrases that include superlative "hype" words, such as "tallest," "widest," "longest," "best," "worst," and "most unusual." Most Americans believe they have the "most advanced health-care system," the "newest technology," the "best sports figures," the "most talented movie stars," and the "most comfortable living conditions."

Given the size, population density, and diversity of the United States, one cannot generalize too much about American culture. Every generalization in this chapter is subject to exceptions, although most people will agree with the descriptions to some degree and on some level. However, we believe the descriptions about the dominant American culture are true for white middle-class European Americans (and many other groups as well) who hold the majority of prestigious positions in the United States. The degree to which people conform to this dominant culture depends on the primary and secondary characteristics of culture discussed in Chapter 1 as well as individual personality differences. We recognize that some Americans do not think there is an American culture and resent any attempt at generalizations. Many foreigners believe that all Americans are rich, everyone lives in fancy apartments or houses, crime is everywhere, everyone drives an expensive car, and that there is no poverty. For the most part, these misconceptions come from the media and Americans who travel overseas.

Heritage and Residence

The United States comprises 3.5 million square miles (6.2 percent of the world's land mass) and a population of nearly 300 million people, which makes it the world's third most populous country. The northernmost point in the United States is Point Barrow, Alaska; the southernmost point is Ka Lee, Hawaii; the easternmost point is West Quoddy, Maine; and the westernmost point is Cape Wrangell, Alaska. The highest point is Mount McKinley, Alaska at 20,320 feet elevation; the lowest point, Death Valley, California, is 282 feet below sea level (Time Almanac, 2001).

When Europeans began settling what is now the United States in the 16th century, approximately 2 million American Indians, who mostly lived in geographically isolated tribes, populated the land. The first permanent European settlement in the United States was St. Augustine, Florida, which was settled by the Spanish in 1565. The first English settlement was Jamestown, Virginia, in 1607. By 1610, the nonnative population in the United States was only 350 people. By 1700, the population increased to 250,900, by 1800 to 5.3 million, and by 1900 to 75.9 million (Time Almanac, 2001). From 1607 until 1890, most immigrants to the United States came from Great Britain, Spain, France, the Netherlands, Germany, Switzerland, Norway, and Sweden and essentially shared a common (northern European) culture. The plantation economy of the South paid for the forced relocation of natives from (primarily western) Africa beginning in 1619 and ending with the American Civil War (1861–1865). This group did not share the common culture, and their acculturation was strongly influenced by their status as slaves.

No limitations were placed on immigrants from Europe until the late 1800s. From 1892 to 1952, most European immigrants to America came through Ellis Island, New York, where they had to prove to officials that they were financially independent. More severe restrictions were placed on other immigrant groups, particularly those from Asia. In the 1960s, immigration policy changed to allow immigrants from all parts of the world without favoritism to or restrictions on ethnicity. Today, the United States includes immigrants or descendents from immigrants from almost every nation and culture of the world. It is the world's premier international nation.

People have been attracted to immigrate to the United States by the allure of its vast resources and economic and personal freedoms, particularly the dogma that "all men are created equal." These immigrants and their descendants achieved enormous material success, which further encouraged immigration.

On July 4, 1776, the original 13 colonies signed the Declaration of Independence, declaring their freedom from Great Britain. The Constitution of the Untied States was ratified in 1789 and included seven articles, which laid the foundation for an independent nation. The Bill of Rights, which comprises the first 10 amendments to the Constitution, was ratified in 1791. It guarantees freedom of religion, freedom of speech and the press, and the right to petition; the right to bear arms; the right to a speedy trial, and other rights and freedoms. Only 17 additional amendments have been made to the Constitution, the last in 1992. The Thirteenth Amendment in 1865 prohibited slavery; the Fourteenth Amendment in 1868 defined citizenship and privileges of citizens; the Fifteenth Amendment in 1870 gave suffrage rights regardless of race or color; and the Nineteenth Amendment in 1920 gave women the right to vote.

The independence of the United States ignited the modern world's first revolutionary war and immediately involved the United States in European politics, with France becoming the United States' first ally. In 1823, the United States declared (in the Monroe Doctrine) that it would not interfere in European affairs and that European nations were not to interfere in the affairs of the Western Hemisphere, thereby encouraging the independence of nations in Latin America. In the 1830s, a war was fought with Mexico, resulting in the annexation of greater Texas. From 1860 until 1865, the North and South fought over the issue of slavery, which resulted not only in the elimination of slavery but also in the industrialization of the North and the establishment of the United States as a major military power. The Spanish-American War (1898) resulted in the United States becoming a colonial power, with the annexation of Spain's last colony in the Western Hemisphere, Cuba, and also its colony in the Philippines. World War I (1914–1918) established the United States as one of the world's superpowers, and World War II (1939–1945) significantly extended U.S. military power. In the postwar period, the ideological differences between the United States and the USSR resulted in the Cold War, which lasted until 1989. Today, U.S. military, cultural, and economic power affect almost every other country on the planet.

The United States is the world's oldest constitutional democracy. It has three branches of government: the executive branch, which includes the Office of the President and the administrative departments; the legislative branch, Congress, which includes both the Senate and the House of Representatives; and the judicial branch, which includes the Supreme Court and the lesser federal courts, including the court of appeals and the district courts. The Supreme Court has nine members appointed by the President and approved by Congress. The Justices serve a life term if they so choose. The President serves a 4-year term and can be re-elected only one time. The President is the Commander-in-Chief of the Armed Forces and oversees the executive departments. The 435 members of the House of Representatives are divided among the states based on the population of each state. Members of the House of Representatives serve 2-year terms. Each state has two senators, regardless of the population of the state. Senators serve 6-year terms. Each of the 50 states has its own constitution establishing, for the most part, a parallel structure to the federal government, with the executive branch headed by a governor, a state congress with representatives and senators, and a state court system.

Reasons for Migration and Associated Economic Factors

The United States has a very large middle-class population and a small, but growing, wealthy population. Approximately 12.7 percent of the population lives in poverty, with higher rates among children (18.9 percent), the elderly (19.9 percent), blacks (26.1 percent), and nonwhite Hispanics (27.1 percent) (Time Almanac, 2001). The social, economic, religious, and political forces of the country of origin play an important role in the development of the ideologies and the worldview of individuals, families, and groups and are often a major motivating force for emigration. The earlier settlers in the United States came for better economic opportunities, because of religious and political oppression, religious freedom, environmental disasters such as earthquakes and hurricanes, and by forced relocation such as slaves and indentured servants. Others have immigrated for educational opportunities and personal ideologies or a combination of factors. Most people immigrate to this country in the hope of a better life; however, the individual or group personally defines this ideology. Understanding the reason for a person's immigration, whether voluntary, sojourner, refugee, or undocumented status, may provide clues to the person's acculturation patterns.

A common practice for many immigrants is to relocate to an area that has an established population with similar ideologies that can provide initial support, serve as cultural brokers, and orient them to their new culture and health-care system. For example, most people of Cuban heritage live in New York and Florida; French Canadians are concentrated in the Northeast; and the Amish are concentrated in Pennsylvania, Indiana, and Ohio. When immigrants settle and work exclusively in predominantly ethnic communities, primary social support is enhanced, but acculturation and assimilation into the wider society may be hindered. Groups without ethnic enclaves in the United States to assist them with acculturation may need extra help in adjusting to their new homeland's language, access to health-care services, living accommodations, and employment opportunities. People who move across cultures voluntarily are likely to experience less difficulty with acculturation than people who are forced to emigrate to a new culture. Some individuals immigrate with the intention of remaining in this country only a short time, making money, and returning home, whereas others immigrate with the intention of relocating permanently. Therefore, it is imperative for health-care providers to assess the reasons behind the individual's migration to understand the implications for culturally competent care.

Educational Status and Occupations

The value placed on formal education differs among cultural and ethnic groups and is often related to their socioeconomic status in their homeland, their reasons for emigrating, or their ability to emigrate. The United States places a high value on education, which has recently become a major issue in presidential elections. Some groups, however, do not stress formal education because it was not needed for employment in their homeland. Consequently, they may become engulfed in poverty, isolation, and enclave identity, which may further limit their potential for formal educational opportunities and planning for the future.

In the United States, preparation in elementary and secondary education varies widely, but all public schools provide the necessary textbooks for students. There is no national curriculum that each school is expected to follow, although there is standardized testing at a national level, which is used in the selection process for admission to institutions of higher education. Each state and local district establishes its own curriculum with little input from the public. Most states require children to attend school until the age of 16, although the child can drop out of school at a younger age with parents' signed permission. The age and circumstances under which the teenager can drop out of school varies somewhat from state to state. Overall, the United States has

the goal of producing a well-rounded individual with a variety of courses and 100 percent literacy. Theoretically, people have the freedom to choose a profession, regardless of gender and background. However, this does not always carry over into practice for many professions. For example, the nursing profession in the United States is predominantly female.

For the most part, private and religious schools are perceived to be better than public schools because they are more demanding; however, parents must pay tuition for their children to attend these schools. Some private schools are very elite, and children must undergo rigid testing to qualify for entrance. Some private schools offer scholarships for poor children, but fail to help them adapt to the elite culture. Thus, when they continue in university settings, they fail to adapt and drop out because of the inability to acculturate. Private and religious schools usually have fewer extracurricular activities such as band, sports, etc. than do public schools. Additionally, in private schools the parents must purchase the child's books; the choices are often restricted according to what the school sees as appropriate for children to read. These choices are usually influenced by religious, cultural, social, and artistic values or the purpose of the private school.

Educational attainment in the United States varies by race, gender, and region of the country. Eighty-four percent of all adults age 25 years and over have completed high school, and 26 percent have completed a bachelor's degree or more. Among women age 25 and over, 84 percent have earned a high school diploma, and 24 percent have completed a bachelor's degree or more. Proportionately, white non-Hispanics have higher educational attainment levels than other groups. High school completion levels are highest in the Midwest (87 percent) and lowest in the South (82 percent) ("Median Age at First Marriage," 2001).

In regard to learning styles, the Western system places a high value on the student's ability to categorize information using linear, sequential thought processes. However, not everyone adheres to this pattern of thinking. For example, many Native Americans have spiral and circular thought patterns that move from concept to concept without being linear or sequential; therefore, they have difficulty placing information in a stepwise methodology (Crow, 1993). When someone is unaware of the value given to such behaviors, he or she may see such individuals as disorganized, scattered, and faulty in their cognitive patterns, resulting in increased difficulty with written and verbal communications.

The American educational system stresses application of content over theory. Most European educational programs emphasize theory over practical application, and Arab education emphasizes theory with little attention given to practical application. As a result, Arab students are more proficient at tests requiring rote learning than at those requiring conceptualization and analysis. Being familiar with the individual's personal educational values and learning modes allows health-care providers, educators, and employers to adjust teaching strategies for clients, students, and employees. Educational materials and explanations must be presented at a level consistent with clients' educational capabilities and within their cultural framework and beliefs.

Immigrants bring job skills from their native homelands and traditionally seek employment in the same or similar trades. Sometimes these job skills are inadequate for the available jobs in the new society; thus, immigrants are forced to take low-paying jobs and join the ranks of the working poor and economically disadvantaged. Immigrants to America are employed in a broad variety of occupations and professions; however, limited experiential, educational, and language abilities of more recent immigrants often restrict employment possibilities. More importantly, experiential backgrounds sometimes encourage employment choices that are identified as high risk for chronic diseases, such as exposure to pesticides and chemicals. Others may work in factories that manufacture hepatotoxic chemicals, in industries with pollutants that increase the risk for pulmonary diseases, and in crowded conditions with poor ventilation that increase the risk for tuberculosis or other respiratory diseases. In some immigrant populations, the country of origin has lost many of its professional and well-educated people. These professional immigrants have difficulty finding work comparable to what they did in their homeland, resulting in a "brain drain" for the home country and underemployment in their new environment.

Knowing and understanding clients' current and previous work background is essential for health screening. For example, newer immigrants who worked in malaria-infested areas in their native country (Egypt, Italy, Turkey, and Vietnam) may need health screening for malaria. Those who worked in mining (Irish and Polish) may need screening for respiratory diseases. Those who lived in overcrowded and unsanitary conditions (refugees and migrant workers) may need to be screened for infectious diseases such as tuberculosis, parasitosis, and respiratory diseases.

Box 2–1 identifies guidelines for assessing the cultural domain *overview, inhabited localities, and topography*.

COMMUNICATION

Perhaps no other domain has the complexities of communication. Communication is interrelated with all other domains and depends on verbal language skills that include the dominant language, dialects, and the contextual use of the language as well as paralanguage variations, such as voice volume, tone, intonations, reflections, and willingness to share thoughts and feelings. Other important communication characteristics include nonverbal communications such as eye contact, facial expressions, use of touch, body language, spatial distancing practices, and acceptable greetings; temporality in terms of past, present, or future orientation of worldview; clock versus social time; and the degree of formality in the use of names. Communication styles may vary between insiders (family and close friends) and outsiders (strangers and unknown health-care providers). Hierarchical relationships, gender, and some religious beliefs affect communication.

BOX 2–1

Overview, Inhabited Localities, and Topography

Overview, Inhabited Localities, and Topography

1 Identify the part of the world from which this cultural or ethnic group originates and describe the climate and topography of the country.

Heritage and Residence

2 Identify where this group predominantly resides and include approximate numbers.

Reasons for Migration and Associated Economic Factors

3 Identify major factors that motivated this group to emigrate.
4 Explore economic or political factors that have influenced this group's acculturation and professional development in America.

Educational Status and Occupations

5 Assess the educational attainment and value placed on education by this ethnic group.
6 Identify occupations that individuals in this group predominantly seek on immigration.

Dominant Language and Dialects

The health-care provider must be aware of the dominant language and the difficulties that dialects may cause when communicating in the client's native language. Most Americans speak only one language. In this monochromic, low contextual culture where most of the message is in the verbal mode, and verbal communication is more important than nonverbal communication, Americans are more likely to miss the more subtle nuances of communication. Accordingly, if a misunderstanding occurs, both the sender and the receiver of the message take responsibility for the miscommunication.

Americans speak *American English*, which differs somewhat in its pronunciation, spelling, and choice of words from English spoken in Great Britain, Australia, and other English-speaking countries. Within the United States, there are several dialects, but generally the differences do not cause a major concern with communications. Aside from people with foreign accents, there are certain areas in the United States where people speak with a dialect; these include the South and Northeast, in addition to local dialects such as "Elizabethan English" and "western drawl." For the most part, these different dialects and accents are not as great as in some other countries; for example, the English spoken in Scotland is utterly unlike the English spoken in Central London. Additionally, there are not as many English accents dialects as there are Spanish accents dialects, for instance. Spanish spoken in Spain differs from the version spoken in Puerto Rico, Panama, or Mexico, which has as many as 50 different dialects within its borders. In such cases, dialects that vary widely may pose substantial problems for health-care providers and interpreters in performing health assessments and in obtaining accurate health data, in turn increasing the difficulty of making accurate diagnoses.

When speaking in a nonnative language, health-care providers must select words that have relatively pure meanings, be certain of the voice intonation, and avoid the use of regional slang and jargon to avoid being misunderstood. Minor variations in pronunciation may change the entire meaning of a word or a phrase and result in inappropriate interventions. For example, in the Spanish language, there are two forms of the verb "to be": *ser* and *estar*. Using the incorrect form can cause a miscommunication, as evidenced by the following situation. A school nurse, who spoke limited Spanish, telephoned the mother of an 8-year-old boy with diarrhea. The nurse used the phrase *es enfermo*, meaning "he is sick" (a permanent condition) instead of *esta enfermo*, meaning "he is sick" (a temporary situation). This subtle distinction in language translation increased the mother's concern and anxiety over her child's illness and resulted in her thinking something was seriously wrong with him.

Given the difficulty of obtaining the precise meaning of words in a language, it is best for health-care providers to obtain someone who can interpret the meaning and message, not just translate the individual words. Here are some guidelines for communicating with non-English-speaking clients.

1 Use interpreters rather than translators. Translators just restate the words from one language to another. An interpreter decodes the words and provides the meaning behind the message.

2 Use dialect-specific interpreters whenever possible.

3 Use interpreters trained in the health-care field.

4 Give the interpreter time alone with the client.

5 Provide time for translation and interpretation.

6 Use same-gender interpreters whenever possible.

7 Maintain eye contact with both the client and interpreter to elicit feedback: read nonverbal cues.

8 Speak slowly without exaggerated mouthing, allow time for translation, use the active rather than the passive tense, wait for feedback, and restate the message. Do not rush; do not speak loudly. Use a reference book with common phrases such as *Roget's International Thesaurus* or *Taber's Cyclopedic Medical Dictionary*.

9 Use as many words as possible in the client's language and nonverbal communication when unable to understand the language.

10 Use phrase charts and picture cards if available.

11 During the assessment, direct your questions to the patient, not to the interpreter.

12 Ask one question at a time and allow interpretation and a response before asking another question.

13 Be aware that interpreters may affect the reporting of symptoms, insert their own ideas, or omit information.

14 Remember that clients can usually understand more than they can express; thus, they need time to think in their own language. They are alert to the health-care provider's body language, and they may forget some or all of their English in times of stress.

15 Avoid the use of relatives, who may distort information or not be objective.

16 Avoid using children as interpreters, especially with sensitive topics.

17 Avoid idiomatic expressions and medical jargon.

18 If an interpreter is unavailable, the use of a translator may be acceptable. The difficulty with translation is omission of parts of the message, distortion of the message, including transmission of information not given by the speaker, and messages not being fully understood.

19 If available, use an interpreter who is older than the patient.

20 Review responses with the patient and interpreter at the end of a session.

21 Be aware that social class differences between the interpreter and the client may result in the interpreter's not reporting information that he or she perceives as superstitious or unimportant.

Those with limited English ability may have inadequate vocabulary skills to communicate in situations where strong or abstract levels of verbal skills are required, such as in the psychiatric setting. Helpful communication techniques with diverse clients include tact, consideration, and respect; gaining trust by listening attentively; addressing the client by preferred name; and showing genuine warmth and openness to facilitate full information sharing. When giving directions, be explicit. Give directions in sequential procedural steps (for example, first, second, third). Do not use complex sentences with conjunctions.

Before trying to engage in more sensitive areas of the health interview, the health-care practitioner may need to start with social exchanges to establish trust, use an open-ended format rather than yes or no closed-response questions, elicit opinions and beliefs about health and symptom management, and focus on facts rather than feelings. An awareness of nonverbal behaviors is essential to establishing a mutually satisfying relationship.

The context within which a language is spoken is an important aspect of communication. The German, English, and French languages are low in context, and most of the message is explicit, requiring many words to express a thought. Chinese and Native American languages are highly contextual, with most of the information either in the physical context or internalized, resulting in the use of fewer words with more emphasis on unspoken understandings. Although many Finns, Chinese, Hopi, and Turkish people speak English primarily in the present tense and do not use the future tense, this practice should not be confused with present temporal orientation. They find it difficult to use the future tense because there is no future tense in their language. Accordingly, health-care providers must listen for the message in context; for example: "I see the doctor tomorrow," "I see the doctor yesterday," or "I see the doctor today."

Voice volume and tone are important paralanguage aspects of communication. Americans and people of African heritage may be perceived as being loud and boisterous because their volume carries to those nearby. Compared to Chinese and Hindus, Americans and African Americans generally talk loudly. Their loud voice volume may be interpreted by Chinese or Hindus as reflecting anger, when in fact a loud voice is merely being used to express their thoughts in a dynamic manner. In contrast, Westerners witnessing impassioned communication among Arabs may interpret the excited speech pattern and shouting as anger, but emotional communication is part of the Arab culture and is usually unrelated to anger. Thus, health-care providers must be cautious about voice tones when interacting with diverse cultural groups so their intentions are not misunderstood. The speed at which people speak varies by region; for example, in parts of Appalachia and the South, people speak more slowly than do people in the northeastern part of the United States.

Cultural Communication Patterns

Communication includes the willingness of individuals to share their thoughts and feelings. Many Americans are willing to disclose very personal information about themselves, including information about sex, drugs, family problems, etc. In fact, personal sharing is encouraged in a wide variety of topics, but not religion as in Central America, politics as in Spain, or philosophical things as discussed in most of Europe. In the United States, having well-developed verbal skills is seen as important, whereas in Japan, the person who has very highly developed verbal skills is seen as having suspicious intentions. Similarly, among many Appalachians, the person who has well-developed verbal skills may be seen as a "smooth talker" and therefore his or her actions may be suspect. In some cultural groups, such as many Asian cultures, individuals are expected to be shy, withdrawn, and diffident—at least in public—whereas in other cultures, such as Jewish and Italian, individuals are expected to be more flamboyant and expressive. Most Appalachians and Mexicans willingly share their thoughts and feelings among family members and close friends, but they may not easily share thoughts, feelings, and health information with "outside" health-care providers until they get to know them. By engaging in small talk and inquiring about family members before addressing the client's health concerns, health-care providers can help establish trust and, in turn, encourage more open communication and sharing of important health information.

Touch, a method of nonverbal communication, has substantial variations in meaning among cultures. For the most part, America is a low-touch society, which has recently been reinforced by sexual harassment guidelines and policies. For many, even casual touching may be seen as a sexual overture and should be avoided whenever possible. People of the same sex (especially men) or opposite sex do not generally touch each other unless they are close friends. However, among most Asian cultures, two people of the same gender can touch each other without it having a sexual connotation. Among Egyptian Americans, touch between opposite sexes is accepted in private and only between husband and wife, parents and children, and adult brothers and sisters; it is less readily accepted from strangers. Mexican Americans, even though they frequently touch family members and friends, tend to be modest during health-care examinations by the opposite gender. Being aware of individual practices regarding touch is essential for effective health assessments.

Personal space needs to be respected when working with multicultural clients and staff. American, Canadian, and British conversants tend to place at least 18 inches of space between themselves and the person with whom they are talking. Arabs require less personal space when talking with each other (Hall, 1990). They are quite comfortable standing closer to each other than Americans; in fact, they interpret physical proximity as a valued sign of emotional closeness. Middle Eastern clients, who stand very close and stare during a conversation, may offend health-care practitioners. These clients may interpret American health-care providers as being cold because they stand so far away. To Germans, who view space as sacred, even the distance between pieces of furniture is not conducive to easy conversation. Doors are used to protect privacy and require a knock and an invitation before entering. In fact, even looking into the room can be perceived as an intrusion of privacy (Hill, 1995). An understanding of personal space and distancing characteristics can enhance the quality of communication among individuals.

Regardless of class or social standing of the conversants, Americans maintain direct eye contact without staring. A person who does not maintain eye contact may be perceived as not listening, not being trustworthy, not caring, or being less than truthful. Among traditional Mexicans, Cubans, Puerto Ricans, Iranians, Egyptians, Italians, and Greeks, sustained eye contact between a child and an older adult may bring on the "evil eye" or "bad eye." In many Asian cultures, a person of lower social class or status should avoid eye contact with superiors or those with a higher educational status. Thus, eye contact must be interpreted within its cultural context to optimize relationships and health assessments.

The use of gestures and facial expressions varies among cultures. Most Americans gesture moderately when conversing and smile easily as a sign of pleasantness or happiness, although one can smile as a sign of sarcasm. A lack of gesturing can mean that the person is too stiff, too formal, or too polite. However, when gesturing to make, emphasize, or clarify a point, one should not raise one's elbows above the head unless saying hello or good-bye. Americans, unlike the Japanese and Chinese, do not normally smile as a form of embarrassment, confusion, or not understanding. For the Japanese and Chinese, happiness hides behind a straight face;

if you are truly happy, you do not need to smile. Additionally, the Cofan Indians of Ecuador rarely smile because showing their teeth may be interpreted as a sign of aggression. This does not mean they do not put on a happy face; they grin broadly with their mouths closed or place a hand over their mouths if the teeth show.

Preferred greetings and acceptable body language also vary among cultural groups. An expected practice for American males and women in business is to extend the right hand when greeting someone for the first time. In northern European countries, it is considered rude and impolite to converse with one's hands in the pockets. In the United States, confidence and competence are associated with a relaxed posture; however, in Korea and Japan, confidence and competence are more closely associated with slightly tense postures (Krebs & Kunimoto, 1994). More elaborate greeting rituals occur in Asian, Arab, and Latin American countries and are covered in individual chapters.

Although many people consider it impolite or offensive to point with one's finger, many Americans do so, and do not see it as impolite. In Iran, beckoning is done by waving the fingers with the palm down, whereas extending the thumb, like thumbs-up, is considered a vulgar sign. Among the Vietnamese, signaling for someone to come by using an upturned finger is a provocation, usually done to a dog. Among the Navajo it is considered rude to point; rather the Navajo shift their lips toward the desired direction.

Temporal Relationships

Temporal relationships, people's worldview in terms of past, present, and future orientation, vary among cultural groups. The American culture is future-oriented, and people are encouraged to sacrifice for today and work to save and invest in the future. The future is important in that people can influence it. Americans generally see fatalism, the belief that powers greater than humans are in control, as negative; but to many others, it is seen as a fact of life not to be judged. For example, the German culture is regarded as a past-oriented society, where laying a proper foundation by providing historical background information can enhance communication. Most people of Central American heritage are more present-oriented, placing great importance on the here and now, not something that may occur in the future or has occurred in the past. Among Brazilians, punctuality, especially in social situations, is not taken seriously. However, for people in many societies, temporality is balanced between past, present, and future in the sense of respecting the past, valuing and enjoying the present, and saving for the future.

Differences in temporal orientation can cause concern or misunderstanding among health-care providers. For example, in a future-oriented culture, a person is expected to delay purchase of nonessential items to afford prescription medications. However, in less future-oriented cultures, the person buys the nonessential item because it is readily available and defers purchasing the prescription medication. The attitude is, why not purchase it now—the prescription medication can be purchased *mañana* (tomorrow or later).

Americans see time as a highly valued resource and do not like to be delayed because it "wastes time." When visiting friends or meeting for strictly social engagements, punctuality is less important, but one is still expected to appear within a reasonable time frame. In the health-care setting if an appointment is made for 9 a.m., the person is expected to be there at 8:45 a.m. so he or she is ready for the appointment and does not delay the health-care provider. Some organizations refuse to see the patient if they are more than 15 to 30 minutes late for an appointment, and a few charge a fee, even though the patient was not seen. In other cultures, the patient is seen whenever they arrive. For immigrants from rural settings, time may be even less important. These individuals may not even own a timepiece or be able to tell time. Expectations for punctuality can cause conflicts between health-care providers and clients, even if one is cognizant of these differences. These details must be carefully explained to individuals when such situations occur. Being late for appointments should not be misconstrued as a sign of irresponsibility or not valuing one's health.

Format for Names

Names are important to individuals, and their format differs among cultures. The American name David Thomas Jones denotes a man whose first name is David, middle name is Thomas, and family surname is Jones. Friends would call him by his first name, David. In the formal setting, he would be called Mr. Jones. Cambodians use the opposite position in sequencing names. For example, the name Pak Pourin denotes a woman whose last name is Pak and whose first name is Pourin. Friends would address her as Pourin. In a formal situation, she would be addressed as Mrs. Pak.

Hispanics may have a more complex system for denoting their full name. For example, a married woman may take her husband's surname while maintaining both her parents' last names, resulting in an extended name such as La Senora Roberta Rodriguez de Malena y Perez. In this example, Mrs. Rodriguez has the first name of Roberta, her husband's surname Rodriguez, her mother's maiden name Malena, and her father's surname Perez. Friends would address her as Roberta, whereas in the formal setting she would be called Mrs. Rodriguez. This extended name format may become even more confusing because one's last name can be, for example, de la Caza. Therefore, a single woman's name might be Angelica (first name) Elena (middle name) de la Caza (family name) y de la Cruz (mother's maiden name). She may choose any name she wants for legal purposes. When in doubt, the health-care provider needs to ask which name the person prefers for record keeping. Such extensive naming formats can create a challenge for health-care workers keeping a medical record when they are unaware of differences in ethnic recording of names.

Box 2–2 identifies guidelines for assessing the cultural domain *communications*.

BOX 2–2

Communications

Dominant Language and Dialects

1 Identify the dominant and other languages spoken by this group.
2 Identify dialects that may interfere with communication.
3 Explore contextual speech patterns of this group. What is the usual volume and tone of speech?

Cultural Communication Patterns

4 Explore the willingness of individuals to share thoughts, feelings, and ideas.
5 Explore the practice and meaning of touch in their society: within the family, between friends, with strangers, with members of the same sex, with members of the opposite sex, and with health-care providers.
6 Identify personal spatial and distancing characteristics when communicating on a one-to-one basis. Explore how distancing changes with friends versus strangers.
7 Explore the use of eye contact within this group. Does avoidance of eye contact have special meanings? How does eye contact vary among family, friends, and strangers? Does eye contact change among socioeconomic groups?
8 Explore the meaning of various facial expressions. Do specific facial expressions have special meanings? How are emotions displayed or not displayed in facial expressions?
9 Are there acceptable ways of standing and greeting outsiders?

Temporal Relationships

10 Explore temporal relationships in this group. Are individuals primarily past-, present-, or future-oriented? How do individuals see the context of past, present, and future?
11 Identify how differences in the interpretation of social time versus clock time are perceived.
12 Explore how time factors are interpreted by this group. Are individuals expected to be punctual in terms of jobs, appointments, and social engagements?

Format for Names

13 Explore the format for a person's names.
14 How does one expect to be greeted by strangers and health-care practitioners?

FAMILY ROLES AND ORGANIZATION

The cultural domain of *family roles and organization* affects all other domains and defines relationships among insiders and outsiders. This domain includes concepts related to the head of the household, gender roles, family goals and priorities, developmental tasks of children and adolescents, roles of the aged and extended family members, individual and family social status in the community, and acceptance of alternative lifestyles such as single parenting, nontraditional sexual orientations, childless marriages, and divorce. Family structure in the context of the larger society determines acceptable roles, priorities, and the behavioral norms for its members.

Head of Household and Gender Roles

An awareness of family dominance patterns (i.e., patriarchal, matriarchal, or egalitarian) is important for determining with whom to speak when health-care decisions have to be made. Among Americans, it is acceptable for women to have a career and for men to assist with child care, household domestic chores, and cooking responsibilities. Both parents work in many families, necessitating placing children in child-care facilities. Recent studies imply that extended hours in child-care facilities leads to increased violence in some children. These findings have prompted some families to reconsider the amount of time their children spend in child-care facilities. For example, a study by the Society for Research in Child Development (2001) conducted with 1364 children over a 10-year period in 10 cities in the United States, suggested that children who spent 30 hours or more per week in day care scored higher on items such as fighting, exhibiting cruel and explosive behavior, arguing, and demanding attention. These conclusions were based on the observations of children's mothers, those caring for them, and kindergarten teachers.

In some families, fathers are responsible for deciding when to seek health care for family members, but mothers may have significant influence on final decisions. Among many Hispanics, the decisions may be egalitarian, but it is the role of the male in the family to be the spokesperson for the family. The health-care provider, when speaking with parents, should maintain eye contact and direct questions to both parents about a child's illness.

Prescriptive, Restrictive, and Taboo Behaviors for Children and Adolescents

Every society has prescriptive, restrictive, and taboo practices for children and adolescents. Prescriptive beliefs are things that children or teenagers *should do* to have harmony with the family and a good outcome in society. Restrictive practices are things that children and teenagers *should not do* to have a positive outcome. Taboo practices are those things that, if done, are likely to cause significant concern or negative outcomes for the child, teenager, family, or community at large.

For most Americans, a child's individual achievement is valued over the family's financial status. This is different from non-Western cultures where attachment to family is more important and the need for children to excel individually is not as important. In most middle- and upper-class American families, children have their own room, television, and telephone, and in many homes, their own computer. At younger ages, rather than having group toys each child has his or her own toys and is taught to share them with others. Americans encourage autonomy in children, and after completing homework assignments (with which parents are expected to help), children are expected to contribute to the family by doing chores such as taking out the garbage, washing dishes, cleaning their own room, feeding and caring for pets, and helping with cooking. They are not expected to help with heavy labor at home except in rural farm communities.

Children are allowed and encouraged to make their own choices, including managing their own money allowance and deciding who their friends might be, although parents may gently suggest one friend might be a better choice than another. American children and teenagers are permitted and encouraged to have friends of the same and opposite gender. They are expected to be well behaved, especially in public. They are taught to stand in line—first come, first served—and to wait their turn. As they reach the teenage years, they are expected to refrain from premarital sex, smoking, recreational drugs, and alcohol until they leave the home. However, this does not always occur and teenage use of these substances remains high. When the child becomes a teenager, most are expected to get a job, such as baby sitting, delivering newspapers, or doing yard work to make their own spending money, which they manage as a way of learning independence. The teenage years are also seen as a time of natural rebellion.

In American society, when young adults become 18 or complete their education, they usually move out of their parents' home (unless they are in college) and live independently or share living arrangements with nonfamily members. More single males (59 percent) than single females (48 percent) over the age of 18 years elect to live with their parents (Time Almanac, 2001). If the young adult chooses to remain in the parents' home, then he or she is expected to pay room and board. However, young adults are generally allowed to return home when they are needed or for financial or other purposes. Individuals over the age of 18 are expected to be self-reliant and independent, which are virtues in the American culture. This differs from other cultures, such as the Japanese and some Hispanic cultures, where children are expected to live at home with their parents until they marry because dependence, not independence, is the virtue.

Adolescents have their own subculture, with its own values, beliefs, and practices that may not be in harmony with those of their major ethnic group. It may be especially important for adolescents to be in harmony with peers and conform to the prevalent choice of music, clothing, hairstyles, and adornment. Thus, role conflicts can become considerable sources of family strain in many more traditional families who may not agree with the American values of individuality, independence, self-assertion, and egalitarian relationships. Many teens may experience a cultural dilemma with exposure outside the home and family.

As outsiders, health-care practitioners in school health can have a significant role in providing factual information regarding issues related to sexuality. Expressing an openness to discuss these sensitive issues in a group or one-on-one format within their cultural context may assist teens to learn more about sexuality and primary prevention. Health-care providers can assist adolescents

and family members to work through these cultural differences by helping them resolve personal conflicts in ways that convey respect for the family's culture. However, in some religions, parental permission may be needed to discuss sexual issues with their children. Discussing personal parenting practices and providing information about disease, illness, and treatment in culturally congruent ways encourages individuals to explore alternative beliefs while continuing to value their own culture.

Family Goals and Priorities

American family goals and priorities are centered on raising and educating children. During this stage in the American culture, young adults make a personal commitment to a spouse or significant other and seek satisfaction through productivity in career, family, and civic interests. In most societies, young adulthood is the time when individuals work on Erikson's developmental tasks of *intimacy versus isolation* and *generativity versus stagnation*. The median age at first marriage in the United States has changed significantly over the last century. In the 1890s, the median age at first marriage for men was 21.6 years and for women 22.0 years. By the 1920s the median age at first marriage for men increased to 22.8 years while it remained relatively stable for women at 20.3 years. By 1998, the age at first marriage for men increased to 26.7 years and to 25 years for women ("Median Age at First Marriage," 2001).

The American culture places a high value on children, and many laws have been enacted to protect children who are seen as the "future of the society." In most Asian cultures, children are desirable and highly valued as a source of family strength, and family members are expected to care for each other more so than in the American culture.

The United States has seen an explosion in its elderly population during the 20th century, up from 3.1 million in 1900 to 34.6 million in 1999 or, stated differently, from 1 in 25 to 1 in 8 people being over the age of 65 years. This population is expected to increase by 74 percent over the next 20 years. In 1990, among those over the age of 100 years, 7901 were males and 29,003 were females (Time Almanac, 2001). The definition of aging varies among cultures and can be defined by age in years, functional abilities, or social mores. In the Korean culture, individuals are considered old and are expected to retire at the age of 60, regardless of their health status. This amount of time allows them to have completed the 60 cycles of the lunar calendar. Within Brazilian-American society, the aged live with one of their children, are included in family activities, and usually accompany their children's family on vacation. The American culture, which emphasizes youth, beauty, thinness, independence, and productivity, contributes to some societal views of the aged as less important members and tends to minimize the problems of the elderly. A contrasting view among some Americans emphasizes the importance of the elderly in society.

Chinese and Appalachian cultures have great reverence for the wisdom of the elderly, and families eagerly make space for them to live with extended families. Children are expected to care for elders when the elders are unable to care for themselves. A great embarrassment may occur to family members when they cannot take care of their elderly family members. Helping the ethnic family to network and find social support, resources, or acceptable long-term-care facilities within the community is a useful strategy for the health-care provider.

The concept of extended family membership varies among societies. The extended family is extremely important in the Hispanic/Latino/Spanish cultures, and health-care decisions are often postponed until the entire family is consulted. The extended family may include biological relatives and nonbiological members who may be considered brother, sister, aunt, or uncle. In some Asian cultures, the influence of grandparents in decision making is considered more important than that of the parents. An accepted practice among Filipinos is for the grandparents to raise the grandchildren so that the parents can work. Grandparents, aunts, and cousins often assume the parental role in African American families, and fellow church members are frequently considered important members of the extended family. A common practice in such cultures is for several generations of a family to live in the same household. The health-care provider can have a significant impact on the health status of the extended family in primary care, home health, acute care, or long-term care.

Americans also place a high value on egalitarianism, nonhierarchical relationships, and equal treatment regardless of their race, color, religion, ethnicity, educational or economic status, sexual orientation, or country of origin. However, these beliefs are theoretical and are not always seen in practice. For example, women still have a lower status than men, especially when it comes to prestigious positions and salaries. Most top-level politicians and corporate executive officers are white men. In 1951, women's earnings were 63.9 percent of men's; in 1998, they were still only 73 percent, down from 74.2 percent in 1997 (Time Almanac, 2001). Subtle classism does exist, as evidenced by comments referring to "working-class men and women." Despite the current inequities, Americans value equal opportunities for all and significant progress has been made in the last 20 years.

Americans are known worldwide for their informality, for treating everyone the same. They call people by their first names very soon after meeting them, whether in the workplace, in social situations, in classrooms, in restaurants, or in places of business. Americans readily talk with waitresses and store clerks and call them by their first names. Most Americans consider this respectful behavior. Unlike many other languages, English no longer has both familiar and formal forms of address; however, formality can be communicated by using the person's last (family) name and title such as Mr., Mrs., Miss, Ms., or Dr. To this end, achieved status is more important than ascribed status. What one has accumulated in material possessions, where one went to school, and one's job position and title are more important than one's family background and lineage. However, among some families in the South and the Northeast, one's

ascribed status has equal importance to achieved status. The United States does not have a caste system or class system, and theoretically one can move readily from one socioeconomic position to another. Most Americans identify themselves by personal achievements, not family lineage. Europeans and Asians are more attentive to status than are Americans. To many Americans, if formality is maintained it may be seen as pompous or arrogant, and some even deride the person who is very formal. However, formality is a sign of respect in many other cultures and is also valued by older Americans.

In cultures governed by rigid caste systems, such as India in the past, one's status is determined by the caste one is born into, regardless of changes in one's socioeconomic status. However, in other societies, such as Korea, not as much attention is given to one's heritage; educational accomplishments give one status. With hard work in American society, a person can climb the socioeconomic scale and gain respect; however, the person can easily fall from high socioeconomic status just as quickly. By using health teachers of the same socioeconomic status as the client, the health-care provider can capitalize on the client's cultural beliefs regarding status when teaching health promotion and disease prevention.

Alternative Lifestyles

The traditional American family is nuclear, with a married man and woman living together with one or more unmarried children. The American family is becoming a more varied community. It includes unmarried people, both men and women, living alone; single people of the same or different genders living together with or without children; single parents with children; and blended families consisting of two parents who have remarried, with children from their previous marriages and additional children from their current marriage. However, in some cultures, the traditional family is extended, with parents, unmarried children, married children with their children, and grandparents all sharing the same living space or at least living in very close proximity. The number of grandchildren living with grandparents has been increasing. In 1990, 2.2 million children lived with their grandparents; however, by 1997, this number increased to 3.9 million. A variety of factors have contributed to this increase: growth in drug use among parents, teen pregnancy, divorce, the rapid rise of single-parent households, child abuse and neglect, death of parents due to AIDS, and incarceration of parents (Time Almanac, 2001).

The sexual revolution of the 1960s marked the beginning of a sharp increase in divorce rates, which passed the 1 million mark by 1975 and hit an all-time high of 5.2 per 1000 marriages in 1979. In the year 1998, the divorce rate per 1000 dropped to 3.5 (Time Almanac, 2001). In some societies, divorce continues to carry a stigma. High levels of marital instability challenge norms and create new patterns of family life.

The newest category of family, domestic partnerships, is sanctioned by over 25 cities or counties in the United States (for example, New York City, San Francisco, Boston, and Minneapolis) and grants some of the rights of traditional married couples to unmarried heterosexual, homosexual, elderly, and disabled couples who share the traditional bond of the family. In Denmark, homosexual marriages are legal, and survivors of same-sex partnerships are granted the right to survivor benefits and the right to inherit their partner's pension, but are not granted the right to adopt children. Courts in New York, New Jersey, Connecticut, Vermont, Minnesota, and California allow gay and lesbian couples to adopt children. Among more rural subcultures, same-sex couples living together may not be as accepted or recognized in the community as they are in larger cities. As gay parents have become more visible, lesbian and gay parenting groups have started in many cities across the United States to offer information, support, and guidance, resulting in more lesbians and gay men considering parenthood through adoption and artificial insemination.

Social attitudes toward homosexual activity vary widely, and homosexual behavior occurs in societies that deny its presence. Homosexual behavior carries a severe stigma in some societies. To discover that one's son or daughter is homosexual is akin to a catastrophic event for Egyptian Americans. In Iran and in some provinces of China, a lesbian or gay man may be killed. As recently as February 2001, a judge in Somalia sentenced two Somali lesbians to death for "exercising unnatural behavior" ("Judge Orders Executions for Lesbian Duo," 2001).

When the health-care provider needs to provide assistance and make a referral for a person who is gay, lesbian, bisexual, or transsexual, a number of options are available. Some referral agencies are local, whereas others are national, with local or regional chapters. Many are ethnically or religiously specific. Some national groups that have links to local and regional organizations include the following:

> Gay, Lesbian, and Straight Education Network, *http://www.glsen.org*
> National Latino(a) Lesbian, Gay, Bisexual, and Transgender Organization, *http://www.lego.org*
> Parents, Families, and Friends of Lesbians and Gays, *http://www.pflag.org*
> National Center for Lesbian Rights, *http://www.info @nclrights.org*
> Log Cabin Republicans, *http://www.lcr.org*
> National Stonewall Democratic Federation, *http://www.stonewalldemocrats.org*
> National Youth Advocacy Coalition, *http://www.nyacyouth.org*
> Family Pride Coalition, *http://www.familypride.org*
> It's Time, America, *http://www.gender.org*
> BINET U.S., *http://www.binetUS.org*
> National Black, Lesbian, and Gay Leadership Forum, *http://www.nblglf.org*

Box 2–3 identifies guidelines for assessing the cultural domain *family roles and organization*.

WORKFORCE ISSUES

Culture in the Workplace

A fourth domain of culture is *workforce issues*. Differences and conflicts that exist in a homogeneous

---

BOX 2–3

Family Roles and Organization

Head of Household and Gender Roles

1 Identify which family members make which types of decisions in the household. Is the overall decision-making pattern patriarchal, matriarchal, or egalitarian?
2 Describe gender-related roles of men and women in the family system.

Prescriptive, Restrictive, and Taboo Behaviors

3 Identify prescriptive, restrictive, and taboo behaviors for children.
4 Identify prescriptive, restrictive, and taboo behaviors for adolescents.

Family Roles and Priorities

5 Describe family goals and priorities emphasized by this culture.
6 Explore developmental tasks in this group.
7 Explore the status and role of the aged in the family.
8 Explore the roles and importance of extended family members.
9 Describe how one gains social status in this cultural system. Is there a caste system?

Alternative Lifestyles

10 Describe how alternative lifestyles and nontraditional families such as single parents, blended families, communal families, same-sex families, and so forth, are viewed by this society.

---

culture may be intensified in a multicultural workforce. Factors that affect these issues include language barriers, degree of assimilation and acculturation, and issues related to autonomy. Moreover, concepts such as gender roles, cultural communication styles, health-care practices of the country of origin, and selected concepts from all other domains affect workforce issues in a multicultural work environment.

Americans are expected to be punctual on their job, with formal meetings, and with appointments. If one is more than a minute or two late, an apology is expected, and if one is late by more than 5 or 10 minutes, a more elaborate apology is expected. When people know they are going to be late for a meeting, the expectation is that they call or send a message indicating that they will be late. The convener of the meeting or teacher in a classroom is expected to start and stop on time out of respect for the other people in attendance. This is in contrast to practices in many other cultures, for example, Panama, where a meeting or class starts when the majority of people arrive. However, in social situations in the United States a person can be 15 or more minutes late, depending on the importance of the gathering. In this instance, an apology is not really necessary or expected; however, most Americans will politely provide a reason for the tardiness.

The American workforce stresses efficiency (time is money), operational procedures on how to get things done, task accomplishment, and proactive problem solving. Intuitive abilities and common sense are not valued as much as technical abilities. The scientific method is valued and everything has to be proven. Americans want to know *why*, not *what*, and will search for a single factor that is the cause of the problem and the reason why something is to be done in a specific way. They are obsessed with collecting facts and figures before they make decisions. Pragmatism is valued. Conversely, the Chinese and Brazilians look at workforce issues from a more holistic perspective, rather than relying on data. In the United States everyone is expected to have a job description, meetings are to have a predetermined agenda (although items can be added at the beginning of the meeting), and the agenda is followed throughout the meeting. Americans prefer to vote on almost every item on an agenda, including approving the agenda itself. Everything is given a time frame and deadlines are expected to be respected. In these situations, American values expect that the needs of individuals are subservient to the needs of the organization. However, in the last decade, with the postmodernist movement, greater credibility and recognition have been given to approaches other than the scientific method.

Most Americans place a high value on "fairness," rely heavily on procedures and policies in the decision-making process, and everyone is expected to have a job description. However, Americans' value for individualism, where the individual is seen as the most important element in society, favors a person's decision to further his or her own career over the needs or wants of the employer. Therefore, individuals frequently demonstrate little loyalty to the organization and leave one position to take a position with another company for a better opportunity. In organizations where people generally conform because of the fear of failure, there is a hierarchical order for decision making, and the person who succeeds is the one with strong verbal skills who conforms to the hierarchy's expectations. This person is well liked and does not stand out too much from the crowd. Frequently, others view the person with a high level of competence who stands out as a threat. Thus, to be successful in the highly technical American workforce, get the facts, control your feelings, have precise and technical communication skills, be informal and direct, and clearly and explicitly state your conclusion.

Clinical professionals trained in their home countries now occupy a significant share of technical and laboratory positions in U.S. health-care facilities. Service employees such as food preparation workers, nurse aides, orderlies, housekeepers, and janitors represent the most culturally diverse component of hospital workforces. These unskilled and semiskilled positions are among the most attainable for new immigrants.

Minority groups employed as professionals are underrepresented among all health-care professions. According to the American Physical Therapy Association, only 0.5 percent of U.S. physical therapists are American Indian or Alaskan Native, 1.3 percent are African American or black, 1.9 percent are Hispanic/Latino, 4.1 percent are Asian/Pacific Islander, and the remainder (92.2 percent) are white (Minority Statistics, 2001). The American Nurses Association found that only 0.5 percent of U.S. registered nurses are Native American or Alaskan Native, 4.2 percent are black, 1.6 percent are Hispanic/Latino, 3.4 percent are Asian/Pacific Islander, and the remainder (89.7 percent) are white ("Distribution by Racial/Ethnic Group," 2001). And according to the American Medical Association (2001), there are 778,000 physicians in the United States; 0.7 percent are Native American or Alaskan Native, 7.9 percent are black, 6.9 percent are Hispanic, 19.4 percent are Asian/Pacific Islander, and 65 percent are white.

The educational preparation of health-care professionals in some countries is not comparable to that of the United States. The vast array of health-care providers in the United States—radiology technicians, physical therapists, occupational therapists, social service workers, electrocardiogram technicians, respiratory therapists, and so on—may not exist in other countries. In Mexico, some Latin American countries, and some other developing countries, nursing education is offered primarily at the high school level. In the Philippines and Australia, a baccalaureate in nursing may not be seen as equivalent to that in the United States because nursing degrees can be a B.A., B.A.N., B.S. or B.S.N. In Australia, all baccalaureate programs are 3 years long, while in Great Britain, most nurses are trained at the diploma level with an accompanying apprenticeship. Moreover, not all nursing programs include psychiatric, community, or obstetric nursing content in the curricula.

Concerns surface about the amount of additional training needed for some emigrating foreign graduates before sitting for the American licensing examination. In eras of nursing shortages, often the sponsoring organization pays for their additional education. Some American-educated health-care providers see this as unfair because they paid for their own education and receive the same salary as foreign-educated health-care providers.

During nursing workforce shortages, American health-care facilities rely on emigrating nurses from the Philippines, Canada, England, Ireland, and other countries to supplement their numbers. Some foreign nurses, such as British and Australian, culturally assimilate into the workforce more easily than others, but still have difficulty with *defensive* charting as is required in the United States. In their socialized health-care system, clients are not likely to initiate litigation (Purnell & Galloway, 1995). Others may have difficulty with the assertiveness expected from American nurses.

Timeliness and punctuality are two culturally based attitudes that can create serious problems in the multicultural workforce. In some situations, conflicts may arise over the issue of reporting to work on time or on an assigned day. The lack of adherence to meeting time demands in other countries is often in direct opposition to the American ethic for punctuality.

Health-care administration and management initiatives to support a diverse work environment may include some of the following: (1) cultural competence and diversity workshops, (2) cultural celebrations, (3) a specific orientation to the changing American health-care system, (4) providing cultural brokers as mentors or preceptors to assist new immigrants in learning about the American workforce, and (5) identifying ways to work more effectively with employees of diverse backgrounds. Orientation classes may need to include topics such as (1) the difference in the length of clients' hospital stays in the United States compared with those in the employees' countries of origin; (2) the diversity in health professionals' responsibilities; (3) the influence of insurance companies on health-care decision making; (4) concerns related to malpractice; and (5) different nursing-care delivery models, such as team nursing, primary nursing, case management, and functional nursing.

Issues Related to Autonomy

Cultural differences related to assertiveness influence how health-care practitioners view each other. Specifically, Asian nurses may not be as assertive with physicians as American nurses. The concept of nurses being dependent on physicians and male administrators is inseparable from the Muslim concept of women being subject to the authority of husbands, fathers, and elder brothers (Harner et al., 1994). Polish nursing is seen as a vocation; therefore, Polish nurses may be unprepared for the level of sophistication and autonomy of American nursing. Educational training for nurses in Pakistan is culturally different from training in America. In Pakistan, "nurses are not socially or culturally prepared to assume the role of decision maker, risk taker, teacher, or change agent" (Harner et al., 1994). These differences can pose problems in the American health-care system.

The Commission on Graduates of Foreign Nursing Schools administers a screening examination for temporary work visas to foreign graduate nurses seeking work. This examination assesses the ability to write and comprehend the English language. It cannot, however, examine the specific nuances of selected language barriers that may cause difficulties in the workplace. One area where problems typically develop is in taking physicians' prescription instructions over the telephone. The newer immigrant health-care professional may have passed the state's professional licensing examination but still need extra time in translating messages and formulating replies.

When individuals speak in their native language at work, it may become a source of contention for both clients and health-care personnel. For example, most non-English-speaking employees do not want to exclude or offend others, but it is easier to speak in their native language to articulate ideas, feelings, and humor among themselves. Negative interpretations of behaviors can be detrimental to working relationships in the health-care environment. Some foreign graduates, with limited aural language abilities, may need to have care instructions written or procedures demonstrated. In addition, health-care employers should provide classes and workshops for all employees who work with multicultural clients and personnel. In addition, English as a Second Language (ESL) classes should be provided to improve communication within the multicultural workforce.

Workforce Issues

Culture in the Workplace

1 Identify specific workforce issues affected by immigration, e.g., education.
2 Describe specific multicultural considerations when working with this culturally diverse individual or group in the workforce.
3 Explore factors influencing patterns of acculturation in this cultural group.
4 Explore native health-care practices and their influence in the workforce.

Issues Related to Autonomy

5 Identify cultural issues related to professional autonomy, superior or subordinate control, religious issues, and gender in the workforce.
6 Identify language barriers with concrete interpretations of the language.

Box 2–4 identifies guidelines for assessing the cultural domain *workforce issues.*

BIOCULTURAL ECOLOGY

The domain *biocultural ecology* identifies specific physical, biological, and physiological variations in ethnic and racial origins. These variations include skin color and physical differences in body habitus, genetic, hereditary, endemic, and topographic diseases; psychological makeup of individuals; and differences in the way drugs are metabolized by the body. No attempt is made here to explain or justify any of the numerous and conflicting views on the genetic and environmental reasons for variations. In this book, observations of physical and genetic variations are identified. These observations may be more accurate with some individuals than with others. Frequently, intraethnic variations are greater than interethnic variations.

Skin Color and Other Biological Variations

Skin coloration is an important consideration for health-care providers because anemia, jaundice, and rashes require different assessment skills in dark-skinned people than in light-skinned people. To assess for oxygenation and cyanosis in dark-skinned people, the practitioner must examine the sclera, buccal mucosa, tongue, lips, nail beds, palms of the hands, and soles of the feet rather than relying on skin tone alone. Jaundice is more easily determined in Asians by assessing the sclera rather than relying on the overall change in skin color. Health-care providers must establish a baseline skin color (by asking a family member or someone known to the individual), use direct sunlight if possible, observe areas with the least amount of pigmentation, palpate for rashes, and compare skin in corresponding areas. People from ethnic groups that are generally fair-skinned, such as Germans, Polish, Irish, and British, to name a few, prolonged exposure to the sun places them at an increased risk for skin cancer.

Variations in body habitus occur among ethnic and racially diverse individuals. For example, the long bones of many blacks are significantly longer and narrower than those of whites (Giger & Davidhizar, 1999). Asians have narrower shoulders and wider hips than other ethnic/racial groups. Additional racial variations include flat nose bridges among Asians, which may be overlooked by opticians when fitting and dispensing eyeglasses. Many Vietnamese children are small by American standards and do not fall within normal ranges on standardized American growth charts. Mandibular tori occur more frequently among Asians, making fitting dentures more difficult. Such biocultural data provide important information for health-care practitioners when assessing health problems geared to the unique attributes of people of diverse cultures. Given diverse gene pools, this type of information is often difficult to obtain.

Diseases and Health Conditions

Some diseases are endemic in specific racial or ethnic groups; that is, they are prevalent in that group. The leading causes of death in Americans of all ethnicities continue to be heart disease, cancer, chronic obstructive lung diseases, unintentional injury, diabetes, and HIV. The incidence varies somewhat among the different ethnic groups. Specific health problems are covered in individual chapters in this book. Cardiovascular disease is the leading killer of both men and women in all racial and ethnic groups in the United States. The causative factors that contribute to the development of cardiovascular disease include: obesity, 54.9 percent; lack of physical activity, 27.7 percent; and smoking, 22.9 percent ("Cardiovascular Disease," 2001). The leading sites for cancer for white male Americans are lung (74.2 percent), prostate (24.4 percent), colon and rectum (23.4 percent), pancreas (9.8 percent), and blood/leukemia (8.6 percent). The most common sites for white female Americans are lung (32.9 percent), breast (27.7 percent), colon and rectum (15.6 percent), ovary (8.2 percent), and pancreas (7.0 percent). Although these same sites account for most cancers in other ethnic and racial groups, the order of occurrence differs. For example, prostate cancer is the highest reported cancer among American Indians, blacks, Filipinos, Japanese, and nonwhite Hispanic men. In women, breast cancer incidence rates are higher in all groups except Vietnamese, for whom cervical cancer rates rank highest. Stomach cancer appears in the top cancers for men and women in Asian populations except for Filipinos and Chinese women ("Current and Accurate Cancer Information," 2001). A more thorough description of the variations in the sites and incidence of cancer among racial and ethnic groups in the United States can be obtained from the National Cancer Institute (National Center for HIV, STD and TB Prevention, 2001) and the Centers for Disease Control.

Almost 16 million Americans have been diagnosed with diabetes mellitus (DM), and there are an additional 5.4 million people in whom the disease is undiagnosed.

More women than men suffer from DM. Additionally, the prevalence of diabetes varies by race and ethnicity. The prevalence of DM among whites is 7.8 percent. However, blacks are 1.7 times as likely to have diabetes as whites; Mexican Americans, 1.9 times as likely; American Indians and Alaskan Natives, 2.8 times as likely. Prevalence rates for Asian and Pacific Islanders in the United States are limited, but DM among Native Hawaiians is twice that of white Americans in Hawaii (National Diabetes Fact Sheet, 2001).

HIV continues as a pandemic trend. An estimated 36 million people are living with HIV/AIDS; 16.4 million are women and 1.4 million are children under the age of 15 years. Worldwide, HIV is increasingly affecting women. The overwhelming majority of people with HIV (95 percent) are from developing countries. Latin America accounts for 1.4 million people with HIV. Brazil having the highest rate in South America, and Honduras has the highest rate in Central America. Nearly 1 million people in the United States have HIV, with the highest concentration in large urban areas. The Caribbean has approximately 390,000 people with HIV; the most affected country is Haiti (National Center for HIV, STD, and TB Prevention, 2001). International health agencies, such as the World Health Organization (WHO), Pan American Health Organization (PAHO), Centers for Disease Control (CDC), and Joint United Nations Programme on HIV/AIDS (UNAIDS) have joined together in partnership for global HIV prevention efforts, with specific programs for selected countries, populations, and cultural groups. A number of world religions, among them Roman Catholicism and Islam, do not believe in the use of condoms because they are contraceptives and because they may encourage promiscuity and sex outside marriage. To them, abstinence is the only option for the control of HIV and AIDS. However, the advent of AIDS is challenging these beliefs ("AIDS Challenges Religious Leaders," 2001). (For more information on AIDS prevention, contact CDC National AIDS Hotline at 1-800-342-AIDS; Spanish 1-800-344-SIDA; Deaf, 1-800-243-7889. The CDC National Prevention Information Network can be contacted at 1-800-458-5231.)

In the United States, more than 65 million people are currently living with an incurable sexually transmitted disease (STD). While extremely common, STDs are difficult to track and many people are not aware they have these infections, resulting in "hidden epidemics" (Cates, 1999). Although syphilis is at an all-time low in the United States, other STDs such as gonorrhea, chlamydia, genital herpes, trichomoniasis, Human Papillomavirus, hepatitis B, and bacterial vaginosis continue to surge through the population. Women bear the greatest burden of STDs, suffering more frequent and more serious complications than men. Roughly one-fourth of these diseases occur in teenagers, with chlamydia and gonorrhea the most prevalent STDs among teenagers and young adults under the age of 25. The incidence of STDs is as much as 30 times higher in the black population of the United States because of poverty, limited access to quality care, health-seeking behaviors, level of drug use, sexual networks, and overall better reporting and surveillance in black communities. STDs affect all racial, ethnic, and cultural groups. Each population needs culturally specific, relevant, and congruent education to decrease the incidence of these diseases. The middle socioeconomic white groups in the United States have responded favorably to educational programs geared to age-specific groups through media and school campaigns. Likewise, other communities have been successful with educational programs geared to the unique needs of the population ("Sexually Transmitted Disease Surveillance," 2000). Some comparisons of each STD with ethnospecific populations, age groups, and gender, can be obtained from the Centers for Disease Control (2001) or the Institute of Medicine (2001).

Illnesses and diseases with an increased incidence in white ethnic groups in the United States include appendicitis, diverticular disease, cancer of the colon, hemorrhoids, varicose veins, cystic fibrosis, rosacea, osteoporosis and osteoarthritis, and phenylketonuria. Many immigrant groups have higher rates of some infectious diseases and illnesses that are not common in the United States. Accordingly, health-care providers should assess newer immigrants for diseases that are common in their homelands. For example, immigrant populations from Egypt may display liver impairment, portal hypertension, esophageal varices, and renal impairment due to bilharzia infection, or infectious blindness and scleral infections due to endemic trachoma. An awareness of populations at risk for specific endemic diseases allows the health professional to provide culturally appropriate screening and education for disease prevention and health promotion. See Appendix for illnesses and diseases and their causes for specific ethnic and cultural groups common in the United States.

The topography of a given country or region may provide the health-care practitioner with essential clues to symptoms requiring investigation. For instance, people who emigrate from mosquito-infested tropical areas such as Brazil, Mexico, Central America, Turkey, and Vietnam may present with chills, fever, lassitude, and splenic enlargement, which are consistent with malaria. Air pollution, which increases the risk for respiratory diseases, may be a significant risk factor for any group that emigrates from or lives in a large city. Knowledge of specific risk factors related to the topography of the client's country of origin and current residence enhances the diagnostic process and ensures accurate assessments.

With increases in globalization, world migration patterns, and climate alterations, health-care providers need to be aware of new and re-emerging illnesses and diseases. As worldwide temperatures increase, algae and zooplankton respond to warming and favor the more toxic cyanobacteria and dino flagellates; as a result shellfish may be toxic to humans. As droughts and then floods occur, brought on by phenomena such as El Niño, new breeding grounds and bursts of activity increase the incidence of cholera, malaria, yellow fever, dengue fever, hanta virus, and Ebola. Additionally, diseases are now being found in areas that normally did not have them; for example, New York and New Jersey have had cases of malaria for the first time. Droughts followed by heavy rain in the southwestern part of the United States resulted in an increase in food for the rodent population, causing an increase in rodent-borne illnesses. Cases of malaria, dengue fever, and cholera in Central America extend for longer time periods than in the past. In perturbed environments, where ecosystems are devoid of genetic and species diversity, and where pesticides eliminate large predators, parasites, pests, and pathogens proliferate, resulting in illness and diseases for which the American health-care system is not prepared.

Within the past 20 years, every continent has had outbreaks of new or re-emerging diseases. North America has had outbreaks of bubonic plague, campylobacteria, cyclospora, salmonella, and Legionnaire's disease. Central and South America have been particularly affected by cholera, yellow fever, malaria, dengue fever, and rabies. Europe has had outbreaks of shigella in Paris, *E. coli* and mad cow disease in Great Britain, and leptospirosis in the Ukraine. Asia has had an increase in dengue fever, anthrax has been seen in Russia and the United States, and avian flu in Hong Kong. Africa has had meningitis in Chad, endemic rates of Ebola in Zaire and the Sudan, and bubonic plague in Malawi and Mozambique. To this end, educators in colleges and health-care organizations need to educate students, staff, and the community about new and re-emerging illnesses as a public health concern.

Variations in Drug Metabolism

Information regarding drug metabolism among racial and ethnic groups has important implications for health-care practitioners when prescribing medications. Besides the effects of smoking (which accelerates drug metabolism), nutritional status, (malnutrition affects drug response), diet (a high-fat diet increases absorption of antifungal medication while a low-fat diet renders the drug less effective), culture (attitudes and beliefs about taking medication), and stress (which affects catecholamine and cortisol levels) on drug metabolism, studies have identified some specific alterations in drug metabolism among diverse racial and ethnic groups. For instance, the Chinese are more sensitive to the cardiovascular effects of propranolol and have an increased absorption of antipsychotics, some narcotics, and antihypertensives than their white American counterparts. Eskimos, American Indians, and Hispanics have an increased risk for developing peripheral neuropathy while taking the drug isoniazid, compared with white Americans, who inactivate the drug more rapidly. African Americans respond better to diuretic therapy than do white ethnic groups. An additional cultural consideration is the difference in the way physicians prescribe medications in various countries. For example, in most Asian countries and Great Britain, the preferred practice is to start out with low dosages of medicines and adjust upward until side effects or therapeutic responses are reached. In the United States, most clinicians start with the maximum dosage and adjust downward as side effects occur (Levy, 1993). Health-care providers need to investigate the literature for ethnic-specific studies regarding variations in drug metabolism, communicate these findings to other colleagues, and educate their

BOX 2–5

Biocultural Ecology

Skin Color and Biologic Variations

1 Identify the skin color and physical variations for this group.
2 Explore any special problems or concerns skin color may pose for health-care practitioners.
3 Identify biologic variations in body habitus or structure.

Diseases and Health Conditions

4 Identify specific risk factors for individuals related to the topography or climate.
5 Identify hereditary or genetic diseases or conditions that are common within this group.
6 Identify endemic diseases specific to this cultural or ethnic group.
7 Identify any diseases or health conditions for which this group has increased susceptibility.

Variations in Drug Metabolism

8 Identify specific variations in drug metabolism, drug interactions, dosages, and related side effects.

clients regarding these side effects. Medication administration is one area where American health-care providers see the importance of culture, ethnicity, and race.

Box 2–5 identifies guidelines for assessing and the cultural domain *biocultural ecology*.

HIGH-RISK BEHAVIORS

Although high-risk behavior exists in all cultures, some groups may not fully understand the implications of certain high-risk health behaviors such as using tobacco, alcohol, or recreational drugs; lack of physical activity; increased calorie consumption; unsafe driving practices; failure to use seat belts and helmets; failure to take precautions against HIV and sexually transmitted diseases.

The incidence of cigarette smoking has been declining in the United States over the last 25 years but continues to remain steady, and it may even be on the increase among newer immigrants. Although black Americans smoke at the same rate as white Americans (28 to 34 percent), they smoke fewer cigarettes, take in 30 percent more nicotine per cigarette, and take nearly 2 hours longer to clear nicotine metabolites from their bloodstream. Fewer black women smoke than white women smoke, 22 versus 25 percent. The data for other ethnic groups indicate lower rates of smoking for Asians compared with white Americans (Perez-Stable et al., 1998); however, the data varies and are inconsistent across studies, suggesting a regional variation.

Alcohol consumption crosses all cultural and socioeconomic groups. There are enormous differences among ethnic and cultural groups around use of and response to alcohol. Even in cultures where alcohol consumption is taboo, it is not ignored. However, alcohol problems are not simply a result of how much people drink. When drinking is culturally approved, it is typically done more by men than women and is more often a social, rather than a solitary, act. The group in which drinking is most frequently practiced is usually composed of same-age social peers (Peele & Brodsky, 2001). Studies on increasing controls on the availability of alcohol to decreasing alcohol consumption, with the premise that alcohol-related problems occur in proportion to per capita consumption, has been disproved in France, Spain, Iceland, and Sweden (Heath, 1995). Furthermore, countries with temperance movements have greater alcohol-related behavior problems than do countries without temperance movements (Peele, 1997).

In countries where drinking alcoholic beverages is integrated into rites and social customs, and where one is expected to have self-control and sociability, there are lower rates of alcohol-related problems than in countries and cultures where ambivalent attitudes toward drinking prevail (Heath, 1995). Additionally, Hilton's (1987) study demonstrated a clear and distinct difference in alcohol abuse rate by socioeconomic status (SES). Higher-SES Americans were more likely to drink, but also more likely to drink without problems. The conclusion of many studies suggests that alcohol-related violence is a learned behavior, not an inevitable result of alcohol consumption. Other studies have correlated per capita alcohol consumption rates with the number of Alcoholics Anonymous (AA) groups per million of population. Countries with the lowest per capita consumption rate of alcohol had higher numbers of AA groups. Countries with the highest per capita consumption rate of alcohol had lower numbers of AA groups; for example, Iceland with a low per capita alcohol consumption rate of 3.9 liters had 784 AA groups, whereas France, with a per capital alcohol consumption rate of 13.2 liters, had 7 AA groups. See Table 2–1. No information was found about the number of people in each group.

When assessing clients' alcohol and recreational drug use, the health-care provider must place these high-risk behaviors within the context of their cultural group. Health-care providers can have a significant impact on behavior-related health problems of alcohol by encouraging moderate drinking, providing educational and counseling materials in a culturally relevant manner, working with the regulators of alcohol manufacturing as well as the beverage industry, and working with elementary and secondary school teachers to promote responsible drinking.

Health-Care Practices

A lack of health promotion and safety practices may be a major threat to the health of some people. For example, obesity is more prevalent among Amish women than non-Amish women in Ohio (Fuchs et al., 1992). Weight gain among the Amish may be related to the importance of food in the culture and the higher rates of pregnancy throughout childbearing years (Wenger, 1991). Health-care providers can assist overweight clients in reducing calorie consumption by identifying healthy choices among culturally preferred foods, altering preparation practices, and reducing portion size.

Table 2–1 *Alcohol Consumption by Country*

Country	Alcohol Consumption (liters per capita)	Number of AA Groups (per million population)
Iceland	3.9	784
Norway	4.0	28
Sweden	5.5	33
Canada	7.1	177
Ireland	7.2	210
United States	7.2	164
United Kingdom	7.6	51
Finland	7.8	110
New Zealand	7.8	102
Australia	8.3	56
Netherlands	8.4	12
Italy	8.6	6
Denmark	9.8	22
Belgium	9.9	53
Portugal	9.9	1
Spain	10.4	8
Switzerland	10.8	22
Austria	11.5	92
Germany	12.6	26
France	13.2	7
Luxembourg	13.6	0

Source: The Stanton Peale Addiction Center. *http://www.stanton-peele.net.*

The ethnocultural practice of self-care using folk and magicoreligious practices before seeking professional care may also have a negative impact on the health status of some individuals. Overreliance on these practices may mean that the health problem is in a more advanced stage when a consultation is sought. Such delays make treatment more difficult and prolonged.

The cultural domain of high-risk behaviors is one area where health-care providers can make a significant impact on clients' health status. High-risk health behaviors can be controlled through ethnic-specific interventions aimed at health promotion and health-risk prevention through educational programs in schools, business organizations, churches, and recreational and community centers, as well as through the use of one-on-one and family counseling techniques. Taking advantage of public communication technology can enhance participation in these programs if they are geared to the unique needs of the individual, family, or community.

Box 2–6 identifies guidelines for assessing the cultural domain *high-risk behaviors*.

NUTRITION

The cultural domain of *nutrition* includes more than having adequate food for satisfying hunger. It also includes the meaning of food to the culture; common foods and rituals; nutritional deficiencies and food limitations; and the use of food for health promotion,

High-Risk Behaviors

High-Risk Behaviors

1 Identify specific high-risk behaviors common among this group.
2 Explore behaviors related to the use of alcohol, tobacco, and recreational drugs and other substances among this group.
3 Explore beliefs and practices related to safe sex.

Health-Care Practices

4 Identify the typical health-seeking behaviors of this group.
5 Assess the level of physical activity in their lifestyle.
6 Assess the use of safety measures such as seat belts and helmets.

restoration, and disease and illness prevention. Understanding a client's food patterns is essential for providing culturally competent dietary counseling. Health-care practitioners may be considered professionally negligent when prescribing, for example, an American diet to a Hispanic or an Asian client whose food choices and meal times may be different from American food patterns.

Meaning of Food

Food and the absence of food—hunger—have diverse meanings among cultures and individuals. Cultural beliefs, values, and types of foods available influence what people eat, avoid, or alter to make food congruent with cultural lifeways; and food offers cultural security and acceptance (Leininger, 1988). Food is not only necessary as a means of survival and relief from hunger, but it also plays a significant role in socialization. It has symbolic meaning for peaceful coexistence and is used to promote healing. It denotes caring or lack of caring, closeness, kinship, and solidarity, and it may be used as an expression of love or anger (Leininger, 1988). When Americans invite a guest to dinner for the first time, the guest frequently brings a gift, although this is not required, and one of the choices is often food. There are no specific rules as to what type of food to bring, but wine, cheese baskets, and candy are usually appropriate. Bread (unless it is a very special bread) and soft drinks are not usually appropriate unless specifically requested.

Common Foods and Food Rituals

American food and preparation practices reflect traditional food habits of early settlers who brought their unique cuisines with them. Accordingly, the "typical American diet" has been brought from elsewhere. Americans vary their meal times and food choices according to the region of the country, urban versus rural residence, and weekdays versus weekends. Additionally, food choices vary by marital status, economic status, climate changes, religion, ancestry, availability, and personal preferences. This chapter will not cover specific foods, preparation practices, and ritual for religious groups found in the United States. Instead, they are covered in specific ethnocultural chapters such as Islamic, Jewish, etc.

Overall, the typical American diet is high in fats and cholesterol and low in fiber, according to the U.S. Department of Agriculture (USDA). The USDA recommends the Food Pyramid, originally adapted in 1950 and revised in 1992. This food pyramid is commonly taught in elementary and secondary education and is used as a guide for teaching healthy eating to the public. Daily recommendations include 6 to 11 servings of bread, cereal, rice, or pasta; 3 to 5 servings of vegetables; 2 to 4 servings of fruit, 2 to 3 servings of milk, yogurt, or cheese; 2 to 3 servings of meat, poultry, fish, dry beans, eggs, and nuts; and limited use of fats, oils, and sweets. However, it has been recognized that specific foods in this pyramid must be adapted for non-American food preferences. Additionally, this pyramid has been questioned by prestigious organizations because it contributes to obesity and overall poor health. Sixty-one percent of Americans are overweight, with 26 percent being obese (30 or more pounds overweight) (USDA, 2001).

Breakfast is usually consumed between 6:00 A.M. and 9:00 A.M., depending on the person's work schedule. On weekends, the time may be delayed 1 or 2 hours or extended into "brunch" at 11:00 A.M. to noon. Favorite foods for people in urban areas and for people doing office-type work are hot or cold cereal; pastry; bagels, either plain or with cream cheese; toast with butter or margarine and/or jelly or preserves; fruit; juice; and coffee or tea. For people doing physical labor and in farming communities, breakfast more likely includes fried, scrambled, or poached eggs; ham, bacon, sausage or scrapple (primarily in the southern United States), fried potatoes; toast with butter or margarine and/or jelly or preserves; juice; and coffee or tea. Children traditionally drink milk with breakfast. Most Americans in the work environment enjoy a midmorning coffee break, although juice, soft drinks, or tea may be consumed instead of coffee.

The noontime meal, typically consumed by 1:00 P.M., is called lunch in urban areas and dinner in rural areas. Urbanites frequently miss lunch completely, carry their lunch to work with them, eat salads or sandwiches, and drink iced beverages such as tea or soft drinks, although many also enjoy hot tea and coffee. Americans like choices and this extends to soft drinks, of which there are a wide variety from which to choose. Unlike in many other countries, Americans can have their soft drink with or without caffeine, diet (artificially sweetened), or regular (with sugar). In farm communities, the noon meal, dinner, is often the largest meal of the day and includes tossed garden salad; meat, such as beef, pork, poultry, or fish; a variety of green or yellow vegetables; a starch such as potatoes, pasta, or rice; bread; a dessert such as cake, pie, cookies, ice cream, or puddings; and choice of beverage. Most people take an afternoon beverage break, to which they are entitled by law. This short break is not as extensive as the afternoon tea that the British and other groups enjoy.

The evening meal, dinner in urban areas or supper in rural areas, is served between 6:00 P.M. and 9:00 P.M., depending on the family's work pattern. Rural people usually eat earlier than urban people. The evening meal is usually the largest meal of the day for most people and includes soup and/or a salad; meat, such as beef, pork, poultry, or fish; a variety of green or yellow vegetables; a starch such as potatoes, pasta, or rice; bread; a dessert such as cake, pie, cookies, ice cream, or puddings; and choice of beverage. People may begin this meal with an appetizer and enjoy wine before or with the meal. Children and some adults might eat a bedtime snack.

Many of the elderly and people living alone do not eat balanced meals, stating they do not have the time to prepare a meal, even though most American homes have labor-saving devices such as stoves, microwave ovens, refrigerators, and dishwashers. For those who are unable to prepare their own meals because of disability or illness, most communities have a Meals on Wheels program where community and church organizations deliver, usually once a day, a hot meal along with a cold meal for later and food for the following morning's breakfast. Other community and church agencies prepare meals for the homeless or collect food, which is delivered to those who have none. When people are ill, they generally prefer toast, tea, juice, and other easily digested foods.

Most cities and towns in the United States have an abundance of fast-food places that have chicken, burgers, and pizza where busy people can "eat and drive" or get food to take home to eat. For the most part, these foods are high in fat and cholesterol, although in some places you can buy heart-healthy foods such as salad.

Socioeconomic status may dictate food selections: for example, hamburger instead of steak, canned or frozen vegetables and fruit rather than fresh, and fish instead of shrimp or lobster. Given the size of the United States and its varied terrain, food choices differ by region: beef in the Midwest, fish in coastal areas, poultry in the South and along the eastern seaboard; vegetables vary by season, climate, and altitude, although larger grocery stores have a wide variety of all types of American and international meats, fruits, and vegetables. Many television stations and major newspapers have large sections devoted to foods and preparation practices, a testament to the value that Americans place on food and diversity in food preparation.

Most table settings include a dinner place for the main entrée, a bread plate, a salad plate and/or a soup bowl, desert plate, and silverware, which includes a knife, entrée fork, salad fork, teaspoon, and soupspoon, if appropriate. At formal dinners, additional plates, wine and water glasses, bowls and silverware are included; the order in which they are placed has special meaning. When in doubt as to which piece of silverware to use, follow the lead of the host or hostess. If you do make a mistake, do not worry, most people will not notice and if they do notice, they will not mind. It is socially taboo to start eating before everyone is seated.

Special occasions and holidays among many cultures are frequently associated with ethnic foods. For example, in the United States, hot dogs are consumed at sports events, and turkey is served at Thanksgiving. Many religious groups are required to fast during specific holiday seasons, such as Ramadan for Muslims and Lent for Catholics. However, health-care providers may need to remind clients that fasting is not required during times of illness or pregnancy.

Given the intraethnic variations of diet, it is important for health professionals to inquire about the specific diets of their clients. Expecting the client to eat according to an American mealtime schedule and to select American foods from an exchange list may be unrealistic for clients of different cultural backgrounds. Counseling about food-group requirements, intake restrictions, and exercise must respect cultural behaviors and individual lifeways. Culturally congruent dietary counseling, such as changing amounts and preparation practices while including ethnic food choices, can reduce the risk for obesity, cardiovascular disease, and cancer. Whenever possible, determining a client's dietary practices should be accomplished during the intake interview.

Dietary Practices for Health Promotion

The nutritional balance of a diet is recognized by most cultures throughout the world. Most cultures have their own distinct theories of nutritional practices for health promotion and disease prevention. Common folk practices and selected diets are recommended during periods of illness and for prevention of illness or disease. For example, many societies such as Iranian, Mexican, Puerto Rican, Chinese, and Vietnamese subscribe to the hot and cold theory of food selection to prevent illness and maintain health. Although each of these ethnic groups has its own specific name for the hot and cold theory of foods, the overall belief is that the body needs a balance of opposing foods.

In the Western health-care system, diets that are low in sodium and fats are prescribed for the prevention and treatment of heart conditions. Diets high in fat are recognized as increasing risks for the development of cardiovascular disease and some types of cancer. Many societies are becoming more health-conscious about reducing fat in their diets. Some Asian cultures prepare very spicy foods, which increase the incidence of stomach cancer, ulcers, and gastrointestinal bleeding. A thorough history and assessment of dietary practices can be an important diagnostic tool to guide health promotion. Although school lunch programs, Meals on Wheels, and church meal plans to name a few, are programs through which the health-care provider can encourage and support families in attaining better nutrition, these programs may not provide optimal nutritional selections.

Nutritional Deficiencies and Food Limitations

Because of limited socioeconomic resources or limited availability of their native foods, immigrants may eat foods that were not available in their home country. These dietary changes may result in health problems when they arrive in a new environment. This is more likely to occur when individuals immigrate to a country where they do not have native foods readily available and do not know which new foods contain the necessary

Nutrition

Meaning of Food

1 Explore the meaning of food to this group.

Common Foods and Food Rituals

2 Identify foods, preparation practices, and major ingredients commonly used by this group.
3 Identify specific food rituals.

Dietary Practices for Health Promotion

4 Identify dietary practices used to promote health or to treat illness in this cultural group.

Nutritional Deficiencies and Food Limitations

5 Identify enzyme deficiencies or food intolerances commonly experienced by this group.
6 Identify large-scale or significant nutritional deficiencies experienced by this group.
7 Identify native food limitations in their new country that may cause special health difficulties.

and comparable nutritional ingredients. Consequently, they do not know which foods to select for balancing their diet. Widespread nutritional deficiencies of many types have occurred with recent immigrants from Southeast Asia, in part because of the time spent in refugee camps, but also because of changes in food habits when immigrating to America. Among the Hindu, the consumption of a single grain such as rice may result in a poor intake of lysine and other essential amino acids.

Enzyme deficiencies exist among some ethnic and racial groups. For example, many Vietnamese Americans are lactose-intolerant and are unable to drink milk or eat dairy products to maintain their calcium needs. By consuming soups and stews made with pureed bones and cooked to an edible consistency, this deficiency can be overcome. In general, the wide availability of foods in this country reduces the risks of these disorders as long as immigrants have the means to obtain culturally nutritious foods. Recent emphasis on cultural foods has resulted in small businesses selling ethnic foods and spices to the general public. The health-care provider's task is to determine how to assist the client and identify alternative foods to supplement the diet when these stores are not financially or geographically accessible.

Box 2–7 identifies guidelines for assessing the cultural domain *nutrition*.

PREGNANCY AND CHILDBEARING PRACTICES

The cultural domain *pregnancy and childbearing practices* includes culturally sanctioned and unsanctioned fertility practices; views toward pregnancy; and prescriptive, restrictive, and taboo practices related to pregnancy, birthing, and the postpartum period.

More traditional, folk, and magicoreligious beliefs surround fertility control, pregnancy, childbearing, and postpartum practices in this cultural domain than in any other. The reason may be the mystique that surrounds the processes of conception, pregnancy, and birthing. Ideas about conception, pregnancy, and childbearing practices are handed down from generation to generation and are acculturated into the society without validation or being completely understood. For some, the success of modern technology in inducing pregnancy in postmenopausal women and others who desire children through in vitro fertilization and the ability to select a child's gender raises serious ethical questions about parenting.

Fertility Practices and Views toward Pregnancy

Commonly used methods of fertility control in the United States include natural ovulation methods, birth control pills, foams, Norplant, the morning-after pill, intrauterine devices, sterilization, vasectomy, prophylactics, and abortion. Although not all of these methods are acceptable to all people, many women use a combination of fertility control methods. The most extreme examples of fertility control are sterilization and abortion. Sterilization in the United States is now strictly voluntary; however, some countries still perform involuntary sterilization to control birth rates and to control conception in people with mental retardation or deformities. Abortion remains a controversial issue in the United States and in other countries. For example, in some countries, women are encouraged to have as many children as possible, and abortion is illegal. However, in China, abortion is commonly used as a means of limiting family size because of China's one couple, one child law. Many Chinese women in China have 5 or 6 abortions in their lifetime because they lack other birth control methods (personal communications with Chinese women in Beijing and Xian, China, 1998).

Although few comprehensive research studies exist regarding the fertility control practices of diverse ethnic, cultural, and racial groups, some are notable. Herold and others (1989) studied the use of fertility control methods among Catholic Puerto Rican women and found that the incidence of pregnancy is higher for Catholic Puerto Ricans than for non-Catholic Puerto Ricans. However, contraceptive use is widespread among the Puerto Rican population regardless of social contexts such as socioeconomic levels, rural versus urban residence, and educational level.

Mosher and Goldscheider (1984) studied 14,000 married women in the United States, white and nonwhite, from Protestant, Catholic, and Jewish backgrounds. Their data showed a dramatic increase in surgical sterilization (from 9 to 23 percent) between 1955 and 1970, with a sharper increase in the use of sterilization among males. This finding implies a much higher use of sterilization in the United States than is found in other industrialized countries. Sterilization increased threefold during this same time among Catholics and doubled among Protestants and Jews. Jewish couples were also more likely to use contraception than Protestants or Catholics. Male sterilization among black couples in all religious groups is rare. Differences in contraceptive choices by race are greater than those by religion. Furthermore, this same study implied that black couples with no religious affiliation were the group least likely to use contraception.

Fertility practices and sexual activity, sensitive topics for many, especially teenagers, is one area in which "outside" health-care practitioners may be more effective than health-care providers known to the client because of the concern about providing intimate information to someone they know. Some of the ways health-care providers can promote a better understanding of and compliance with practices related to family planning include the following: using videos in the native language and videos and pictures of native ethnic people, using material written at the individual's level of education, and providing written instructions in both English and the native language. Health-care providers should avoid family planning discussions on the first encounter; such information may be better received on subsequent visits when some trust has developed. Approaching the subject of family planning obliquely may make it possible to discuss these topics more successfully.

Prescriptive, Restrictive, and Taboo Practices in the Childbearing Family

Most societies have prescriptive, restrictive, and taboo beliefs for maternal behaviors and the delivery of a healthy baby. Such beliefs affect sexual and lifestyle behaviors during pregnancy, birthing, and the immediate postpartum period. Prescriptive practices are things that the mother should do to have a good outcome (healthy baby and pregnancy). Restrictive belief practices are those things that the mother should not do to have a positive outcome (healthy baby and delivery). Taboo practices are those things that, if done, are likely to harm the baby or mother.

A prescriptive belief among Americans is that women are expected to seek preventive care, eat a well-balanced diet, and get adequate rest to have a healthy pregnancy and baby. The American health-care system encourages women to breast-feed, and many places of employment have made arrangements for women to breast-feed while working. A restrictive belief among Americans is that pregnant women should refrain from being around loud noises for prolonged periods of time. Taboo behaviors during pregnancy among Americans are smoking, drinking alcohol, high caffeine intake, and taking recreational drugs—practices that are sure to cause harm to the mother and baby.

Among the Navajo a restrictive belief is that clothes should not be purchased for the infant before birth because preparing for the infant is forbidden by Indian tradition. Thus, when an expectant woman does not prepare for the birth of her baby, it does not mean that she does not care about herself or her baby. A taboo belief among some populations is that a pregnant woman should not reach over her head because the baby may be born with the umbilical cord around its neck. A restrictive belief among Indians in Belize and Panama is that permitting the father to be present in the delivery room and seeing the mother or baby before they have been cleaned can cause harm to the baby or mother. Because the father is absent from the delivery room or does not want to see the mother or baby immediately after birth does not mean that he does not care about them. However, in the American culture, in which the father is often encouraged to take prenatal classes with the expectant mother and provide a supportive role in the delivery process, fathers with opposing beliefs may feel guilty if they do not comply.

In the American culture under the Family Medical Leave Act, women and men are guaranteed maternity/paternity leave of up to 90 days if their employer hires more than 50 people. Most women, but few men, take advantage of this opportunity. The woman's female relatives, mother, sisters, and aunts provide assistance to the new mother until she is able to care for herself and baby. Additional cultural beliefs carried over from cultural migration and American diversity include the following:

If you wear an opal ring during pregnancy, it will harm the baby.
Birth marks are caused by eating strawberries or seeing a snake and being frightened.
Congenital anomalies can occur if the mother sees or experiences a tragedy during her pregnancy.
Nursing mothers should eat a bland diet to avoid upsetting the baby.
The infant should wear a band around the abdomen to prevent the umbilicus from protruding and becoming herniated.
A coin, key, or other metal object should be put on the umbilicus to flatten it.
Cutting a baby's hair before baptism can cause blindness.
Raising your hands over your head while pregnant may cause the cord to wrap around the baby's neck.
Moving heavy items can cause your "insides" to fall out.
If the baby is physically or mentally abnormal, God is punishing the parents.

In some other cultures, the postpartum woman is prescribed a prolonged period of recuperation in the hospital or at home, something that may not be feasible in the United States because of the shortened length of confinement in the hospital after delivery. Among the Vietnamese, the head is considered sacred, and it is taboo to touch the head of the mother or the infant. Even removal of vernix from the infant's head can cause distress.

The health-care provider must respect cultural beliefs associated with pregnancy and the birthing process when making decisions related to the health care of pregnant women, especially those practices that do not cause harm to the mother or baby. Most cultural practices can be integrated into preventive teaching in a manner that promotes compliance.

Box 2–8 identifies guidelines for assessing the cultural domain *pregnancy and childbearing practices*.

BOX 2–8

Pregnancy and Childbearing Practices

Fertility Practices and Views Toward Pregnancy

1 Explore cultural views and practices related to fertility control.
2 Identify cultural practices and views toward pregnancy.

Prescriptive, Restrictive, and Taboo Practices in the Childbearing Family

3 Identify prescriptive, restrictive, and taboo practices related to pregnancy, such as foods, exercise, intercourse, and avoidance of weather-related conditions.
4 Identify prescriptive, restrictive, and taboo practices related to the birthing process, such as reactions during labor, presence of men, position for delivery, preferred types of health practitioners, or place of delivery.
5 Identify prescriptive, restrictive, and taboo practices related to the postpartum period, such as bathing, cord care, exercise, foods, and roles of men.

DEATH RITUALS

The cultural domain *death rituals* includes how the individual and the society view death and euthanasia, rituals to prepare for death, burial practices, and bereavement. Death rituals of ethnic and cultural groups are the least likely to change over time and may cause concerns among health-care personnel. Some staff may not understand the value of customs that they are not familiar with, such as the ritual washing of the body. Death practices, beliefs, and rituals vary significantly among cultural and religious groups. To avoid cultural taboos, health professionals must become knowledgeable about unique practices related to death, dying, and bereavement.

Death Rituals and Expectations

For many American health-care providers educated in a culture of mastery over the environment, death is seen as one more disease to conquer and when this does not happen, death becomes a personal failure. Thus, for many, death does not take a natural course because it is "managed" or "prolonged," making it difficult to die with dignity. Accordingly, death and responses to death are not easy topics for many Americans to verbalize. Instead, many euphemisms are used rather than verbalizing that the person died: for example, "He passed on or passed away," "She is no longer with us," and "He went to visit the Grim Reaper." The American cultural belief in self-determination and autonomy extends to people making their own decisions about end-of-life care. Mentally competent adults have the right to decide what medical treatment and interventions they wish to extend life, such as artificial life support and artificial feeding.

Among Americans, the belief is that a dying person should not be left alone, and accommodations are usually made for a family member to be with the dying person at all times. Health-care personnel are expected to care for the family as much as for the patient during this time. Most people are buried or cremated within 3 days of the death, but extenuating circumstances may lengthen this period to accommodate family and friends who must travel a long distance to attend a funeral or memorial service. The family can decide if the deceased will have an open casket for viewing the deceased by family or friends, or if the casket will remain closed.

Significant variations in burial practices occur with other ethnocultural groups in the United States. The tradition among Orthodox Jews is to bury their deceased before sundown the next day and have post-death rituals that last for several days. Other groups have elaborate ceremonies in commemoration of the dead, such as a *velorio* among Mexican Americans, which may last for days. To some people, these rituals look like a celebration; in reality it is a celebration of the person's life. In Greek Orthodox culture, there are successive stages of mourning that include memorial services 40 days after burial and then at 3 months and 6 months, with yearly rituals thereafter. When Muslims approach death, they may wish to face Mecca and recite passages from the Qur'an; the health-care provider needs to determine the direction of Mecca and position the bed accordingly. Whether in the hospital, extended-care facility, or at home in the community, the furniture may need to be rearranged to accomplish this important ritual.

Responses to Death and Grief

Over the last decade, American society, medical and otherwise, has launched a major initiative to help patients die as comfortably as possible without pain. As a result, more people are choosing to remain at home or to enter a hospice for end-of-life care, where their comfort needs are better met. One of the requirements for entering a hospice in the United States is that the patient must sign documents indicating that he or she does not want extensive life-saving measures performed. However, African Americans are less receptive to hospice care (Neubauer & Hamilton, 1990); they are also less likely than white Americans to desire assisted death, wanting to be given every treatment available to them (O'Brien et al., 1997). When death does occur, most Americans conservatively control their grief, although women are usually more expressive than men. For many, especially men, they are expected to be stoic in their reactions to death, at least in public. Generally, tears are shed, but loud wailing and uncontrollable sobbing rarely occur. The belief is that the person has progressed to a better existence and does not have to undergo the pressures of life on Earth.

The expression of grief in response to death varies among cultural groups. For example, in Hindu culture, loved ones are expected to suffer the grief of death in silence with little display of emotion (Miller & Supersad, 1991). Bereavement time for Chinese people may be a week or longer, depending on the relationship of the family member to the deceased and the degree of acculturation. The family of a deceased Chinese American

Death Rituals

Death Rituals and Expectations

1 Identify culturally specific death rituals and expectations.
2 Explain death rituals and mourning practices.
3 What are specific burial practices, such as cremation?

Responses to Death and Grief

4 Identify cultural responses to death and grief.
5 Explore the meaning of death, dying, and the afterlife.

may need extra leave time to fulfill their cultural obligations. These variations in the grieving process may cause confusion for health-care providers, who may perceive some clients as overreacting and others as not caring. The behaviors associated with the grieving process must be placed in the context of the specific ethnocultural belief system in order to provide culturally competent care. Caregivers should encourage ethnically specific bereavement practices when providing support to family and friends. Bereavement support strategies include being physically present, encouraging a reality orientation, openly acknowledging the family's right to grieve, permitting varied behavioral responses to grief, acknowledging the patient's pain, giving the client and family permission to grieve, assisting them to express their feelings, encouraging interpersonal relationships, promoting interest in a new life, and making referrals to other resources such as a priest, minister, rabbi, or pastoral care person with the patient's or family's permission.

Box 2–9 identifies guidelines for assessing the cultural domain *death rituals*.

SPIRITUALITY

The domain *spirituality* involves more than formal religious beliefs related to faith and affiliation and the use of prayer. For some people, religion has a strong influence over and shapes nutrition practices, health-care practices, and other cultural domains. Spirituality includes all behaviors that give meaning to life and provide strength to the individual. Furthermore, it is difficult to distinguish religious beliefs from cultural beliefs because for some, especially the very devout, religion guides the dominant beliefs, values, and practices even more than their culture.

Spirituality, a component of health related to the essence of life, is a vital human experience that is shared by all humans. Spirituality helps provide balance among the mind, body, and spirit. Trained and folk religious leaders provide comfort to both the patient and family. Spirituality does not have to be scientifically proven and is patterned unconsciously from a person's worldview. Accordingly, people may deviate somewhat from the majority view or position of their formally recognized religion.

Dominant Religion and Use of Prayer

Many groups settled in America for religious freedom. Today, most practice one of the many Judeo-Christian religions: Baptist, Catholic, Church of Latter-Day Saints (Mormon), Episcopal, Jewish, Lutheran, Methodist, Seventh-Day Adventist, and so on. Furthermore, specific religious groups are concentrated regionally in the United States, with Baptists in the South, Lutherans in the North and Midwest, and Catholics in the Northeast, East, and Southwest. Within this context, there is a separation of church and state, and the United States government cannot support any particular religion or prevent people from practicing their chosen religion. However, this does not include cults or extremist groups, which usually devote themselves to esoteric ideals and fads. Even though there is a separation of church and state in the United States, many public events and ceremonies open with a prayer, and phrases such as "one nation under God" are often heard. American money still has the phrase "in God we trust." Most people see these religious symbols as harmless rituals. Instead of speaking to "religious values," politicians speak to "family values" as a way of getting around religious principles. However, these issues are subject to debate from time to time. Unlike in many countries that support a specific church or religion and where people discuss their religion frequently and openly, religion is not an everyday topic of conversation for most Americans.

The health-care practitioner, who is aware of the client's religious practices and spiritual needs, is in a better position to promote culturally competent health care. The practitioner must demonstrate an appreciation of and respect for the dignity and spiritual beliefs of clients by avoiding negative comments about religious beliefs and practices. Clients may find considerable comfort in speaking with religious leaders in times of crisis and serious illness.

Prayer takes different forms and different meanings. Some people pray daily and may have altars in their homes. Others may consider themselves devoutly religious and only say prayers on special occasions or in times of crisis or illness. Among the Amish, faith-related behavior includes corporate (group) worship, prayer, and singing, which help build conformity and maintain harmony within the group. Prayer is a significant source of strength for Muslims, who pray five times a day. Health-care providers may need to make special arrangements for individuals to say prayers in accordance with their belief systems.

Meaning of Life and Individual Sources of Strength

What gives meaning to life varies among and within cultural groups. To some people, their formal religion may be the most important facet of fulfilling their spirituality needs, whereas for others, religion may be replaced as a driving force by other life forces and worldviews. Among other people, family is the most important social entity and is extremely important in helping meet their spiritual needs. For others, what gives meaning to life is good health and well-being. For a few, spirituality may include work or money.

A person's inner strength comes from different sources. Among the Navajo, the inner self is dependent on being in harmony with one's surroundings. For Christians, a belief in God may give personal strength. For most people, spirituality includes a combination of these factors. Knowing these beliefs allows health-care providers to assist individuals and families in their quest for strength and self-fulfillment.

Spiritual Beliefs and Health-Care Practices

Spiritual wellness brings fulfillment from a lifestyle of purposeful and pleasurable living that embraces free choices, meaning in life, satisfaction in life, and self-esteem. For example, when Navajo Indians are not in harmony with their surroundings and experience insomnia from anxieties, the Blessing Way Ceremony, ritual dancing, and herbal treatments, combined with prayers and songs are performed for total body healing and the return of spirits to the body (Wilson, 1983). Practices that interfere with a person's spiritual life can hinder physical recovery and promote physical illness.

Health-care providers should inquire if the person wants to see a member of the clergy even if they have not been active in church. Religious emblems should not be removed as they provide solace to the person and removing them may increase or cause anxiety. A thorough assessment of spiritual life is essential for the identification of solutions and resources that can support other treatments.

Box 2–10 identifies guidelines for assessing the cultural domain *spirituality*.

HEALTH-CARE PRACTICES

Another domain of culture is *health-care practices*. The focus of health care includes traditional, magicoreligious, and biomedical beliefs; individual responsibility for health; self-medicating practices; and views toward mental illness, chronicity, rehabilitation, organ dona-

---

BOX 2–10

Spirituality

Religious Practices and Use of Prayer

1 Identify the influence of the dominant religion of this group on health-care practices.
2 Explore the use of prayer, meditation, and other activities or symbols that help individuals reach fulfillment.

Meaning of Life and Individual Sources of Strength

3 Explore what gives meaning to life for individuals.
4 Identify the people's sources of strength.

Spiritual Beliefs and Health-Care Practices

5 Explore the relationship between spiritual beliefs and health practices.

tion, and transplantation. In addition, responses to pain and the sick role are shaped by specific ethnocultural beliefs. Significant barriers to health care may be shared among cultural and ethnic groups.

Health-Seeking Beliefs and Behaviors

For centuries people's health has been maintained by a wide variety of healing and medical practices. Currently, the United States is undergoing a paradigm shift: from one that places high value on curative and restorative medical practices, with sophisticated technological care, to one of health promotion and wellness, illness and disease prevention, and increased personal responsibility. Most believe that the individual, the family, and the community have the ability to influence their health. However, among other populations, good health may be seen as a divine gift from God, with individuals having little control over health and illness.

The primacy of patient autonomy is generally accepted as an enlightened perspective in American society. To this end, advance directives are an important part of medical care. Accordingly, patients can specify their wishes concerning life and death decisions before entering an inpatient facility. The advance directive allows the patient to name a family member or significant other to speak for the patient and make decisions when or if the patient is unable to do so. The patient can also have a living will that outlines the person's wishes in terms of life-sustaining procedures in the event of a terminal illness. Each inpatient facility has these forms available and will ask the patient what his or her wishes are. Patients may sign these forms at the hospital or elect to bring their own forms. The acceptance of advanced directives and living wills is not uniform across ethnocultural groups. Only 12 percent of African Americans, 13 percent of Korean Americans, 47 percent of Mexican Americans, and 69 percent of white Americans favor advance directives (McKinley et al., 1996; Hanson & Rodgman, 1996).

Undergoing surgery is always a major concern and decision for most people. Attitudes about surgery also vary among ethnocultural groups. For example, many Hispanics, as well as others, believe that undergoing surgery for cancer will cause the cancer to spread (Morgan et al., 1995); they are less likely to believe that surgery for breast cancer will cure the disease (Fulton et al., 1995).

Most countries and cultural groups engage in preventive immunization for children. Guidelines for immunizations were developed largely as a result of the influence of the WHO. Specific immunization schedules and the ages at which they are prescribed vary widely among countries and can be obtained from the Website of the WHO (*http://www.who.int.gov*). Campaigns since the early 1970s in the United States have resulted in an increase in immunization rates for children. In 1999, 78 percent of children age 19 to 35 months had completed the combined series of vaccinations for DPT, polio, measles, and *Haemophilus* influenza type b (Hib), up from 69 percent in 1994. Some still consider this unsatisfactory because other countries have higher immunization rates ("America's Children," 2001). However, some religious groups, such as Christian Scientists, do not believe in immunizations. Beliefs like this, which restrict optimal child health, have resulted in court battles with various outcomes.

Some societies do not have the sophisticated technology and resources needed to facilitate health promotion. For example, pap smears are new in Egypt, and mammograms are not offered, encouraged, or even known in some societies. Thus, the health-care provider's first step may be to assess a person's previous knowledge and experience related to preventive and acute-care practices.

Responsibility for Health Care

The United States is moving to a paradigm where people take increased responsibility for their health. In a society where individualism is valued, people are expected to be self-reliant. In fact, people are expected to exercise some control over disease, including controlling the amount of stress in their life. If someone does not maintain a healthy lifestyle and then gets sick, some believe it is the person's own fault. Unless someone is very ill, he or she should not neglect social and work obligations.

The health-care delivery system of the country of origin may shape the client's and employee's beliefs regarding personal responsibility for health care. In the United States everyone, regardless of socioeconomic or immigration status, can receive acute-care services. However, they will be charged a fee for the service, and they may not be able to get nonacute follow-up care unless they can prove they are able to pay for the service. Even if they are covered by health insurance, an insurance company representative may need to approve the visit and then have a list of procedures, medicines, and treatments for which it will pay. However, Great Britain and Canada have free health care at the point of entry to the health-care system, with reimbursement coming from the government. Individuals who did not need health insurance in their native country may not realize the importance of having health insurance in the United States.

A large number of the working poor cannot afford to purchase basic economic essentials for the family, and thus cannot even consider the purchase of health insurance. Health-care providers should not assume that clients who do not have health insurance or practice health prevention do not care about their health. The health-care provider must assess clients individually and provide culturally congruent education regarding health promotion and disease prevention activities.

A potential high-risk behavior in the self-care context includes self-medicating practices. Self-medicating behavior in itself may not be harmful, but when combined with or used to the exclusion of prescription medications, it may be detrimental to the person's health. A common practice with prescription medications is for people to take medicine until the symptoms disappear and then discontinue the medicine prematurely. This practice commonly occurs with antihypertensive medications and antibiotics.

Each country has some type of control over the purchase and use of medications. The United States is more restrictive than many countries and provides warning labels and directions for the use of over-the-counter medications. In many countries, pharmacists may be consulted before physicians for fever-reducing and pain-reducing medicines. In parts of Central America, a person can purchase antibiotics, intravenous fluids, and a variety of medications over the counter; most stores sell medications, and vendors sell drugs in street corner shops and on public transportation systems. People who are accustomed to purchasing medications over the counter in their native country frequently see no problem in sharing their medications with family and friends. To help prevent contradictory or exacerbated effects of prescription medication and treatment regimens, health-care providers should ask about clients' self-medicating practices. One cannot ignore the ample supply of over-the-counter medications in American pharmacies, the numerous television advertisements for self-medication, and media campaigns for new medications, encouraging viewers to ask their doctor or health-care provider about this particular medication.

Folk Practices

Some societies favor traditional, folk, or magicoreligious health-care practices over biomedical practices, and use some or all of them simultaneously. For many, what is considered alternative or complementary health-care practices in one country may be mainstream medicine in another society or culture. In the United States, interest has increased in alternative and complementary health practices. The U.S. government has an Office of Alternative Medicine at the National Institutes of Health that has awarded millions of dollars in grants to bridge the gap between traditional and nontraditional therapies.

As an adjunct to biomedical treatments, many people use acupuncture, acupressure, acumassage, herbal therapies, and other traditional treatments. Some cultural groups, for example, Hispanics, commonly visit traditional healers because modern medicine is viewed as inadequate. Examples of folk medicines include covering a boil with axle grease, wearing copper bracelets for arthritis pain, mixing wild turnip root and honey for sore throat, and drinking herbal teas. Native American traditions include ceremonial dances and songs. The Chinese subscribe to the yin-and-yang theory of treating illnesses, and Hispanic groups believe in the hot-and-cold theory of foods for treating illnesses and disease. Traditional schools of pharmacy in Brazil grow, sell, and teach courses on folk remedies. Most Americans practice folk medicine in some form; they may use family remedies passed down from previous generations.

An awareness of combined practices when treating or providing health education to individuals and families helps ensure that therapies do not contradict each other, intensify the treatment regimen, or cause an overdose. At other times, they may be harmful, conflict with, or potentiate the effects of prescription medications. It is essential to inquire about the full range of therapies being used, such as food items, teas, herbal remedies, nonfood substances, over-the-counter medications, and medications prescribed or loaned by others. Many times

these traditional, folk, and magicoreligious practices are and should be incorporated into the plans of care for clients. However, health-care providers must ask clients about these practices so that conflicting treatment modalities are not used. If clients perceive that the health-care provider does not accept their beliefs, they may be less compliant with prescriptive treatment and less likely to share their use of these practices.

Barriers to Health Care

In order for people to receive adequate health care, a number of considerations need to be addressed.

Availability: Is the service available and at a time when needed. For example, no services exist after 6 p.m. for someone who needs suturing of a minor laceration. Clinic hours coincide with clients' work hours, making it difficult to schedule appointments for fear of work reprisals.

Accessibility: Transportation services may not be available, or rivers and mountains may make it difficult for people to obtain needed health-care services when no health-care provider is available in their immediate region. It can be difficult for a single parent with four children to make three bus transfers to get one child immunized.

Affordability: The service is available, but the client does not have financial resources.

Appropriateness: Maternal and child services are available, but what might be needed are geriatric and psychiatric services.

Accountability: Are health-care providers accountable for their own education and do they learn about the cultures of the people they serve?

Adaptability: A mother brings her child to the clinic for an immunization. Can she get a mammogram at the same time or must she make another appointment?

Acceptability: Are services and client education offered in a language preferred by the client?

Awareness: Is the client aware that needed services exist in the community? The service may be available, but if clients are not aware of it, the service will not be used.

Attitudes: Adverse subjective beliefs and attitudes from caregivers means that the client will not return for needed services until the condition is more compromised. Do health-care providers have negative attitudes about patients' home-based traditional practices?

Approachability: Do clients feel welcomed? Do health-care providers and receptionists greet patients in the manner in which they prefer? This includes greeting patients with their preferred names.

Alternative practices and practitioners: Do biomedical providers incorporate clients' alternative or complementary practices into treatment plans?

Additional services: Are child- and adult-care services available if a parent must bring children or an aging parent to the appointment with them?

Health-care providers can help reduce some of these barriers by calling an area ethnic agency or church for assistance, establishing an advocacy role, involving professionals and laypeople from the same ethnic group as the client, and using cultural brokers. If all of these elements are in place and used appropriately, they have the potential of generating culturally responsive care.

Cultural Responses to Health and Illness

In the United States, significant research has been conducted on patients' responses to pain, which has been called the "fifth vital sign." Most Americans believe that patients should be made comfortable and not have to tolerate high levels of pain. Accrediting bodies, such as the Joint Commission for Accreditation of Healthcare Organizations (JCAHO), survey organizations to assure that patients' pain levels are assessed and that appropriate interventions are instituted. Beliefs regarding pain are one of the oldest culturally related research areas in health care. A 1969 study revealed that Irish Americans are stoic in their responses to pain, while Jewish Americans and Italian Americans are more vocal (Zborowski, 1969). The Navajo regard pain and discomfort as a way of life (Bell, 1994), and many Filipinos view pain as part of life and an opportunity to atone for past transgressions; thus, they may be tolerant and stoic while experiencing pain (Mattson & Lew, 1991). Astute observations and careful assessments must be completed to determine the level of pain a person can and is willing to tolerate. Health-care practitioners must investigate the meaning of pain to each person within a cultural explanatory framework to interpret diverse behavioral responses and provide culturally competent care. The health-care provider may need to offer and encourage pain medication and explain that it will help the healing progress. Research needs to be conducted in the areas of ethnic pain experiences and management of pain.

The manner in which mental illness is perceived and expressed by a cultural group has a direct effect on how individuals present themselves, and consequently on how health-care providers interact with these people. In some societies, such as American and Asian, mental illness may be seen by many as not being as important as physical illness. Mental illness is culture-bound; what may be perceived as a mental illness in one society may not be considered a mental illness in another. The landmark study by Jewell (1952) demonstrated how a Navajo Indian was misdiagnosed with schizophrenia when, in actuality, the Navajo was reacting in a manner expected of him in his culture.

Among most Asian American groups mental illness or emotional difficulty is considered a disgrace and taboo (Yamamoto et al., 1993). As a result, the family is likely to keep the mentally ill person at home as long as they can. This practice may be reinforced by the belief that all individuals are expected to contribute to the household for the common good of the family, and when a person is unable to contribute, further disgrace occurs.

Filipinos may not readily accept professional mental health care but are open to support and advice from family and friends. In Korea, mentally disturbed children are stigmatized, and the lack of supportive services may cause families to abandon their loved ones because of the cost of long-term care and the family's desire and desperate need for support. Such children are kept from the public eye in hope of saving the family from stigmatization. Koreans in the United States may hold these same values.

Here are some points to keep in mind in order to provide culturally congruent mental health services for these clients.

1 Avoid emphasizing the independence of children and adolescents on the first encounter.

2 Explore the cultural normative approach to shame and guilt (Sue & Sue, 1990).

3 Maintain formality and conversational distance (Chung, 1992; Yamamoto, 1986).

4 Do not expect an open public discussion of emotional problems (Sue & Sue, 1990).

5 Expect somatization of emotional problems (Ho, 1992; Hughes, 1993).

6 Consider the first session a crisis because of the delay in seeking treatment (Fujii et al., 1993; Gaw, 1993).

7 Avoid discussion of hospitalization and seek alternative care services if possible (Fujii et al., 1993; Yamamoto, 1986).

8 Provide concrete and tangible advice. The Asian client does not expect psychotherapy on the first session (Sue & Sue, 1990).

9 On the first encounter, avoid sensitive issues such as sexual practices (Gaw, 1993; Kim, 1993).

The physically and mentally handicapped may be treated differently in diverse cultures. In previous decades, physically handicapped individuals in the United States were seen as less desirable than those who did not have a handicap. If the handicap was severe, the person was sometimes hidden from the public's view. In 1992, the Americans with Disabilities Act went into effect, protecting handicapped individuals from discrimination.

In the United States, rehabilitation and occupational health services focus on returning individuals with handicaps to productive lifestyles in society as soon as possible. The goal of the American health-care system is to rehabilitate everyone: criminals, people with alcohol and drug problems, as well as those with physical conditions. Among Greek Americans and Egyptian Americans, rehabilitation programs that include drastic changes in lifestyles are more appealing when the clients and their families are convinced that programs are scientifically supported. To establish rapport, health-care practitioners working with clients suffering from chronic disease must avoid assumptions regarding health beliefs and provide rehabilitative health interventions within the scope of cultural customs and beliefs. Failure to respect and accept clients' values and beliefs can lead to misdiagnosis, lack of cooperation, and alienation of clients from the health-care system.

Sick role behaviors are culturally prescribed and vary among ethnic societies. Traditional American practice calls for fully disclosing the health condition to the client, but Filipino families prefer to be informed of the bad news first, and then slowly break the news to the sick family member. The sick role may not be readily accepted by Italian Americans and Polish Americans; some individuals may keep an illness hidden from the family until it reaches a more advanced stage. Given the ethnocultural acceptance of the sick role, health-care providers must assess each client and family individually and incorporate culturally congruent therapeutic interventions to return the client to an optimal level of functioning.

Blood Transfusions and Organ Donation

Most Americans and most, but not all, religions favor organ donation and transplantation and blood or blood products transfusions. Jehovah's Witnesses do not believe in blood transfusions. Christian Scientists, Orthodox Jews, Greeks, and some Spanish-speaking societies choose not to participate in organ donation or autopsy because of their belief that they will suffer in the afterlife or that the body will not be whole on resurrection (Perkins et al., 1993). Many African Americans are less receptive than white Americans to organ donation because of suspicion of the medical establishment and fear that their organs may be taken prematurely (Warren et al., 1995). Additionally, some African Americans prefer that their organs go to other African Americans. (Information about kidney transplants can be found at the National Kidney Foundation's Website, *http://www.kidney.org*). Health-care providers may need to assist clients in obtaining a religious leader to support them in making decisions regarding organ donation or transplantation.

Some people will not sign donor cards because the concept of organ donation and transplantation is not customary in their homelands. Health-care professionals should provide information regarding organ donation on an individual basis, be sensitive to individual and family concerns, explain procedures involved with organ donation and procurement, answer questions factually, and explain involved risks. A key to successful marketing approaches for organ donation is cultural awareness.

Box 2–11 identifies guidelines for assessing the cultural domain *health-care practices*.

HEALTH-CARE PRACTITIONERS

The domain *health-care practitioners* includes the status, use, and perceptions of traditional, magicoreligious, and biomedical health-care providers. It is interconnected with communications, family roles and organization, and spirituality. In addition, the gender of the health-care provider may be significant for some people.

Traditional versus Biomedical Practitioners

Most people combine the use of biomedical health-care practitioners with traditional practices, folk healers, and magicoreligious healers. The health-care system abounds with individual and family folk practices for curing or treating specific illnesses. A significant percent of all care is delivered outside the perimeter of the formal health-care arena. Many times herbalist-prescribed thera-

---

BOX 2–11

Health-Care Practices

Health-seeking Beliefs and Behaviors

1 Identify predominant beliefs that influence health-care practices.
2 Describe health promotion and prevention practices.

Responsibility for Health Care

3 Describe the focus of acute-care practice (curative or fatalistic).
4 Explore who assumes responsibility for health care in this culture.
5 Describe the role of health insurance in this culture.
6 Explore practices associated with the use of over-the-counter medications.

Folklore Practices

7 Explore combinations of magicoreligious beliefs, folk and traditional beliefs that influence health-care behaviors.

Barriers to Health Care

8 Identify barriers to health care such as language, economics, accessibility and geography for this group.

Cultural Responses to Health and Illness

9 Explore cultural beliefs and responses to pain that influence interventions. Does pain have a special meaning?
10 Describe beliefs and views about mental illness in this culture.
11 Differentiate between the perceptions of mentally and physically handicapped in this culture.
12 Describe cultural beliefs and practices related to chronicity and rehabilitation.
13 Identify cultural perceptions of the sick role in this group.

Blood Transfusion and Organ Donation

14 Describe the acceptance of blood and blood products, organ donation, and organ transplantation among this group.

---

pies are handed down from family members and may have their roots in religious beliefs. Traditional and folk practices often contain elements of historically rooted beliefs.

The American practice is to assign staff to patients regardless of gender differences, although often an attempt is made to provide a same-sex health-care provider when intimate care is involved, especially when the patient and caregiver are of the same age. However, health-care providers should recognize and respect differences in gender relationships when providing culturally competent care, because not all ethnocultural groups accept care from someone of the opposite sex. For example, many Hispanics are traditionally quite modest, even with health-care providers and, as a result, may feel uncomfortable and refuse care provided by someone of the opposite sex. Because any open display of affection is taboo, Hindu women may be especially modest and generally seek out female health-care providers for gynecologic examinations. Health-care providers need to respect clients' modesty by providing adequate privacy and assigning a same-sex caregiver whenever possible. In providing care to a Hasidic male client, a female caregiver should only touch him when providing care, and then preferably with gloves. Therapeutic touch is inappropriate with these clients.

Status of Health-Care Providers

Health-care practitioners are perceived differently among ethnocultural groups. Individual perceptions of selected practitioners may be closely associated with previous contact and experiences with health-care providers. In many Western societies, health-care providers, especially physicians, are viewed with great respect, although recent studies show that this is declining among some groups. Although many nurses in the United States do not believe they have respect, public opinion polls usually place clients' respect of nurses higher than that of physicians. The advanced practice role of registered nurses is gaining respect as more of them have successful careers and the public sees them as equal or preferable to physicians and physician assistants in many cases.

Within Iranian culture, the physician may rely more on physiological cues than technology for a diagnosis. When physicians order many tests or ask clients what they think the problem is, the client may view them as incompetent (Lipson & Meleis, 1985). Immigrant doctors from Iran may misunderstand the assertive behavior of American nurses, and immigrant Iranian nurses may be considered not as assertive as they should be in the American culture. Many people from the Middle East perceive older male physicians as being of higher rank and more trustworthy than younger health professionals (Lipson & Meleis, 1985). Chinese Americans are taught from a very early age to respect elders and to show deference to nurses and physicians, regardless of gender or age.

Evidence suggests that respect for professionals is correlated with their educational level. For example, Project 2000 in Great Britain proposes that requiring baccalaureate nursing programs to move from hospitals to university settings will raise the status of women in British society and elevate the standards of nursing practice. In Australia, paramedics and policemen are held in higher regard than nurses. In most cultures, the nurse is expected to defer to physicians. In many countries, the nurse is viewed more as a domestic than as a professional person, and it is only the physician who commands respect.

Nurses in the United States, however, are held in high regard. This may be related to factors such as the completion of high school or an equivalency examination before entering a nursing program, the rigorous licensing examination required before practicing

BOX 2–12

Health-Care Practitioners

Traditional Versus Biomedical Care

1 Explore the roles of traditional, folk/traditional, and magicoreligious practitioners and their influence on health practitioners.
2 Describe the acceptance of health-care practitioners in providing care to each gender. Does the age of the practitioner make a difference?

Status of Health-Care Providers

3 Explore perceptions of health-care practitioners with this group.
4 Identify the status of health-care providers in this society.
5 Describe how different health-care practitioners view each other.

the profession; baccalaureate, master's, and doctoral-level program of study, and the impact of nursing interventions on health-care outcomes. Some countries do not have programs leading to a master's or doctorate in nursing.

In some cultures, folk and magicoreligious health-care providers may be deemed superior to biomedically educated physicians and nurses. It may be that folk, traditional, and magicoreligious health-care providers are well known to the family and provide more individualized care. In such cultures, practitioners take time to get to know clients as individuals and engage in small talk totally unrelated to the health-care problem to accomplish their objectives. Establishing satisfactory interpersonal relationships is essential for improving health care and education in these ethnic groups.

Box 2–12 identifies the guidelines for assessing the cultural domain *health-care practitioners*.

REFERENCES

AIDS challenges religious leaders. (2001). *The Washington Post,* August 8, p. A10.

America's children: Key national indicators of well-being. (2001). Federal Interagency Forum on Child and Family Statistics. Retrieved August 12, 2001, from http://www.childstats.gov.

American Medical Association. (2001). http://www.ama-assn.org.

Bell, R. (1994). Prominence of women in Navajo healing beliefs and values. *Nursing and Health Care, 15*(1), 232–242.

Campinha-Bacote, J. (1999). *The process of cultural competence in the delivery of health-care services: A culturally competent model of care* (3rd ed.). Cincinnati, OH: Transcultural C.A.R.E. Associates.

Cates, W. (1999). Estimates of the incidence and prevalence of sexually transmitted diseases in the United States. *Sexually Transmitted Diseases, 26*(supp): S2–S7

Cardiovascular disease. (2001). Centers for Disease Control, http://www.cdc.gov.

Chung, D. (1992). Asian cultural communications: A comparison with mainstream American culture. In D. K. Chung et al. (Eds.), *Social work practice with Asian Americans* (pp. 27–44). Newbury Park, CA: Sage.

Crow, K. (1993). Multiculturalism and pluralistic thought in nursing education: Native American world view and the nursing academic world view. *Journal of Nursing Education, 32*(5), 198–204.

Current and accurate cancer information. (2001). National Cancer Institute. Retrieved August 11, 2001, from http://www.cancernet. nci.nih.gov.

Distribution by racial/ethnic group. (2001). American Nurses Association. Retrieved August 13, 2001, from http://www.nursingworld.org.

Fuchs, J., et al. (1992). Update on the search for DNA markers linked to manic-depressive illness in Old Order Amish. *Journal of Psychiatric Research, 26*(4), 305–308.

Fulton, J., et al. (1995). *Public Health Reports, 110,* 476–482.

Fujii, J., et al. (1993). Psychiatric care of Japanese Americans. In A. Gaw (ed.), *Culture, ethnicity, and mental illness* (pp. 305–345). Washington, DC: American Psychiatric Press.

Gaw, C. (1993). Psychiatric care of Chinese Americans. In A. Gaw (Ed.): *Culture, ethnicity, and mental illness* (pp. 245–280). Washington, DC: American Psychiatric Press.

Giger, J. N., & Davidhizar, R. E. (1999). *Transcultural nursing: Assessment and intervention* (3rd ed.). St. Louis: Mosby.

Hall, E. (1990). *The silent language.* New York: Anchor Books.

Hanson, L., & Rogdman, E. (1996). The use of living wills at the end of life: A national study. *Archives of Internal Medicine, 156,* 1018–1022.

Harner, R., et al. (1994). Community-based nursing education in Pakistan. *Journal of Continuing Education in Nursing, 25*(3), 130–132.

Heath, D. (1995). An anthropological view of alcohol and culture in international and perspective. In D. B. Heath (Ed.), *International handbook on alcohol and culture* (pp. 328–347). Westport, CT: Greenwood Press.

Herold, J. M., et al. (1989). Catholicism and fertility in Puerto Rico. *American Journal of Public Health, 79*(9), 1258–1262.

Hill, R.(1995). *We Europeans.* Brussels, Belgium: Europublications.

Hilton, M. (1987). Demographic characteristics and the frequency of heavy drinking as predictors of drinking problems. *British Journal of Addiction, 82,* 913–925.

Ho, M. (1992). *Minority children and adolescents in therapy.* Newbury Park, CA: Sage.

Hughes, C. (1993). Culture in clinical psychiatry. In A. Gaw (ed.), *Culture, ethnicity, and mental illness* (pp. 347–357). Washington, DC: American Psychiatric Press.

Institute of Medicine. (2001). http://www.iom.org.

Jewell, D. (1952). A case of a "psychotic" Navajo Indian male. *Human Organization, 11,* 32–36.

Judge orders executions for lesbian duo. (2001). *Washington Blade,* February 23.

Kim, L. (1993). Psychiatric care of Korean Americans. In A. Gaw (ed.), *Culture, ethnicity, and mental illness* (pp. 347–357). Washington, DC: American Psychiatric Press.

Krebs, G., & Kunimoto, Y. (1994). *Effective communication in multicultural health-care settings.* Thousand Oaks, CA: Intercultural Press.

Leininger, M. E. (1988). Transcultural eating patterns and nutrition: Transcultural nursing and anthropological perspectives. *Holistic Nursing Practice, 3*(1), 16–25.

Levy, R. (1993). Ethnic and racial differences in response to medications: Preserving individualized therapy in managed pharmaceutical programmes. *Pharmaceutical Medicine, 7,* 139–165.

Lipson, J. G., & Meleis, A. I. (1985). Culturally appropriate care: The case of immigrants. *Topics in Clinical Nursing, 7*(3), 48–56.

Mattson, S., & Lew, L. (1991). Culturally sensitive prenatal care for Southeast Asians. *Journal of Obstetric, Gynecological, and Neonatal Nursing, 12*(1), 48–54.

McKinley, E., et al. (1996). Differences in end-of-life decision-making among black and white ambulatory cancer patients. *Journal of General Internal Medicine, 11,* 651–656.

Median age at first marriage. (2001). Bureau of the Census. Retrieved June 4, 2001, from http://www.census.gov.

Miller, W. S., & Supersad, J. W. (1991). East Hindu Americans. In J. N. Giger and R. E. Davidhizar (Eds.), *Transcultural nursing: Assessment and intervention* (pp. 437–464). St. Louis, MO: Mosby.

Minority statistics. (2001). American Physical Therapy Association. Retrieved August 12, 2001, from http://www.apta.org.

Morgan, C., et al. (1995). Beliefs, knowledge, and behavior about cancer among urban Hispanics. *Journal of the National Cancer Institute, 18,* 57–63.

Mosher, W. D., & Goldscheider, C. (1984). *Studies in Family Planning, 15*(3), 101–111.

National Center for HIV, STD, and TB Prevention. (2001). Centers for Disease Control. http://www.cdc.gov.

National diabetes fact sheet. (2001). Centers for Disease Control. Retrieved August 12, 2001, from *http://www.cdc.gov.*

National Kidney Foundation. (2002). http://www.kidney.com.

Newbauer, B., & Hamilton, C. Racial differences in attitudes toward hospice care. *Hospice Journal, 16,* 37–48.

O'Brien, L., et al. (1997). Tube feeding among nursing home residents. *Journal of General Internal Medicine, 12,* 354–371.

Peele, S. (1997). Utilizing culture and behavior in epidemiological models of alcohol consumption and consequences for Western nations. *Alcohol and Alcoholism, 32,* 51–64.

Peele, S., & Brodsky, A. (2001). Alcohol and society. Retrieved August 21, 2001, from http://www.peele.net.

Perez-Stable, E., et al. (1998). Nicotine metabolism and intake in Black and White smokers. *Journal of the American Medical Association, 280*(2), 152–156.

Perkins, H., et al. (1993). Autopsy decisions: The possibility of conflicting cultural attitudes. *Journal of Clinical Ethics, 4,* 145–154.

Purnell, L., & Galloway, W. (1995). What to do if called upon to testify. *Accident and Emergency Nursing, 17*(4), 246–249.

Sexually transmitted disease surveillance. (2001). Centers for Disease Control. Retrieved August 7, 2001, from http://www.cdc.gov.

Society for Research in Child Development. (2001). http://www.child-stats.gov.

Sue, D. W., & Sue, D. (1990). *Counseling the culturally different: Theory and practice* (2nd ed.). New York: John Wiley.

Time almanac. (2001). Boston: Time Inc.

U.S. Department of Agriculture. (2001). *http://www.nal.usda.gov.*

Warren, J., et al. (1995). Organ-limited autopsies: Obtaining permission for postmortem examination of the urinary tract, *Archives of Pathology Laboratory Medicine, 119,* 440–443.

Wenger, A. F. Z. (1991). The culture care theory and the Old Order Amish. In M. M. Leininger (Ed.), *Culture care diversity and universality: A theory of nursing* (pp. 147–178). New York: National League for Nursing.

Wilson, U. (1983). Nursing care of the American Indian patient. In M. S. Orque, B. Block, & L.S.A. Monrroy (Eds.), *Ethnic nursing care: A multicultural approach* (pp. 47–63). St. Louis, MO: Mosby.

Yamamoto, J. (1986). Therapy for Asian Americans and Pacific Islanders. In C. Wilkinson (Ed.), *Ethnic psychiatry* (pp. 89–141). New York: Plenum.

Yamamoto. J., et al. (1993). Cross-cultural psychotherapy. In A. Gaw (ed.), *Culture, ethnicity, and mental illness* (pp. 101–124). Washington, DC: American Psychiatric Press.

Zborowski, M. (1969). *People in pain.* San Francisco: Jossey-Bass.

Chapter 3

People of African American Heritage

CATHRYN L. GLANVILLE

Overview, Inhabited Localities, and Topography

OVERVIEW

African Americans are one of the largest ethnic groups in the United States. Statistics from the U.S. Census Bureau reveal that there are approximately 34,333,000 African Americans in the United States, which represents 12.1 percent of the total population (U.S. Department of Commerce, Bureau of the Census, 2001).

African Americans are mainly of African ancestry; however, many have non-African ancestors as well. In fact, African Americans encompass a gene pool of over 100 racial strains (Goddard, 1990). African Americans have been identified as "Negro," "colored," "black," "black American," and "people of color." Depending on their cohort group, some African Americans may prefer to identify themselves differently. For example, younger blacks may prefer the term **African American**, whereas elderly African Americans may use the terms *Negro* and **colored**. In contrast, middle-aged African Americans refer to themselves as *black* or *black American*. These different descriptors can cause confusion for those who are attempting to use the politically correct term for this ethnic group. In addition, we still see such organizational titles as the National Black Nurses Association, National Center for the Advancement of Blacks in the Health Professions, and the National Association for the Advancement of Colored People, which clearly depict the differences in how African Americans prefer to be identified. Therefore, it is culturally sensitive to ask African Americans what they prefer to be called.

Because there is much diversity among African Americans, health-care providers must be aware of intraethnic or intracultural variation within this ethnic group. Intraethnic or intracultural variation implies that there is more variation within an ethnic group than across ethnic groups. Factors such the primary and secondary characteristics of culture (see Chapter 1) are but a few variables that contribute to the diversity of the African American population. Thus, in order to avoid stereotyping, the health-care provider must assess and plan interventions for African Americans on an individual basis.

HERITAGE AND RESIDENCE

African Americans are largely the descendants of Africans who were brought forcibly to this country as slaves between 1619 and 1860. The literature contains many conflicting reports of the exact number of slaves that arrived in this country. Varying estimates reveal that from 3.5 to 24 million slaves landed in the Americas during the slave trade era (Curtin, 1969). Many slaves who were brought to the American colonies and early United States came from the west coast of Africa, from the Kwa- and Bantu-speaking people. *A Rap on Race* (Mead & Baldwin, 1971) provides a description and interpretation of life in America for blacks. Furthermore, the legacy of African American heritage and history of slavery is often passed on from generation to generation through black folk tales and lived experiences (see, for example, Taulbert, 1969).

African American slaves were settled mostly in Southern states, and currently over 50 percent of African Americans still live in the South; 19 percent live in the North and Northeast, 9 percent in the West, and 19 percent in the Midwest. The highest concentration of African Americans can be found in metropolitan areas, with over 2 million in New York City and over 1 million in Chicago (U.S. Department of Commerce, Bureau of the Census, 2001). There are also major African-American communities in 11 other cities: Atlanta, Georgia; Washington, D.C.; Baltimore, Maryland; Jackson, Mississippi; Gary, Indiana; Newark, New Jersey; Detroit, Michigan; Memphis, Tennessee; Birmingham, Alabama; Richmond, Virginia; and New Orleans, Louisiana (Louisiana Department of Health and Hospitals, 2001).

REASONS FOR MIGRATION AND ASSOCIATED ECONOMIC FACTORS

The Civil War ended slavery and, particularly in the state of South Carolina, the Reconstruction Act allowed blacks the right to vote and participate in state government (Davis, 1976). However, most blacks in the South were denied their civil rights and were segregated. Thus, African Americans lived in poverty and encountered many hardships. After the Civil War, more African Americans migrated from southern rural areas to northern urban areas. Blacks migrated because of a lack of security for life and property. They were unable to get out of debt and support their families in spite of having good crops. Also, World War II was a major catalyst in fostering migration to urban and northern areas, which provided them with greater economic opportunities and brought African Americans and European Americans into close contact for the first time. Jaynes and Williams (1989) reported that during the 1940s, a net outmigration from the South totaled approximately 1.5 million African Americans (15 percent of the South's black population). Although the migration was viewed as a positive move, many blacks encountered all the problems of fragmented urban life, racism, poverty, and covert segregation.

EDUCATIONAL STATUS AND OCCUPATIONS

Before 1954, educational opportunities for African Americans were compromised. School systems were segregated and blacks were victims of inferior facilities. In fact, in 1910 almost one-third of all blacks were illiterate (Blum et al., 1981). However, in 1954, the Supreme Court decision in *Brown v. Board of Education of Topeka* ruled against the segregation of blacks and whites in the public school systems.

Conant (1961) described the plight of black Americans in segregated schools and, to some extent, predicted the long-term social consequences of such a system. His predictions have been borne out in inadequate job opportunities and poor wages, resulting in poverty. Poverty has had a ripple effect on African American communities often leading to poorly educated individuals, high dropout rates from school, and drug and alcohol abuse (Ladner & Gourdine, 1992). In many African American communities this oppressive environment contributes to the existing alcohol and drug problems and dropout rate among African Americans, which has been reported as high as 61 percent (Braithwaite, et al., 2000).

Despite these devastating occurrences, most African American families place a high value on education. Hines and Boyd-Franklin (1982) stated that the African American family views education as the process most likely to ensure work security and social mobility. Families often make great sacrifices so at least one child can go to college. In African American families it is not uncommon to see cooperative efforts among siblings to assist each other financially to obtain a college education. For example, as the older child graduates and becomes employed, that child then assists the next sibling who, in turn, assists the next one. This continues until all of the children who attend college have graduated.

Before the civil rights movement, a major emphasis for blacks in higher education was vocational. The thinking was that if African Americans could learn a trade or vocation, they could become self-sufficient and improve their economic well-being. Preparation for vocational careers is evidenced in the name, mission, and goals of two of the reknown historically black institutions, Hampton University and Tuskegee University, formerly known as Hampton Institute and Tuskegee Normal and Industrial Institute. Although African Americans have successfully completed a variety of majors in universities, there are significant differences in the ethnic, racial, and gender makeup of those obtaining higher degrees. For example, between 1977 and 1993, 55 percent of African Americans awarded doctorates were women. In 1995, there was a disproportionately higher number of black women than black men in the labor force (Albers, 1999). Today, African Americans continue to be underrepresented in managerial and professional positions, especially professional nursing (National Advisory Council on Nursing Education and Practice, 1996). African Americans represent a large segment of blue-collar workers employed in service occupations (U.S. Department of Health and Human Services, 1990). One reason for this disproportionate representation in professional and managerial positions is thought to be discrimination in employment and job advancement. In 1961, President Kennedy established the Committee on Equal Employment Opportunity to protect minorities from discrimination in employment. However, most African Americans still believe that job discrimination is a major variable contributing to problems they encounter in obtaining better jobs or successful career mobility. With the dismantling of affirmative-action programs, based on misinterpretation of their purpose, this view will, perhaps, continue to gain support.

Most working-class African Americans do not typically advance to the higher socioeconomic levels (Goddard, 1990). Because they are overrepresented in the working class, they are more likely to be employed in hazardous occupations, resulting in occupation-related diseases and illness. For example, Michaels (1993) reported that African American males are at a higher risk for developing cancer, which is related to their high representation in the steel and tire industries. According to Clark (1999), genetic factors of greatest importance in the work environment are probably race and gender. Implications are that health-care providers must not only assess African American clients for occupation-related diseases, such as cancer, and stress-related diseases, such as hypertension, but must also be familiar with the government's *Healthy People 2010* goals for the health and safety of individuals in the work environment (U.S. Department of Health and Human Services, 1997).

Communications

DOMINANT LANGUAGE AND DIALECTS

The dominant language spoken among African Americans is English. However, many people have referred to the informal language of African Americans as **black English.** This term is incorrect because black English is not a language, but rather a dialect in which the pronunciation of words may be different. For example, some African Americans may pronounce *th* as *d*. Therefore, the word *these* may be pronounced "dese." Health-care professionals must not stereotype African Americans as speaking only in black English because most African Americans are articulate and competent in the formal English language.

Pidgin is another form of communication found in the African American population. Pidgin dates to the slavery era, when African slaves from different tribes were forced to develop their own form of communication. Pidgin is a form of communication that occurs when two groups do not have a common language and are forced to develop a third language (pidgin), which is a combination of their respective languages. When a pidgin becomes the first language of a group of speakers it is termed a *creole* language. **Gullah** is a creole language spoken by African Americans who live on or near the sea islands off Georgia and South Carolina. African Americans in Mississippi, Alabama, and Louisiana, especially in New Orleans, speak Gullah. After the Civil War, the Georgia and South Carolina sea islands, such as Sapelo and Hilton Head, were left to the freed slaves, who developed their own culture. Today, their descendants still speak Gullah, a dialect derived from several West African languages. It is not uncommon for African Americans who see themselves as high minority, high mainstream to use black English when conversing with each other. According to Murray and Zentner (2001), black English provides a framework for communicating unique cultural ideas. Allender and Spradely (2001) maintain that it symbolizes racial pride and identity. In all situations, it is important for health-care providers to refrain from assuming that clients who use dialects are poorly educated or lack intelligence.

CULTURAL COMMUNICATION PATTERNS

Many African Americans tend to be high-keyed, animated, confrontational, and interpersonal (Mindess, 1999), expressing their feelings openly to trusted friends or family. What transpires within the family is viewed as private, and not appropriate for discussion with strangers. A common phrase that reflects this perspective is, "Don't air your dirty laundry." The volume of African Americans' voices is often louder than those in some other cultures. Health-care providers must not misunderstand this attribute: people may not necessarily be reflecting anger, but merely expressing their thoughts in a dynamic manner.

Humor is a form of communication that serves as a tool to release of hostile, angry feelings and reduce stress and may ease racial tension. **The dozens,** a social game in which African Americans use humor, is a joking relationship between two African Americans in which each in turn is, by custom, permitted to tease or make fun of the other. Oftentimes the joking is loud and can be mistaken for aggressive communication if not understood within the context of the African American culture.

African American speech is dynamic and expressive. Body movements are involved when communicating with others. Facial expressions can be very demonstrative. Touch is another form of nonverbal communication seen when African Americans are interacting with relatives and extended family members. African Americans are reported to be comfortable with a closer personal space than other ethnic groups. Maintaining direct eye contact can be misinterpreted as aggressive behavior by some African Americans. Health-care providers must consider these nonverbal behaviors when providing care to African American clients.

TEMPORAL RELATIONSHIP

In general, African Americans are more present- than past- or future-oriented. However, the past or future may be valued in specific subgroups of African Americans, such as the elderly, who place greater emphasis on the past than on the present. In contrast, younger and middle-aged African Americans are more present-oriented, with evidence of becoming more future-oriented, as indicated by the value placed on education.

Some African Americans are more relaxed about time. It is more important to make an appointment than to be on time for the appointment. What they see as important is the fact that they are there, even though they may arrive one to two hours late. Therefore, flexibility in timing appointments may be necessary for African Americans, who have a circular sense of time rather than the dominant culture's linear sense of time (Murray & Zentner, 2001).

FORMAT FOR NAMES

Most African Americans prefer to be greeted formally as Mr., Mrs., Ms., or Miss. They prefer their surname, because the "family name" is highly respected and connotes pride in their family heritage. However, African Americans do not use such formal names when they interact among themselves. It is common for an African American youth to address an unrelated African American who lives in the community as uncle, aunt, or cousin. It is also common to find adult African Americans called names different from their Christian or legal name. The health-care provider should greet the African American client by the last name and appropriate title.

Family Roles and Organization

HEAD OF HOUSEHOLD AND GENDER ROLES

Just as apartheid altered family life for blacks in South Africa, slavery altered family life, structure, functions, and processes in African American families. Strong family bonds were terminated and there was a loss of family identity because slave owners defined family life. Families were often separated, and fathers or older children were sold to other plantations. Although today it is common to find a patriarchal system in African American families, a high percentage of families still have a matriarchal system and live below the poverty line. The head of the household is either a single mother or a grandmother. Ladner and Gourdine (1992) stated, "single parenting and poverty are viewed as the causal factor in de-stabilizing the African-American family" (p. 208). Other contributing factors are the absence (Heady, 1996) and plight of black males, who have high unemployment rates and low life expectancy. Poverty and incarceration are three times higher among black males than among their white counterparts. Furthermore, a number of incarcerated black males have left children behind, thus increasing the number of black children who lack male role models and must be cared for by the mother.

A single head of household is accepted without associated stigma in African American families. When women are unable to provide emotional and physical support for their children, grandmothers, aunts, and extended or augmented families readily provide assistance or take responsibility for the children.

Because African American families are pluralistic in nature, gender roles and childrearing practices vary widely depending on ethnicity, socioeconomic class, rural versus urban location, and educational achievement. The diverse family structure extends the care of family members beyond the nuclear family to include relatives and nonrelatives. Dual employment of many middle-class African American families requires cooperative teamwork. Many family tasks such as cooking, cleaning, child care, and shopping are shared, requiring flexibility and adaptability of roles.

One important trend noted today is that a growing number of African American grandparents are functioning in primary parental roles. For example, 44 percent of all children living with grandparents today are African American. Approximately 66 percent of these children have grandparents as the primary caregivers.

Because many African American families, especially those with a single head of household, are matrifocal in nature, the health-care provider must recognize women's importance in decision making and disseminating health information. Also, the health-care provider must focus on, and work with the strengths of African American families, especially single-parent families. Hill (1997) states that many African American families headed by single women are economically disadvantaged; however, such families should not be compared or equated with broken or intact families.

PRESCRIPTIVE, RESTRICTIVE, AND TABOO ROLES FOR CHILDREN AND ADOLESCENTS

Given African Americans' strong work and achievement orientation, they value self-reliance and education for their children. A dichotomy might exist here, because many parents do not expect to get full benefit from their efforts because of discrimination. Thus, families tend to be more protective of their children and act as a buffer between their children and the outside world.

Respectfulness, obedience, conformity to parent-defined rules, and good behavior are stressed for children. The belief is that a firm parenting style, structure, and discipline is necessary to protect the child from danger outside of the home. In violence-ridden communities, mothers try to keep young children off the streets and encourage them to engage in productive activities. Adolescents are assigned household chores as part of their family responsibility or seek employment for pay when they are old enough, thus learning "survival skills."

By 1999, the rate of teen pregnancy dropped from 15 percent in 1981 to approximately 12.5 percent (National Center for Health Statistics, 1999). Although there has been a decline in the incidence of teen pregnancy, it continues to be a problem in the African American community because of poor pregnancy outcomes such as premature and low-birth-weight infants and obstetrical complications. Furthermore, the teenage mother is expected to assume primary responsibility for her child where the extended family becomes a strong support system. Premarital teenage pregnancy is not condoned in African American families; rather, it is accepted after the fact. In other instances the infant may be informally adopted and someone other than the mother may become the primary caregiver.

FAMILY ROLES AND PRIORITIES

African American families share a wide range of characteristics, family values, goals, and priorities. An example of a strong family value is the level of respect bestowed upon the elders within the African American community. Within this community, the elders, especially grandmothers, are respected for their insight. The role of the grandmother is one of the most central roles in the African American family. Grandmothers are frequently the economic support of African American families, and they often play a critical role in child care. It is common to see African American children raised by grandparents; this has contributed to an increase in the number of skipped generational families seen in the African American community.

Boyd-Franklin (1989) stated that it is essential to understand the role of the extended family in the lives of African Americans. There are several African American extended-family models. Billingsley (1968) divided them into four major types: subfamilies, families with secondary members, augmented families, and nonblood relatives. **Subfamily** members include nieces, nephews, cousins, aunts, and uncles. **Secondary members** consist of peers of the primary parents, older relatives of the primary parents, and parents of the primary parents.

In an **augmented family,** the head of household raises children who are not his or her own relatives. Nonblood relatives are individuals who are unrelated by blood ties, but who are closely involved with the family functioning.

Social status is important within the African American community. Certain occupations receive higher esteem than others. For example, African American physicians and dentists tend to have privileged positions. Ministers and clergy also receive respect within the African American community.

African Americans who move up the socioeconomic ladder often find themselves caught between two worlds. They have their roots in the African American community, but at times they find themselves interacting more within the European American community. Other African Americans refer to these individuals as "oreos"—a derogatory term that means "black on the outside, but white on the inside." Furthermore, Frazier (1957) argues that African American families who achieve upper-middle-class and middle-class status—the so-called **black bourgeoisie**—perpetuate a myth of "Negro society." According to Frazier (1957), this term describes behavior, attitudes, and values of a make-believe world created by middle- and upper-class African Americans in order to escape feelings of inferiority in American society.

ALTERNATIVE LIFESTYLES

Lesbian and gay relationships undoubtedly occur as frequently among African Americans as in other ethnic groups. Acceptance of same-sex relationships varies between and among families. Personal disclosure to friends and family may jeopardize relationships, thereby forcing some to remain closeted. There is an ongoing debate about the pros and cons of legitimizing lesbian and gay families especially when children are involved. Opponents of this family form believe that parental behavior has a profound effect on children's gender identities and establishing family values (Bender, 1998).

Workforce Issues

CULTURE IN THE WORKPLACE

African Americans adhere to a strong work ethic, but often experience ethnic or racial tension. *Ethnic or racial tension* is defined as a "negative workplace atmosphere motivated by prejudicial attitudes about cultural background and/or skin color" (Stevens, et al., 1992, pp. 759–760). Employers and employees must increase their sensitivity and awareness of cultural nuances and issues that create ethnic or racial tension in the workplace environment (Lowenstein & Glanville, 1995).

Although an African American axiology reflects a strong emphasis on spirituality, there is an economic-driven emphasis on materialism. African Americans feel a need to acculturate into mainstream society to survive in the workforce. Bell and Evans (1981) identify four different interacting styles within the African American culture. The *acculturated interpersonal* style occurs when African American people make a conscious or subcon-

scious decision to reject the values, beliefs, practices, and general behaviors associated with their own ethnic group. Acculturated African Americans become sensitive to punctuality, timeliness, and adoption of other values of European Americans. In contrast, the *culturally immersed* African American rejects all values and behaviors except those held by his or her own culture. This person is often labeled "militant" or "difficult to work with." In the *traditional interacting* style, African Americans neither reject nor accept their ethnic identity. They do not disclose and are referred to as the "easy-to-get-along-with" African Americans. Their motto is "Don't rock the boat." The *bicultural interacting* style demonstrates the pride that African Americans have for their identity, history, and cultural traditions, while still feeling comfortable in the mainstream. The bicultural African American's values integrate living and ethnic diversity.

ISSUES RELATED TO AUTONOMY

Some African American men may experience a difficult time in taking direction from European American supervisors or bosses. This difficulty stems from the era of slavery when African Americans were considered the property of their master. Many African Americans continue to be frustrated at their lower-level positions and the absence of African American leadership in many workplaces. Lowenstein and Glanville (1995) found that along with historical circumstances, culture and politics affect the employment of blacks in the health-care industry often relegating African Americans to nonskilled roles. Today there continue to be a large number of blacks working as nursing assistants, LPNs, or technicians. Thus, if the professional nurse who directs and supervises nonprofessional workers lacks cultural sensitivity toward other ethnic groups, the stage is set for cultural conflict.

Because the dominant language of African Americans is English, they usually have no difficulty communicating verbally with others in the workforce. However, some people may view African Americans who exclusively speak black English as poorly educated or unintelligent. This misinterpretation may affect employment and job promotion where verbal skills are more valued. In addition, nonverbal communications of African Americans are sometimes misunderstood and are often labeled as more aggressive than assertive because of intonation and body movements.

Biocultural Ecology

SKIN COLOR AND OTHER BIOLOGIC VARIATIONS

Goddard (1990) stated that African Americans encompass a gene pool of over 100 racial strains. Therefore, skin color among African Americans can vary from light to very dark. Assessing the skin of most African American clients requires different clinical skills from those for assessing people with white skin. For example, pallor in dark-skinned African Americans can be observed by the absence of the underlying red tones that give the brown and black skin its "glow" or "living color." Lighter-skinned African Americans appear more yellowish brown, whereas darker-skinned African Americans appear ashen.

To assess such conditions as inflammation, cyanosis, jaundice, and petechiae may require natural light and the use of different assessment skills. Health-care professionals cannot rely solely on their usual observational skills. African Americans exhibiting inflammation or petechiae must be assessed by palpation of the skin for warmth, edema, tightness, or induration. To assess for cyanosis in dark-skinned blacks, the health-care professional needs to observe the oral mucosa or conjunctiva. Jaundice is assessed more accurately in dark-skinned persons by observing the sclera of the eyes, the palms of the hands, and the soles of the feet, which may have a yellow discoloration.

African Americans have a tendency toward the overgrowth of connective tissue associated with the protection against infection and repair after injury. Keloid formation is one example of this tendency toward overgrowth of connective tissue. Diseases such as lymphoma and systemic lupus erythematosus occur in African Americans secondary to this overgrowth of connective tissue.

Bone density is a biologic variation noted among African Americans. African Americans have a higher bone density than European Americans, Asians, and Hispanics. In addition, their long bones are longer. African Americans also experience a lower incidence of osteoporosis.

Certain skin conditions are gender-specific among some African Americans. Pseudofolliculitis ("razor bumps") is more common among African American males, whereas melasma ("mask of pregnancy") is more common among darker-skinned African American females during pregnancy. African Americans also experience a disproportionate amount of pigment discoloration, with vertiligo being the most common. This is an autoimmune disease that not only causes skin discoloration but is also associated with diabetes and thyroid disorders. If left untreated, it can cause skin cancer (Simmons-O'Brien, 1997).

Birthmarks are more prevalent in African Americans. Birthmarks occur in 20 percent of the African American population as compared to the 1 to 3 percent in other ethnic groups (Giger & Davidhizar, 1999). One example is mongolian spots, which are found more often in African American newborns, but disappear over time.

The pathophysiology of hypertension in African Americans is related to volume expansion, decreased rennin, and increased intracellular concentration of sodium and calcium. Genetically, African Americans are more prone than whites to retain sodium. This variance is attributed to salt sensitivity. Therefore, a high intake of sodium; an overweight, sedentary lifestyle; smoking; alcohol; and high stress levels are associated with increased blood pressure, which is cited as one of the most common health problems among African Americans (Saunders, 1997).

DISEASES AND HEALTH CONDITIONS

During the past 15 to 20 years, significant improvements have occurred in the health status of Americans. Life expectancy has increased to a 75.6-year average for white males and 79 years for white females (Clark, 1999). Close examination of the health-illness statistics reveals that African Americans have a lower life expectancy with a 65-year average for males and 74 years for females.

While the race gap with lower quality of care among racial and ethnic minorities has been documented for some time, previous research attributed much of the problem to lack of access to care. However, the Institute of Medicine's (IOM) study on health care among people who have health insurance found that racial and ethnic minorities received lower quality health care than whites. A panel of the IOM cited subtle racial prejudice and differences in the quality of health plans as possible reasons for increased disparities ("Minorities Get Inferior Care, Even If Insured," 2002). Thus, disparities in health care among African Americans and other disenfranchised groups is multifactoral in nature.

Although there has been a decline in leading causes of death such as accidents, cancer, infant mortality, and cardiovascular diseases, the adjusted death rates for African Americans is higher than for whites (Helvie, 1998). Other causes of death among African Americans are homicide, cirrhosis, malnutrition, chemical dependency, and diabetes. When examining the relationship of social characteristics such as education, income, and occupation to health indicators, African Americans have worse indicators when compared to whites (Navarro, 1997). African Americans are at greater risk for many diseases, especially those associated with low income, stressful life conditions, lack of access to primary health care, and negating health behaviors. Examples of such behaviors are violence, poor dietary habits, lack of exercise, and lack of importance placed on seeking primary health care early. In terms of primary health care, the delays in seeking early treatment may be associated with perceived health status or perceived risk of acquiring a particular disease (Edleman & Mandle, 1998).

Of the 34 million African Americans living in the United States, 50 percent are women. Thirty percent of this female population lives in poverty and has limited access to health care because of a lack of health insurance. The leading causes of death among African American women are cancer, stroke, chronic obstructive pulmonary disease, pneumonia, unintentional injuries, diabetes, suicide, and HIV/AIDS. Alcohol, illicit drug use, and depression are also leading causes of death for African American women (Collins, 1996).

Because African Americans are concentrated in large inner cities, they are at risk for being victims of violence. In fact, the leading cause of death among young African American males is homicide. This violence has been referred to as "black-on-black" violence. Brownstein (1995) indicates that young black men are murdered by other black men at 10 times the rate of white men between the ages of 20 to 29. The situation led the NAACP to refer to the black male as an endangered species. Gangs are more prevalent in larger cities, which only increase the likelihood of the occurrence of violence in African American communities.

Living in urban industrial areas also exposes African Americans to pollution, which puts them at increased risk for developing diseases associated with environmental hazards. Seemingly, minorities suffer the most from environmental pollution and benefit the least from environmental cleanup programs. In 1993, the federal Environmental Protection Agency found evidence that racial and ethnic minorities were disproportionately located near superfund sites, areas where hazardous waste and chemicals deleteriously affect people's health and the local ecosystem. Currently, efforts are directed toward environmental justice in order to ensure that no particular part of the population is burdened by negative effects of pollution (American Public Health Association, 1999).

In addition to the exposure to harmful environmental conditions, African Americans suffer from certain genetic conditions. Sickle cell disease is the most common genetic disorder among the African American population. However, sickle cell disease is also found among people from geographic areas where malaria is endemic, such as the Caribbean, the Middle East, the Mediterranean region, and Asia. Sickle cell disease represents several hemoglobinopathies that include sickle cell anemia, sickle cell hemoglobin C disease, and sickle cell -thalassemia. In addition to sickle cell disease, glucose-6-phosphate dehydrogenase deficiency, which interferes with glucose metabolism, is another genetic disease found in African Americans.

Finally, in addition to environmental hazards and genetic conditions, AIDS contributes to the lower life expectancy of African Americans compared to European Americans. The number of African Americans with AIDS approximated the number of reported cases seen in the white population (Ward & Duchin, 1998). According to the Centers for Disease Control, a larger percentage of African Americans are infected with HIV and are dying from AIDS than other ethnic groups in the United States.

In summary, health conditions and health status for most African Americans are below average. Health-care providers must provide culturally congruent health education, prevention practices, and screening aimed at improving their health status and reducing their risks.

VARIATIONS IN DRUG METABOLISM

Most clinical drug trials are conducted on European-American men. More recently, clinical trials have included European-American women. However, specific ethnic groups, regardless of gender, continue to be underrepresented in research studies regarding clinical drug trials. African Americans are among the underrepresented groups.

According to Saunders (1997), research conducted at the University of Maryland reveals that African Americans and other minorities do not always respond to drugs in the same manner as European Americans. Examples of drugs that African Americans respond to or metabolize differently are alcohol, antihypertensives, beta blockers, psychotropic drugs, and caffeine. Side effects of psychotropic and antidepressant drugs vary

among ethnic groups. Campinha-Bacote (1991) reported that African American psychiatric clients experience a higher incidence of extrapyramidial effects with haloperidol decanoate than European Americans. African Americans are also more susceptible to tricyclic antidepressant (TCA) delirium than European Americans. For example, Strickland, et al. (1991) reported that for a given dose of a TCA, African Americans show higher blood levels and a faster therapeutic response. As a result, African Americans experience more toxic side effects from a TCA than do European Americans. Glazer, Morganstern and Doucette (1993) reported from their research that African Americans are twice as likely to develop tardive dyskinesia than their white counterparts. Health-care providers must make extended efforts to observe African American clients for side effects related to tricyclics and other psychotropic medications.

Cultural factors, such as a health-care professional's personal beliefs about a specific ethnic group, may also account for how a drug is prescribed (Levy, 1993). For example, African Americans are at a higher risk of misdiagnosis for psychiatric disorders and, therefore, may be treated inappropriately with drugs.

Eye color is another genetic variation related to difference in response to a specific drug. For example, light eyes dilate wider in response to mydriatic drugs than do dark eyes. This difference in response to a mydriatic drug must be taken into consideration when treating African Americans.

High-Risk Behaviors

High-risk behaviors among African Americans can be inferred from the high incidences of HIV/AIDS and other sexually transmitted diseases, teenage pregnancy, violence, unintentional injuries, smoking, alcoholism, drug abuse, sedentary lifestyle, and delayed seeking of health care. Community health workers can have a significant impact on these detrimental practices by providing health education at community affairs located in African American communities. The goals of health education are to change high-risk health behaviors and improve decision making (Edleman & Mandel, 1998). Examples of effective methods for changing behaviors are mutual goal setting and behavior contracts. Another strategy for changing high-risk behaviors is a teaching module using a culturally appropriate Afrocentric approach to early screening for breast and cervical cancer (Baldwin, 1996).

Efforts to change high-risk behaviors are not always successful. According to Edleman and Mandel (1998), health-care professionals must understand influential factors affecting decision making regarding health behaviors. These factors include values, attitudes, beliefs, religion, previous experiences with the health-care system, and life goals.

HEALTH-CARE PRACTICES

Because a significant proportion of African Americans are poor and live in inner cities, they tend to concentrate on day-to-day survival. Health care often takes second place to basic needs of the family, such as food and shelter. In addition, the role of the family has an impact on the health-seeking behaviors of African Americans. African Americans have strong family ties; when an individual becomes ill, that individual is frequently taught to seek health care from the family rather than from health-care professionals. This cultural practice may contribute to the failure of African Americans to seek treatment at an early stage. Screening programs may best be initiated in community and church activities where the entire family is present.

Nutrition

MEANING OF FOOD

Food is used as a way to celebrate special events, holidays, and birthdays. Food is a symbol of both health and wealth and is usually offered to guests when they enter or leave an African American household. One is expected to accept the "gift" of food. Health-care providers must be sensitive to the meaning attached to food, because if individuals reject the food, they are also perceived as rejecting the giver of the food. Food may have a negative meaning attached to it when referred to in conjunction with perceived **witchcraft**. It is thought that witchcraft promotes intentional poisoning through food. Thus, many African Americans find it important to watch carefully what they eat and who gives them food.

COMMON FOODS AND FOOD RITUALS

African American diets are frequently high in fat, cholesterol, and sodium. African Americans eat more animal fat, less fiber, and fewer fruits and vegetables than the rest of American society. Their diet is referred to as **soul food**. The term *soul food* comes from the need for African Americans to "express the group feeling of soul" (Bloch 1983, p. 95). Salt pork (**fatback** or "fat meat") is a key ingredient in the diet of many African Americans. Salt pork is inexpensive and therefore more frequently purchased. However, a person with "high blood" (a term often used for high blood pressure) should avoid or reduce salt intake, pork, red meats, and fried foods. Thus, a diet of liver, greens, eggs, fruits and vegetables, vinegar, lemon, and garlic are recommended to remedy "low blood."

In the African American community, it is common for African Americans to view individuals who are at an ideal body weight as "not having enough meat on their bones." African Americans believe that it is important to have meat on your bones to be able to afford to lose weight during times of sickness. Therefore, being overweight is seen as positive in this ethnic group.

A significant variation is sometimes seen in eating patterns among African American infants. African American parents are encouraged by their elders to begin feeding solid foods, such as cereal, at an early age (usually before 2 months). The cereal is mixed with the formula and is given to the infant in a bottle. African Americans believe that giving only formula is starving the baby and that the infant needs "real food" to sleep through the night. Health-care providers working with family planning and child-care clinics can provide factual knowledge regarding the deleterious effects of giving infants solid foods at an early age.

DIETARY PRACTICES FOR HEALTH PROMOTION

Some African Americans believe that too much red meat causes high blood pressure, which is thought to cause strokes. Some foods, such as milk, vegetables, and meat, are referred to as "strength foods." However, religious affiliations may lead an African American individual to engage in a diet that does not include such foods. For example, a Muslim *halal* diet is similar to a Jewish kosher diet (no pork or pork products are allowed). Also Muslims refuse pork-based insulin. They consider these products to be filthy and believe that "you are what you eat."

NUTRITIONAL DEFICIENCIES AND FOOD LIMITATIONS

Lactose intolerance occurs in 75 percent of the African American population. Low levels of thiamine, riboflavin, vitamins A and C, and iron seen among African Americans are mostly associated with a poor diet secondary to a low socioeconomic status. African Americans' major food preferences are generally available in the United States. "Southern food" is a common preference among European American subcultures as well as African Americans.

Pregnancy and Childbearing Practices

FERTILITY PRACTICES AND VIEWS TOWARD PREGNANCY

Historically, African American families have been large, especially in rural areas. A large family was viewed as an economic necessity and African American parents depended on their children to support them when they could no longer work. However, as families moved to cities, they soon found that large families could become an economic burden. To some extent, this shifted attention to family planning. Billingsly (1968) indicated that among lower income African American families, reproduction and sex are not separated from one another. Furthermore, sex, like religion, was a personal choice, or personal freedom, over which whites had no control. Billingsly (1968) also points out that perhaps the suspicion some African Americans have about using birth control may be due to their idea that birth control takes away their personal freedom. In addition, there are some African Americans who perceive birth control as "African American genocide" or a way of limiting the growth of the African American community (Spector, 2000), or as having a dangerous effect on one's body.

Although oral contraceptives may be the most popular choice of birth control among African Americans who use birth control, religious beliefs also play a role in choices made. For example, African American Catholics may choose the rhythm method over other birth control methods. There are also many views within African American communities regarding the issue of pregnancy versus abortion. Many African Americans who oppose abortion do so because of religious or moral beliefs. Others oppose abortion because of moral, cultural, or Afrocentric beliefs. Such beliefs may cause a delay in making a decision so that it is no longer safe to have an abortion.

PRESCRIPTIVE, RESTRICTIVE, AND TABOO PRACTICES IN THE CHILDBEARING FAMILY

African American women usually respond to pregnancy in the same manner as other ethnic groups, based on their satisfaction with self, economic status, and career goals. The African American family network guides many of the practices and beliefs of the pregnant woman, including the common practice of geophagia. One theory of geophagy, the eating of earth or clay, is that this natural craving alleviates several mineral deficiencies and that the unborn child "needs" this supplement. However, geophagy can lead to a potassium deficiency, constipation, and anemia, and although it is a common practice among many African Americans, some are unaware that the practice exists. The elders in the family provide advice and counseling about what should and should not be done during pregnancy.

Some African Americans claim that the baby signals what it wants to the mother via a food craving, and if the mother does not consume the specific food, the child is marked (birth-marked) with that particular food. Health-care providers need to provide factual information regarding the consequences of eating nonfood substances that may be harmful to the mother or fetus.

Certain practices are believed to be taboo during pregnancy. For example, some African Americans believe that pregnant women should not take pictures because it may cause a stillbirth; nor should they have their picture taken because it captures their soul. Some also believe that it is not wise to reach over their heads if they are pregnant because the umbilical cord will wrap around the baby's neck. Another taboo concerns the purchase of clothing for the infant. It is thought to be bad luck to purchase clothes for the unborn baby.

Snow (1993) reported several home practices related to initiating labor in pregnant African American women. Taking a ride over a bumpy road, ingesting castor oil, eating a heavy meal, or sniffing pepper are all thought to induce labor. If a baby is born with the amniotic sac (referred to as a "veil") over its head or face, the neonate is thought to have special powers. In addition, certain children are thought to have received special powers from God: those born after a set of twins, those born with a physical problem or disability, or a child who is the seventh son in a family.

The postpartum period for the African American woman is greatly extended. It is believed that during the postpartum period the mother is at greater risk than the baby. She is cautioned to avoid cold air and is encouraged to get adequate rest to restore the body to normal. Postpartum practices for child care can involve the use of a bellyband or a coin. These objects, when placed on top of the infant's umbilical area, are believed to prevent the umbilical area from protruding outward.

Death Rituals

DEATH RITUALS AND EXPECTATIONS

For most African Americans, death does not end the connection among people, especially family. Relatives communicating with the deceased's spirit are one example of this endless connection. Snow (1993) studied African American families in the southern United States and noted interesting rituals regarding spirits of the deceased. If one passes an infant over the casket of the deceased who has died a sudden or violent death, this protects the infant from the deceased victim's "haunting spirits."

In addition, some African Americans believe in "voodoo death," which is a belief that illness or death may come to an individual via a supernatural force (Campinha-Bacote, 1992). Voodoo is more commonly known as "root work," "hex," "fix," "conjuring," "tricking," "mojo," "witchcraft," "spell," "black magic," or "hoodoo" (Campinha, 1986). However, Western medicine has a different explanation for voodoo death. Lex (1974) gave a comprehensive explanation of voodoo death in her three phases of "tuning." She noted that in the third stage, both the parasympathetic and sympathetic nervous systems are stimulated. This view is in contrast to Cannon's (1957) and Richter's (1957) explanations of "magical death." Cannon explained magical death in terms of the response of the autonomic nervous system to extreme emotion. Richter believes that this is due to an excessive response in the parasympathetic nervous system related to feelings of helplessness.

African Americans do not believe in rushing to bury the deceased. Therefore, it is common to see the burial service held 5 to 7 days after death. It is important to allow time for relatives who live far away to attend the funeral services.

RESPONSES TO DEATH AND GRIEF

Waters (2000) conducted a research study examining end-of-life directives among African Americans. Findings suggest that African Americans are less likely to know about or complete advance directives. This is attributed, in part, to the fact that end-of-life decisions are usually made by the family. However, implications of findings from the study suggest a need for culturally relevant discussion and education in the African American community.

African Americans believe that the body must be kept intact after death. For example, it is common to hear an African American say, "I came into this world with all my body parts, and I'll leave this world with all my body parts!"

One response to hearing about a death of a family member or close member in the African American culture is **falling out,** which is manifested by sudden collapse and paralysis and the inability to see or speak. However, the individual's hearing and understanding remain intact. Health-care providers must understand the African American culture to recognize this condition as a cultural response to the death of a family member or other severe emotional shock, and not as a medical condition requiring emergency intervention.

Some African Americans are less likely to express grief openly and publicly. However, they do express their feelings openly during the funeral. Funeral services encourage emotional expression and catharsis by incorporating religious songs into the ceremony as well as by providing visual display of the body.

Spirituality

DOMINANT RELIGION AND USE OF PRAYER

Religion and religious behavior is an integral part of the African American community (Fig. 3–1). African American churches have played a major role in the development and survival of African Americans. As clearly stated by Lincoln (1974):

> To understand the power of the black Church, it must first be understood that there is no disjunction between the black Church and the black community . . . whether one is a church member or not is beside the point in any assessment of the importance and meaning of the black Church. (pp. 115–116)

African Americans take their religion seriously, and they expect to receive a message in preaching that helps them in their daily lives. Brown and Gary (1994) found that religious involvement is associated with positive mental health. Furthermore, most African Americans expect to take an active part in religious activities. Participation may involve group singing, creating original words to songs, spontaneous testimony of a personal spiritual view, or expression of deep emotion (Roberson, 1985). Roberson further stated that singers might be

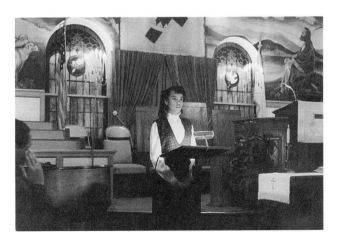

FIGURE 3–1 For many African Americans spirituality is a significant force for promoting well-being.

encouraged with cries of "sing it, sister" or "that's all right" (p. 89).

Most African American Christians are affiliated with the Baptist and Methodist denomination. However, many other denominations and distinct religious groups are represented in African American communities within the United States. These include African Methodist Episcopal, Jehovah's Witnesses, Church of God in Christ, Seventh-Day Adventists, Pentecostal, Apostolic, Presbyterian, Lutheran, Roman Catholic, Nation of Islam, and other Islamic sects (Boyd-Franklin, 1989).

African Americans strongly believe in the use of prayer for all situations they may encounter. They also use prayer for the sake of others who are experiencing problems. "Prayers reflect the trust and faith one has in God" (Roberson 1985, p. 106). African Americans also believe in the **laying on of hands** while praying. It is believed that certain individuals have the power to heal the sick by placing hands on them. African Americans may pray in a language that is not understood by anyone but the person reciting the prayer. This expression of prayer is referred to as **speaking in tongues.**

MEANING OF LIFE AND INDIVIDUAL SOURCES OF STRENGTH

Most African Americans' inner strength comes from trusting in God. Some African Americans believe that whatever happens is "God's will." Because of this belief, African Americans may be perceived to have a fatalistic view of life. For example, Snow (1993) reported that African Americans trust in "Doctor Jesus" and believe that sickness and pain are forms of weakness that come directly from Satan. Therefore, for African Americans, having faith in God is a major source of inner strength.

SPIRITUAL BELIEFS AND HEALTH-CARE PRACTICES

African Americans consider themselves spiritual beings, and sickness is viewed as a separation between God and man. Furthermore, God is thought to be the supreme healer, thus health-care practices center on religious and spiritual activities such as going to church, praying daily, laying on of hands, and speaking in tongues. In addition, because religion is a very important part of health and illness, some African Americans may associate illness or disorders in children with the sins of their parents. In this instance, they believe that healing can only occur through the prayers of a faith healer.

Health-Care Practices

HEALTH-SEEKING BELIEFS AND BEHAVIORS

According to Snow (1974), many African Americans are pessimistic about human relationships and believe that it is more natural to do evil than to do good. Snow concluded that some African Americans' belief systems emphasize three major themes:

1 The world is a very hostile and dangerous place to live.

2 The individual is open to attack from external forces.

3 The individual is considered to be a helpless person who has no internal resources to combat such an attack and, therefore, needs outside assistance.

Because most African Americans tend to be suspicious of health-care professionals, they may see a physician or nurse only when absolutely necessary. Some older African Americans continue to use the *Farmers' Almanac* to choose what is thought to be good times for medical and dental procedures.

RESPONSIBILITY FOR HEALTH CARE

The African American population believes in natural and unnatural illnesses. Natural illness occurs in response to normal forces from which individuals have not protected themselves. Unnatural illness is the belief that harm or sickness can come to you via a person or spirit. In treating an unnatural illness, African Americans seek clergy or a folk healer or pray directly to God. In general, health is viewed as harmony with nature, whereas illness is seen as a disruption in this harmonic state due to demons, "bad spirits," or both.

Individuals commonly use home remedies, consult folk healers (root doctors), and also receive treatment from Western health-care professionals. To render services that are effective and culturally acceptable to African Americans, health-care providers must do a thorough cultural assessment and also become partners with the African American community. Strategies such as focus groups can provide health-care professionals with insight into health-care practices acceptable to African Americans.

African Americans may use home remedies to maintain their health and treat specific health conditions. When taking prescribed medications, it is common for African Americans to take the medications differently from the way they are prescribed. For example, in treating hypertension, African Americans may take their antihypertensive medication on an "as-needed" basis. This self-medicating practice may contribute to the high mortality and morbidity among African Americans from hypertension. However, there are other strategies, when combined with medical treatment modalities, that are effective in treating African Americans with hypertension; for example, relaxation techniques such as transcendental meditation (Barnes, et al., 1997).

FOLK PRACTICES

African Americans, like most ethnic groups, engage in folk medicine. The history of African American folk medicine has its origin in slavery. Slaves had a limited range of choices in obtaining health care. Although they were expected to inform their masters immediately when they were ill, slaves were reluctant to submit themselves to the harsh prescriptions and treatments of 18th- and 19th-century European American physicians (Savitt, 1978). They preferred self-treatment or treatment by friends, older relatives, or "folk doctors." This led to a dual system: "white medicine" and "black medicine"

(Savitt, 1978). Snow (1993) studied hundreds of folk practices used by African Americans. One example is the belief that drinking a glass half-filled with an alcoholic beverage and half-filled with fish blood can cure alcoholism. This is believed to give an undesirable taste and cause nausea and vomiting when subsequent alcoholic drinks are taken.

BARRIERS TO HEALTH CARE

Some African Americans experience economic barriers to health-care services. Needed health-care services may not be affordable for those in lower socioeconomic groups. Although some services may be accessible and available for African Americans, they may not be culturally relevant. For example, a health-care professional may prescribe a strict American Diabetic Association diet to a newly diagnosed diabetic African American client without taking into consideration the dietary habits of this person. Therefore, therapeutic interventions developed by health-care professionals may be underutilized or ignored.

Some African Americans fear that health-care providers may take risks with their clients' lives when rendering care. Thus, there is a general distrust of health-care professionals, practitioners, and the health-care system. Another barrier is the unequal distribution or underrepresentation of ethnic minority health-care providers. In the absence of adequate representation, minority populations are less likely to access and use health-care services.

CULTURAL RESPONSES TO HEALTH AND ILLNESS

African Americans often perceive pain as a sign of illness or disease. Therefore, it is possible that if they are not experiencing severe and/or immediate pain, a regimen of regularly prescribed medicine may not be followed. One example is in the treatment of hypertension. African Americans may take their antihypertensive drugs or diuretics only when they experience head or neck pain. This cultural practice interferes with successful and effective treatment of hypertension. In other cases, some African Americans believe, as part of their spiritual and religious foundation, that suffering and pain are inevitable and must be endured, thus contributing to their high tolerance levels for pain. Prayers and the laying on of hands are thought to free the person from all suffering and pain, and people who still experience pain are considered to have little faith.

In addition to religious beliefs, low educational levels among African Americans may limit their access to information about the etiology and treatment of mental illness. Some African Americans hold a stigma against mental illness. The high frequency of misdiagnosis among African Americans contributes to their reluctance to trust mental health professionals. For example, Adebimpe (1981) reported that over the years a major diagnostic issue has been the high frequency of the diagnosis of schizophrenia among African American clients. Specifically, African Americans are more likely to report hallucinations when suffering from an affective disorder, which may lead to the misdiagnosis of schizophrenia.

Close family and spiritual ties within the African American family allow one to enter the sick role with ease. Extended and nuclear family members willingly care for sick individuals and assume their role responsibilities without hesitation. Sickness and tragedy bring African American families together, even in the presence of family conflict.

BLOOD TRANSFUSIONS AND ORGAN DONATION

While blood transfusions are generally accepted (unless the African American client belongs to a religious group such as Jehovah's Witnesses that does not permit this practice), low levels of organ donation among African Americans may be related to social practices, religious beliefs, and cultural expectations. Plawecki and Plawecki (1992) reported five reasons for the low level of organ donation among African Americans: lack of information about kidney transplantation, religious fears and superstitions, distrust of health-care providers, fear that donors would be declared dead prematurely, and racism (African Americans prefer to give their organs to other African Americans). Also, some African Americans thought originally that in order to get to heaven, they needed all of their body parts. However, the Congress of National Black Churches wants more African Americans to become donors. In May 1998, the Congress decided to make organ and tissue donation a top-priority health issue (Associated Press, 1998).

Health-Care Practitioners

TRADITIONAL VERSUS BIOMEDICAL PRACTITIONERS

Physicians are recognized as heads of the health-care team, with nurses having lesser importance. However, as nurses are becoming more educated, African Americans are holding them in higher regard. Most health professionals have a healthy respect for each group's profession and consult them in their specialty areas.

Among the African American community, folk practitioners can be spiritual leaders, grandparents, elders of the community, voodoo doctors, or priests. Voodoo doctors are consulted for specific illnesses. Another reason for consulting voodoo doctors is to remove a hex. An individual may place a hex on a person because of resentment of achievement, sexual jealousy, love, or envy (Ness & Wintrob, 1981). Someone they know personally usually victimizes hexed persons. A hex can be placed on the victim by using a piece of the individual's hair, fingernails, blood, or some other personal belonging of the victim. The victims usually seek help from a voodoo or conjure doctor to have the hex removed with magicoreligious powers.

While some individuals may prefer a health provider of the same gender for urologic and gynecologic conditions, generally gender is not a major concern in selec-

tion of a health-care provider. Men and women can provide personal care to the opposite sex. On occasion, young men prefer that another man or older women give personal care. With current emphasis on women's health and responses of women to illness and treatment regimens, some African American women prefer female primary-care physicians. The health-care provider should respect these wishes when possible.

STATUS OF HEALTH-CARE PROVIDERS

Western health-care professionals do not generally regard folk practitioners with high esteem. However, as homeopathic and alternative medicine increases in importance in preventive health, these practitioners are likely to gain more respect. Folk practitioners are respected and valued in the African American community and frequently used by African Americans of all socioeconomic levels. Many African Americans perceive health-care professionals as outsiders, and they resent them for telling them what their problems are or telling them how to solve them (Underwood, 1994). Generally, most African Americans are suspicious and cautious of health-care practitioners they have not heard of or do not know. Because interpersonal relationships are highly valued in this group, it is important to initially focus on developing a sound, trusting relationship.

CASE STUDY Mr. and Mrs. Evans are an African American couple who retired from the school system last year. Both are 65 years of age and reside on 20 acres of land in a large rural community approximately 5 miles from a Superfund site and 20 miles from two chemical plants. Members of their household consist of their two daughters, Anna, age 40 years, and Dorothy, age 42 years; their grandchildren, ages 25, 20, 19, and 18; and their 2-year-old great-grandson. Anna and Dorothy and their children all attended university.

Mr. Evans' mother and three of his nieces and nephews live next door. Mr. Evans' mother has brothers, sisters, other sons and daughters, grandchildren, and great-grandchildren who live across the road on 10 acres of land. Mr. Evans has other immediate and extended family who live on 80 acres adjacent to his mother. All members of the Evans family own the land on which they live.

Mrs. Evans has siblings and extended family living on 70 acres of land adjacent to Mr. Evans' family who live across the road. Mr. and Mrs. Evans also have family living in Chicago, Detroit, New York, San Francisco, and Houston. Once a year, the families come together for a reunion. Every other month, local family members come together for a social hour. The family believes in strict discipline with lots of love. It is common to see adult members of the family discipline the younger children regardless of who the parents are.

Mr. Evans has hypertension and diabetes. Mrs. Evans has hypertension. Both are on medication. Their daughter Dorothy is bipolar, and is on medication. Within the last 5 years Mr. Evans has had several relatives diagnosed with lung cancer and colon cancer. One of his maternal uncles died last year from lung cancer. Mrs. Evans has indicated on her driver's license that she is an organ donor.

Sources of income for Mr. And Mrs. Evans are their pension from the school system and Social Security. Dorothy receives SSI because she is unable to work any longer. Mr. Evans and his brothers must assume responsibility for their mother's medical bills and medication. Although she has Medicare parts A and B, many of her expenses are not covered.

Mr. and Mrs. Evans, all members of their household, and all other extended family in the community attend a large Baptist church in the city. Several family members, including Mr. and Mrs. Evans, sing in the choir, are members of the usher board, teach Bible classes, and do community ministry.

STUDY QUESTIONS

1 Describe the organizational structure of this family and identify strengths and limitations of this family structure.

2 Describe and give examples of what you believe to be the family's values about education.

3 Discuss this family's views about childrearing.

4 Discuss the role that spirituality plays in this family.

5 Identify two religious or spiritual practices in which members of the Evans family may engage for treating hypertension, diabetes, and mental illness.

6 Identify and discuss views that Dorothy and her parents may have about mental illness and medication.

7 To what extent are members of the Evans family at risk for illnesses associated with environmental hazards?

8 Susan has decided to become an organ donor. Describe how you think the Evans family will respond to her decision.

9 Discuss views that African Americans have about advanced directives.

10 Name two dietary health risks for African Americans.

11 Identify five characteristics to consider when assessing the skin of African Americans.

12 Describe two taboo views that African Americans may have about pregnancy.

REFERENCES

Adebimpe, V. (1981). Overview: White norms in psychiatric diagnosis of black American patients. *American Journal of Psychiatry, 138*(3), 279–285.

Albers, C. (1999). *Sociology of families.* Thousand Oaks, CA: Pine Forge Press.

Allender, J., & Spradley, B. (2001). *Community health nursing: Concepts and practice.* Philadelphia: Lippincott.

American Public Health Association (1999). More research needed to guide policy on environmental justice. *Nation's Health, 29*(3), 4.

Black ministers push organ donation. (1998, August 2). *Associated Press News Journal,* p. A9

Baldwin, D. (1996). Model for describing low-income African-American women's participation in breast and cervical cancer early detection and screening. *Advances in Nursing Science 19*(2), 21–42.

Barnes, V., Alexander, C., & Staggers, F. (1997). Stress, stress reduction, and hypertension in African Americans: An updated review. *Journal of National Medical Association, 89*(7), 464–476.

Bell, P., & Evans, J. (1981). Counseling the black client. Minneapolis, MN: Hazelden Education Materials.

Bender, D. (1998). *The family: Opposing viewpoints.* San Diego: Greenhaven Press.

Billingsley, A. (1968). *Black families in White America.* Upper Saddle River, NJ: Prentice Hall.

Bloch, B. (1983). Nursing care of black patients. In M. Orque, B. Bloch, and L. Monrroy (Eds.), *Ethnic nursing care* (pp. 82–108). St. Louis: C. V. Mosby.

Blum, J., Morgan, E., Rose, W., Schlesinger, A., Stampp, K., & Woodward, C. (1981). *The national experience.* New York: Harcourt Brace Jovanovich.

Boyd-Franklin, N. (1989). *Black families in therapy.* New York: Guilford Press.

Braithwaite, R., Taylor, S., & Austin, J. (2000). *Building health coalitions in the black community.* Thousand Oaks, CA: Sage Publications.

Brown, D., & Gary, L. (1994). Religious involvement and health status among African-American males. *Journal of the National Medical Association, 86*(11), 825–831.

Brownstein, R. (1995, Nov. 6). Why are so many black men in jail? Numbers in debate equal a paradox. *Los Angeles Times,* p. A5.

Campinha J. (1986). Consideration of the cultural belief systems of individuals experiencing conjure illness by public health nurses and emergency room nurses: An exploratory study. Unpublished doctoral dissertation, University of Virginia, Charlottesville.

Campinha-Bacote, J. (1991). Community mental health services for the underserved: A culturally specific model. *Archives of Psychiatric Nursing, 5*(4), 29–35.

Campinha-Bacote, J. (1992). Voodoo illness. *Perspectives in Psychiatric Nursing, 28*(1), 11–19.

Cannon, W. (1957). Voodoo death. *Psychosomatic Medicine 19*(3), 183–190.

Clark, M. J. (1999). Nursing in the community: Dimensions of community health nursing. Stamford, CT: Appleton & Lange.

Collins, J. (1996). *African-American women's health and social issues* (2nd ed.). Westport, CT: Auburn House.

Conant, J. (1961). *Slums and suburbs.* New York: New American Library Publishers.

Curtin, P. (1969). *The Atlantic slave trade.* Milwaukee: University of Wisconsin Press.

Davis, M. (1976). *South Carolina's blacks and Native Americans.* Columbia, SC: State Human Affairs Commission.

Edleman, C., & Mandel, C. (1998). *Health promotion throughout the lifespan* (3rd ed.). St. Louis. C. V. Mosby.

Frazier, E. (1957). Race and culture contacts in the modern world. Boston: Beacon Press.

Giger, J., & Davidhizar, R. (1999). *Transcultural nursing: Assessment and intervention* (2nd ed.). St. Louis: C. V. Mosby.

Glazer, W. M., Morganstern, H., & Doucette, J. T. (1993). Predicting the long-term risk of tardive dyskinesia in outpatients maintained on neuroleptic medications. *Journal of Clinical Psychiatry, 54*(4), 133–139.

Goddard, L. (1990). *An Afrocentric model of prevention for African-American high-risk youth.* Oakland, CA: Institute for the Advanced Study of Black Family Life and Culture.

Heady, M. (1996; May 15). Holistic plan urged to aid black males. *Los Angeles Times,* p. A12.

Helvie, C. (1998). *Advanced practice nursing in the community.* Thousand Oaks, CA: Sage.

Hill, R. (1997, July 7). Sociologist taught strength of black family. *Baltimore Sun Times,* p. 2B

Hines, P., & Boyd-Franklin, N. (1982). Black families. In M. McGoldrick, J. Pearce, and J. Giordano (Eds.), *Ethnicity and family therapy* (pp. 84–105). New York: Guilford Press.

Jaynes, D., & Williams, R. (1989). *A common destiny: Blacks and American society.* Washington, DC: National Academy Press.

Ladner, J., & Gourdine, R. (1992). Adolescent pregnancy in the African-

American community. In R. Braithwaite and S. Taylor (Eds.), *Health issues in the black community* (pp. 206–221). San Francisco: Josey-Bass.

Levy, R. (1993). Ethnic and racial differences in response to medicines: Preserving individualized therapy in managed pharmaceutical programmes. *Pharmaceutical Medicine, 7,* 139–165.

Lex, B. (1974). Voodoo death: New thoughts on an old explanation. *American Anthropologist, 76,* 818–823.

Lincoln, C. (1974). *The black church since Frazier.* New York: Schocken Books.

Louisiana Department of Health and Hospitals (2001). *Louisiana Health Report Card.* New Orleans, LA: Louisiana Auxiliary Enterprises.

Lowenstein, A., & Glanville, C. L. (1995). Cultural diversity and conflict in the health care workplace. *Nursing Economics, 13*(4) 203–209.

Mead, M., & Baldwin, J. (1971). *A rap on race.* NY: Dell Publishing.Michaels, D. (1993). Occupational cancer in the black population: The health effects of job discrimination. *Journal of the National Black Medical Association, 75,* 1014–1018.

Mindess, A. (1999). *Reading between the signs.* Yarmouth, ME: Intercultural Press.

Minorities get inferior care, even if insured. (2002, March 21). *New York Times.* Retrieved March 21, 2001, from *http*://www.nytimes.com.

Murrary, R., & Zentner, J. (2001). *Health promotion strategies through the lifespan.* Upper Saddle River, NJ: Prentice Hall.

National Center for Health Statistics (1999). *Health US 1999, with socioeconomic status and health chartbook.* Hyattsville, MD: Author.

National Advisory Council on Nurse Education and Practice (1996). *Report to the secretary of the Department of Health and Human Services on the basic registered nurse workforce.* Washington, DC: Author.

Navarro, V. (1997). Race or class versus race and class: Mortality differentials in the US. In P. R. Lee and C. L. Estes (Eds.), *The nation's health* (pp. 32–36). Sudbury, MA: Jones & Barlett.

Ness, R., & Wintrob, R. (1981). Folk healing: A description of synthesis. *American Journal of Psychiatry, 138*(11), 1477–1481.

Plawecki, H., & Plawecki, J. (1992). Improving organ donation rates in the black community. *Journal of Holistic Nursing, 10*(1), 34–46.

Richter, C. (1957). On the phenomenon of sudden death in animals and man. *Psychosomatic Medicine, 23*(3) 191–198.

Roberson, M. (1985). The influence of religious beliefs on health choices of Afro-Americans. *Topics in Clinical Nursing, 7*(3), 57–63.

Saunders, E. (1997). High blood pressure: A call to action for African–Americans. *Baltimore Sun.* p. 3.

Savitt, T. (1978). *Medicine and slavery.* Chicago: University of Illinois Press.

Simmons-O'Brien, E. (1997). Higher risk: African Americans suffer disproportionately from a number of conditions. *Baltimore Sun.* p. 7.

Snow, L. (1974). Folk medical beliefs and their implications for care of patients. *Annals of Internal Medicine, 81,* 82–96.

Snow, L. (1993). *Walkin' over medicine.* Boulder, CO: Westview Press.

Spector, R. (2000). *Cultural diversity in health and illness* (5th ed.). Stamford, CT: Appleton & Lange.

Stevens, P., Hall, J., & Meleis, A. (1992). Examining vulnerability of women clerical workers from five ethnic/racial groups. *Western Journal of Nursing Research, 14*(6), 754–774.

Strickland, T. L., Ranganath, V., Lin, K-M, Poland, R. E., Mendoza, R., & Smith, M. W. (1991). Psychopharmacologic considerations in the treatment of black American populations. *Psychopharmacology Bulletin, 27*(4), 441–448.

Taulbert, C. (1969). *Once upon a time when we were colored.* Tulsa, OK: Counsel Oak Books.

Underwood, S. (1994). Increasing the participation of minorities and other at-risk groups in clinical trials. *Innovations in Oncology Nursing, 10*(4), 106.

U.S. Department of Commerce, Bureau of the Census. (2001). www.census.com.

U.S. Department of Commerce, Bureau of Census. (1993). *We the American blacks.* Washington, DC: U.S. Government Printing Office.

U.S. Department of Health and Human Services. (1997). *Healthy people 2010: National health promotion and disease prevention objectives.* Washington, DC: Author.

U.S. Department of Health and Human Services, Bureau of Health Professions, Division of Health Professions Analysis (1990). *Minorities and women in health fields.* DHHS Publication No.HRSA-P-DV-90–3. Washington, DC: Author.

Ward, J., & Duchin, J. (1998). The epidemiology of HIV and AIDS in the United States. *AIDS Clinical Review* 12(1), 1–45.

Waters, C. (2000). End-of-life directives among African Americans: A need for community-centered discussion and education. *Journal of Community Health Nursing, 17*(1), 25–37.

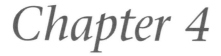

Chapter 4

The Amish

ANNA FRANCES Z. WENGER and MARION R. WENGER

Overview, Inhabited Localities, and Topography

OVERVIEW

As dusk gathers on the hospital parking lot, a man first ties his horse to the hitching rack and then helps a matronly figure wrapped in a shawl as dark as his own greatcoat down from the carriage. On their mother's heels, a flurry of children dressed like undersized replicas of their parents turn their wide eyes toward the fluorescent-lit glass façade of the reception area, a glimmering beacon from the world of high-technology health care. Their excitement is muted by their father's soft-spoken rebuke in a language more akin to German than English, and in a hush, the Amish family crosses a cultural threshold—into the workaday world of health-care professionals.

This Amish family appears to come from another time and place. Those familiar with the health-care needs of the Amish know the profound cultural distance they have bridged in seeking professional help. Others, only marginally acquainted with Amish ways, may ask why this group dresses, acts, and talks like visitors to the North American cultural landscape of the 21st century. Amish are "different" by intention and by conviction. That is to say, for most of the ways in which they depart from the norm for contemporary American culture, they cite a reason related to their understanding of the biblical mandate to live a life separated from a world they see as unregenerate or sinful.

As noted in the primary and secondary characteristics of culture in the introduction to cultural diversity in

Chapter 1, dissimilar appearance, behavior, or both may signal deeper underlying differences in the Amish culture. Noting these differences does not, of necessity, lead to better acceptance or deeper understanding of attitudes and behaviors. Appearances can be misleading. For example, the Amish family's arrival at the hospital by horse and carriage might suggest a general taboo against modern technological conveniences. In fact, most Amish homes are not furnished with electric and electronic labor-saving devices and appliances. But that does not preclude their openness to using state-of-the-art medical technology if it is perceived as necessary to promoting their health.

This minority group's exotic features of dress and language may disguise true motivations regarding health-seeking behaviors, which they share in common with the larger, or majority, culture. To enable such clients to attain their own standard of health and well-being, health-care professionals need to look beyond the superficial appearance and to listen more carefully to the cues they provide.

HERITAGE AND RESIDENCE

It is as important to locate the Amish topographically according to cultural and religious coordinates as well as by the geographical areas they inhabit. The hospital visit scene just portrayed could have taken place in any one of a number of towns across the American Midwest and the eastern seaboard, but the basic circumstances surrounding the interaction with professional caregivers and the cultural assumptions underlying it are the same. For the Amish, seeking help from health-care professionals requires them to go outside their own people and, in so doing, to cross over a significant "permeable boundary" that delimits their community in cultural-geographic terms.

Today's Amish live in rural areas in a band of over 20 states stretching westward from Pennsylvania, Ohio, and Indiana as far as Montana, with some scattered **settlements** as far south as Florida and as far north as the province of Ontario, Canada (Huntington, 2001). About 75 percent of their estimated total population of over 175,000 is concentrated in Pennsylvania, Ohio, and Indiana (Kraybill, 2001). The **Old Order Amish**, so-called for their strict observance of traditional ways that distinguishes them from other, more progressive "plain folk," are the largest and most notable group among the Amish. As such, they constitute an ethnoreligious cultural group in modern America with roots in Reformation-era Europe.

REASONS FOR MIGRATION AND ASSOCIATED ECONOMIC FACTORS

The Amish emerged after 1693 as a variant of one stream of the **Anabaptist** movement that originated in Switzerland in 1525 and spread to neighboring German-speaking lands. The Amish embraced, among other essential Anabaptist tenets of faith, the baptism of adult believers as an outward sign of membership in a voluntary community with an inner commitment to live peaceably with all. The Amish parted ways with the larger Anabaptist group, now known as Mennonites, over the Amish propensity to strictly avoid community members whom they excluded from fellowship in their church (Hostetler, 1993). The Amish name is derived from the surname of Jacob Ammann, a 17th-century Anabaptist who led the Amish division from the Anabaptists in 1693 (Hüppi, 2000). Similarly, the name Mennonite is derived from the given name of Menno Simons, a former Catholic priest, who was a key leader of the Anabaptist movement in Europe.

Anabaptists were disenfranchised and deported, and their goods expropriated, for their refusal to bear arms as a civic service and to accept the authority of the state church in matters of faith and practice. Their attempts at radical discipleship in a "free church," following the guidelines of the early church as set forth in the New Testament, resulted in conflict with Catholic and Protestant leaders. After experiencing severe persecution and martyrdom in Europe, the Amish and related groups emigrated to America in the 17th and 18th centuries. There are no Amish living in Europe today, the last survivors having been assimilated into other religious groups (Hostetler, 1993). As a result, the Amish, unlike many other ethnic groups in the United States, have no larger reference group in their former homeland to which their customs, language, and lifeways can be compared.

Denied the right to hold property in their homelands, the Amish sought not only religious freedom but also the opportunity to buy farmland where they could live out their beliefs in peace. In their communities, the Amish have transplanted and preserved a way of life that bears the outward dress of preindustrial European peasantry. In modern industrial America, they have persisted in social isolation based on religious principles, a paradoxically separated life of Christian altruism. Living for others entails a caring concern for members of their in-group, a community of mutuality, but it also calls them to reach out to others in need outside their immediate Amish household of faith (Hostetler, 1993).

Although the Amish value inner harmony, mutual caring, and a peaceable life in the country, it would be a mistake to see Amish society as an idyllic, pastoral folk culture, frozen in time and serenely detached from the dynamic developments all around them. Since the mid-19th century, Amish communities have experienced inner conflicts and dissension as well as outside pressures to conform and modernize. Over time, the Amish have continued to adapt and change, but at their own pace, accepting innovations selectively.

One cost of controlled, deliberate change has been the loss of some members through factional divisions over "progressive" motivations, both religious and material. The influence of revivalism led to religious reform variants, which introduced Sunday schools, missions, and worship in meetinghouses instead of homes. Others who were impatient to use modern technology such as gasoline-powered farm machinery, telephones, electricity, and automobiles also split off from the main body of the most conservative traditionalists, now called the Old Order Amish. Some variant groups were named after their factional leaders (for example, Egli and Beachy Amish); some were called Conservative Amish Mennonites; and others, The New Order Amish. Today, these progressives stand somewhere between the parent body, the Mennonites, and the Old Order Amish (technically Old Order Amish Mennonites), hereafter simply referred to as the Amish (Hostetler, 1993). This latter group, the (Old Order) Amish, which has been widely researched and reported on, provides the observational basis for this present culture study.

EDUCATIONAL STATUS AND OCCUPATIONS

The controversy over schooling of Amish children is a good example of a policy issue that attracts public attention. Amish parents assume primary responsibility for child rearing, with the constant support of the extended family and the church community to reinforce their teaching. On the family farm, parents and older siblings model work roles for younger siblings. Corporate worship and community religious practices nurture and shape their faith. Learning how to live and to prepare for death is more important in the Amish tradition than acquiring special skills or knowledge through formal education or training (Hostetler & Huntington, 1992).

The mixed-grade, one-room schoolhouses (Fig. 4–1), typical of rural America before 1945, were acceptable to the Amish because the schools were more amenable to local control. With the introduction of consolidated high schools, however, the Amish resisted secondary education, particularly compulsory schooling mandated by state and federal agencies, and raised objections both on principle and on scale. To illustrate the latter, the amount of time required by secondary education and the distances required to bus students out of their home communities were cited as problems. But probably more

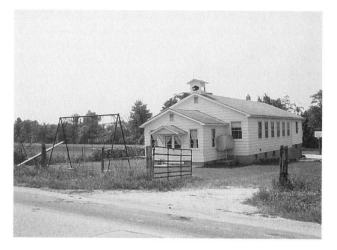

FIGURE 4–1   A one-room Amish schoolhouse in Indiana. (Photograph by Joel Wenger.)

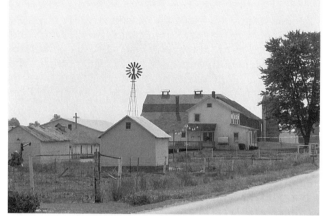

FIGURE 4–2   An Amish farm. The windmill in the background is usually used to pump water. (Photograph by Joel Wenger.)

crucial was the understanding that the high school promised to socialize and instruct the young in a value system that was antithetical to the Amish way of life. For example, in the high school, individual achievement and competition were promoted, rather than mutuality and caring for others in a communal spirit. On pragmatic grounds, Amish parents objected to "unnecessary" courses in science, advanced math, and computer technology, which seemed to have no place and little relevance in their tradition (Meyers, 1993).

The Amish response to this perceived threat to their culture was to build and operate their own private elementary schools. Their right to do so was litigated but finally upheld in the U.S. Supreme Court in the 1972 *Wisconsin v. Yoder* ruling. Today, school-aged children are encouraged to attend only eight grades, but Amish parents actively support local private and public schools.

The Amish rejection of higher learning for their children means that only the rare individual may pursue professional training and still remain Amish. Health-care professionals, by definition, are seen as outsiders who mediate information on health promotion, make diagnoses, and propose therapies across cultural boundaries. To the extent that they do so with sensitivity and respect for Amish cultural ways, they are respected, in turn, and valued as an important resource by the Amish.

Throughout the three centuries of Amish history in North America, their principal and preferred occupations have been agricultural work and farm-related enterprises (Fig. 4–2). So naturally they settled on good farmland in their earliest immigration to North America over 250 years ago. Those who work away from the home farm (for example, young women who have learned quantity cookery at the many church and family get-togethers) may find jobs in restaurants or use skills learned in household chores to work for wages in child care or housecleaning. Young men who bring craft skills from the farm may practice carpentry or cabinet-making in the construction industry. Jobs away from home increase contacts with non-Amish people and test the strength of the many sociocultural bonds that

tie young people to the Amish culture. Given the enticements of the majority culture to change, perhaps it is remarkable that so many Amish find their way back to full membership in the culture that nurtured them.

Communication

DOMINANT LANGUAGES AND DIALECTS

Like most people, the Amish vary their language usage depending on the situation and the individuals being addressed. American English is only one of three language varieties in their repertoire. For the Amish, English is the language of school, of written and print communications, and above all, the language used in contacts with most non-Amish outsiders, especially business contacts. Because English serves a useful function as the contact language with the outside world, Amish schools all use English as the language of instruction, with the strong support of parents, since elementary schooling offers the best opportunity for Amish children to master the language. But within Amish homes and communities, use of English is discouraged in favor of the vernacular **Deitsch**, or Pennsylvania German. Because all Amish except preschool children are literate in their second language, American English, language usage helps to define their cultural space (Hostetler, 1993).

The first language of most Amish is *Deitsch*, an amalgamation of several upland German dialects that emerged from the interaction of immigrants from the Palatinate and Upper Rhine areas of modern France, Germany, and Switzerland. Their regional linguistic differences were resolved in an immigrant language better known in English as "Pennsylvania German." Amish immigrants who later moved more directly from the Swiss Jura and environs to Midwestern states (with minimal mixing in transit with *Deitsch*-speakers) call their home language *Düütsch*, a related variety with marked Upper Alemannic features. Today, *Deitsch* and *Düütsch* both show a strong admixture of vocabulary borrowed from English, while the basic structure remains clearly German. Both have practically the same functional distribution (Wenger, 1970).

Deitsch is spoken in the home and in conversation with fellow Amish and relatives, especially during *visiting,* a popular social activity by which news is disseminated orally. It is important to note that *Deitsch* is primarily a spoken language. Some written material has been printed in Pennsylvania German, but Amish seldom encounter it in this form. Even Amish publications urging the use of *Deitsch* in the family circle are printed in English, by default the print replacement for the vernacular, the spoken language ("What is in a language?", 1986).

Health-care providers can expect all their Amish clients of school age and older to be fluently bilingual. They can readily understand spoken and written directions and answer questions presented in English, although their own terms for some symptoms and illnesses may not have exact equivalents in *Deitsch* and English. Amish clients may be more comfortable consulting among themselves in *Deitsch,* but generally they intend no disrespect for those who do not understand their mother tongue.

Although of limited immediate relevance for health-care considerations, the third language used by the Amish deserves mention in this cultural profile to complete the scope of their linguistic repertoire. Amish proficiency in English varies according to the type and frequency of contact with non-Amish, but it is increasing. The use of Pennsylvania German is in decline outside the Old Order Amish community. Its retention by Amish, despite the inroads of English, has been related to their religious communities' persistent recourse to *Hochdeitsch,* or Amish High German, their so-called third language, as a sacred language (Huffines, 1994).

Amish do not use Standard Modern High German, but an approximation, which gives access to texts printed in an archaic German with some regional variations. Rote memorization and performance for certain ceremonial and devotional functions, and for selected texts from the Luther Bible, the Ausbund hymnal, and devotional literature are a part of public and private prayer and worship among the Amish. Such restricted nonproductive use of a third language hardly justifies the term "trilingual," because it does not comprise a fully developed range of discourse. However, Amish High German provides a situational-functional complement to their other two languages (Enninger & Wandt, 1982). Its retention is one more symbol of a consciously separated way of life that reaches back to its European heritage.

Within a highly contextual subculture like the Amish, the base of shared information and experience is proportionately larger. As a result, less overt verbal communication is required than in the relatively low-contextual American culture, and more reliance is placed on implicit, often unspoken understandings. Amish children and youth may learn adult roles in their society more through modeling, for example, than through explicit teaching. The many and diverse kinds of multigenerational social activities on the family farm provide the optimal framework for this kind of enculturation.

Although this may facilitate the transmission of traditional, or accepted, knowledge and values within a high-context culture, this same information network may also impede new information imparted from the outside, which entails some behavior changes. Wenger (1988, 1991c) suggested that nurses and other health-care providers should consider role modeling as a teaching strategy when working with Amish clients. Later on, a brief example of the promotion of inoculation is presented to illustrate how public health workers can use culture-appropriate information systems to achieve fuller cooperation among the Amish.

In a final note on language and the flow of verbal information, health-care providers should be aware that much of what passes for "general knowledge" in our information-rich popular culture is screened, or filtered out of, Amish awareness. The Amish have severely restricted their own access to print media, permitting only a few newspapers and periodicals. Most have also rejected the electronic media, beginning with radio and television, but also including entertainment and information applications of film and computers. On the other hand, the Amish are openly curious about the world beyond their own cultural horizons, particularly regarding various literature that deals with health and quality-of-life issues. They especially value the oral and written personal testimonial as a mark of the efficacy of a particular treatment or health-enhancing product or process. Wenger (1988, 1994) identified testimonials from Amish friends and relatives as a key source of information in making choices about health-care providers and products.

CULTURAL COMMUNICATION PATTERNS

Fondness and love for family members is held deeply but privately. Some nurses have observed the cool, almost aloof behavior of Amish husbands who accompany their wives to a maternity center, but it would be premature to assume that it reflects a lack of concern. The expression of joy and suffering is not entirely subdued by dour or stoic silence, but Amish are clearly not outwardly demonstrative or exuberant. Amish children, who can be as delightfully animated as any other children at play, are taught to remain quiet throughout a worship service lasting more than 2 hours. They grow up in an atmosphere of restraint and respect for adults and elders. But privately, Amish are not so sober as to lack a sense of humor and appreciation of wit.

Beyond language, much of the nonverbal behavior of Amish is also symbolic. Many of the details of Amish garb and customs were once general characteristics without any particular religious significance in Europe, but in the American setting, they are closely regulated and serve to distinguish the Amish from the dominant culture as a self-consciously separate ethnoreligious group (Kraybill, 2001).

It is precisely in the domain of ideas held to be normative for the religious aspects of Amish life that they find their English vocabulary lacking. The key source texts in *Hochdeitsch* and the oral interpretation of them in *Deitsch* are crucial to an understanding of two German values, which have an important impact on Amish nonverbal behavior. **Demut**, German for humility, is a priority value, the effects of which may be seen in details such as the height of the crown of an Amish man's hat, as well as in very general features such as the modest and unassuming bearing and demeanor usually shown by Amish people in public. This behavior is reinforced by frequent verbal warnings against its opposite, **Hochmut**, pride or arrogance, which is to be avoided (Hostetler, 1993).

The second term, **Gelassenheit**, is embodied in behavior more than it is verbalized. *Gelassenheit* is treasured not so much for its contemporary German connotations of passiveness, even of resignation, as for its earlier religious meanings, denoting quiet acceptance and reassurance, encapsulated in the biblical formula "godliness with contentment" (1 Tim. 6:5). The following Amish paradigm for the good life flows from the calm assurance found through inner yielding and foregoing one's ego for the good of others:

1 One's life rests secure in the hands of a higher power.

2 A life so divinely ordained is therefore a good gift.

3 A godly life of obedience and submission will be rewarded in the life hereafter (Kraybill, 2001).

A combination of these inner qualities, an unpretentious, quiet manner, and modest outward dress in plain colors lacking any ornament, jewelry, or cosmetics, presents a striking contrast to contemporary fashions, both in clothing styles and in personal self-actualization. Amish public behavior is consequently seen as deliberate, rather than rash, deferring to others instead of being assertive or aggressive, avoiding confrontational speech styles, and public displays of emotion in general.

Health-care workers should greet Amish clients with a handshake and a smile. Amish use the same greeting both among themselves and with outsiders, but little touching follows the handshake. Younger children are touched and held with affection, but older adults seldom touch socially in public. Therapeutic touch, on the other hand, appeals to many Amish and is practiced informally by some individuals who find communal affirmation for their gift of **warm hands**. This concept is discussed further in the section on health-care practices.

In public, the avoidance of eye contact with non-Amish may be seen as an extension, on a smaller scale, of the general reserve and measured larger body movements related to a modest and humble being. But in one-on-one clinical contacts, Amish clients can be expected to express openness and candor with unhesitating eye contact.

Among their own, Amish personal space may be collapsed on occasions of crowding together for group meetings or travel. In fact, Amish are seldom found alone, and a solitary Amish person or family is the exception rather than the rule. But Amish are also pragmatic, and in larger families, physical intimacy cannot be avoided in the home where childbearing and care of the ill and dying are accepted as normal parts of life. Once health-care professionals recognize that Amish prefer to have such caregiving within the home and family circle, professionals will want to protect modest Amish clients who feel exposed in the clinical setting.

TEMPORAL RELATIONSHIPS

So much of current Amish life and practice has a traditional dimension reminiscent of a rural American past that it is tempting to view the Amish culture as "backward-looking." In actuality, Amish self-perception is very much grounded in the present, and historical anteceents or reasons for current consensus have often been lost to common memory. On the other hand, the Amish existential expression of Christianity focused on today is clearly seen as a preparation for the afterlife. So one may say that Amish are also future-oriented, at least in a metaphysical sense, although not as it relates to modern, progressive, or futuristic thought.

After generations of rural life guided by the natural rhythms of daylight and seasons, the Amish manage the demands of clock time in the dominant culture. They are generally punctual and conscientious about keeping appointments, although they may seem somewhat inconvenienced by not owning a telephone or car. These communication conveniences, deemed essential by the dominant American culture, are viewed by the most conservative Amish as technological advances that could erode the deeply held value of community, where face-to-face contacts are easily made. Therefore, telephones and automobiles are generally owned by nearby non-Amish neighbors and used by Amish only when it is deemed essential, such as for reaching health-care facilities.

Because the predominant mode of transportation for the Amish is horse and carriage, travel to the doctor's office, a clinic, or a hospital requires the same adjustment as any other travel outside their rural community to shop, trade, or attend a wedding or funeral. The latter three reasons for travel are important means of reinforcing relationship ties, and on these occasions the Amish may use hired or public transportation. Taking time out of normal routines for extended trips related to medical treatments is not uncommon, such as a visit to radioactive mines in the Rocky Mountains or to a laetrile clinic in Mexico to cope with cancer (Wenger, 1988).

FORMAT FOR NAMES

Using first names with Amish people is appropriate, particularly because generations of intermarriage have resulted in a large number of Amish who share only a limited number of surnames. So it is preferable to use John or Mary during personal contacts rather than Mr. or Mrs. Miller, for example. In fact, within Amish communities, with so many Millers, Lapps, Yoders, and Zooks, given names like Mary and John are overused to the extent that individuals have to be identified further by nicknames, residence, a spouse's given name, or a patronymic, which may reflect three or more generations of patrilineal descent. For example, a particular John Miller may be known as "Red John," or "Gap John," or "Annie's John," or "Sam's Eli's Roman's John" (Hostetler, 1993).

During an interview with an Amish mother and her 5-year-old son, Wenger (1988) asked the child where he was going that day. The boy replied that he was going to play with Joe Elam John Dave Paul, identifying his age-mate Paul with four preceding generations. This little boy was giving useful everyday information while at the same time, unbeknown to him, keeping oral history alive. The patronymics also illustrate the cultural value placed on intergenerational relationships and help to create a sense of belonging that embraces several generations. Thus, one can see that medical record keeping can be a challenge where an extensive Amish clientele is served.

Family Roles and Organization

HEAD OF HOUSEHOLD AND GENDER ROLES

From the time of marriage, the young Amish man's role as husband is defined by the religious community he belongs to. Titular patriarchy is derived from the Bible: man is the head of the woman as Christ is the head of the church (I Cor. 3). This patriarchal role in Amish society is balanced or tempered by realities within the family, where the wife and mother is accorded high status and respect for her vital contributions to the success of the family. Practically speaking, husband and wife may share equally in decisions regarding the family farming business. In public, the wife may assume a retiring role, deferring to her husband, but in private they are typically partners. However, it is best to listen to the voices of Amish women themselves as they reflect on their values and roles within Amish family and their shared ethnoreligious cultural community.

Traditionally, the highest priority for the parents is child rearing, a charge laid on them by the church. With a completed family of seven children, the Amish mother must contribute physically and emotionally to the burgeoning growth in Amish population. She also has an important role in providing for family food and clothing needs, as well as a major share in child nurturing. Amish society expects the husband and father to contribute guidance, provide a role model, and discipline the children. This shared task of parenting takes precedence over other needs, including economic or financial success in the family business. On the family farm, all must help out as needed but, in general, field and barn work and animal husbandry are primarily the work of men and boys, whereas food production and preservation, clothing production and care, and management of the household are mainly the province of women.

PRESCRIPTIVE, RESTRICTIVE, AND TABOO BEHAVIORS FOR CHILDREN AND ADOLESCENTS

Children and youth represent a key to the vitality of the Amish culture. Babies are welcomed as a gift from God, and the high birth rate is one factor in their growth in population. Another is the surprisingly high retention of youth, an estimated 75 percent or more, who choose as adults to remain in the Amish way. Before and during elementary school years, parents are more directive as they guide and train their children to assume responsible, productive roles in Amish society.

Young people over age 16 may be encouraged to work away from home to gain experience, but their wages are still sent home to the parental household. Some experimentation with non-Amish dress and behavior among Amish teenagers is tolerated during this period of relative leniency, but the expectation is that an adult decision to be baptized before marriage will call young people back to the discipline of the church, as they take on fully adult roles.

FAMILY GOALS AND PRIORITIES

The Amish family pattern is referred to as the **freindschaft**, the dialectical term used for the three-generational family structure. This kinship network includes consanguine relatives consisting of the parental unit and the households of married children and their offspring. All members of the family personally know their grandparents, aunts, uncles, and cousins, with many Amish knowing their second and third cousins as well.

Individuals are identified by their family affiliation. Children and young adults may introduce themselves by giving their father's first name or both parents' names so they can be placed geographically. Families are the units that make up church districts, and the size of church districts are measured by the number of families, rather than by the number of church members. This extended-family pattern has many functions. Families visit together frequently, thus learning to anticipate caring needs and preferences. Health-care information often circulates through the family network, even though families may be geographically dispersed. Wenger (1988) found that informants referred to *freindschaft* when discussing the factors influencing the selection of health-care options. "The functions of family care include maintaining *freindschaft* ties, bonding family members together intergenerationally, and living according to God's will by fulfilling the parental mandate to prepare the family for eternal life" (Wenger, 1988: 134).

As grandparents turn over the primary responsibility for the family farm to their children, they continue to enjoy respected status as elders, providing valuable advice and sometimes material support and services to the younger generation. Many nuclear families live on a farm with an adjacent grandparent's cottage, which promotes frequent interactions across generations. Grandparents provide child care and help in rearing grandchildren and, in return, enjoy the respect generally paid by the next generations. This emotional and physical proximity to older adults also facilitates elder care within the family setting. In an ethnonursing study on care in an Amish community, Wenger (1988) reported that an informant discussed the reciprocal benefits of having her grandparents living in the attached **daadihaus** and her own parents living in a house across the road. Her 3-year-old daughter could go across the hall to spend time with her great-grandfather which, the mother reported, was good for him in that he was needed, while the small child benefited from learning to know her great-grandfather, and the young mother gained some time to do chores. There is no set retirement age among the Amish, and grandmothers also continue in active roles as advisers and assistants to younger mothers.

Assuming full adult membership and responsibility means the willingness to put group harmony ahead of personal desire. In financial terms, it also means an obligation to help others in the brotherhood who are in need. This mutual aid commitment also provides a safety net, which allows Amish to rely on others for help in emergencies. Consequently, the Amish do not need federal pension or retirement support; they have their own informal "social security" plan. Amish of varying degrees of affluence enjoy approximately the same social status, and extremes of poverty and wealth are uncommon. Property damage or loss and unusual health-care expenses are also covered to a large extent by an informal brotherhood alternative to commercial insurance coverage. The costs of high-technology medical care present a new and severe test of the principle of mutual aid or "helping out," which is almost synonymous with the Amish way of life.

ALTERNATIVE LIFESTYLES

There is little variation from the culturally sanctioned expectations for parents and their unmarried children to live together in the same household while maintaining frequent contact with the extended family. Unmarried children live in the parents' home until marriage, which usual takes place between the ages of 20 and 30. Some young adults may move to a different community to work and would then live as a boarder with another Amish family. Being single is not stigmatized, although almost all Amish do marry. Single adults are included in the social fabric of the community with the expectation that they will want to be involved in family-oriented social events.

Individuals of the same gender do not live together except in situations where their work may make it more convenient. For example, two female schoolteachers may live together in an apartment or in a home close to the Amish school where they teach. There are no available statistics on the incidence of homosexuality in Amish culture. Isolated incidents of homosexual practice may come to the attention of health professionals, but homosexual lifestyles do not fit with the deeply held values of Amish family life and procreation.

Pregnancy before marriage does not usually occur, and it is viewed as a situation to be avoided. When it does occur, in most Amish families the couple would be encouraged to consider marriage. If they are not yet members of the church, they need to be baptized and to join the church before being married. While not condoning pregnancy before marriage, the families and the Amish community support the young couple about to have a child. If the couple chooses not to marry, the young girl is encouraged to keep the baby and her family helps raise the child. Abortion is an unacceptable option. Adoption by an Amish family is an acceptable alternative.

Workforce Issues

CULTURE IN THE WORKPLACE

In every generation except the present one, the Amish have worked almost exclusively in agriculture and farm-related tasks. Their large families were ideally suited to labor-intensive work on the family farm. As the number of family farms has been drastically reduced because of competition from agribusinesses that use mechanized and electronically controlled production methods, few options are available for Amish youth.

Traditionally, the Amish have placed a high value on hard work, with little time off for leisure or recreation. Productive employment for all is the ideal, and the intergenerational family provides work roles appropriate to the age and abilities of each person. But prospects began to narrow with the increased concentration of family farms in densely settled Amish communities as their population increased.

In addition, several cultural factors combine to limit the opportunities for young Amish to adapt to new work patterns. Amish children, who are encouraged to attend school only through eight grades, lack a basis for vocational training in work areas other than agriculture. Amish avoidance of compromising associations with "worldly" organizations, such as labor unions, restricts them to nonunion work, which often pays lower hourly rates. Work off the family farm, at one time a good option for unmarried youth, has become an economic necessity for some parents, although it is considered less acceptable for social reasons. Fathers who "work away," sometimes called "lunchpail daddies," have less contact with children during the workday, which in turn has an impact on the traditional father's modeling role and places more of the responsibility for child rearing on stay-at-home mothers. This shift in traditional parental roles is the source of some concern, although the effects are not yet clear.

ISSUES RELATED TO AUTONOMY

As described previously, external and internal factors have converged in the late 20th century to cause doubt about the continued viability of compact Amish farming communities. Exorbitant land prices triggered group outmigrations and resettlement in states to the west and south. The declining availability of affordable prime arable land in and around the centers of highest Amish population density is due in part to their non-Amish neighbors' land-use practices, especially in areas of suburban sprawl. A powerful internal force is at work as well in the population growth rate among the Amish, now well above the national average. So, contrary to popular notions that such a "backward" subculture is bound to die out, the Amish today are thriving. Population growth continues even without a steady influx of new immigrants from the European homeland or significant numbers of new converts to their religion or way of life (Kraybill, 2001).

The resulting pressures to control the changes in their way of life while maintaining its religious basis, particularly the high value placed on in-group harmony, have challenged the Amish to develop adaptive strategies. One outcome is an increasingly diversified employment base, with a trend toward cottage industries and related retail sales, as well as toward wage labor to generate cash needed for higher taxes and increasing medical costs.

Another recent development includes a shift from traditional multigenerational farmsteads, as some retirees and crafts workers employed off the farm have begun to relocate to the edges of country towns. In summary, pressures to secure a livelihood within the Amish tradition have heightened awareness of the tension field within which the Amish coexist with the surrounding majority American culture.

Because English is the language of instruction in schools and is used with business contacts in the outside world, there is generally no language barrier for the Amish in the workplace. English vocabulary that is lacking in their normative ideas for religious aspects of Amish life is rarely a concern in the workplace.

Biocultural Ecology

SKIN COLOR AND OTHER BIOLOGIC VARIATIONS

Most Amish are descendants of 18th-century southern German and Swiss immigrants; therefore, their physical characteristics vary, as do those of most Europeans, with skin variations ranging from light to olive tones. Hair and eye colors vary accordingly. No specific health-care precautions are relevant to this group.

DISEASES AND HEALTH CONDITIONS

Since 1962, several hereditary diseases have been identified among the Amish. The major findings of the genetic studies have been published by Dr. Victor McKusick of the Johns Hopkins University (McKusick, 1978). Because Amish tend to live in settlements with relatively little domiciliary mobility, and because they keep extensive genealogical and family records, genetic studies are more easily done than with more mobile cultural groups. Many years of collaboration between the Amish and a few geneticists from the Johns Hopkins Hospital have resulted in mutually beneficial projects (Hostetler, 1993). The Amish received printed community directories, and geneticists compiled computerized genealogies for the study of genetic diseases that continue to benefit society in general.

The Amish are essentially a closed population with exogamy occurring very rarely. However, they are not a singular genetically closed population. The larger and older communities are consanguineous, meaning that within the community the people are related through bloodlines by common ancestors. Several consanguine groups have been identified where relatively little intermarriage occurs between the groups. "The separateness of these groups is supported by the history of the immigration into each area, by the uniqueness of the family names in each community, by the distribution of blood groups, and by the different hereditary diseases that occur in each of these groups" (Hostetler, 1993: 328). These diseases are one of the indicators of distinctiveness among the groups.

Hostetler (1993) cautions that although inbreeding is more prevalent in Amish communities than in the general population, inbreeding does not inevitably result in hereditary defects. Through the centuries in some societies, marriages between first and second cousins were relatively common without major adverse effects. However, in the Amish gene pool there are several recessive tendencies that in some cases are limited to specific Amish communities where the consanguinity coefficient (degree of relatedness) is high for the specific genes. Of at least 12 recessive diseases, 4 should be noted here (Hostetler, 1993; McKusick, 1978; Troyer, 1994).

Dwarfism has long been recognized as obvious in several Amish communities. Ellis–van Creveld syndrome, known in Europe and named for a Scottish and a Dutch physician, is especially prevalent among the Lancaster County, Pennsylvania, Amish (McKusick et al., 1964). This syndrome is characterized by short stature and an extra digit on each hand, with some individuals having a congenital heart defect and nervous system involvement resulting in a degree of mental deficiency. The Lancaster County Amish community, the second largest Amish settlement in the United States, is the only one where Ellis–van Creveld syndrome is found. The lineage of all affected people has been traced to a single ancestor, Samuel King, who immigrated in 1744 (Troyer, 1994).

Cartilage hair hypoplasia, also a dwarfism syndrome, has been found in nearly all Amish communities in the United States and Canada, and is not unique to the Amish (McKusick et al., 1965). This syndrome is characterized by short stature and fine, silky hair. There is no central nervous system involvement, and therefore no mental deficiency. However, most affected individuals have deficient cell-mediated immunity, thus increasing their susceptibility to viral infections (Troyer, 1994).

Pyruvate kinase anemia, a rare blood cell disease, was described by Bowman and Procopio in 1963. The lineage of all affected individuals can be traced to Jacob Yoder (known as "Strong Jacob"), who immigrated to Mifflin County, Pennsylvania, in 1792 (Hostetler, 1993; Troyer, 1994). This same genetic disorder was found later in the Geauga County, Ohio, Amish community. Notably, the families of all those who were affected had migrated from Mifflin County, Pennsylvania, and were from the "Strong Jacob" lineage. Symptoms usually appear soon after birth, with the presence of jaundice and anemia. Transfusions during the first few years of life and eventual removal of the spleen can be considered cures.

Hemophilia B, another blood disorder, is disproportionately high among the Amish, especially in Ohio. Ratnoff (1958) reported on an Amish man who was treated for a ruptured spleen. It was discovered that he had grandparents and 10 cousins who were hemophiliacs; 5 of the cousins had died from hemophilia. Research studies on causative mutations indicated a strong probability that a specific mutation may account for much of the mild hemophilia B in the Amish population (Ketterling et al., 1991).

Through the vigilant and astute observations of some public health nurses known to these authors, a major health-care problem was noted in a northern Indiana Amish community. A high prevalence of phenylketonuria (PKU) was found in the Elkhart-Lagrange Amish settlement (Martin, Davis, & Askew, 1965). Those affected are unable to metabolize the amino acid phenylalanine, resulting in high blood levels of the substance and, eventually, severe brain damage if the disorder is untreated. Through epidemiologic studies, the health department found that 1 in 62 Amish were affected, whereas the ratio in the general population was 1 in 25,000 at that time. Through the leadership of these nurses, the county and the state improved case funding for PKU and health-care services for affected families throughout Indiana.

In recent years, a biochemical disorder called glutaric aciduria has been studied. Dr. Holmes Morton, a Harvard-educated physician who has chosen to live and work among the Amish in Lancaster County, Pennsylvania, made house calls, conducted research at his own expense because funding was not forthcoming, and established a clinic in the Amish community to screen, diagnose, and educate people to care for individuals afflicted with the disease (Allen, 1989). By observing the natural history of glutaric aciduria type I, the researchers postulated that the onset or progression of neurological disease in Amish clients can be prevented by screening individuals at risk; restricting dietary protein; and thus limiting protein catabolism, dehydration, and acidosis during illness episodes.

Dr. Morton was well received in the Amish community, with many people referring friends and relatives to him. When he noted the rapid onset of the symptoms and the high incidence among the Amish, he did not wait for them to come to his office. He went to their homes and spent evenings and weekends driving from farm to farm, talking with families, running tests, and compiling genealogical information (Wolkomir & Wolkomir, 1991). In 1991, he built a clinic with the help of donations, in part the result of an article in the *Wall Street Journal* about the need for this nonprofit clinic. Hewlett-Packard donated the needed spectrometer that cost $80,000, local companies provided building materials, and an Amish couple donated the building site. Although volunteers helped to build the clinic, a local hospital provided temporary clinic space lease-free because the community recognized the very important contribution Morton was making, not only to the Amish and the advancement of medical science but also to the public health of the community.

A countywide screening program is now in place. Health-care professionals are able to recognize the onset of symptoms. Research continues on this metabolic disorder, its relationship to cerebral palsy in the Amish population, and the biochemical causes and methods of preventing spastic paralysis in the general population. However, education remains a highly significant feature of any community health program. Nurses and physicians need to plan for family and community education about genetic counseling, screening of newborns, recognition of symptoms during aciduric crises in affected children, and treatment protocols.

Extensive studies of manic-depressive illnesses have been conducted in the Amish population. At first, there seemed to be evidence of a link between the Harvey-*ras*-1 oncogene and the insulin locus on chromosome 11. Studies on non-Amish families (Foroud et al., 2000) and more extensive studies on Amish families have revealed new information on the genome, although the locus for the bipolar disorder has not yet been found (Ginns et al., 1992; Kelsoe et al., 1989, 1993; Law et al., 1992; Pauls, Morton, & Egeland, 1992). Attempts have been made to gain knowledge about the affective response the Amish have to their ethnoreligious cultural identity and experience. Reiling (1998) studied the relationship between Amish self-identity and mental health.

The incidence of alcohol and drug abuse, which can complicate psychiatric diagnoses, is much lower among the Amish than in the general North American population, thus contributing to the importance of the Amish sample. Although the incidence of bipolar affective disorder is not found to be higher in the Amish, some large families with several affected members continue to contribute to medical science by being subjects in the genetic studies. Because the Old Order Amish descend from 30 pioneer couples whose descendants have remained genetically isolated in North America, have relatively large kindred groups with multiple living generations, and generally live in close geographic proximity, they are an ideal population for genetic studies (Kelsoe et al., 1989).

VARIATIONS IN DRUG METABOLISM

No drug studies specifically related to the Amish were found in the literature. However, given the genetic disorders common among selected populations of Amish, this is one area where more research needs to be conducted.

High-Risk Behaviors

Amish are traditionally agrarian and prefer a lifestyle that provides intergenerational and community support systems to promote health and mitigate against the prevalence of high-risk behaviors. Genetic studies using Amish populations are seldom confounded by use of alcohol and other substances. However, health professionals should be alert to potential alcohol and recreational drug use in some Amish communities, especially among young unmarried men. There tends to be tolerance for young adult men straying from the Amish way of life and "sowing their wild oats" before becoming baptized church members and before marriage. Although this may be considered a high-risk behavior, it is not prevalent in all communities, nor is it promoted in any. Parents confide in each other and sometimes in trusted outsiders that this errant behavior causes many heartaches, although at the same time they try to be patient and keep contact with the youth so they may choose to espouse the Amish lifeways.

Another lifestyle pattern that poses potential health risks is nutrition. Amish tend to eat high-carbohydrate and high-fat foods with a relatively high intake of refined sugar. Wenger (1994) reported that in an ethnonursing study on health and health-care perceptions, informants talked about their diet being too high in "sweets and starches" and knowing they should eat more vegetables. The prevalence of obesity was found to be greater among Amish women than for women in general in the state of

Ohio (Fuchs et al., 1990). In this major health-risk survey of 400 Amish adults and 773 non-Amish adults in Ohio, it was found that the pattern of obesity in Amish women begins in the 25-year-old and older cohort, with the concentration occurring between the ages of 45 and 64. An explanation for the propensity for weight gain among the Amish may be related to the central place assigned to the consumption of food in their culture and the higher rates of pregnancy throughout their childbearing years (Wenger, 1994).

HEALTH-CARE PRACTICES

Most Amish are physically active, largely due to their chosen agrarian lifestyle, and farming as a preferred occupation. Physical labor is valued, and men as well as women and children help with farm work. Household chores and gardening, generally considered to be women's work, require physical exertion, particularly because the Amish do not choose to use electrically operated appliances in the home, or machinery, such as riding lawn mowers, that conserve human energy. Nevertheless, many women do contend with a tendency to be overweight. In recent years, it is not uncommon to find Amish women seeking help for weight control from Weight Watchers and other similar weight-control support groups.

Farm and traffic accidents are an increasing health concern in communities with a dense Amish population. In states such as Indiana, with relatively high concentrations of Amish who drive horse-drawn vehicles (Fig. 4–3), blinking red lights and large red triangles are required by law to be attached to their vehicles. Jones (1990) reported on a study of trauma by examining hospital records of Amish clients admitted to one hospital in mideastern Ohio. Transportation-related injuries were the largest group, with many of those involving farm animals. Falls from ladders and down hay holes resulted in orthopedic injuries, but no deaths. Amish families need to be encouraged to monitor their children who operate farm

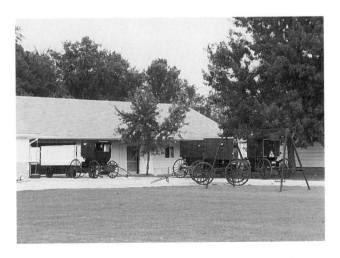

FIGURE 4–3   Amish buggies parked outside a home. Note the reflective safety triangle attached to the back of the rightmost buggy in the picture. These are usually required by law in areas that have large Amish populations. (Photograph by Joel Wenger.)

equipment and transportation vehicles and to teach them about safety factors. Concern about accidents is evident in Amish newsletters, many of which have a regular column reporting accidents and asking for prayers or expressing gratitude that the injuries were not more severe, that God had spared the person, or that the community had responded in caring ways (Wenger, 1988).

Nutrition

MEANING OF FOOD

Among the Amish, food is recognized for its nutritional value. Most Amish prefer to grow their own produce for economic reasons and because for generations they have been aware of their connections with the earth. They believe that God expects people to be the caretakers of the earth and to make it flourish.

The Amish serve food in most social situations since food also has a significant social meaning. Because visiting has a highly valued cultural function, many occasions occur during most weeks for Amish to visit family, neighbors, and friends, especially those within their church district. Some of these visits are planned when snacks or meals are shared, sometimes with the guests helping to provide the food. Even if guests come unexpectedly, it is customary in most Amish communities for snacks and drinks to be offered.

COMMON FOODS AND FOOD RITUALS

Typical Amish meals include meat; potatoes, noodles, or both; a cooked vegetable; bread; something pickled (for example, pickles, red beets); cake or pudding; and coffee. Beef is usually butchered by the family and then kept in the local commercially owned freezer for which they pay a rental storage fee. Some families also preserve beef by canning, and most families have chickens and other fowl, such as ducks or geese, which they raise for eggs and for meat. Amish families still value growing their own foods and usually have large gardens. A generation ago, this was an unquestioned way of life, but an increasing number of families living in small towns and working in factories and construction own insufficient land to plant enough food for the family's consumption.

Snacks and meals in general tend to be high in fat and carbohydrates. A common snack is large, home-baked cookies about 3 inches in diameter. Commercial non-Amish companies have recognized large soft cookies as a marketable commodity and have advertised their commercially made products as "Amish" cookies, even though no Amish are involved in the production. Other common snacks are ice cream (purchased or home-made), pretzels, and popcorn.

When Amish gather for celebrations such as weddings, birthdays, work bees, or quiltings, the tables are usually laden with a large variety of foods. The selection, usually provided by many people, includes several casseroles, noodle dishes, white and sweet potatoes, some cooked vegetables, few salads, pickled dishes, pies, cakes, puddings, and cookies. Hostetler (1993) provides a detailed ethnographic description of the meaning and practices surrounding an Amish wedding, including the food preparation, the wedding dinner and supper, and the roles and functions of various key individuals in this most important rite of passage that includes serving food.

In communities where tourists flock to learn about the Amish, many entrepreneurs have used the Amish love of wholesome simple foods to market their version of Amish cookbooks, food products, and restaurants that more aptly reflect the Pennsylvania German or Dutch influence of communities such as Lancaster County, Pennsylvania. Many of these bear little resemblance to authentic Amish foods, and some even venture to sell "Amish highballs" or "Amish sodas" (Hostetler, 1993). Some Amish families help to satisfy the public interest in their way of life by serving meals in their homes for tourists and local non-Amish. But most Amish view their foods and food preparation as commonplace and functional, not something to be displayed in magazines and newspapers. Because many Amish are wary of outsiders' undue interest, health professionals need to discuss nutrition and food as a part of their lifeways to promote healthy nutritional lifestyles.

In Amish homes, a "place at the table" is symbolic of belonging (Hostetler, 1993). Seating is traditionally arranged with the father at the head and boys seated youngest to oldest to his right. The mother sits to her husband's left with the girls also seated youngest to oldest or placed so that an older child can help a younger one. The table is the place where work, behavior, school, and other family concerns are discussed. During the busy harvesting season, preference is given to the men and boys who eat and return to the fields or barn. At mealtimes, all members of the household are expected to be present unless they are working away from home or are visiting at a distance, making it difficult to return home.

Sunday church services, which for the Old Order Amish are held in their homes or barns, are followed by a simple meal for all who attended church (Fig. 4–4). The church benches, which are transported from home to home wherever the church service is to be held, are set up with long tables for serving the food. In many communities, some of the benches are built so they can quickly be converted into tables. Meals become ritualized so the focus is not on what is being served but rather on the opportunity to visit together over a simple meal. In one community, an Amish informant who had not attended services because of a complicated pregnancy told the researcher that she missed the meal, which in that community consisted of bread, butter, peanut butter, apple butter, pickles, pickled red beets, soft sugar cookies, and coffee (Wenger, 1988).

Pregnancy and Childbearing Practices

FERTILITY PRACTICES AND VIEWS TOWARD PREGNANCY

Children are viewed as a gift from God and are welcomed into Amish families. Estimates place the aver-

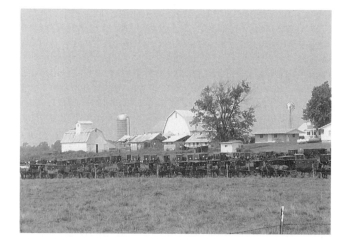

FIGURE 4–4   Buggies parked in a field on an Amish farm where people have gathered for a Sunday church service and noon meal. (Photograph by Joel Wenger.)

age number of live births per family at seven (Hostetler & Huntington, 1992). The Amish fertility pattern has remained constant during the past 100 years, while many others have declined. Household size varies from families with no children to couples with 15 or more children (Huntington, 1988). Even in large families, the birth of another child brings joy because of the core belief that children are "a heritage from the Lord," and another member of the family and community means another person to help with the chores (Hostetler, 1993).

Having children has a different meaning in Old Order Amish culture than in the dominant American culture. In a study on women's roles and family production, the authors suggested that women in Amish culture enjoy high status despite the apparent patriarchal ideology because of their childbearing role and their role as producers of food. A large number of children benefit small labor-intensive farms and, with large families, comes an apparent need for large quantities of food. Interpretation of this pragmatic view of fertility should always be moderated with recognition of the moral and ethical core cultural belief that children are a gift from God, given to a family and community to nurture in preparation for eternal life.

Scholars and researchers of long-term acquaintance with Old Order Amish agree that the pervasive Amish perception of birth control is that it interferes with God's will and thus should be avoided (Kraybill, 2001). Nevertheless, fertility control does exist, although the patterns are not well known and very few studies have been reported. Wenger (1980) discussed childbearing with two Amish couples in a group interview, and they conceded that some couples do use the rhythm method. In referring to birth control, one Amish father stated, "It is not discussed here, really. I think Amish just know they shouldn't use the pill" (Wenger, 1980, p. 5). Three physicians and three nurses were interviewed, and they reported that some Amish do ask about birth control methods, especially those with a history of difficult perinatal histories and those with large families. Some Amish women do use intrauterine devices, but this practice is uncommon. Most Amish women are reluctant to ask physicians and nurses and, therefore, should be counseled with utmost care and respect because this is a topic that generally is not discussed, even among themselves. Approaching the subject obliquely may make it possible for the Amish woman or man to sense the health professional's respect for Amish values and thus encourage discussion. "When you want to learn more about birth control, I would be glad to talk to you" is a suggested approach.

PRESCRIPTIVE, RESTRICTIVE, AND TABOO PRACTICES IN THE CHILDBEARING FAMILY

Amish tend to have their first child later than do non-Amish. In a retrospective chart review examining pregnancy outcomes of 39 Amish and 145 non-Amish women at a rural hospital in southern New York State, it was found that Amish had their first child an average of one year later than non-Amish couples (Lucas et al., 1991). The Amish had a narrower range of maternal ages and had proportionately fewer teenage pregnancies. All subjects received prenatal care, with the Amish receiving prenatal care from Amish lay midwives during the first trimester.

In some communities, Amish have been reputed to be reluctant to seek prenatal health care. Professionals who gain the trust of the Amish learn that they want the best perinatal care, which fits with their view of children being a blessing (Miller, 1997). However, they may choose to use Amish and non-Amish lay midwives who promote childbearing as a natural part of the life cycle. In a study of childbearing practices as described by Amish women in Michigan, Miller (1997) learned that they prefer home births, they had "limited formal knowledge of the childbirth process" (p. 65), and health-care professionals were usually consulted only when there were perceived complications. Although many may express privately their preference for perinatal care that promotes the use of nurse-midwifery and lay midwifery services, home deliveries, and limited use of high technology, they tend to use the perinatal services available in their community. In ethnographic interviews with informants, Wenger (1988) found that grandmothers and older women reported greater preference for hospital deliveries than did younger women. The younger women tend to have been influenced by the increasing general interest in childbirth as a natural part of the life cycle and the deemphasis on the medicalization of childbirth. Some Amish communities, especially those in Ohio and Pennsylvania, have a long-standing tradition of using both lay midwifery and professional obstetric services, often simultaneously.

In Ohio, the Mt. Eaton Care Center developed as a community effort in response to retirement of an Amish lay midwife known as Bill Barb (identified by her spouse's name as discussed in the section on communication). She provided perinatal services, including labor and birth, with the collaborative services of a local Mennonite physician who believed in providing culturally congruent and safe health-care services for this Amish population. At one point in Bill Barb Hochstetler's 30-year practice, the physician moved a trailer with a telephone onto Hochstetler's farm so that he could be called in case of an emergency (Huntington, 1993). Other sympathetic physicians also delivered babies at Bill Barb's home. After state investigation, which coincided with her intended retirement, Hochstetler's practice was recognized to be in a legal gray area. The Mt. Eaton Care Center became a reality in 1985 after careful negotiation with the Amish community, Wayne County Board of Health, Ohio Department of Health, and local physicians and nurses. Physicians and professional nurses and nurse-midwives, who are interested in Amish cultural values and health-care preferences, provide low-cost, safe, low-technology perinatal care in a homelike atmosphere.

Because the Amish want family involvement in perinatal care, outsiders may infer that they are open in their discussion of pregnancy and childbirth. In actuality, most Amish women do not discuss their pregnancies openly and make an effort to keep others from knowing about them until physical changes are obvious. Mothers do not inform their other children of the impending birth of a sibling, preferring for the children to learn of it as "the time comes naturally" (Wenger, 1988). This fits with the Amish cultural pattern of learning through observation that assumes intergenerational involvement in life's major events. Anecdotal accounts exist of children being in the house, though not physically present, during birth. Fathers are expected to be present and involved, although some may opt to do farm chores that cannot be delayed, such as milking cows.

Amish women do participate in prenatal classes, often with their husbands. The women are interested in learning about all aspects of perinatal care but may choose not to participate in sessions when videos are used. Prenatal class instructors should inform them ahead of time when videos or films will be used, so they can decide whether to attend. For some Amish where the **Ordnung** (the set of unwritten rules prescribed for the church district) is more prescriptive and strict, the individuals may be concerned about being disobedient to the will of the community. Even though the information on the videos may be acceptable, the type of media is considered unacceptable.

Amish have no major taboos or requirements for birthing. Men may be present, and most husbands choose to be involved. However, they are likely not to be demonstrative in showing affection verbally nor physically. This does not mean they do not care; it is culturally inappropriate to show affection openly in public. The laboring woman cooperates quietly, seldom audibly expressing discomfort.

Given the Amish acceptance of a wide spectrum of health-care modalities, the nurse or physician should be aware that the woman in labor might be using herbal remedies to promote labor. Knowledge about and a respect for Amish health-care practices alerts the physician or nurse to a discussion about simultaneous treatments that may be harmful or helpful. It is always better if these discussions can take place in a low-stress setting before labor and birth.

As in other hospitalizations, the family may want to spend the least allowable time in the hospital. This is generally related to the belief that birth is not a medical condition and because most Amish do not carry health insurance. In their three-generational family, and as a result of their cultural expectations for caring to take place in the community, many people are willing and able to assist the new mother during the postpartum period. Visiting families with new babies are expected and generally welcomed. Older siblings are expected to help care for the younger children and to learn how to care for the newborn. The postpartum mother resumes her family role managing, if not doing, all the housework, cooking, and child care within a few days after childbirth. For a primiparous mother, her mother often comes to stay with the new family for several days to help with care of the infant and give support to the new mother.

The day the new baby is first taken to church services is considered special. People who had not visited the baby in the family's home want to see the new member of the community. The baby is often passed among the women to hold as they become acquainted and admire the newcomer.

Death Rituals

DEATH RITUALS AND EXPECTATIONS

Amish customs related to death and dying have dual dimensions. On the one hand, they may be seen as holdovers from an earlier time when, for most Americans, major life events such as birth and death occurred in the home. On the other hand, Amish retention of such largely outdated patterns is due to distinctively Amish understandings of the individual within and as an integral part of the family and community. Today, when 70 percent of elderly Americans die in hospitals and nursing homes, some still reflect nostalgically on death as it should be and as in fact it used to be, in the circle of family and friends, a farewell with familiarity and dignity. In Amish society today, this is still a reality in most cases. As physical strength declines, the expectation is that the family will care for the aging and the ill in the home. Hostetler's brief observation that Amish prefer to die at home (1993) is borne out by research findings. Tripp-Reimer and Schrock (1982) reported from their comparative study of the ethnic aged that 75 percent of the Amish surveyed expressed a preference for living with family, 25 percent preferred living at home with assistance, and none would choose to live in a care facility, even if bedfast.

Clearly, these preferences are motivated by more than a wish to dwell in the past or unwillingness to change with the times. The obligation to help others, in illness as in health, provides the social network that supports Amish practices in the passage from life to death. In effect, it is a natural extension of caregiving embraced as a social duty with religious motivation. The Amish accept literally the biblical admonition to "bear one another's burdens," and this finds expression in communal support for the individual, whether suffering, dying, or bereaved. Life's most intensely personal and private act becomes transformed into a community event.

Visiting in others' homes is, for the Amish, a normal and frequent reinforcement of the bonds that tie individuals to extended family and community. As a natural extension of this social interaction, visiting the ill takes on an added poignancy, especially during an illness believed to be terminal. Members of the immediate family are offered not only verbal condolences but many supportive acts of kindness as well. Others close to them prepare their food and take over other routine household chores to allow them to focus their attention and energy on the comfort of the ailing family member.

RESPONSES TO DEATH AND GRIEF

Ties across generations, as well as across kinship and geographic lines, are reinforced around death as children witness the passing of a loved one in the intimacy of the home. Death brings many more visitors into the home of the bereaved, and the church community takes care of accommodations for visitors from a distance as well as funeral arrangements. The immediate family is thus relieved of responsibility for decision making, which otherwise may add distraction to grief. In some Amish settlements, a wakelike "sitting up" through the night provides an exception to normal visiting patterns. The verbal communication with the bereaved may be sparse, but the constant presence of supportive others is tangible proof of the Amish commitment to community. The return to normal life is eased through these visits by the resumption of conversations.

Apart from the usual number of visitors who come to pay their respect to the deceased and survivors, the funeral ceremony is as simple and unadorned as the rest of Amish life. A local Amish cabinetmaker frequently builds a plain wooden coffin. In the past, interment was in private plots on Amish farms, contrasting with the general pattern of burial in a cemetery in the churchyard of a rural church. Because Amish worship in their homes and have no church buildings, they also have no adjoining churchyards. An emerging pattern is burial in a community cemetery, sometimes together with other Mennonites.

Grief and loss are keenly felt, although verbal expression may seem muted, as if to indicate stoic acceptance of suffering. In fact, the meaning of death as a normal transition is embedded in the meaning of life from the Amish perspective. Parents are exhorted to nurture their children's faith because life in this world is seen as a preparation for eternal life.

Spirituality

DOMINANT RELIGION AND USE OF PRAYER

Amish settlements are subdivided into church districts similar to rural parishes with 30 to 50 families in each district. Local leaders are chosen from their own religious community and are generally untrained and unpaid. Authority patterns are congregationalist, with local consensus directed by local leadership, designated as bishops, preachers, and deacons, all of whom are male. No regional or national church hierarchy exists to govern internal church affairs, although a national committee may be convened to address external institutions of government regarding issues affecting the broader Amish population.

In addition to Sunday services, silent prayer is always observed at the beginning of a meal, and in many families, a prayer also ends the meal. Children are taught to memorize prayers from a German prayer book for beginning and ending meals and for silent prayer. The father may say an audible amen or merely lift his bowed head to signal the time to begin eating.

MEANING OF LIFE AND INDIVIDUAL SOURCES OF STRENGTH

Outsiders, who are aware of the Amish detachment from the trappings of our modern materialistic culture, may be disappointed to discover in their "otherworldliness" something less than a lofty spirituality. Amish share the earthy vitality of many rural peasant cultures and a pragmatism born of immediate life experiences, not distilled from intellectual pursuits such as philosophy or theology. Amish simplicity is intentional, but even in austerity there is a relish of life's simpler joys rather than a grim asceticism.

If death is a part of life and a portal to a better life, then individuals are well advised to consider how their lives prepare them for life after death. Amish share the general Christian view that salvation is ultimately individual, preconditioned on one's confession of faith, repentance, and baptism. These public acts are undertaken in the Amish context as part of preparing to assume fully one's adult role in a community of faith. In contrast with the ideals of American individualism, however, the Amish surrender much of their individuality as the price of full acceptance as members of that community. In practical, everyday terms, the religiously defined community is inextricably intertwined with a social reality, which gives it its distinctive shape.

For the Amish, the importance of conformity to the will of the group can hardly be exaggerated. To maintain harmony within the group, individuals often forgo their own wishes. In terms of faith-related behavior, outsiders sometimes criticize this "going along with" the local congregational group as an expression of religiosity, rather than spirituality. The frequent practice of corporate worship, including prayer and singing, helps to build this conformity. It is regularly tested in "counsel" sessions in the congregational assembly where each individual's commitment to the corporate religious contract is reviewed before taking communion (Kraybill, 2001).

SPIRITUAL BELIEFS AND HEALTH-CARE PRACTICES

As seen in earlier sections on communication among Amish and their socioreligious provenance, many symbols of Amish faith point to the separated life, which they live in accordance with God's will. Over time, they have chosen to embody their faith rather than verbalize it. As a result, they seldom proselytize among non-Amish and nurture among themselves a noncreedal,

often-primitive form of Christianity that emphasizes "right living." Their untrained religious leaders offer unsophisticated views of what that entails based on their interpretation of the Bible. Most members are content to submit to the congregational consensus on what right living means, with the assumption that it is based on submission to the will of a loving, benevolent God, an aspect of their spirituality that is seldom articulated (Kraybill, 2001).

Although the directives of religious leaders are normative for many types of decisions, this appears not to be the case for health-care choices (Wenger, 1991b). When choosing among health-care options, families usually seek counsel from religious leaders, friends, and extended family, but the final decision resides with the immediate family. Health-care providers need to be aware of the Amish cultural context and may need to adjust the normal routines of diagnosis and therapy to fit Amish clients' socioreligious context.

Health-Care Practices

HEALTH-SEEKING BELIEFS AND BEHAVIORS

Amish believe that the body is the temple of God and that human beings are the stewards of their bodies. This fundamental belief is based on the Genesis account of creation. Medicine and health care should always be used with the understanding that it is God who heals. Nothing in the Amish understanding of the Bible forbids them from using preventive or curative medical services. A prevalent myth among health-care professionals in Amish communities is that Amish are not interested in preventive services. Although it is true that many times the Amish do not use mainstream health services at the onset of recognized symptoms, they are highly involved in the practices of health promotion and illness prevention.

Although the Amish, as a people, have a reputation for honesty and forthrightness, they may withhold important medical information from medical professionals by neglecting to mention folk and alternative care being pursued at the same time. When questioned, some Amish admit to being less than candid about using multiple therapies, including herbal and chiropractic remedies because they believe that "the doctor wouldn't be interested in them." Making choices among folk, alternative, and professional health-care options does not necessarily indicate a lack of confidence or respect for the latter, but rather reflects the belief that one must be actively involved in seeking the best health care available (Wenger, 1994).

RESPONSIBILITY FOR HEALTH CARE

The Amish believe that it is their responsibility to be personally involved in promoting health. As in most cultures, health-care knowledge is passed from one generation to the next through women. In the Amish culture, men are involved in major health-care decisions and often accompany the family to the chiropractor, physician, or hospital. Grandparents are frequently consulted about treatment options. In one situation, a scheduled consultation for a 4-year-old was postponed until the maternal grandmother was well enough after a cholecystectomy to make the 3-hour automobile trip to the medical center.

A usual concern regarding responsibility for health care is payment for services. Many Amish do not carry any insurance, including health insurance. However, in most communities, there is some form of agreement for sharing losses caused by natural disasters as well as catastrophic illnesses. Some have formalized mutual aid, such as the Amish Aid Society. Wenger (1988) found that her informants were opposed to such formalized agreements and wanted to do all they could to live healthy and safe lives, which they believed would benefit their community in keeping with their Christian calling. Many hospitals have been astounded by the Amish practice of paying their bills despite financial hardship. Because of this generally positive community reputation, hospitals have been willing to set up payment plans for the larger bills.

Active participation was found to be a major theme in Wenger's (1991b, 1994, 1995) studies on cultural context, health, and care. The Amish want to be actively involved in health-care decision making, which is a part of daily living. "To do all one can to help oneself" involves seeking advice from family and friends, using herbs and other home remedies, and then choosing from a broad array of folk, alternative, and professional health-care services. One informant, who visited an Amish healer while considering her physician's recommendation that she have a computerized axial tomography (CAT) scan to provide more data on her continuing vertigo, told the researcher, "I will probably have the CAT scan, but I am not done helping myself and this [meaning the healer's treatment] may help and it won't hurt." In this study, health-care decision making was found to be influenced by three factors: (1) type of health problem, (2) accessibility of health-care services, and (3) perceived cost of the service. When the Amish use professional health-care services, they want to be partners in their health care and want to retain their right to choose from all culturally sanctioned health-care options.

Caring within the Amish culture is synonymous with being Amish. "It's the Amish way" translates into the expectation that members of the culture be aware of the needs of others and thus fulfill the biblical injunction to bear one another's burdens. Caring is a core value related to health and well-being. Care is expressed in culturally encoded expectations that they can best describe in their dialect as **abwaarde**, meaning "to minister to someone by being present and serving when someone is sick in bed." A more frequently used term for helping is **achtgewwe**, which means "to serve by becoming aware of someone's needs and then to act by doing things to help." Helping others is expressed in gender-related and age-related roles, *freindschaft* (the three-generational family), church district, community (including non-Amish), Amish settlements, and worldwide. No outsiders or health-care providers can be expected to understand fully this complex caring network, but health-care providers can learn about it in the local setting by establishing trust in relationships with their Amish clients.

When catastrophic illness occurs, the Amish community responds by being present, helping with chores, and relieving family members so that they can be with the afflicted person in the acute-care hospital. Some do opt to accept medical advice regarding the need for high-technology treatment, such as transplants or other high-cost interventions. The client's family seeks prayers and advice from the bishop and deacons of their church and their family and friends, but the decision is generally a personal or family one.

Amish engage in self-medication. Although most Amish regularly visit physicians and use prescription drugs, they also use herbs and other nonprescription remedies, often simultaneously. When discussing the meaning of health and illness, Wenger (1988, 1994) found that her Amish informants considered it their responsibility to investigate their treatment options and to stay personally involved in the treatment process rather than to relegate their care to the judgment of the professional physician or nurse. Consequently, they seek testimonials from other family members and friends about what treatments work best. They may also seek care from Amish healers and other alternative-care practitioners, who may suggest nutritional supplements. One informant told how she would take "blue cohosh" pills with her to the hospital when she was in labor because she believed that they would speed up the labor.

Because of the Amish practice of self-medication, it is essential that health-care providers inquire about the full range of remedies that are being used. For the Amish client to be candid, the provider must develop a context of mutual trust and respect. Within this context, the Amish client can feel assured that the professional wants to consider and negotiate the most advantageous yet culturally congruent care for them.

FOLK PRACTICES

The Amish, like many other cultures, have an elaborate health-care belief system that includes traditional remedies passed from one generation to the next. They also use alternative health care that is shared by other Americans, though often not sanctioned by medical and other health-care professionals. Although the prevalence of specific health-care beliefs and practices, such as use of chiropractic, Western medical and health-care science, reflexology, iridology, osteopathy, homeopathy, and folklore, is influenced mainly by *freindschaft* (Wenger, 1991b), variations depend on geographic region and the conservatism of the Amish community.

Herbal remedies include those handed down by successive generations of mothers and daughters. One elderly grandmother showed the researcher the cupboard where she kept some cloths soaked in a herbal remedy and shared the recipe for it. She stated that the cupboard was where she remembers her grandmother keeping those same remedies when her grandmother lived in the *daadihaus,* the grandparents' cottage attached to the family farmhouse where her daughter and son-in-law live. She also confided that, although she prepared the herb-soaked cloths for her daughters when they married, she thinks they opt for more modern treatments, such as herb pills and prescription drugs. This is a poignant example of the effect of modern health care on a highly contextual culture.

"Of all Amish folk health care, **brauche** has claimed the most interest of outsiders, who are often puzzled by its historical origins and contemporary application" (Wenger, 1991a: 87). *Brauche* is a folk-healing art that was practiced in Europe around the time of the Amish immigration to North America and is not unique to the Amish, but is a common healing art used among Pennsylvania Germans. As with some other European practices, the Amish have retained *brauche* in some communities. In other communities, the practice is considered suspect, and it has been the focus of some church divisions.

Brauche is sometimes referred to as sympathy curing or powwowing. It is unrelated to American Indian powwowing, and the use of this English term to refer to the German term *brauche* is unclear. In most literary descriptions of sympathy curing, it refers to the use of words, charms, and physical manipulations for treating some human and animal maladies. In some communities, the Amish refer to *brauche* as "warm hands," the ability to feel when a person has a headache or a baby has colic. Informants describe situations where some individuals can "take" the stomach ache from the baby into their own bodies in what is described by researchers as transference. Wenger (1991b, 1994) stated that all informant families volunteered information about *brauche*, using that term or "warm hands" to describe folk healing. One informant asked the author if she could "feel" it, too.

A few folk illnesses have no Western scientific equivalents. The first is **abnemme**, which refers to a condition where the child fails to thrive and appears puny. Specific treatments given to the child may include incantations. Some of the older people remember these treatments, and some informants remember having been taken to a healer for the ailment. The second is **aagwachse**, or *livergrown,* meaning "hide-bound" or "grown together," once a common ailment among Pennsylvania Germans (Hostetler, 1993). Symptoms include crying and abdominal discomfort that is believed to be caused by jostling in rough buggy rides. Wenger (1988) reported accompanying an informant with her newborn baby to an Amish healer, and the woman carried the baby on a pillow because she believed the baby to be suffering from *aagwachse*. As stated previously, Amish clients are more likely to discuss folk beliefs and practices with professionals if the nurse or physician gives cues that it is acceptable to do so.

BARRIERS TO HEALTH CARE

Barriers to health care include delay in seeking professional health care at the onset of symptoms, occasional overuse of home remedies, and a prevailing perception that health-care professionals are not interested in, or may disapprove of, the use of home remedies and other alternative treatment modalities. Additionally, some families may live far from professional health-care services, making travel by horse and buggy difficult or inad-

visable. Because in some Amish communities, such as the Old Order Amish, telephones are not permitted in the home, there may be delays in communication with Amish clients. Finally, the cost of health care without health insurance can deter early access to professional care, which could result in more complex treatment regimens.

CULTURAL RESPONSES TO HEALTH AND ILLNESS

The Amish are unlikely to display pain and physical discomfort. The health-care provider may need to remind the Amish client that medication is available for pain relief if they choose to accept it.

Community for the Amish means inclusion of people who are chronically ill or "physically or mentally different." Amish culture approaches these differences as a community responsibility. Children with mental or physical differences are sometimes referred to as "hard learners," who are expected to go to school and be incorporated into the classes with assistance from other student "scholars" and parents. A culturally congruent approach is for the family and others to help engage those with differences in work activities, rather than to leave them sitting around and getting more anxious or depressed.

Hostetler (1993) states that "Amish themselves have developed little explicit therapeutic knowledge to deal with cases of extreme anxiety" (p. 332). They do seek help from trusted physicians, and some are admitted to mental health centers or clinics. However, the mentally ill are generally cared for at home whenever possible. Studies of clinical depression and manic-depressive illness were discussed in the section on biocultural ecology.

As previously mentioned, when individuals are sick, other family members take on additional responsibilities. Little ceremony is associated with being sick, and members know that to be healthy means to assume one's role within the family and community. Caring for the sick is highly valued, but at the same time, receiving help is accompanied by feelings of humility. Amish newsletters abound with notices of thanks from individuals who were ill. A common expression is, "I am not worthy of it all." A care set identified in one research study is that giving care is a privilege and an obligation and that receiving care involves both expectation and humility (Wenger, 1991b). The sick role is mediated by very strong values related to giving and receiving care.

The Amish culture also sanctions time out for illness when the sick are relieved of their responsibilities by others who minister to their needs. A good analogy to the communal care of the ill is found in the support offered by family and church members at the time of bereavement, as noted in the section on dying. The informal social support network is an important factor in the individual's sense of well-being. An underlying expectation, however, is that healthy individuals will want to resume active work and social roles as soon as their recovery permits. With reasonable adjustments for age and physical ability, it is understood that a healthy person is actively engaged in work, worship, and social life of the family and community (Wenger, 1994). Work and rest are kept in balance, but for the Amish, the accumulation of days or weeks of free time or time off for vacation outside the framework of normal routines and social interactions is a foreign idea.

In a study of Amish women's construction of health narratives, Nelson (1999) found that the "collective descriptions [of] health included a sense of feeling well and the physical ability to complete one's daily work responsibilities" (p. vi). Women's health traditions included the use of herbal and other home remedies and consulting lay practitioners. In general, health values and beliefs are influenced by cultural group membership and personal developmental history.

BLOOD TRANSFUSIONS AND ORGAN DONATION

There are no cultural or religious rules or taboos that prohibit Amish from accepting blood transfusions or organ transplantation and donation. In fact, with the genetic presence of hemophilia, blood transfusion has been a necessity for some families. Anecdotal evidence is available regarding individuals who have received heart and kidney transplants, although no research reports or other written accounts were found. Thus, some Amish may opt for organ transplantation after the family seeks advice from church officials, extended family, and friends, but the patient or immediate family generally make the final decision.

Health-Care Practitioners

TRADITIONAL VERSUS BIOMEDICAL PRACTITIONERS

Amish usually refer to their own healers by name rather than by title, although some say *brauch-doktor* or **braucher**. In some communities, both men and women provide these services. They may even specialize, with some being especially good with bed-wetting, nervousness, women's problems, or livergrown. Some set up treatment rooms and people come early in the morning and wait long hours to be seen. They do not charge fees but do accept donations. A few also treat non-Amish clients. In some communities, Amish folk healers use a combination of treatment modalities, including physical manipulation, massage, *brauche,* herbs and teas, and reflexology. A few have taken short courses in reflexology or therapeutic massage. In a few cases, their practice has been reported to the legal authorities by individuals in the medical profession or others who were concerned about the potential for illegal practice of medicine. Huntington (1993) chronicled several cases, including those of Solomon Wickey and Joseph Helmuth, both in Indiana. Both men continue to practice with some carefully designed restrictions.

STATUS OF HEALTH-CARE PROVIDERS

For the Old Order Amish, health-care practitioners are always outsiders because thus far this sect has been unwilling to allow their members to attend medical, nursing, or other health-related professional schools or to seek higher education in general. Therefore, the Old Order Amish must learn to trust individuals outside their culture for health care and medically related scientific knowledge. Hostetler (1993) contends that the Amish live in a state of flux when securing health-care services. They rely on their own tradition to diagnose and sometimes treat illnesses, while simultaneously seeking technical and scientific services from health-care professionals.

Most Amish consult within their community to learn about physicians, dentists, and nurses with whom they can develop trusting relationships. For more information on this practice, see the Amish informants' perceptions of caring physicians and nurses in Wenger's (1994, 1995) chapter and article on health and health-care decision making. Amish prefer professionals who discuss their health-care options, giving consideration to cost, need for transportation, family influences, and scientific information. They also like to discuss the efficacy of alternative methods of treatment, including folk care. When asked, many Amish, like others from diverse cultures, claim that professionals do not want to hear about nontraditional health-care modalities that do not reflect dominant American health-care values.

Amish hold all health-care providers in high regard. Health is integral to their religious beliefs, and care is central to their worldview. They tend to place trust in people of authority when they fit their values and beliefs. Because Amish are not sophisticated in their knowledge of physiology and scientific health care, the health-care professional who gains their trust should bear in mind that because the Amish respect authority, they may unquestioningly follow orders. Therefore, health-care providers should make sure that their clients understand instructions. Role modeling and other concrete teaching strategies are recommended to enhance understanding.

An excellent database on Amish and health can be found on the Internet at *http://ublib.buffalo.edu/units/hsl/ resources/guides/amishbibweb.html.*

CASE STUDY Elmer and Mary Miller, both 35 years old, live with their five children in the main house on the family farmstead in one of the largest Amish settlements in Indiana. Aaron and Annie Schlabach, aged 68 and 70, live in the attached grandparents' cottage. Mary is the youngest of their eight children, and when she married, she and Elmer moved into the grandparents' cottage with the intention that Elmer would take over the farm when Aaron wanted to retire.

Eight years ago they traded living space, and now Aaron continues to help with the farm work, despite increasing pain in his hip, which the doctor advises should be replaced. Most of Mary and Elmer's siblings live in the area, though not in the same church district or settlement. Two of Elmer's brothers and their families recently moved to Tennessee, where farms are less expensive and where they are helping to start a new church district.

Mary and Elmer's fifth child, Melvin, was born 6 weeks prematurely and is 1 month old. Sarah, age 13, Martin, age 12, and Wayne, age 8, attend the Amish elementary school located 1 mile from their home. Lucille, age 4, is staying with Mary's sister and her family for a week because baby Melvin has been having respiratory problems, and their physician told the family he will need to be hospitalized if he does not get better within 2 days.

At the doctor's office, Mary suggested to one nurse, who often talks with Mary about "Amish ways," that Menno Martin, an Amish man who "gives treatments," may be able to help. He uses "warm hands" to treat people and is especially good with babies because he can feel what is wrong. The nurse noticed that Mary carefully placed the baby on a pillow as she prepared to leave.

Elmer and Mary do not carry any health insurance, and are concerned about paying the doctor and hospital bills associated with this complicated pregnancy. In addition, they have an appointment for Wayne to be seen at Riley Children's Hospital, 3 hours away at the University Medical Center in Indianapolis, for a recurring cyst located behind his left ear. Plans are being made for a driver to take Mary, Elmer, Wayne, Aaron, Annie, and two of Mary's sisters to Indianapolis for the appointment. Because it is on the way, they plan to stop in Fort Wayne to see an Amish healer who gives nutritional advice and does "treatments." Aaron, Annie, and Elmer have been there before, and the other women are considering having treatments, too. Many Amish and non-Amish go there and tell others how much better they feel after the treatments.

They know their medical expenses seem minor in comparison to the family who last week lost their barn in a fire and to the young couple whose 10-year-old child had brain surgery after a fall from the hayloft. Elmer gave money to help with the expenses of the child and will go to the barn raising to help rebuild the barn. Mary's sisters will help to cook for the barn raising, but Mary will not help this time because of the need to care for her newborn.

The state health department is concerned about the low immunization rates in the Amish communities. One community health nurse, who works in the area where Elmer and Mary live, has volunteered to talk with Elmer, who is on the Amish school board. The nurse wants to learn how the health department can work more closely with the Amish and also learn more about what the people know about immunizations. The county health commissioner thinks this is a waste of time, and that what they need to do is let the Amish know that they are creating a health hazard by neglecting or refusing to have their children immunized.

STUDY QUESTIONS

1 Develop three open-ended questions or statements you would use in learning from Mary and Elmer what health and caring mean to them and to the Amish culture.

2 List four or five areas of perinatal care that you would want to discuss with Mary.

3 Why do you think Mary placed the baby on a pillow as she was leaving the doctor's office?

4 If you were the nurse to whom Mrs. Miller confided her interest in taking the baby to the folk healer, how would you learn more about their simultaneous use of folk and professional health services?

5 List three items to discuss with the Millers to prepare them for their consultation at the medical center.

6 If you were preparing the reference for consultation, what would you mention about the Millers that would help to promote culturally congruent care at the medical center?

7 Imagine yourself participating in a meeting with state and local health department officials and several local physicians and nurses to develop a plan to increase the immunization rates in the counties with large Amish populations. What would you suggest as ways to accomplish this goal?

8 Discuss two reasons many Old Order Amish choose not to carry health insurance.

9 Name three health problems with genetic links that are prevalent in some Amish communities.

10 How might health-care providers use the Amish values of the three-generational family and their visiting patterns in promoting health in the Amish community?

11 List three Amish values to consider in prenatal education classes.

12 Develop a nutritional guide for Amish women who are interested in losing weight. Consider Amish values, daily lifestyle, and food production and preparation patterns.

13 List three ways in which Amish express caring.

REFERENCES

Allen, F. (1989, September 20). Country doctor: How a physician solved the riddle of rare disease in children of Amish. *Wall Street Journal*, pp. 1, A16.

Bowman, H. S., & Procopio, J. (1963). Hereditary non-sperocytic hemolytic anemia of the pyruvate kinase deficient type. *Annals of Internal Medicine, 58*, 561–591.

Enninger, W., & Wandt, K-H. (1982). Pennsylvania German in the context of an Old Order Amish settlement. *Yearbook of German-American Studies, 17,* 123–143.

Foroud, T., Casteluccio, P., Kollar, D., Edenberg, H., Miller, M., et al. (2000). Suggestive evidence of a locus on chromosome 10p using the NIMH genetics initiative bipolar affective disorder pedigrees. *American Journal of Medical Genetics, 96*(1), 18–23.

Fuchs, J. A., Levinson, R., Stoddard, R., Mullet, M., & Jones, D. (1990). Health risk factors among Amish: Results of a survey. *Health Education Quarterly, 17*(2), 197–211.

Ginns, E. D., Egeland, J., Allen, C., Pauls, D., & Falls, K. (1992). Update on the search for DNA markers linked to manic-depressive illness in the Old Order Amish. *Journal of Psychiatric Research, 26*(4), 305–308.

Hostetler, J. A. (1993). *Amish society*, 4th ed. Baltimore, MD: Johns Hopkins University Press.

Hostetler, J. A., & Huntington, G. E. (1992). *Amish children: Education in the family, school, and community*, 2d ed. Dallas: Harcourt Brace Jovanovich.

Huffines, M. L. (1994). Amish languages. In J. R. Dow, W. Enninger, & J. Raith (Eds.), *Internal and external perspectives on Amish and Mennonite life 4: Old and new world Anabaptist studies on the language, culture, society and health of Amish and Mennonites* (pp. 21–32). Essen, Germany: University of Essen.

Huntington, G. E. (1988). The Amish family. In C. Mindel & R. Haberstein (Eds.), *Ethnic families in America*, 3rd ed. (pp. 367–399). New York: Elsevier.

Huntington, G. E. (1993). Health care. In D. B. Kraybill (Ed.), *The Amish and the state*. Baltimore, MD: Johns Hopkins University Press.

Huntington, G. E. (2001). *Amish in Michigan*. East Lansing, MI: Michigan State University Press.

Hüppi, J. (2000). Research note: Identifying Jacob Ammann. *Mennonite Quarterly Review, 74*(10), 329–339.

Jones, M. W. (1990). A study of trauma in an Amish community. *Journal of Trauma, 30*(7), 899–902.

Kelsoe, J. R., Ginns, E. D., Egeland, J. A., et al. (1989). Re-evaluation of the linkage relationship between chromosome 11p loci and the gene for bipolar affective disorder in the Old Order Amish. *Nature, 342*, 338–342.

Kelsoe, J. R., Kristobjanarson, H., Bergesch, P., Shilling, S., Hutch, S., et al. (1993). A genetic linkage study of bipolar disorder and 13 markers on chromosome 11 including the D2 dopamine receptor. *Neuropsychopharmocology, 9*(4), 293–307.

Ketterling, R. P., Bottema, C. D., Koberl, D. D., Setsuko Ii, & Sommer, S. S. (1991). T^{296}M, a common mutation causing mild hemophilia B in the Amish and others: Founder effect, variability in factor IX activity assays, and rapid carrier detection. *Human Genetics, 87*, 333–337.

Kraybill, D. B. (2001). *The riddle of Amish culture*, rev. ed. Baltimore, MD: Johns Hopkins University Press.

Law, A., Richard, C. W., III, Cottingham, R. W., Jr., Lathrop, M. G., Cox, D. R., & Myers, R. M. (1992). Genetic linkage analysis of bipolar affective disorder in an Old Order Amish pedigree. *Human Genetics, 88*, 562–568.

Lucas, C. A., O'Shea, R. M., Zielezny, M. A., Freudenheim, J. L., & Wold, J. F. (1991). Rural medicine and the closed society. *New York State Journal of Medicine, 91*(2), 49–52.

Martin, P. H., Davis, L., & Askew, D. (1965). High incidence of phenylketonuria in an isolated Indiana community. *Journal of the Indiana State Medical Association, 56*, 997–999.

McKusick, V. A. (1978). *Medical genetics studies of the Amish: Selected papers assembled with commentary*. Baltimore, MD: Johns Hopkins University Press.

McKusick, V. A., Egeland, J. A., Eldridge, D., & Krusen, E. E. (1964). Dwarfism in the Amish I. The Ellis-van Creveld syndrome. *Bulletin of the Johns Hopkins Hospital, 115*, 306–330.

McKusick, V. A., Eldridge, D., Hostetler, J. A., Ruanquit, U., & Egeland, J. A. (1965). Dwarfism in the Amish II. Cartilage hair hypoplasia. *Bulletin of the Johns Hopkins Hospital, 116*, 285–326.

Meyers, T. J. (1993). Education and schooling. In D. Kraybill (Ed.), *The Amish and the state* (pp. 87–106). Baltimore, MD: Johns Hopkins University Press.

Miller, N. L. (1997). Childbearing practices as described by Old Order Amish women. Doctoral dissertation, Michigan State University. *Dissertation Abstracts International*, UMI 1388555.

Nelson, W. A. (1999). *A study of Amish women's construction of health narratives*. Unpublished doctoral dissertation, Kent State University.

Pauls, D. L., Morton, L. A., & Egeland, J. A. (1992). Risks of affective illness among first-degree relatives of bipolar and Old Order Amish probands. *Archives of General Psychiatry, 49*, 703–708.

Ratnoff, O. D. (1958). Hereditary defects in clotting mechanisms. *Advances in Internal Medicine, 9*, 107–179.

Reiling, D. M. (1998). An explanation of the relationship between Amish identity and depression among Old Order Amish. Doctoral dissertation, Michigan State University. *Dissertation Abstracts International*, UMI 9985454.

Tripp-Reimer, T., & Schrock, M. (1982). Residential patterns of ethnic aged: Implications for transcultural nursing. In C. Uhl & J. Uhl (Eds.), *Proceedings of the Seventh Annual Transcultural Nursing Conference* (pp. 144–153). Salt Lake City: University of Utah, Transcultural Nursing Society.

Troyer, H. (1994). Medical considerations of the Amish. In J. R. Dow, W. Enninger, & Raith, J. (Eds.), *Internal and external perspectives on Amish and Mennonite life 4: Old and new world Anabaptist studies on the language, culture, society and health of the Amish and Mennonites* (pp. 68–87). Essen, Germany: University of Essen.

Wenger, A. F. (1980, October). *Acceptability of perinatal services among the Amish*. Paper presented at a March of Dimes symposium, Future Directions in Perinatal Care, Baltimore, MD.

Wenger, A. F. Z. (1988). The phenomenon of care in a high-context culture: The Old Order Amish. Doctoral dissertation, Wayne State University. *Dissertation Abstracts International, 50/02B*.

Wenger, A. F. Z. (1991a). Culture-specific care and the Old Order Amish. *Imprint, 38*(2), 81–82, 84, 87, 93.

Wenger, A. F. Z. (1991b). The culture care theory and the Old Order Amish. In M. M. Leininger (Ed.), *Cultural care diversity and universality: A theory of nursing* (pp. 147–178). New York: National League for Nursing.

Wenger, A. F. Z. (1991c). The role of context in culture-specific care. In P. L. Chinn (Ed.), *Anthology of caring* (pp. 95–110). New York: National League for Nursing.

Wenger, A. F. Z. (1994). Health and health-care decision-making: The Old Order Amish. In J. R. Dow, W. Enninger, & Raith, J. (Eds.), *Internal and external perspectives on Amish and Mennonite life 4: Old and New World Anabaptists studies on the language, culture, society and health of the Amish and Mennonites* (pp. 88–110). Essen, Germany: University of Essen.

Wenger, A. F. Z. (1995). Cultural context, health and health-care decision making. *Journal of Transcultural Nursing, 7*(1), 3–14.

Wenger, M. R. (1970). *A Swiss German dialect study: Three linguistic islands in Midwestern USA*. Ann Arbor, MI: University Microfilms.

What is in a language? (1986, February). *Family Life*, p. 12.

Wolkomir, R., & Wolkomir, J. (1991, July). The doctor who conquered a killer. *Readers Digest, 139*, 161–166.

Chapter 5

People of Appalachian Heritage

LARRY D. PURNELL

Overview, Inhabited Localities, and Topography

OVERVIEW

Appalachia, a region rich in coal, timber, and natural beauty, comprises 406 counties in 13 states—Georgia, Alabama, Mississippi, Virginia, West Virginia, North Carolina, South Carolina, Kentucky, Tennessee, Ohio, Maryland, New York, and Pennsylvania. In addition, the region is divided into Southern Appalachia, Central Appalachia, and Northern Appalachia. West Virginia is the only state entirely within Appalachia. Most of the Appalachian region is rugged, mountainous terrain that is partially responsible for its residents' values and traditions. The population of 22.3 million is relatively stable because of limited out-migration (Appalachian Regional Commission [ARC], 2001). The term *Appalachian* is used in this chapter to describe the people born in the region and their descendants who live in or near the Appalachian mountain range.

In some areas of Appalachia, substandard secondary and tertiary roads, as well as limited public bus, rail, and airport facilities, prevent easy access to the area. No Standard Metropolitan Statistical Area (SMSA) exists in the entire state of West Virginia. Difficulty in accessing the area is partially responsible for continued geographic and sociocultural isolation. Even though the Appalachian region includes several large cities, many people live in small settlements; rugged roads separate communities and thus help to preserve their identity. The rugged terrain can significantly delay ambulance

response time and is a deterrent to people who need health care when the health condition is severe. This is one area where telehealth innovations can provide needed services.

HERITAGE AND RESIDENCE

Appalachians generally characterize themselves according to their family name and by their country of origin, such as German, Scotch-Irish, Welsh, French, or British, the primary groups who settled the region between the 17th and 19th centuries. Most Appalachians can identify a family link with Native Americans who populated the area before them. It is important to remember that migrating into the area does not make one an Appalachian. Historically, the population has been predominantly white. Appalachians cannot be distinguished from other white cultural and ethnic groups by their outward appearance—name, skin color, or dress—and as a result they are an invisible or neglected minority. However, similarities in beliefs and practices, tempered by the primary and secondary characteristics of culture (see Chapter 1), give them a unique and rich ethnic identity. Like many disenfranchised groups, the people of Appalachia have been described in stereotypically negative terms (e.g., "poor white trash") that in no way represent the people or the culture as a whole. They are also known as mountaineers, hillbillies, isolationists, and Elizabethans. The media perpetuate these stereotypes with cartoon strips such as "Li'l Abner" and "Snuffy Smith," television programs such as the *Beverly Hillbillies*, and stories of the feuding Hatfields and McCoys and the Whites and Garrards. Interestingly, these feuds were among the wealthy families over salt deposits and land

and among families who had high political profiles. Failure of the courts to intervene and a propensity of Appalachians to "handle things themselves" perpetuated the feuds.

The reality of Appalachian existence is a deep-seated work ethic, a low cost of living, and a high quality of life. Appalachians are loyal, caring, family-oriented, religious, hardy, independent, honest, patriotic, and resourceful.

Other groups in the region who may identify with Appalachian culture include Native Americans, African Americans, and Melungeons, who are of mixed African American, Native American, Middle Eastern, Mediterranean, and white ethnic descent (Costello, 2000). With the increase in immigration to the United States within the last 30 years, the Appalachian region is becoming more ethnically and culturally diverse.

REASONS FOR MIGRATION AND ASSOCIATED ECONOMIC FACTORS

Initially, people came to Appalachia for religious freedom, space for themselves, and personal control over interactions with the outside world. As mining and timber resources were depleted and farmland eroded, Appalachians migrated to larger urban areas seeking employment. Here, they have felt alone and have sometimes become depressed because of their separation from family and friends. Many are afraid of urban centers because they are alien environments and have high crime rates and a stressful environment. Often, they are afraid to leave their homes at night, continuing to live in isolation. Those who remain in urban settings become bicultural, adapting to urban life while retaining, as much as possible, their traditional culture.

The limited opportunities for employment in Appalachia often require wage earners to leave their families to seek work elsewhere, only returning home to maintain close ties with kinfolks as resources allow. Their migration pattern is regional, where individuals from one area primarily migrate to the same urban areas as their relatives and friends; a pattern that is common with many immigrants. This practice helps decrease depression and feelings of isolation, and provides a support network of family and friends that is important for Appalachian culture, and serves as a network for obtaining employment in new locations.

Appalachian migration patterns reflect the economic conditions found in the area as well as some of the cultural values of home, connection to the land, and the importance of the family. Working-age individuals move to make their living where they can and return to the area to retire. Because of these patterns, Appalachia has the highest existing aging population and the highest population of the aged returning to the region. The pattern of returning home to retire has given rise to challenges for health-care delivery with the aging population. The Appalachian concept of "home" is associated with the land and the family, not a physical structure. The average Appalachian does not move far from the family of origin.

For generations, the region has been a symbol of poverty in a land of wealth and opportunity. During the 1960s, the ARC appropriated funds for building roads to attract industry and provided loans for residents to start their own businesses. In many areas of Central Appalachia, the unemployment rate and the number of people living in poverty have been above the national average, while the per capita income has remained below the national average. Eight of the 13 states in Appalachia have an unemployment rate higher than the national average of 4.8 percent, and the national poverty rate of 12.6 percent is exceeded by 10 of the 13 states in Appalachia. The average per capita income rate in Appalachia is $20,872. Not one state in Appalachia achieves the national per capita income of $25,288. However, one must realize that the cost of living in much of the area is also lower than in many other parts of the United States (ARC, 2001).

EDUCATIONAL STATUS AND OCCUPATIONS

The original immigrants to this area were highly educated when they arrived, but limited access to formal education resulted in isolation of later generations and fewer educational opportunities. Despite the value placed on education, this led to a disparity in educational facilities. Knowledge of the larger society and educational opportunities that could be made available to Appalachians continues to be depressed. Thus, there is a dichotomy between those who are poorly educated and those who are extremely well educated.

Because isolationism results in a cultural lag, IQ scores of children from Appalachia are sometimes lower than in the rest of the population, which has access to larger schools and live in urban settings, with increased stimuli. However, with television and the Internet, this cultural lag is not as great as it was in previous decades. Factors such as improved mobility, access to better schools with qualified teachers, increased employment opportunities in some regions, and greater use of technology with access to the Internet, are responsible for improving socioeconomic conditions and better performance on standard IQ tests.

Education beyond elementary levels is not considered important by some Appalachians because it is not viewed as necessary to earning a living in their traditional occupations. In addition, many Appalachian parents do not want their children influenced by mainstream middle-class American values.

However, fewer children drop out of school today than in previous decades. Because of the high cultural and social value placed on cars and trucks, several states in Appalachia have laws that grant driving privileges upon completion of schooling; this has lowered dropout rates significantly.

Parents who value higher education encourage their children to seek quality education at the best institutions possible, although little change has occurred in the graduation rate from college, which has remained at 36 percent, compared with 45 percent for non-Appalachian counterparts (ARC, 2001). Unfortunately, the highly educated who return to the area are often unable to secure suitable employment.

Because educational levels of individuals within the Appalachian regions vary, it is essential for health-care providers to assess the educational preparation and occupational status of individuals when providing health teaching. Educational materials and explanations must be presented at levels consistent with clients' capabilities. If materials are presented at a level that is not understandable to clients, providers may be seen as being "stuck-up" or "putting on airs."

Communication

DOMINANT LANGUAGE AND DIALECTS

The dominant language of the Appalachian region is English, with many words derived from 16th-century Saxon and Gaelic. Some insular groups in Appalachia speak Elizabethan English, which has its own distinct vocabulary and syntax; this can cause communication difficulties with practitioners who are not familiar with the dialect. Some examples of variations in pronunciation for words are *allus* for "always," and *fit* for "fight." Word meanings that may be different include *poke* or *sack* for "paper bag," and *sass* for "vegetables." The Appalachian region is also noted for its use of strong preterits such as *clum* for "climbed," *drug* for "dragged," and *swelled* for "swollen." Plural forms of monosyllabic words are formed like Chaucerian English, which adds *es* to the word, for example: "post" becomes *postes,* "beast" becomes *beastes,* "nest" becomes *nestes,* and "ghost" becomes *ghostes.* Many people, especially in the nonacademic environment, drop the *g* on words ending in *ing.* For example, "writing" becomes *writin',* "reading" becomes *readin',* and "spelling" becomes *spellin'.* In addition, vowels may be pronounced with a diphthong that can cause difficulty to one unfamiliar with this dialect; hence, *poosh* for "push," *boosh* for "bush," *warsh* for "wash," *hiegen* for "hygiene," *deef* for "deaf," *welks* for "welts," *whar* for "where," *hit* for "it," *hurd* for "heard," and *your'n* for "your." However, when the word is written, the meaning is apparent. Comparatives and superlatives are formed by adding a final *er* or *est,* making the word "bad" become *badder* and "preaching" become *preachin'est* (Wilson, 1989).

If health-care practitioners are unfamiliar with the exact meaning of a word, it is best to ask clients to elaborate. Otherwise, miscommunication can occur and possibly result in an incorrect diagnosis. The health-care practitioner may want to have the person write the words (if the person has writing skills) to help prevent errors in communication and improve compliance with health prescriptions and treatments.

Once outsiders learn the Appalachian dialect and become accustomed to the accent, the language barrier is minimized. Word meanings may differ, but this usually does not present a major problem. Because the Appalachian dialect tends to be very concrete, exposure to this dialect is necessary so that misunderstandings do not occur. Negative interpretations of Appalachian behaviors by non-Appalachian professionals can be detrimental to health-care working relationships.

Cultural Communications Patterns

Appalachians practice the ethic of neutrality, which helps shape communication styles, their worldview, and other aspects of the Appalachian culture. Four dominant themes affect communication patterns in the Appalachian culture: (1) avoiding aggression and assertiveness, (2) not interfering with others' lives unless asked to do so, (3) avoiding dominance over others, and (4) avoiding arguments and seeking agreement (Barnett et al., 1994).

Because Appalachians tend to accept others and do not want to judge others, they may use fewer adjectives and adverbs when speaking and writing. Thus, many Appalachians may be less precise in describing emotions, be more concrete in conversations, and answer questions in a more direct manner. Accordingly, the health-care provider may need to use more open-ended questions when obtaining health information and eliciting opinions and beliefs about health-care practices; otherwise, Appalachian clients are likely to give a yes or no answer without expanding or clarifying their answers.

Appalachians are private people who do not want to offend others; nor do they easily trust or share their thoughts and feelings with *outsiders.* They are more likely to say what they think the listener wants to hear rather than what the listener should hear. In addition, because of past experiences with large mining and timber companies, many Appalachians dislike authority figures and institutions that attempt to control behavior. Individualism and self-reliant behavior are idealized; personalism and individualism are admired; and people are accepted on the basis of their personal achievements, qualities, and family lineage.

Appalachians' perceptions of themselves and their families influence many aspects of their communication styles. Families are more than genetic relationships, and have been described by some to include brothers, sisters, aunts, uncles, parents, grandparents, in-laws, and out-laws. This perception of community transcends the concept of self as "I." The use of the pronoun "we" throughout speech patterns recognizes the concept of self. "We can make it," "We will survive," "We will be there" may refer only to the person speaking.

The interactions in an Appalachian community are illustrated by this statement from a key informant in the Counts and Boyle (1987) Genesis Project, which lasted from 1985 to 1994. Miss Ruth, a 94-year-old native Appalachian, was interviewed in the house in which she was born. She had had her appendix removed in the living room of this same house by a traveling nurse. After returning from a trip to Africa (she had a doctorate and liked to travel, but always returned home), Miss Ruth described the concept of "neighboring" as a double-edged sword. The positive side is that when you are sick, everyone comes around to take care of you; however, on the negative side, when you try to do something quietly, everyone knows about it.

Appalachians may be sensitive to direct questions about personal issues. Sensitive topics are best approached with indirect questions and suggestions because individuals are often very sensitive to hints of criticism. Traditionally, Appalachians are taught to deny anger and not complain. Information should be gathered in the context of broader relationships with respect for the ethic of equality, which implies more horizontal than hierarchical relationships, allowing cordiality to precede information sharing. Starting with sensitive issues may invite ineffectiveness; thus, the health-care provider may need to "sit a spell" and "chat" before getting down to the business of collecting health information. To establish trust, the health-care provider must show interest in the client's family and other personal matters, drop hints instead of give orders, and solicit the client's opinions and advice. This increases self-worth and self-esteem and helps to establish the trust that is needed for effective working relationships. Health-care providers from outside the community must be attuned to these cultural patterns. Understanding the relationships between Appalachian people and authority figures that have resulted from historical inequities will help health providers to accept these differences.

Because traditional Appalachians like personal space, they are more likely to stand at a distance when talking with people in both social and health-care situations. This physical distancing has its origins in religious persecution endured by this group in the earlier part of the century and has been perpetuated by isolationism, which encourages family members to become the main contact for individuals.

Traditional Appalachians may perceive direct eye contact, especially from strangers, as aggression or hostility. Staring is considered to be bad manners. Because direct eye contact is considered impolite, they may avoid it when communicating their needs to outsider health-care providers.

To communicate effectively with Appalachian clients, nonverbal behavior must be assessed within the contextual framework of the culture. Many Appalachians are comfortable with silence, and when talking with health-care providers who are outsiders, they are likely to speak without emotion, facial expression, or gestures and avoid telling unpleasant news to avoid hurting someone's feelings. Health-care providers who are unfamiliar with the culture may interpret these nonverbal communication patterns as not caring. Within this context, the health-care provider needs to allow sufficient time to develop rapport by dropping hints instead of giving orders.

TEMPORAL RELATIONSHIPS

The traditional Appalachian culture is "being"-oriented (i.e., living for today) as compared with "doing"-oriented (i.e., planning for the future). A being orientation not only opposes progress, it also may mean ignoring expert advice and "accepting one's lot in life."

With the potential for economic and cultural lags among Appalachians, other problems may be more pressing and "just getting by" may be the most important activity. Health-care providers must realize that the emphasis on illness prevention in our current society is still relatively new for many Appalachians. For those engulfed in poverty and isolation, the trend is to live for today, relying on tradition for things that cannot be controlled. This worldview is common with present-oriented societies, in which some higher power is in charge of life and its outcomes, but it is a deterrent to preventive health services. With a fatalistic view, where individuals have little or no control over nature and the time of death is "predetermined by God," one frequently hears expressions such as "I'll be there, God willing and if the crick (creek) don't rise." As communication systems such as televisions, satellite dishes, and the Internet become more commonplace, temporal relationships are becoming more future-oriented.

For the traditional Appalachian, life is unhurried and body rhythms control activities, not the clock. One may come early or late for an appointment and still expect to be seen. If individuals are not seen because they are late for an appointment and are asked to reschedule, they may not return because they may feel rejected by the health-care provider. Many Appalachians are hesitant to make appointments because "somethin' better might come up." Appalachians who live outside the area usually talk about, and sometimes even dwell upon, "home" in a nostalgic way. To some, this might seem like a glorification of a past temporal orientation. However, this author believes it is nostalgia for "the way things used to be." Most people do not want to return to the harshness of life of past generations.

FORMAT FOR NAMES

Although the format for names in Appalachia follows the standard given name plus family name, individuals address nonfamily members by their last name. A common practice that denotes neighborliness with respect is to call a person by his or her first name with the title Miss (pronounced "miz" similar to "Ms.," when referring to women, whether single or married) or Mr.; for example, Miss Lillian or Mr. Bill. Miss Lillian may or may not be married. There is also a need to provide a link with both families of origin. Many times Appalachians refer to a married woman as "she was [born] a . . . ," thus linking the families and enhancing the feeling of continuity.

To communicate effectively with traditional Appalachians, health-care providers must not ignore speech patterns; they must clarify any differences in word meanings, translate medical terminology into everyday language using concrete terms, explain not only what is to be done but also why, and ask clients to repeat instructions to assure understanding. Adopting an attitude of respect and flexibility demonstrates interest and helps bridge barriers imposed by health-care providers' personal ideologies and cultural values. Throughout history, Appalachians have enjoyed storytelling, a practice that still continues; accordingly, some individuals may respond better to verbal instructions and education, with reinforcement from videos rather than printed communications.

Family Roles and Organization

HEAD OF HOUSEHOLD AND GENDER ROLES

In previous decades, gender roles were more clearly defined: Men were supposed to do physical work, to support the family financially, and to provide transportation. Women took care of the house and assumed responsibility for child rearing. Self-made individuals and families were idealized. The traditional Appalachian household continues to be patriarchal, with many families becoming more egalitarian in belief and in practice, especially if the woman makes more money than the man. Women are providers of emotional strength; older women have a lot of clout in health-care matters and are usually responsible for preparing herbal remedies and folk medicines. Older women have a higher status in the community than men, who in turn have a higher status than younger women. With the advent of better access to education and improved transportation throughout the Appalachian region, more women are working outside the home, thus creating an environment where gender roles are becoming more egalitarian.

PRESCRIPTIVE, RESTRICTIVE, AND TABOO BEHAVIORS FOR CHILDREN AND ADOLESCENTS

Children are important to the Appalachian culture. Large families are common, and children are usually accepted regardless of their negative behaviors in school or with authority figures. Publicly, parents impose strict conformity for fear of community censure and their own parental feelings of inferiority; however, permissive behavior at home is unacceptable, and hands-on physical punishment, to a degree that some perceive as abuse, is common. For Appalachian children who have problems with school performance, the most effective approach for increasing performance is to provide individualized attention rather than group support or attention, which is congruent with the ethic of neutrality. To be effective in changing negative behavior, it is necessary to emphasize positive points.

As children progress into their teens, mischievous behavior is accepted but not condoned. Continuing formal education may not be stressed because many teens are expected to get a job to help support the family. Children are seen as being important, and to many, having a child, even at an early age, means fulfillment. Motherhood increases the woman's status in the church and in the community. In previous generations, it was not uncommon for teenagers to marry by the age of 15, and some as early as 13. Children, single or married, may return to their parents' home, where they are readily accepted, whenever the need arises.

Many teens in Appalachia may be in a cultural dilemma with exposure to other beliefs outside the home and family. Health-care providers can assist adolescents and family members in working through these cultural differences by helping them to resolve personal conflicts by promoting self-awareness that conveys respect for the family's culture; by discussing personal parenting practices; and by providing information about disease, illness, and treatments in culturally congruent ways.

FAMILY GOALS AND PRIORITIES

Appalachian families take great pride in being independent and doing things for themselves. Even though economics may permit paying others to do some tasks, great pride is taken in being able to do for oneself. This is an area where I can still strongly relate to my Appalachian roots. Even though I have reached a financial position where I can pay someone to do chores on my home and farm, I continue to take pride in doing them myself. For many, family priorities include men getting a job to make a living and women bearing children. Traditionally, nuclear and extended families are important in the Appalachian culture, so family members frequently live in close proximity. Relatives are frequently sought for advice on child rearing and most other aspects of life.

Elders are respected and honored in the Appalachian family. Grandparents frequently care for grandchildren, especially if both parents work. This form of child care is readily accepted and is an expectation in large extended families. Elders usually live close to or with their children when they are no longer able to care for themselves. The physical structure of the home is designed to assist aging parents in maintaining function. Many adult children do not consider nursing home placement because it is the equivalent of a death sentence. Migration of children out of the home area may force many elderly people to relocate outside their home area to be with their children. A dilemma occurs because they have an equally strong Appalachian value of attachment to place and family. As a compromise, some practice "snow birding"—leaving their home in the winter and moving in with their children, then returning to their home in the summer. It is not unusual for adult children to drive 3 to 5 hours on days off work to spend time with and help maintain their elderly parents in their home in Appalachia.

One's obligation to extended family outweighs the obligations to school or work. The nuclear family feels a personal responsibility for nieces and nephews, and readily takes in relatives when the need arises. This extended family is important regardless of the socioeconomic level. Upon migration to urban areas, the nuclear family becomes dominant because extended family is usually left behind in Appalachia. This strong sense of family, where the family distrusts outsiders and values privacy, can be a deterrent to getting involved in community activities or joining self-help group activities.

The Appalachian family network can be a rich resource for the health-care provider when health teaching and assistance with personalized care is needed. For programs with Appalachians to be effective, support must begin with the family, specifically the grandmothers and immediate neighborhood activities. The health-care provider must respect each person as an individual and be nonbureaucratic in nature. The family, rather than the individual, must be considered as the basic treatment unit.

Social status is gained from having the respect of family and friends. Formal education and position do not gain one respect, which has to be earned by proving that one is a good person and "living right." Living right is based on the ethic of neutrality and on being a good "Christian person." Having a job, regardless of what the work might be, is as important as having a prestigious position. Families are very proud of their family members and let the entire community know about their accomplishments. Migration to the city may result in mixed views toward one's status. Monetary gain does not improve one's status. However, skills and character traits that allow one to achieve financial comfort are given high status.

ALTERNATIVE LIFESTYLES

Alternative lifestyles are usually readily accepted in the Appalachian culture. Single and divorced parents are readily accepted into the extended family. Same-sex couples and families living together are accepted, but rarely discussed. Such acceptance is congruent with the ethic of neutrality, the Appalachian need for privacy, not interfering with other's lives unless asked to do so, avoiding arguments, and seeking agreement, even though agreement may be implied rather than spoken.

Workforce Issues

CULTURE IN THE WORKPLACE

Because many Appalachians value family, reporting to work may become less of a priority when a family member is ill or other family obligations are pressing. When family illnesses occur, many Appalachian individuals willingly quit their jobs to care for family members. For many, the preferred work pattern is to work for a while, take time off, and then return to work. Work patterns may change for some Appalachians, but the reality for Appalachians is a deep-seated work ethic. Liberal leave policies for funerals and family emergencies are essential for a positive work environment among traditional Appalachians.

Because personal space is important, many Appalachians use a greater distance when communicating in the workplace. This practice should not interfere with positive working relationships when both parties understand each other's cultural behaviors. Appalachians prefer to work in a harmonious environment that fosters cooperation and agreement in decision making. Professionals who come from outside the area may have difficulty establishing rapport in the workplace because of "outsidedness," not because they are foreigners.

Appalachian individuals usually wish to maintain independent lifestyles. Although they want progress, they also wish to remain isolated from the mainstream. More traditional groups may be slower to assimilate values of middle-class society into their work habits.

ISSUES RELATED TO AUTONOMY

A lack of leadership is not uncommon among traditional Appalachians because ascribed status is more important than achieved status and because there is an attempt to keep hierarchal relationships to a minimum. The Appalachian ethic of neutrality and values of individualism and nonassertiveness, with a strong people orientation, may pose a dichotomous perception at work for outsiders who may not be familiar with the Appalachian way of life. However, when conflicts occur, mutual collaboration for seeking agreement is consistent with their ethic of neutrality. In addition, because many Appalachians align themselves more closely with horizontal rather than hierarchical relationships, they are sometimes reluctant to take on management roles. When Appalachians do accept management roles, they take great pride in their work and in the organization as a whole. This is one case where the working manager may have more respect than someone in a straight management position.

Most middle-class Americans gain self-actualization through work and personal involvement with doing. Appalachians seek fulfillment through kinship and neighborhood activities of being. To foster positive and mutually satisfying working relationships, organizations should capitalize on individual strengths such as independence, sensitivity, and loyalty, which are recognized values in the Appalachian culture. Many Appalachians prefer to work at their own pace, devising their own work rules and methods for getting the job done. Some local factories and health-care facilities that hire managers and administrators from outside the region provide educational seminars about the Appalachians' worldview, work culture, and way of life to foster cultural sensitivity.

Biocultural Ecology

SKIN COLOR AND OTHER BIOLOGIC VARIATIONS

Since its first settlement, the Appalachian region has had a predominantly white population with little variation over time. Some individuals can trace their heritage to a mixture of white ancestry and Cherokee or Apalachee Indian. A few blacks, a distinct minority of 3.2 percent, may identify themselves as Appalachian (ARC, 2001). The influence of Native Americans can be seen in skin color. Those of Scotch-Irish background and others with light skin tones need to take precautions and protect themselves from the harmful effects of the sun because they are at increased risk for skin cancer.

DISEASES AND HEALTH CONDITIONS

Many Appalachians live in cities in seriously degraded conditions, inadequate sewage and plumbing systems, lack of refrigeration, and environmental problems stemming from industrial pollution. The predominant occupations—farming, textile manufacturing, mining, furniture making, and timbering—place residents at increased risk for respiratory diseases such as black lung, brown lung, emphysema, and tuberculosis. The incidence of other health conditions such as hypochromic anemia, otitis media, cardiovascular diseases, female obesity, non-insulin-dependent diabetes mellitus, and parasitic infections are greater than the national norm. White Appalachian residents have a 20 percent greater chance of dying from heart disease between the ages of 35 and 64 than other white Americans because of their limited access to healthy foods and recreational facilities, and because of lack of access to medical care (Centers for Disease Control, 2001). One of the areas in the United States with the highest rate of disability is Appalachia (McCoy, Davis, & Hudson, 1994).

Children are at greater risk for sudden infant death syndrome, congenital malformations, and infections. The infant mortality rate throughout the Appalachian region varies greatly. Although the overall infant mortality rate in Appalachia is 7.7 per 100 live births, which is lower than the national average of 7.9, the states of Alabama, Mississippi, and North Carolina have an infant mortality rate that exceeds the national rate (ARC, 2001). Only 70 percent of children are immunized, compared to 90 percent for the nation as a whole. The area also has a higher than the national average for childhood injuries due to burns, trauma, poisoning, child neglect, and abuse (*Voices of Appalachia Healthy Start Project,* 2001). Cancer, suicide, and accidents in some parts of Appalachia are significantly greater than the national average. The higher rate of cancer in Appalachia prompted the National Cancer Institute in 1999 to create the Appalachian Leadership Initiative on Cancer (ALIC) to help communities challenge cancer at the grassroots level. Significant progress has been made on screening for cervical and breast cancer among low-income older women (National Institutes of Health, 1995). An effective success strategy used by ALIC is storytelling, a strong tradition in Appalachia.

Educational information presented in a nonjudgmental manner can have a significant impact on the health of Appalachian clients. The presentation of health and educational material needs to include the entire family and be linked with improvement in function in order to be taken seriously. Clients generally prefer verbal rather than printed material to obtain health-related information.

VARIATIONS IN DRUG METABOLISM

The literature reports no studies specific to the pharmacodynamics of drug interactions among Appalachians. Given the diverse gene pool of many residents, the health-care professional needs to observe each individual for adverse drug interactions.

High-Risk Behaviors

Compared with non-Appalachians, Appalachians are less concerned about their overall health and risks associated with smoking (McCoy, Davis, & Hudson, 1994). Their use of smokeless tobacco is the highest in the country. Underage use of alcohol is widespread among teens.

There continues to be a low rate of exercise and a diet that is high in fats and refined sugars (Ramsey & Glenn, 1998). The Appalachian definition of health encompasses three levels: body, mind, and spirit. This definition precludes viewing disease as a problem unless it interferes with one's functioning. Consequently, many conditions are denied or ignored until they progress to the point of decreasing function. (Nutrition practices are covered more extensively later in the chapter.)

HEALTH-CARE PRACTICES

A 10-step pattern of health-seeking behaviors has been identified among Appalachians.

1 At the onset of symptoms, Appalachians typically implement self-care practices that are usually learned from mothers.

2 When the symptoms persist, they call their mother, if she is available.

3 If the mother is unavailable, they call the female in their kin network who is perceived as knowledgeable regarding health. If a nurse is available, they may seek the nurse's advice.

4 If relief is not achieved, they use over-the-counter (OTC) medicine they have seen advertised on television for symptoms that most closely match their own.

5 If that is ineffective, they use some of "Mable's medicine" (she lives down the road, had similar symptoms, and did not finish her medicine).

6 Next, they ask the local pharmacist for a recommendation; this usually marks the first encounter with a professional health provider. (Of course, they usually do not tell the pharmacist that they tried Mable's medicine.) The pharmacist may strongly suggest that they see a health-care provider; however, on their insistence, the pharmacist may recommend another OTC medication.

7 When no relief is achieved, they seek a local health-care provider, who may or may not speak understandable English. The provider treats them to the best of his or her ability.

8 If the condition does not resolve itself, the local health-care provider refers them to a specialist in the area.

9 The specialist treats the condition to the best of his or her ability.

10 If unsuccessful, the specialist refers them to the closest tertiary medical center.

These 10 steps may not always follow the sequence presented here; some steps may be skipped, and not all steps are always completed. Moreover, the time frame around these 10 steps may be several years. Often by the time typical Appalachians are referred for definitive treatment, compensatory reserves have been depleted and they die at large medical centers. The story is then passed on in the "holler": "So-and-So went to [Hospital X] and died." This pattern leads to a significant mistrust of large medical centers and continued reluctance to use these facilities effectively.

Health-care providers can have a significant impact on improving a client's health-seeking behaviors by providing information early in this pattern. Nurses especially can help to reverse this pattern because they are viewed as knowledgeable, nonjudgmental, and respectful of Appalachian lifestyles.

Nutrition

MEANING OF FOOD

As with most ethnic and cultural groups, food has meaning beyond providing nutritional sustenance. To many Appalachians, wealth means having plenty of food for family, friends, and social gatherings. One should drink plenty of fluids and eat plenty to have a strong body. A strong body is a healthy body.

COMMON FOODS AND FOOD RITUALS

Many Appalachians, especially those living in rural areas, eat wild game, which includes muskrat, groundhog, rabbit, squirrel, duck, turkey, and venison. Wild game traditionally has a lower fat content than meat raised for commercial purposes. However, consistent with traditional practices from previous decades, most parts of both wild and domesticated animals are eaten. High-cholesterol organ meats such as tongue, liver, heart, lungs (called lights), and brains are considered delicacies. Bone marrow is used to make sauces, and stomach, intestines (chitlins or chitterlings), pigs' feet, tail, and ribs are also commonly eaten. Low-fat game meat is usually breaded and fried with lard or animal fat, negating the overall gains from these low-fat meat sources. Most diets include sweet prepackaged drinks, Kool-Aid with added sugar, very sweet iced tea, and soda.

Food preparation practices may increase dietary risk factors for cardiac disease because many recipes contain lard and meats are preserved with salt. Other common foods in particular regions of Appalachia that may be unfamiliar to nonnative Appalachians are sweet potato pie; molasses candy; apple beer; gooseberry pie; pumpkin cake; and pickled beans, fruit, corn, beets, and cabbage, all of which are high in sodium. Frying foods with bacon grease or lard is a common practice. Fried green tomatoes, biscuits, and thick gravies are favorites.

Appalachians celebrate Thanksgiving, Christmas, other national and religious holidays, and many other occasions with food. In rural areas, people celebrate with food when game and livestock are slaughtered because this is usually an extended-family or community affair. The value of self-reliance is enhanced during the "cannin" season when foodstuffs are preserved. Canning becomes a social or family occasion and is an excellent avenue for health teaching if the health-care provider is willing to participate and learn. Additional celebrations with food occur during times of death and grieving, when friends and participants bring dishes specifically prepared for the occasion.

DIETARY PRACTICES FOR HEALTH PROMOTION

Many Appalachians believe that good nutrition has an effect on one's health. In one study with rural Appalachians, young mothers were asked what it meant to eat well for good health. They referred to "taking fluids" and "eating right," but they were unable to describe healthy eating patterns any further. In a study by Hansen and Resick (1990), the respondents had no real knowledge of healthy nutrition for primary prevention.

Many believe that the sooner a baby can take food other than milk, the healthier it will be. Babies from the first month are fed grease, sugar, and coffee to promote hardiness. I fondly remember as a child being fed teaspoons of bacon grease so I would be sure to grow up strong and healthy. Another family with whom I lived saved the skin from fried chicken for me to eat because I was too thin. The Women, Infants, and Children program, commonly known as WIC, has done much to change some of these practices. Health-care providers have a rich opportunity to provide primary education in healthy eating practices. Factual information that describes health risks with early feeding of solid foods may help prevent later nutritional allergies in children.

The severity of hypertension in one community was decreased significantly when a health-care provider participated in the "cannin" of beans and showed the residents that the beans would remain crisp with a "tige of vinegar" rather than a "pile of salt." It is essential for health-care providers to assess each person's specific food practices and preparation in order to provide effective dietary counseling for health promotion and wellness. Health-care providers in clinics and school settings have an excellent opportunity to have a positive impact on the nutritional status of individuals and families. School breakfast and lunch programs, Meals on Wheels, and church-sponsored meal plans are some of the ways in which health-care providers can encourage and support families in attaining better nutrition practices.

NUTRITIONAL DEFICIENCIES AND FOOD LIMITATIONS

Many rural and urban Appalachian children replace meals with snacks. The most common snacks are candy, salty foods, desserts, and carbonated beverages. Many adolescents skip breakfast and lunch entirely, preferring to eat snack foods. This pattern of snacking can result in deficiencies in vitamin A, iron, and calcium.

There are no specific food limitations or enzyme deficiencies among Appalachians. With subsistence farming and commercial farms from nearby areas, all foods for a healthy diet are readily available during the growing season. Even though the climate is ideal for growing a large variety of vegetables, I rarely see broccoli, cauliflower, or asparagus as vegetables of choice in the mountainous regions of Appalachia. Limitations may come from lack of readily accessible grocery stores and lack of financial ability to purchase nutritious foods.

Pregnancy and Childbearing Practices

FERTILITY PRACTICES AND VIEWS TOWARD PREGNANCY

Birth outcomes among some regions of Appalachia are poorer than among middle-class white groups in rural, suburban, and urban populations. In one study comparing birth outcome among rural, rural-adjacent, and urban women, rural women had the worst birth outcomes overall; rural-adjacent women had the best birth outcomes of the three groups, yet were the youngest, least educated, least likely to be married, and least likely to be privately insured (Hulme & Blegen, 1999). Contraceptive practices of Appalachians follow the general pattern of the U.S. population. Methods include birth control pills, condoms, and tubal ligation; abortion is an individual choice. A popular belief among many is that taking laxatives facilitates an abortion. A disproportionate number of teenage pregnancies occur at a younger age among Appalachians compared with non-Appalachians.

Fertility practices and sexual activity, both sensitive topics for many teenagers, are areas in which outsiders unknown to the family may be more effective than health-care practitioners who are known to the family. To be effective, counseling by the health-care provider must be accomplished within the cultural belief patterns of this group and must be approached in a nonhierarchical manner, preferably with a health-care provider of the same gender.

PRESCRIPTIVE, RESTRICTIVE, AND TABOO PRACTICES IN THE CHILDBEARING FAMILY

The literature reports no specific research or studies related to prescriptive, restrictive, or taboo practices during pregnancy. Pregnant women subscribe to the belief that to have a healthy baby they need to eat well and take care of themselves. Other beliefs include the following: Boys are carried higher and the mother's belly appears pointy, whereas girls are carried low. Picture taking can cause a stillbirth. Reaching over one's head can cause the cord to strangle the baby. Wearing an opal ring during pregnancy may harm the baby. Being frightened by a snake or eating strawberries or citrus fruit can cause birthmarks. And if the mother experiences a tragedy, a congenital anomaly may occur. If the mother craves a particular food during her pregnancy, then she should eat that food or the baby will have a birthmark similar to the craved food. Childbearing is a family affair. The birthing mother is expected to accept childbirth as a short, intense, natural process that will bring her closer to the earth and must be endured.

The literature reports no specific studies on beliefs related to postpartum practices. When a new baby is born, relatives and extended family members gather to assist the new mother with household chores until she is able to complete them herself. Some newborns wear a band around the abdomen to prevent umbilical hernias and an **asafetida bag** around the neck to prevent or ward off contagious disease. The health-care professional providing pregnancy counseling to the Appalachian family needs to demonstrate an openness to discuss cultural differences.

Death Rituals

DEATH RITUALS AND EXPECTATIONS

When a death is expected, family and friends may stay through the night and prepare food for the event. Because death is such an important occasion in Appalachia, many factories give workers 3 days' funeral leave for deaths of extended family members. After a death, extended family and friends may spend the night with the deceased's immediate family to prevent loneliness.

Deaths in Ohio are frequently published in West Virginia newspapers with a notice that the individual will be returned to the mountains for burial. Funeral services serve an important social function and are usually simple in Appalachia. This is a time when extended family and friends come together for services that can last for 3 hours. The length of time for a service varies according to the age of the deceased. The service for an elderly person is usually longer than for a younger person. The body is displayed for hours, either in the home or at the church, so that all those who wish to view the body can do so. At the end of the service, all who wish to view the body again can, with the closest relative being the last to view the body. Funerals can be an interesting experience for outsiders unfamiliar with the specific religious service. Many Appalachian families go to funeral homes that specialize in personal services to the Appalachian culture. Urban Appalachian areas have funeral homes that specialize in long-distant transport for burial. These funeral homes are familiar with Appalachian customs and meet their culturally specific requirements.

The deceased is usually buried in his or her best clothes. Some individuals have a custom-made set of clothes in which to be buried and may even design their own funeral services. A common practice is to bury the deceased with personal possessions. At the funeral home, the person's favorite chair, a picture of the deceased, or other personal items may be displayed. Flowers are more important than donations to a charity. Cremation is an acceptable practice, and what to do with the ashes is a personal decision. After the funeral services are completed, elaborate meals are served either in the home or at the church. Services are accompanied by singing before, during, and after the service. Cemeteries throughout Appalachia show frequent visitations and give a sense of place and relationship to the land. Plots are carefully tended with displays of flowers, wreaths, and flags. Other beliefs regarding burial practices include placing graveyards on hillsides for fear that graves may be flooded out in low-lying areas. If the body is exhumed and reburied, it is believed that the person may not go to heaven.

RESPONSES TO DEATH AND GRIEF

Clergy help families through the grieving process by providing counseling and support to family members. Although it is reported that Appalachians are particularly good at working through the grieving process, this author believes that this is a false perception because of the high value placed on stoicism in the culture.

Spirituality

DOMINANT RELIGION AND USE OF PRAYER

The original inhabitants of Appalachia were mostly Protestant and Episcopalian. Central organization of churches was difficult in the wilderness; thus, people individualized their chosen church structure. Today the predominant religions in the Appalachian region are Baptist, Methodist, Presbyterian, Holiness, Pentecostal, and Episcopalian. There are a few Roman Catholics and Jehovah's Witnesses. Many different religious groups in Appalachia call themselves Baptists. These sects are quite diverse with important central beliefs. Most of these sects have a strong belief in autonomy at the local level. As a result, many divisions have occurred within and among churches to accommodate more personal beliefs and philosophies. Regardless of the denomination, most churches in the region stress fundamentalism in religious practices and use the King James version of the Bible.

Many small churches have lay preachers instead of trained ministers. Most believe that to be a preacher, a person must have a divine calling, not something one consciously chooses, and that a person needs to have been moved to this calling. Thus, a minister may or may not be a preacher. Many of the Baptist faiths believe that baptism must be done in a river, pond, or lake so that the body can be submerged. Another practice, feet washing, where men wash men's feet and women wash women's feet, demonstrates humility. Many fundamentalist churches segregate women and children on one side of the church and men on the other side. Some denominations believe in divine healing, and the region is full of examples to testify to its effectiveness.

Two or more weekly services are common, and revival meetings are customary. Revivals tend to be lively, allowing individuals to shout out when the spirit moves them. Some denominations speak in tongues and believe in visions. Stringed music is played in some churches.

Some freewill churches, for example, Holiness Church, preach against attending movies, ball games, and social functions where dancing occurs. Other sects believe in handling poisonous snakes, though this is rare; it is believed that the snake will not bite those who have faith. A few people get snake bites and usually heal themselves, but a few deaths occur each year after snake handling. Some ingest strychnine in small doses during religious services to increase sensory stimuli. This practice can precipitate convulsions if ingested in large enough amounts. Fire handling is still practiced by some groups, again with the belief that the hot coals will not burn those who have faith.

Prayer for many Appalachians is a primary source of strength. Prayer is personally designed around specific church and religious beliefs and practices, which vary widely throughout the region and between and among churches of similar faith. More religiously devout individuals pray daily whether or not they attend church formally. Religious beliefs are often of a more spiritual nature and not tied to the tenets of any singular faith. They are part of the harmony of the mountains and being at one with life. Churches in many parts of Appalachia serve as the social centers of the community.

MEANING OF LIFE AND INDIVIDUAL SOURCES OF STRENGTH

Meaning in life comes from the family and "living right," which is defined by each person and usually means living right with God and in the beliefs of a chosen church. Religion tends to be less focused on institutional rituals and ceremonies and consists more of personalized beliefs in God, Christ, and church. Because life in the mountainous regions can often be harsh, religious beliefs and faith make life worth living in a grim situation. The church provides a way of coping with the hurts, pains, and disappointments of a sometimes hostile environment and becomes a source for celebration and a social outlet.

Common themes that give Appalachians strength are family, traditionalism, personalism, self-reliance, religiosity, a worldview of being, and not having undue concern about things that one cannot control, such as nature and the future. Appalachians believe that rewards come in another life, where God repays one for kind deeds done on earth.

SPIRITUAL BELIEFS AND HEALTH-CARE PRACTICES

Within the context of *fatalism* comes the belief that what happens to the individual is largely a result of God's will. Appalachians may not seek health care until symptoms of illness are well advanced. This practice is described more thoroughly under "High-Risk Behaviors," discussed earlier in this chapter. Forming partnerships between health-care providers and faith-related organizations for health promotion and illness and disease prevention has strong potential for improving the health-status of Appalachians. Health-care practitioners who are aware of clients' religious practices and spirituality needs are in a better position to promote culturally competent health care and to incorporate nonharmful practices into clients' care plans. Practitioners must indicate an appreciation and respect for the dignity and spiritual beliefs of Appalachians without expressing negative comments about differing religious beliefs and practices.

Health-Care Practices

HEALTH-SEEKING BELIEFS AND BEHAVIORS

Beliefs that influence health-care practices for many Appalachians are derived from concepts such as family, fatalism, traditionalism, self-reliance, individualism, and the ethic of neutrality. Even though many Appalachians believe that much of health is due to God's will, the concept of self-reliance can foster good health practices through self-care. Many may not see formal biomedical health-care practitioners until self-medicating and folk remedies have been exhausted. Appalachians, compared with non-Appalachians, are less likely to use the emergency room or to have private physicians (Obermiller & Handy, 1994). For many, when they do seek formal health care, the condition has become severe, takes longer to treat, and has a less favorable outcome. The 10 steps in the pattern of health care, described earlier, illustrate this influence. Health information on the Appalachian client should be gathered in the context of broader family relationships and cordiality that precedes information sharing. Health-care providers must consider the family rather than the individual as the basic unit for treatment. Because direct approaches are frowned upon, health-care providers need to approach sensitive topics indirectly. Many Appalachians expect the health-care provider to establish an advocacy role and to understand and accept their cultural differences; thus, it is best to involve professionals from the same backgrounds, if they are available.

Obermiller and Oldendick (1994) surveyed a large sample of Northern Appalachians and asked what they thought was responsible for good health. Sixty-four percent stated that good health is due to self-care; 39 percent, family relationships; 36 percent, heredity; 26 percent, luck; 22 percent, God's will; and 6 percent, physicians. Seventy percent of those in the study believed that death is predetermined. Approaching clients' beliefs and health responses in a nonjudgmental manner avoids defensiveness and enhances respect for health-care providers. Recognizing and encouraging positive self-care activities can accomplish effective health-care education.

RESPONSIBILITY FOR HEALTH CARE

When Appalachians enter the biomedical health-care arena, many feel powerless regarding their own health, abdicate responsibility for their own care, expect that the physician will take over their care completely, have high expectations and unrealistic dependence on the health-care system, and abandon self-reliance activities (Counts & Boyle, 1987). In addition, emergency rooms and formal health-care organizations are perceived as impersonal, sometimes drastic, and frequently ineffective.

A major health concern for many Appalachians is the state of the **blood**, which is described as being thick or thin, good or bad, and **high** or **low**; these conditions can be regulated through diet (Tripp-Reimer & Freidl, 1977). Venereal disease and Rh-negative blood fall into the category of bad blood. Sour foods can also cause bad blood. Appalachian men report a greater number of backaches, and women report a greater number of headaches, than the rest of society (Horton, 1984).

The primary focus on health for many Appalachians is self-care. Self-care is primarily perceived as an individual responsibility, and care is focused within the family rather than within the community. Because many Appa-

lachians value the ability to respond to, and cope with, events of daily life, many home remedies, treatments, and active consultation with family members are sought before seeking outside help (Counts & Boyle, 1987). Good health is feeling well and being able to meet one's obligations. Care within the medical system is used when the condition is perceived as serious, does not respond to self-care, or has a high potential for death. Furthermore, because self-reliance activities and nature predominate over people, many believe that it is best to let nature heal. Health-care providers should give explanations and instructions within the context of the Appalachian culture to make them more acceptable to clients and families. When elderly Appalachians go to a physician, many expect immediate help. Physicians who dispense medications in their offices are seen as helpful. If physicians give prescriptions to the individuals, this may be interpreted as rejection. If the health-care provider gives a tube of ointment for the client to apply, it is not seen as helpful. However, if the health-care provider applies the ointment, it is seen as helpful.

Health-care providers can assist Appalachian clients by reinforcing their preferred coping methods and strategies when they are ill. The five most frequently used coping methods are helping, thinking positively, worrying about the problem, trying to find out more about the problem, and trying to handle things one step at a time. The five most effective coping strategies were talking the problem over with friends, praying, thinking about the good things in life, trying to handle things one step at a time, and trying to see the good side of the situation (Hunsucker, Flannery, & Frank, 2000). Using churches, grange halls, and meeting places for the entire family is an effective way of working with Appalachians at the community level.

FOLK PRACTICES

A strong belief in folk medicine is a traditional part of the Appalachian culture. Using herbal medicines, poultices, and teas is common practice among individuals of all socioeconomic levels. Table 5–1 presents a reference guide for the health-care practitioner with the major ingredients and conditions for which the folk treatments are used. These treatments can be adjusted to accommodate prescription therapies or education regarding folk treatments. Information in this table has been derived from the *Foxfire* series, the author's background and experience, and health-care professionals at a cultural diversity conference in northern Appalachia. Note that specific amounts are not given, and in many cases the amounts vary from person to person, according to the geographic region and local family practices. Local names are given rather than scientific names because this is how the residents identify them. Many folk and traditional practices were learned from the Cherokee and Apalachee Indians living in the region, and have been passed down from generation to generation. Although many of these home remedies are not harmful, some may have a deleterious effect when used to the exclusion of, or in combination with, prescription medications. This should be evident from the 10-step

Table 5–1 Health Conditions and Appalachian Folk Medicine Practices

Health Condition	Folk Medicine Practices
Arthritis	Make tea from boiling the roots of ginseng. Drink the tea or rub it on the arthritic joint.
	Mix roots of ginseng and goldenseal in liquor and drink it. Ginseng is used heavily by many Koreans and was exported to Korea in the 18th and 19th centuries.
	Eat large amounts of raw fruits and vegetables.
	Carry a buckeye around in your pocket.
	Drink tea from the stems of the barbell plant.
	Drink a mixture of honey, vinegar, and moonshine (or other liquor).
	Drink tea made from alfalfa seeds or leaves.
	Drink tea made from rhubarb and whiskey.
	Place a magnet over the joint to draw the arthritis out of the joint.
Asthma	Drink tea from the bark of wild yellow plum trees, mullein leaves, and alum. Take every 12 hrs.
	Combine gin and heartwood of a pine tree. Take twice a day.
	Suck salty water up your nose.
	Smoke or sniff rabbit tobacco.
	Swallow a handful of spiderwebs.
	Smoke strong tobacco until you choke.
	Drink a mixture of honey, lemon juice, and whiskey.
	Inhale smoke from ginseng leaves.
Bedbugs/chiggers	Apply kerosene liberally to all parts of the body. *Caution:* Kerosene can cause significant irritation to sensitive skin, especially when exposed to sunlight.
Bleeding	Place a spiderweb across the wound. This is also used in rural Scotland.
	Put kerosene oil on the cut.
	Place soot from the fireplace into a cut. Be sure to wash out the soot after bleeding is stopped or the area will scar.
	Apply a mixture of honey and turpentine on the bleeding wound.
	Apply a mixture of soot and lard on the wound.
	Place a cigarette paper over the wound.
	Put pine resin over the cut.
	Place kerosene oil on the wound. *Caution:* If used in large doses, kerosene will burn the skin.
High blood pressure (not to be mistaken for high blood)	Drink sasparilla tea.
	Drink a half cup of vinegar.
Blood builders	Drink tea from the bark of a wild cherry tree.
	Combine cherry bark, yellowroot, and whiskey. Take twice each day.
	Eat fried pokeweed leaves.
Blood purifiers	Drink tea from burdock root.
	Drink tea from spice wood.
Blood tonic	Take a teaspoonful of honey and a tiny amount of sulfur.
	Take a teaspoon of molasses and a tiny amount of sulfur.
	Drink tea made from bloodroot.
	Soak nails in a can of water until they become rusty. Drink the rusty water.
Boils or sores	Apply a poultice of walnut leaves or the green hulls with salt.
	Apply a poultice of the houseleek plant.
	Apply a poultice of rotten apples.
	Apply a poultice of beeswax, mutton tallow, sweet oil, oil of amber, oil of spike, and resin.
	Apply a poultice of kerosene, turpentine, Vaseline, and lye soap.
	Apply a poultice of heart leaves, lard, and turpentine.
	Apply a poultice of bread and milk.
	Apply a poultice of slippery elm and pork fat.
	Apply a poultice of flaxseed meal.
	Apply a poultice of beef tallow, brown sugar, salt, and turpentine.

Table 5–1 Health Conditions and Appalachian Folk Medicine Practices (Continued)

Health Condition	Folk Medicine Practices
Burns	Apply a poultice of baking soda and water.
	Place castor oil on the burn.
	Apply a poultice of egg white and castor oil.
	Place a potato on the burn.
	Wrap the burn in a gauze and keep moist with salt water.
	Place linseed oil on the burn.
	Apply a poultice of lard and flour.
	Put axle grease on the burn. This is also a practice with some Germans in Minnesota.
Chapped hands and lips	Apply lard, grease, or tallow from pork or mutton.
Chest congestion	Apply poultice to the chest made of kerosene, turpentine, and lard. Make sure the poultice is not applied directly to the chest but rather on top of a cloth.
	Apply mutton tallow directly to the chest.
	Apply a warm poultice of onions and grease.
	Rub pine tar on the chest.
	Chew leaves and stems of peppermint.
	Drink a combination of ginger and sugar in hot water.
	Make a mixture of rock candy and whiskey. Take several teaspoons several times each day.
	Drink tea made from ginger, honey, and whiskey.
	Drink tea made from pine needles.
	Put goose grease on your chest.
	Drink red pepper tea.
	Eat roasted onions.
	Drink brine from pickles or kraut.
	Make tea from boneset, rosemary, and goldenrod.
	Make tea from the butterfly weed.
Colic	Make tea from calamus root and catnip. (Calamus is a suspected carcinogen.)
	Tie an asafetida bag around the neck.
	Drink baking soda and water.
	Chew and swallow the juice of camel root.
	Massage stomach with warm castor oil.
	Drink ginseng tea.
Constipation	Take two tablespoons of turpentine.
	Combine castor oil and mayapple roots.
	Take castor oil or Epsom salts.
Croup	Have child wear a bib containing pine pitch and tallow.
	Apply cloth to the chest saturated with groundhog fat, turpentine, and lamp oil.
	Drink juice from a roasted onion.
	Apply to the back a poultice made from mutton tallow and beeswax.
	Eat a spoonful of sugar with a drop of turpentine.
	Eat honey with lemon or vinegar.
	Eat onion juice and honey.
Diarrhea	Drink water from boiling the ladyslipper plant.
	Place soot in a glass of water, let the soot settle to the bottom of the glass, and drink the water.
	Drink tea made from blackberry roots.
	Drink tea from red oak bark.
	Drink blackberry or strawberry juice.
	Drink tea made from strawberry or blackberry leaves.
	Drink tea made out of willow leaves.
	Drink the juice from the bark of a white oak tree or a persimmon tree.
Earache	Place lukewarm salt water in the ear.
	Put castor oil or sweet oil in the ear.
	Put sewing machine oil in the ear.

(Continued on following page)

Table 5–1 Health Conditions and Appalachian Folk Medicine Practices (Continued)

Health Condition	Folk Medicine Practices
Earache	Place a few drops of urine in the ear.
	Place cabbage juice in the ear.
	Blow smoke from tobacco in the ear.
	Place a Vicks-soaked cotton ball in the ear.
Eye ailments	Place a few drops of castor oil in the eye.
	Drop warm salty water in the eye.
	Drink tea made from rabbit tobacco or snakeroot.
Fever	Drink tea made from the butterfly weed, wild horsemint, or feverweed.
	Mash garlic bulbs and place in a bag tied around the pulse points.
	Drink water from wild ginger.
Headache	Drink tea made of ladyslipper plants.
	Tie warm fried potatoes around your head.
	Take Epsom salts.
	Tie ginseng roots around your head.
	Place crushed onions on your head.
	Rub camphor and whiskey on your head.
Heart trouble	Drink tea made from heartleaf leaves or bleeding heart.
	Eat garlic.
Kidney trouble	Drink tea made from peach leaves or mullein roots.
	Drink tea made from corn silk or arbutus leaves.
Liver trouble	Drink tea made from lion's tongue leaves.
	Drink tea made from the roots of the spinet plant.
Poison Ivy	Urinate on the affected area.
	Take a bath in salt water and then apply Vaseline.
	Wash the area with bleach.
	Wash the area with the juice of the milkweed plant.
	Apply a poultice of gunpowder and buttermilk.
	Apply baking soda to wet skin.
Sore throat	Gargle with sap from a red oak tree.
	Eat honey and molasses.
	Eat honey and onions.
	Drink honey and whiskey.
	Tie a poultice of lard of cream with turpentine and Vicks to your neck.
	Apply a poultice of cottonseed to your throat.
	Swab your throat with turpentine.

pattern health-seeking behaviors among Appalachians presented in the section on health-care practices.

Because ingredients in some of these herbal medicines can have serious side effects, especially if taken in large quantities, health-care providers must become familiar with folk medicines used by Appalachians as part of client assessments. Health-care providers must ascertain if individuals intend to use folk medicines simultaneously with prescription medications and treatment regimens so that these remedies can be incorporated into the plan of care so that dialogue can be undertaken to prevent adverse effects. Health-care providers who integrate folk medicine into allopathic prescriptions have a greater chance of improving clients' compliance with health prescriptions and interventions. Health-care providers must remember that today's scientific medicine may be traditional or folk medicine to the next generation.

BARRIERS TO HEALTH CARE

Barriers to health care for Appalachians are numerous, and center on accessibility, affordability, adaptability, acceptability, appropriateness, and awareness. Bureaucratic forms foster fear and suspicion of health-care providers, which can lead to confusion, distrust, and negative stereotyping by both parties. Some individuals fear "being cut on" or "going under the knife" and feel that a hospital is a place where you go to give birth or die.

The rugged terrain and distance to health-care facilities, especially specialty services, is a deterrent to accessing services when there is no public transportation system. Even though the ARC has sponsored road-building campaigns in the mountainous regions of Appalachia since 1965, transportation problems continue to exist in parts of the region (see Fig. 5–1). The high rate of unem-

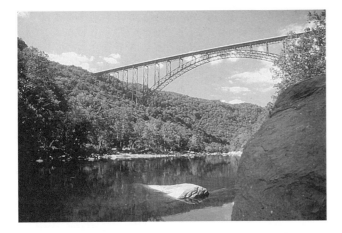

FIGURE 5–1 Before the construction of the New River Gorge bridge, many people were isolated from health care. (Courtesy of West Virginia Division of Tourism and Parks.)

ployment in Appalachia means that many people cannot afford basic health care. A disproportionate number of Appalachians, especially those who are self-employed, unemployed, or underemployed do not have health insurance. For some who do not believe in owing money, seeing a health-care provider may be postponed until the condition is severe. If services can be offered on a sliding scale, more people may be willing to access the services. Offering transportation on a regular schedule and by appointment may improve access. Health-care facilities are closing in some areas related to decreasing employment opportunities necessitating people moving from the area and the national trend for downsizing. These changes have necessitated that some individuals relocate, and make it more difficult for those people remaining to obtain needed services.

A shortage of health-care providers frequently means that the care is not even available locally. Because the physician shortage in Appalachia has been greater than the nurse shortage, nurses have historically delivered most primary care. When physicians are sought in outlying rural areas, they make their fee payment schedules more flexible, they dispense drugs, and they give injections in their offices. For many, a "being" orientation blocks prevention and enhances a crisis orientation. Prevention services have not been stressed in the past and are not perceived as important by many.

Even when services are available, people may not feel they are delivered in an appropriate manner. Outsiders may be seen as disrespectful of Appalachian ways and self-care practices. Patients may be especially sensitive to criticism. If the provider uses language that the patient does not understand, the provider may be perceived as "stuck up." Many Appalachians do not like the impersonal care delivered in clinics and therefore shop around for a private health-care provider whom they feel meets their personal needs. "Sittin' for a spell and engagin' in small talk" with the patient before an examination or treatment will help assure return visits for follow-up care.

When health-care facilities have limited hours or are not adaptable, patients may not return for scheduled appointments. For example, a mother may bring her child in for an immunization. If the mother has a health problem and perhaps needs a Pap smear, she may be willing to have the test performed. However, if she is given an appointment to return at a later date, she may not keep the appointment because it is too far to travel for a nonurgent problem. If services are not available during evening hours, people may be afraid of taking time off during regular work hours to access services for fear of losing their job.

CULTURAL RESPONSES TO HEALTH AND ILLNESSES

Appalachians generally take care of their own; their view is to accept the person as a "whole individual." Thus, those with mental impairments or physical handicaps are readily accepted and not turned away. The mentally handicapped are not crazy, but rather have "bad nerves," they are "quite turned," or "odd turned." Appalachians may label certain behaviors as "lazy," "mean," "immoral," "criminal," or "psychic" and recommend punishment by either the social group or the legal system, or tolerance of these behaviors (Flaskerud, 1980).

Traditional Appalachians believe that disability is a natural and inevitable part of the aging process. Their culture of being discourages the use of rehabilitation as an option. To establish trust and rapport when working with Appalachian clients with chronic diseases, health-care providers must avoid assumptions regarding health beliefs and provide health maintenance interventions within the scope of cultural customs and beliefs.

Individual responses to pain cannot be classified among Appalachians. The Appalachian background is too varied, and no studies regarding cultural beliefs about pain could be found in the literature. For many Appalachians, pain is something that is to be endured and accepted stoically. However, when a person becomes ill or has pain, personal space collapses inward, and the person expects to be waited on and to be cared for by others. A belief among many is that if one places a knife or axe under the bed or mattress of a person in pain, the knife will help cut the pain. This practice occurs with childbearing and other conditions that cause pain. The author is aware of an Appalachian woman who requested to have a knife or axe placed under the bed or mattress postoperatively to help cut (or decrease) the pain associated with surgery. The author offered a small pocketknife or butter knife to place under the bed. Both were unacceptable; the pocketknife was too small and the butter knife was too dull to be of any use. A sharp meat-cutting knife from the dietary department was deemed appropriate because it was both large enough and sharp enough to help cut the pain.

BLOOD TRANSFUSIONS AND ORGAN DONATION

Appalachians generally do not have any specific rules or taboos about receiving blood, donating organs, or undergoing organ transplantation. These decisions are largely one's own, but advice is usually sought from family and friends.

Health-Care Practitioners

TRADITIONAL VERSUS BIOMEDICAL PRACTITIONERS

For decades, both lay and trained nurses have provided significant health-care services, including obstetrics, in this mountainous region. Grannies and trained midwives have provided obstetric services throughout the history of the region. Folk practitioners are primarily older women, but may be men. Grannies and herb doctors are trusted and known to the individual and the community for giving more personalized care.

The entire Appalachian area has a shortage of health personnel, especially a shortage of physicians. As a result, nurses have delivered the bulk of health care in some areas of Appalachia. The physician shortage today is not as severe as it was 10 years ago (Myers, Russell, & Baldwin, 1999).

The Frontier Nursing Service, started by Mary Breckenridge, is one of the oldest and most well-known nurse-run clinics in the United States, and is a notable example of nurses taking the initiative to provide health care in Appalachia. It was started in one of the most rural areas of Appalachia in response to a lack of physicians and the high birth and child mortality rates in the area. Many Appalachians prefer to go to *insider* health-care professionals, especially in the more rural areas, because the system of payment for services is accepted on a sliding scale and, in some communities, even an exchange of goods for health services exists. One nurse-practitioner in private practice states that the only time she locks her car is when the zucchini are "in." If she does not, when she gets in her car after a clinic session, she has no room to drive because of all the "presents" of the large vegetable.

Locally respected Appalachians are engaged to facilitate acceptance of outside programs and of the staff who participate at the grassroots level in planning and initiating programs. For Appalachian clients to become more accepting of biomedical care, it is important for health-care providers to approach individuals in an unhurried manner consistent with their relaxed lifestyle, to engage clients in decision making and care planning, and to use locally trained support staff whenever possible.

STATUS OF HEALTH-CARE PROVIDERS

Most herbal and folk practitioners are highly respected for their treatments, mostly because they are well known to their people and trusted by those who need health care. Physicians and other health-care professionals are frequently seen as outsiders to the Appalachian population and are therefore mistrusted. This initial mistrust is rooted in outsider behaviors that exploited the Appalachian people and took their land for timbering and coal mining in earlier generations. Trust for an outsider is gained slowly. Once the person gets to know and trust the health-care provider, the provider is given much respect. Trust and respect for health-care providers depend more on personal characteristics and personal behavior than on knowledge.

Appalachians prefer home-based nurses, health-care workers, and social workers. To obtain full cooperation, the health-care provider needs to ask clients what they consider to be the problem before devising a plan of care; otherwise, the clients may resent the health-care provider. It is equally important to decrease language barriers by decoding the jargon of the health-care environment.

CASE STUDY Leona Sperry, age 74, lost her husband, a preacher, to emphysema two months ago. Since that time she has been living alone on a limited income from her husband's Social Security. Mrs. Sperry states that she has lived in the same West Virginia community all of her life, just like her parents and grandparents. She is known in the community as Miss Leona, and is respected for her knowledge of folk medicine and "deliverin' babies," which she has done as long as she can remember, just like her mother and grandmother. All but one of her nine children live within 50 miles. Miss Leona does her own cooking, bakes biscuits and bread twice a week, and makes large pots of meat stew so she does not have to cook every day. A farmer neighbor supplies her with milk, eggs, and meat in trade for using the land from her small farm to pasture his cattle. Even though she only went to the third grade, she enjoys reading stories in the *Reader's Digest*, which she keeps on her bedside table. She also enjoys talking on the telephone with her children and sister, who lives about 5 miles away. Miss Leona lives on top of a hill and has to cross a footbridge to get to her home. Her driveway ends at the footbridge, requiring her to carry her groceries up a steep incline with many steps. Sometimes a neighbor or the postman delivers her groceries when her children are unable to bring them to her.

Miss Leona's granddaughter, a nurse who lives out of the area, called the Visiting Nurse Association and requested that someone see her grandmother. Miss Leona tells the visiting nurse that she has had arthritis in her hands, hips, and knees for many years. She has also suffered from "low blood" all her life. Now she has other health problems as well, and some chest congestion, which is not responding to her usual treatment. Her most recent health concern, she says, is "heart problems," which her physician, Dr. Adi, tells her is from her high-fat diet. However, Miss Leona believes her heart problems were brought on by her husband's death because she did not have them until after he died. Her physician also gave her a jar of salve to put on a leg wound caused by an insect bite, which became infected when she scratched it in her sleep.

On her last visit to her physician a month ago, he referred her to a heart specialist at a medical center 50 miles from her home. He also wanted her to make an appointment with an arthritis specialist. So far, she has not made an appointment with either specialist because she does not know when one of her children will be available to take her to the medical center. Besides, she says her children have their own families and jobs and she does not like to bother them with her problems. In addition, she tells you that she is looking forward to her 16-year-old granddaughter, who is 3 months pregnant, coming to live with her in a couple of months. After all, she misses being a midwife.

She admits not using the salve given to her by Dr. Adi because he told her to apply the salve according to the instructions on the jar. She has been drinking the brine from her home-canned pickles for her "low blood," drinking ginseng tea for her arthritis, and applying a poultice made from bacon grease on the leg wound. She tells you that she does not want to return to Dr. Adi because she cannot understand him, he does not listen to her, and he did not help her when she last saw him. She explains that she is a good "Christianwoman," has lived right all her life, and does not interfere with her neighbors' lives. She rarely misses Sunday church services because all her neighbors go to the same Baptist church and she "allus" has plenty of volunteers to carry (take) her to the church.

STUDY QUESTIONS

1 Why do the members of her community call Mrs. Sperry by the name Miss Leona?

2 What can the nurse do to assist Miss Leona to decrease the barriers to needed health care?

3 What might Dr. Adi do to ensure a more trusting relationship with Miss Leona?

4 What historical precedence is there for distrust of "outsiders" in Appalachia?

5 What evidence do you see of the "ethic of neutrality" in this case study?

6 What is the difference between a minister and a preacher as practiced by Baptists in Appalachia?

7 What do Appalachians mean by the term "low blood"? What are some folk treatments for this condition?

8 What advice would you give Miss Leona about her folk remedies?

9 What might you do to encourage Miss Leona to make appointments with the specialists recommended by Dr. Adi?

10 How might you help Miss Leona eat a more nutritious diet?

11 What strategies might you encourage for Miss Leona to cope with her "heart problems" that began after her husband died?

12 What kind of prenatal advice would you give the granddaughter when she comes to live with Miss Leona?

REFERENCES

Appalachian Regional Commission. (2001). Available at http://www.arc.gov.

Barnett, D., Bauer, A., Baker, B., Ehrhardt, K. E., & Stoller, S. (1994). A case for naturalistic assessment and intervention in an urban Appalachian community. In K. M. Borman & P. J. Obermiller (Eds.), *From mountain to metropolis: Appalachian migrants in American cities* (pp. 94–104). Westport, CT: Greenwood Publishing Group.

Centers for Disease Control. (2001). http://www.cdc.gov.

Costello, C. (2000, May 30). Beneath myth, Melungeons find roots of oppression: Appalachian descendants embrace heritage. *The Washington Post*, p. A4.

Counts, M. M., & Boyle, J. S. (1987). Nursing, health, and policy within a community context. *Advances in Nursing Science, 9*(3), 12–23.

Flaskerud, J. H. (1980). Perceptions of problematic behavior by Appalachians, mental health professionals and lay non-Appalachians. *Nursing Research, 29*(3), 140–149.

Hansen, M. M., & Resick, L. K. (1990). Health beliefs, health care, and rural Appalachian subcultures from an ethnographic perspective. *Family and Community Health, 13*(1), 1–10.

Hulme, P., & Blegen, M. (1999). Residential status and birth outcomes: Is the rural/urban distinction adequate? *Public Health Nursing, 16*(3), 176–181.

Hunsucker, S., Flannery, J., & Frank, D. (2000). Coping strategies of rural families of critically ill patients. *Journal of the American Academy of Nurse Practitioners, 12*(4), 123–127.

Horton, C. F. (1984). Women have headaches, men have backaches: Patterns of illness in an Appalachian community. *Social Science Medicine, 19*(6), 647–654.

McCoy, J., Davis, M., & Hudson, R. (1994). Geographic patterns of disability in the United States. *Social Security Bulletin, 57*(1), 25–26.

Myers, W., Russell, J., & Baldwin, F. (1999). A conversation on rural health care. *Appalachia, 32*(2), 16–21.

National Institutes of Health. (1995). Appalachian initiative lowers breast cancer. NIH Publication No. 95-3999. Washington, DC.

Obermiller, P., & Handy, J. (1994). Health education strategies for urban blacks and Appalachians. In K. Borman & P. Obermiller (Eds.), *From mountain to metropolis: Appalachian migrants in American cities* (pp. 61–71). Westport, CT: Greenwood Publishing Group.

Obermiller, P., & Oldendick, R. (1994). Urban Appalachian health concerns. In K. Borman & P. Obermiller (Eds.), *From mountain to metropolis: Appalachian migrants in American cities* (pp. 51–60). Westport, CT: Greenwood Publishing Group.

Ramsey, P., & Glenn, L. (1998). Risk factors for heart disease in rural Appalachia. *Family and Community Health 20*(4), 71–82.

Tripp-Reimer, T. (1982). Barriers to health care: Variations in interpretation of Appalachian client behavior by Appalachian and non-Appalachian professionals. *Western Journal of Nursing Research, 4*(2), 179–191.

Tripp-Reimer, T. and Freidl, M. C. (1977). Appalachians: A neglected minority. *Nursing Clinics of North America, 12*(1), 41–54.

Voices of Appalachia Health Start Project. (2001). Whitley County Public Health Department. Available at http://www.wcphd.com.

Wilson, C. M. (1989). Elizabethan America. In W. K. Neil (Ed.), *Appalachian images in folk and popular cultures* (pp. 205–216). London: UMI Press.

Chapter 6

People of Arab Heritage

ANAHID DERVARTANIAN KULWICKI

Overview, Inhabited Localities, and Topography

OVERVIEW

Arabs trace their ancestry and traditions to the nomadic desert tribes of the Arabian Peninsula. They share a common language, **Arabic**, and most are united by **Islam**, a major world religion that originated in seventh-century Arabia. Despite these common bonds, even Arab residents of a single Arab country are characterized by diversity in thought, attitude, and behavior. Country of origin, degree of development and urbanization, rural versus urban upbringing, education, social class, and religion shape the Arab, influencing thinking, attitudes, and behaviors. Indeed, a poor tradition-bound farmer from rural Yemen may appear to have little in common with an educated professional from cosmopolitan Beirut. Additional factors such as refugee status, time since arrival, **ethnic identity**, disparity between cultures, economic status, employment status, social support, and English language skills influence the immigration experience and the Arab American's adjustment to life in America.

The September 11, 2001, al Qaeda terrorist attack on the United States has increased negative comments about Arabs by some people. Health-care providers need to understand that few Arab Americans support the terrorist attacks and they must not pigeonhole people by their cultural background.

The diversity among Arabs makes presenting a representative account of Arab Americans a formidable task. Three related difficulties include author bias; data based on subgroups of Arabs and Arab Americans; and a limited amount of literature describing Arab Americans. Zogby

(1990) attributed this scarcity to the Arab American community's "invisibility." The earliest Arab immigrants arrived as part of the great wave of immigrants at the end of the 19th century and beginning of the 20th century. They were predominantly Christians from the region that is present-day Lebanon and Syria, and like most newcomers of the period, they valued assimilation and were rather easily absorbed into mainstream U.S. society. Arab Americans tend to disappear in national studies because they are counted as white in census data, rather than as a separate ethnic group. Therefore, to portray Arab Americans as fully as possible, including the large numbers of new arrivals since 1965, literature that describes Arabs is used to supplement research completed by groups studying Arab Americans residing in Michigan and the San Francisco Bay area of California. An underlying assumption is that the attitudes and behaviors of first-generation immigrants are similar in some aspects to those of their counterparts in the Arab world.

Islamic doctrines and practices are included because most post-1965 Arab American immigrants are **Muslims**. Religion, whether official Islam, Christianity, or a local folk variant, is an integral part of everyday Arab life. Historically Christians, Muslims, and Jews share a common religious background, and the three prophets are descendants from the same father, Abraham. Moses, the messenger of Judaism, and Jesus, the messenger of Christianity, are believed to be descendants of Isaac; whereas, Mohammed, the messenger of Islam, is believed to be a descendant of Abraham's eldest son, Ishmael. Moreover, because Arabism and Islam are so intrinsically interwoven and because Islam has some elements of Christianity, Arabs, whether Christian or Muslim, share some basic traditions and beliefs. Consequently, knowledge of religion is critical to understanding the Arab American client's cultural frame of reference and for providing care that considers specific religious beliefs and practices of devout Arab Muslim clients.

HERITAGE AND RESIDENCE

Arab Americans are defined as immigrants from the 22 Arab countries of North Africa and Southwest Asia: Algeria, Bahrain, Comoros, Djibouti, Egypt, Iraq, Jordan, Kuwait, Lebanon, Libya, Mauritania, Morocco, Oman, Palestine, Qatar, Saudi Arabia, Somalia, Sudan, Syria, Tunisia, United Arab Emirates, Yemen. In 1994, the Arab American Institute estimated that there were 3 million Arab Americans, though this number is undoubtedly greater today. Arab immigration has been described as occurring in two waves (Zogby, 1990), which are distinct with respect to immigrants' characteristics. First-wave immigrants and their descendants typically reside in urban centers of the Northeast: New York; Washington, D.C.; Boston; Bergen-Passaic counties, New Jersey; Pittsburgh; Philadelphia; and Nassau-Suffolk counties, New York. Second-wave Arab American immigrants have settled in cities in the Midwest and West; they outnumber U.S.-born Arab Americans in Illinois (Chicago) and California. Detroit-Dearborn, Michigan, is one of the two largest, and perhaps most visible, Arab American communities (Zogby, 1990). Houston, Texas, and Cleveland, Ohio, are also among the top 10 cities for Arab Americans (El-Badry, 1994).

REASONS FOR MIGRATION AND ASSOCIATED ECONOMIC FACTORS

First-wave immigrants came to the United States between 1887 and 1913 seeking economic opportunity and perhaps the financial means to return home and buy land or set up shop in their ancestral villages. While most of these first Arab Americans engaged in pack peddling, others worked in the textile, steel, and auto industries (Vincent-Barwood, 1986). Most of the immigrants were male, illiterate (44 percent), and unskilled mountain or rural immigrants who became successful peddlers (Naff, 1980). About half of today's Arab Americans were from Greater Syria, now known as Lebanon and Syria, and most were Christian.

Second-wave immigrants entered the United States after World War II; the numbers increased dramatically after the Palestinian-Israeli conflict erupted and the passage of the Immigration Act of 1965 (Naff, 1980). Unlike the more economically motivated Lebanese-Syrian Christians, most second-wave immigrants are refugees from nations beset by war and political instability—chiefly, occupied Palestine, Jordan, Iraq, Yemen, Lebanon, and Syria. Included in this group are a large number of professionals and individuals seeking educational degrees who have subsequently remained in the United States. Most are Muslims with a political consciousness and sense of ethnic identity unknown to first-wave immigrants (Zogby, 1990). Second-wave Arab immigrants are younger at the time of arrival; 47 percent are under age 25 years, while a small percentage (5.9 percent) are age 65 years or older. Almost half (46.5 percent) of Arab Americans age 18 and older speak a language other than English (Zogby, 1990).

EDUCATIONAL STATUS AND OCCUPATIONS

Because Arabs favor professional occupations, education, as a prerequisite to white-collar work, is valued. Not surprisingly, both U.S.- and foreign-born Arab Americans are more educated than the average American (Zogby, 1990). Michigan's Arab Americans fare better in terms of socioeconomic status than African Americans, Latinos, and Native Americans. One-fourth of Michigan's Arab population age 25 years and older hold a university degree (Office of Minority Health [OMH], 2001). In contrast, literacy rates among adults in the Arab world vary from 44 percent in Yemen to 88 percent in Lebanon and Jordan. Literacy rates among women also vary, ranging from 23.7 percent in Yemen to 84 percent in Lebanon where women often earn university degrees (Arab Human Development Report, 2000).

In comparison with Americans, Arab Americans are more likely to be self-employed and much more likely to be in managerial and professional specialty occupations (Zogby, 1990). Nearly 25 percent are involved in retail trade. Conversely, Arab Americans are less likely to be involved in farming, forestry, fishing, precision production, crafts, or work as operators and fabricators.

Arab Americans have the highest mean income when compared to other ethnic groups in the United States. Despite the affluence of Arab Americans as a group, their poverty rate is substantially higher than the American national average because of the differences between U.S.- and foreign-born Arab Americans. Whereas U.S.-born Arab Americans tend to be employed and prosperous, foreign-born Arab Americans are more likely to be unemployed and poor (Zogby, 1990).

Communication

DOMINANT LANGUAGE AND DIALECTS

Arabic is the official language of the Arab world. Modern or classical Arabic is a universal form of Arabic used for all writing and formal situations ranging from radio newscasts to lectures. Dialectal or colloquial Arabic, of which each community has a variety, is used for everyday spoken communication. Arabs often mix Modern Standard Arabic and colloquial Arabic according to the complexity of the subject and the formality of the occasion. The presence of numerous dialects with differences in accent, inflection, and vocabulary may create difficulties in communication between Arab immigrants from Syria and Lebanon and Arab immigrants from Iraq and Yemen.

The Arab person's speech is likely to be characterized by repetition and gesturing, particularly when involved in serious discussions. Arabs may be loud and expressive when involved in serious discussions to stress their commitment and their sincerity in the subject matter. Observers witnessing such impassioned communication may assume that Arabs are argumentative, confrontational, or aggressive.

English is a common second language in Egypt, Jordan, Lebanon, Yemen, Bahrain, and Kuwait. Despite this, and the finding that 83.7 percent of Arab-born U.S. Census respondents report speaking English "well" (Zogby, 1990), there is ample evidence that language and communication pose formidable problems in American health-care settings. For example, Kulwicki and Miller (1999) report that 66 percent of respondents using a community-based health clinic spoke Arabic at home and only 30.2 percent spoke both English and Arabic. Even English-speaking Arab Americans report difficulty in expressing their needs and understanding health-care providers.

Health-care providers have cited numerous interpersonal and communication problems, including erroneous assessments of patient complaints, delayed or failed appointments, reluctance to disclose personal and family health information, and in some cases, noncompliance with medical treatments (Kulwicki, 1996; Kulwicki, Miller, & Schim, 2000) and a tendency to exaggerate when describing complaints (Sullivan, 1993).

CULTURAL COMMUNICATION PATTERNS

Arab communication has been described as highly nuanced, with more communication contained in the context of the situation than in the actual words spoken. Arabs value privacy and resist disclosure of personal information to strangers, especially, when it relates to familial disease conditions. Conversely, among friends and relatives, Arabs express feelings freely. These patterns of communication become more comprehensible when interpreted within the Arab cultural frame of reference. Many personal needs may be anticipated without the individual having to verbalize them because of close family relationships. The family may rely more on unspoken expectations and nonverbal cues than overt verbal exchange.

Arabs need to develop personal relationships with a health-care provider before sharing personal information. Because meaning may be attached to both compliments and indifference, manner and tone are as important as what is said. Arabs are sensitive to the courtesy and respect they are accorded, and good manners are important in evaluating a person's character. Therefore greetings, inquiries about well-being, pleasantries, and a cup of tea or coffee precede business. Conversants stand close together, maintain steady eye contact, and touch (only between members of the same sex) the other's hand or shoulder. Sitting and standing properly is critical; to do otherwise is taken as a lack of respect. Within the context of personal relationships, verbal agreements are considered more important than written contracts. Keeping promises is considered a matter of honor.

Substantial efforts are directed at maintaining pleasant relationships and preserving dignity and honor. Hostility in response to perceived wrongdoing is warded off by an attitude of **maalesh**, "never mind, it doesn't matter." Individuals are protected from bad news for as long as possible and are then informed as gently as possible.

When disputes arise, Arabs hint at their disagreement or simply fail to follow through. Alternatively, an intermediary, someone with influence, may be used to intervene in disputes or present requests to the person in charge. Mediation saves face if a conflict is not settled in one's favor and reassures the petitioner that maximum influence has been employed (Nydell, 1987).

Guidelines for communicating with Arab Americans include the following:

1 Employ an approach that combines expertise with warmth. Minimize status differences, as Arab Americans report feeling uncomfortable and self-conscious in the presence of authority figures. Pay special attention to the person's feelings. Arab Americans perceive themselves as sensitive, with the potential for being easily hurt, belittled, and slighted (Reizian & Meleis, 1987).

2 Take time to get acquainted before delving into business. If sincere interest in the person's home country and adjustment to American life is expressed, he or she is likely to enjoy relating such information, much of which is essential to assessing risk for traumatic immigration experience (see "Barriers to Health Care") and understanding the person's cultural frame of reference. Sharing a cup of tea does much to give an initial visit a positive beginning (Kulwicki, 1996; Lipson & Meleis, 1985).

3 Nurses may need to clarify role responsibilities regarding history taking, performing physical examinations, and providing health information for newer immigrants. Although recent Arab American immigrants may now recognize the higher status of nurses in the United States, they are still accustomed to nurses' functioning as medical assistants and housekeepers (see "Status of Health-Care Providers").

4 Perform a comprehensive assessment. Explain the relationship of the information needed for physical complaints.

5 Interpret family members' communication patterns within a cultural context. Recognize that a spokesperson may answer questions directed to the client, and that the family members may edit some information that they feel is inappropriate (Kulwicki, 1996). Family members can also be expected to act as the client's advocates; they may attempt to resolve problems by taking appeals "to the top" or by seeking the help of an influential intermediary.

6 Convey hope and optimism. The concept of "false hope" is not meaningful to Arabs because they regard God's power to cure as infinite. The amount and type of information given should be carefully considered.

TEMPORAL RELATIONSHIPS

First-generation Arab immigrants may believe in predestination; that is, God has predetermined the events of one's life. Accordingly, individuals should work hard to make the best of life while acknowledging that God has ultimate control over all that happens. Consequently, plans and intentions are qualified with the phrase **inshallah**, "if God wills," and blessings and misfortunes are attributed to God rather than to the actions of individuals.

Throughout the Arab world, there is nonchalance about punctuality except in cases of business or professional meetings; otherwise, the pace of life is more leisurely than in the West. Social events and appointments tend not to have a fixed beginning or end. Although certain individuals may arrive on time for appointments, the tendency is to be somewhat late. However, for most Arab Americans who belong to professional occupations or who are in the business field, punctuality and respecting deadlines and appointments are considered important (Kulwicki, 2001).

FORMAT FOR NAMES

Etiquette requires shaking hands on arrival and departure. However, when an Arab man is introduced to an Arab woman, the man waits for the woman to extend her hand. Devout Muslim men may not shake hands with women.

Titles are important and are used in combination with the person's first name (e.g., Mr. Khalil or Dr. Ali). Some may prefer to be addressed as mother (Um) or father (Abu) of the eldest son (e.g., Abu Khalil, "father of Khalil").

Family Roles and Organization

HEAD OF HOUSEHOLD AND GENDER ROLES

Arab Muslim families are characterized by a strong patrilineal tradition (Aswad, 1999). Women are subordinate to men, and young people are subordinate to older people. Consequently, within his immediate family, the man is the head of the family and his influence is overt. In public, a wife's interactions with her husband are formal and respectful. However, behind the scenes, she typically wields tremendous influence, particularly in matters pertaining to the home and children. A wife may sometimes be required to hide her power from her husband and children to preserve the husband's view of himself as head of the family.

Within the larger extended family, the older male figure assumes the role of decision maker. Women attain power and status in advancing years, particularly when they have adult children. The bond between mothers and sons is typically strong, and most men make every effort to obey their mother's wishes, and even her whims (Nydell, 1987).

Gender roles are clearly defined and regarded as a complementary division of labor. Men are breadwinners, protectors, and decision makers, whereas women are responsible for the care and education of children and for maintenance of a successful marriage by tending to their husbands' needs.

Although women in more urbanized Arab countries such as Lebanon, Syria, Jordan, and Egypt often have professional careers, with some women advocating for women's liberation, the family and marriage remain primary commitments for the majority. Most educated women still consider caring for their children as their primary role after marriage. Arab women value modesty, especially, among devout Muslim Arabs where modesty is expressed with their attire. For example, many Muslim women view the **hijab**, "covering the body except for one's face and hands," as offering them protection in situations where the sexes mix, because it is a recognized symbol of Muslim identity and good moral character.

Ironically, many Americans associate the *hijab* with oppression rather than protection. Similarly, the authority structure and division of labor within Arab families are often misinterpreted, fueling common stereotypes of the overtly dominant Arab male and the passive and oppressed Arab woman. Thus, by extension, conservative Arab Americans perceive the stereotypical understanding of the submissive role of women as a criticism to the Arab culture and family values (Kulwicki, 2000).

PRESCRIPTIVE, RESTRICTIVE, AND TABOO BEHAVIORS FOR CHILDREN AND ADOLESCENTS

In the traditional Arab family, the roles of the father and mother as they relate to the children are quite distinct. Typically, the father is the disciplinarian, whereas the mother is an ally and mediator, an unfailing source of love and kindness. Although some fathers feel that it is advantageous to maintain a degree of fear, family relationships are usually characterized by affection and sentimentality. Children are dearly loved, indulged, and included in all family activities.

Among Arabs, raising children so they reflect well on the family is an extremely important responsibility. A child's character and successes (or failures) in life are attributed to upbringing and parental influence. Because of the emphasis on familialism rather than individualism within the Arab culture, conformity to adult rules is favored. Correspondingly, child-rearing methods are oriented toward accommodation and cooperation. Family reputation is important; children are expected to behave in an honorable manner and not bring shame to the family. Child-rearing patterns also include great respect toward parents and elders. Children are raised to not question elders and to be obedient to older brothers and sisters (Kulwicki, 1996). Methods of discipline include physical punishment and shaming. Children are made to feel ashamed because others have seen them misbehave, rather than to experience guilt arising from self-criticism and inward regret.

While adolescence in the West is centered on acquiring a personal identity and completing the separation process from family, Arab adolescents are expected to remain enmeshed in the family system. Family interests and opinions often influence career and marriage decisions. Arab adolescents are pressed to succeed academically, in part because of the connections between professional careers and social status.

Conversely, behaviors that would bring family dishonor, such as academic failure, sexual activity, illicit drug use, and juvenile delinquency, are avoided. For girls in particular, chastity and decency are required. Adolescence in North America may provide more opportunities for academic success and more freedom in making career choices than their counterparts in the Arab countries. Cultural conflicts between American values and Arab values often cause significant conflicts for Arab American families (Aswad & Gray, 1996). Arab American parents cite a variety of concerns related to conflicting values regarding dating, after-school activities, drinking, and drug use (Eisonlohr, 1996).

FAMILY GOALS AND PRIORITIES

The family is the central socioeconomic unit in Arab society. Family members cooperate to secure livelihood, rear children, and maintain standing and influence within the community. Family members live nearby, sometimes intermarry (first cousins), and expect a great deal from one another regardless of practicality or ability to help. Loyalty to one's family takes precedence over personal needs. Maintenance of family honor is paramount.

Within the hierarchical family structure, older family members are accorded great respect. Children, sons in particular, are held responsible for supporting elderly parents. Therefore, regardless of the sacrifices involved, the elderly parents are almost always cared for within the home, typically until death.

Responsibility for family members rests with the older men of the family. In the absence of the father, brothers are responsible for unmarried sisters. In the event of a husband's death, his family provides for his widow and children. In general, family leaders are expected to use influence and render special services and favors to kinsmen.

Although educational accomplishments (doctoral degrees), certain occupations (medicine, engineering, law), and acquired wealth contribute to social status, family origin is the primary determinant. Certain character traits such as piety, generosity, hospitality, and good manners may also enhance social standing.

ALTERNATIVE LIFESTYLES

Most adults marry. Although the Islamic right to marry up to four wives is sometimes exercised, particularly if the first wife is chronically ill or infertile, most marriages are monogamous and for life. Recent studies have reported that 2 to 5 percent of Arab Muslim marriages are polygamous (Kulwicki, 2000). Whereas homosexuality occurs in all cultures to some extent, it is stigmatized among Arab cultures. In some Arab countries, it is considered a crime; fearing family disgrace and ostracism, gays and lesbians remain closeted (Global Gayz, 2002). However, in recent years Arab American gays and lesbians have been active in gay and lesbian organizations, and some have been outspoken and publicly active in raising community awareness about gay and lesbian rights in Arab American communities.

Workforce Issues

CULTURE IN THE WORKPLACE

Cultural differences that may have an impact on work life include beliefs regarding family, gender roles, one's ability to control life events, maintaining pleasant personal relationships, guarding dignity and honor, and the importance placed on maintaining one's reputation. Arabs and Americans may also differ in attitudes toward time, instructional methods, patterns of thinking, and the amount of emphasis placed on objectivity. However, because many second-wave professionals were educated in the United States, and thereby socialized to some extent, differences are probably more characteristic of less educated, first-generation Arab Americans.

Stress is a common denominator in recent studies of first-generation immigrants. Sources of stress include separation from family members, difficulty adjusting to American life, marital tension, and intergenerational conflict, specifically coping with adolescents socialized in American values through school activities (Cainkar, 1996; Eisonlohr, 1996; Seikaly, 1999). In addition, issues related to discrimination have been reported as a major source of stress among Arab Americans in their work environment. Arab Americans are keenly aware of the misperceptions Americans hold about Arabs, such as notions that Arabs are inferior, backward, sinister, and violent. In addition, the American public's ignorance of mainstream Islam, and the stereotyping of Muslims as fanatics, extremist, and confrontational, burden Arab American Muslims.

Muslim Arab Americans face a variety of challenges as they practice their faith in a secular American society. For example, Islamic and American civil law differ on matters such as marriage, divorce, banking, and inheritance. Individuals who wish to attend Friday prayer services and observe religious holidays frequently encounter job-related conflicts. Children are often torn between fulfilling Islamic obligations regarding prayer, dietary restrictions, and dress and hiding their religious identity in order to fit into the American public school culture.

ISSUES RELATED TO AUTONOMY

Whereas American workplaces tend to be dominated by deadlines, profit margins, and maintaining one's competitive edge, a more relaxed, cordial, and relationship-oriented atmosphere prevails in the Arab world. Friendship and business are mixed over cups of sweet tea to the extent that it is unclear where socializing ends and work begins. Managers promote optimal performance by using personal influence and persuasion, and performance evaluations are based on personality and social behavior as well as job skills.

Significant differences also exist in workplace norms. In the United States, position is usually earned, laws are applied equally, work takes precedence over family, honesty is an absolute value, facts and logic prevail, and direct and critical appraisal is regarded as valuable feedback. In the Arab world, position is often attained through one's family and connections, rules are bent, family obligations take precedence over the demands of the job, subjective perceptions often dictate actions, and criticism is often taken personally as an affront to dignity and family honor (Nydell, 1987). In Arab offices, supervisors and managers are expected to praise their emploees to assure them that their work is noticed and appreciated. Whereas such direct praise may be somewhat embarrassing for Americans, Arabs expect and want praise when they feel they have earned it (Nydell, 1987).

Biocultural Ecology

SKIN COLOR AND OTHER BIOLOGIC VARIATIONS

Although Arabs are uniformly perceived as swarthy, and while many do, in fact, have dark or olive skin, they may also have blonde or auburn hair, blue eyes, and fair complexions. Because color changes are more difficult to assess in dark-skinned people, pallor and cyanosis are best detected by examination of the oral mucosa and conjunctiva.

DISEASES AND HEALTH CONDITIONS

The major public health concerns in the Arab world include trauma related to motor vehicle accidents, maternal-child health, and control of communicable diseases. The incidence of infectious diseases such as tuberculosis, malaria, trachoma, typhus, hepatitis, typhoid fever, dysentery, and parasitic infestations varies between urban and rural areas and from country to country. For example, disease risks are relatively low in modern urban centers of the Arab world, but quite high in the countryside where animals such as goats and sheep virtually share living quarters, open toilets are commonplace, and running water is not available. Schistosomiasis (also called bilharzia), infecting about one-fifth of Egyptians, has been called Egypt's number one health problem. Its prevalence is related to an entrenched social habit of using the Nile River for washing, drinking, and urinating. Similarly, outbreaks of cholera and meningitis are continuous concerns in Saudi Arabia during the Muslim pilgrimage season. In Jordan, where contagious diseases have declined sharply, emphasis has shifted to preventing accidental death and controlling noncommunicable diseases such as cancer and heart disease. Correspondingly, seat-belt use, smoking habits, and pesticide residues in locally grown produce are major issues. Campaigns directed at improving children's health include hepatitis B vaccinations and dental health programs.

Glucose-6-phosphate dehydrogenase (G-6-PD) deficiency, sickle cell anemia, and the thalassemias are extremely common in the eastern Mediterranean region, probably because carriers enjoy an increased resistance to malaria (Hamamy & Alwan, 1994). High consanguinity rates—roughly 30 percent of marriages in Iraq, Jordan, Kuwait, and Saudi Arabia are between first cousins—and the trend of bearing children up to menopause also contribute to the prevalence of genetically determined disorders in Arab countries (Hamamy & Alwan, 1994).

With modernization and increased life expectancy, multifactorial disorders—hypertension, diabetes, and coronary heart disease—have also emerged as major problems in eastern Mediterranean countries (Kulwicki, 2001). In many countries, cardiovascular disease is a major cause of death. In Lebanon, the increased frequency of familial hypercholesterolemia is a contributing factor. Individuals of Arabic ancestry are also more likely to inherit familial Mediterranean fever, a disorder characterized by recurrent episodes of fever, peritonitis, or pleurisies, either alone or in some combination.

The extent to which these conditions affect the health of Arab Americans is limited. However, a Wayne County Health Department (1994) project, a telephone survey including Arabs residing in the Detroit area, identified cardiovascular disease as one of two specific risks based on the high prevalence of cigarette smoking, high-cholesterol diets, obesity, and sedentary lifestyles. Although the prevalence of hypertension was lower in the Arab community than in the rest of Wayne County, Arab respondents were less likely to report having their blood pressure checked. In fact, lower rates for appropriate testing and screening, such as cholesterol testing and uterine and breast cancer screening, were considered the second area of major risk for this group of Arab Americans. The Michigan Department of Public Health (MDPH, 1995) report indicated that the age-adjusted death rates for Arab females, compared to other whites, was higher from heart disease, about the same from cancer, and lower from strokes. The age-adjusted death rate for Arab females from coronary heart disease (81.6 per 100,000) was lower than the goal set by the Public Health Service for Healthy People 2000 (no more than 100 cases per 100,000 population). However, the age-adjusted death rate for Arab males from coronary heart disease was higher (273 per 100,000) when compared to white males (212 per 100,000). The age-adjusted death rate from cancer was about the same among Arab males and white males.

The rate of infant mortality in the Arab world is very high, ranging from 24 per 1000 births in Syria to 108 per 1000 births in Iraq. In Bahrain the infant mortality is low: 8.5 per 1000 births (World Health Organization, 2001b). Recent figures for Michigan show a lower infant mortality rate for Arab Americans (6.2 per 1000 births) than for white infants (7.8 per 1000), and much lower than for African American infants (MDPH, 1995).

VARIATIONS IN DRUG METABOLISM

Information describing drug disposition and sensitivity in Arabs is limited. Between 1 and 1.4 percent of Arabs are known to have difficulty metabolizing debrisoquine and substances that are metabolized similarly: antiarrhythmics, antidepressants, beta-blockers, neuroleptics, and opioid agents. Consequently, a small number of Arab Americans may experience elevated blood levels and adverse effects when customary dosages of antidepressants are prescribed. Conversely, typical codeine dosages may prove inadequate because some individuals cannot metabolize codeine to morphine to promote optimal analgesic effect (Levy, 1993).

High-Risk Behaviors

Despite Islamic beliefs discouraging tobacco use, smoking remains deeply ingrained in Arab culture. For many Arabs, offering cigarettes is a sign of hospitality. Consistent with their cultural heritage, Arab Americans are characterized by higher smoking rates and lower quitting rates than European Americans (Rice & Kulwicki, 1992).

According to the Wayne County Health Department (1994) report, middle-aged Arab American men (53.3 percent) and women (42.2 percent), and older women (49.1 percent) are most likely to smoke. Young women (18.7 percent) are least likely to be cigarette smokers.

Islamic prohibitions do appear to influence patterns of alcohol consumption and attitudes toward drug use (Wayne County Health Department, 1994). Ninety percent of the Arab respondents in the survey reported that they abstain from drinking alcohol. None reported heavy drinking, with a limited number reporting binge drinking (2.2 percent) and driving under the influence of alcohol (1.4 percent). All respondents believed that occasional use of cocaine entails "great" risk, with most saying the same about occasional use of marijuana.

The actual risk for, and incidence of, human immunodeficiency virus (HIV) infection and acquired immunodeficiency syndrome (AIDS) in Arab countries and among Arab Americans is low. However, an increase in the rate of infection was noticed among many Arab countries during the early 1990s, followed by a steady decline between 1997 and 1998. For instance, approximately 400,000 cases of AIDS were reported in eastern Mediterranean countries (WHO, 2001a). The reported number of individuals having AIDS in the Arab countries varies, and may not be an accurate reflection of the real incidence due to restrictions placed on HIV/AIDS research by some Arab countries. The largest number of AIDS cases is seen in Djibouti (1783) and Saudi Arabia (394); the lowest numbers of individuals with AIDS are found in Palestine (32), Syria (53), Jordan (71), Iraq (108), Lebanon (147), Egypt (209), and Yemen (156) (WHO 2001a).

Despite the reported low rate of HIV/AIDS among Arab Americans (approximately 10 of 400 individuals), 4 percent of the Arab American respondents surveyed by Kulwicki and Cass (1994) reported that they were at high risk for AIDS. In addition, the sample demonstrated less knowledge of primary routes of transmission and more misconceptions regarding unlikely modes of transmission than other populations surveyed.

Cultural norms of modesty for Arab women are also a significant risk related to reproductive health among Arab Americans. For example, the rate of breast cancer screening among Arab women was 50.8 percent, compared to 71.2 percent for other women in Michigan. The rate of cervical pap smears was 59.9 percent, and the rate of mammogram screenings was 51.2 percent (Kulwicki, 2000). Arab American women may be at a higher risk for domestic violence, especially new immigrants, because of the higher rates of stress, poverty, poor

spiritual and social support, and isolation from family members due to immigration (Kulwicki, 2001).

Sedentary lifestyle and high fat intake among Arab Americans places them at higher risk for cardiovascular diseases. For instance, 43 percent of the participants surveyed by Wayne County Health Department indicated that they had been told that their cholesterol level was high (OMH, 2001). Studies in Arab countries and in Michigan have also reported higher rates of cardiovascular disease and diabetes among Arabs and Arab Americans.

HEALTH-CARE PRACTICES

According to the Wayne County Health Department (1994), Arab Americans' risk in terms of safety is mixed. Factors enhancing safety include low rates of gun ownership and high recognition of the risks associated with having guns in the house. Conversely, lower rates of fire escape planning and seat-belt usage for adults and older children (car seats are generally used for younger children), as well as higher rates of physical assaults, threaten their safety.

In most health areas surveyed in Michigan, education and income were important determinants of risk for people of Arab descent. Socioeconomic status was also a strong indicator in accessing health-care services. The Wayne County Health Department (1994) indicated that 37.2 percent of the adult Arab respondents were not covered by health insurance. Use of health-care services for prenatal care was, however, higher among Arab American females than other ethnic groups in Michigan (MDPH, 1995). Physical or mental disability among Arab Americans in Michigan was almost equal to white Americans.

Nutrition

MEANING OF FOOD

Sharing meals with family and friends is a favorite pastime. Offering food is also a way of expressing love and friendship, hospitality, and generosity. For the Arab woman, whose primary role is caring for her husband and children, the preparation and presentation of an elaborate midday meal is taken as an indication of her love and caring. Similarly, in entertaining friends, the types and quantity of food served, often several entrees, is a measure of one's hospitality and esteem for one's guests. Honor and reputation are based on the manner in which guests are received. In return, family members and guests express appreciation by eating heartily.

COMMON FOODS AND FOOD RITUALS

Although cooking and national dishes vary from coun-try to country and seasoning from family to family, Arabic cooking shares many general characteristics. Familiar spices and herbs such as cinnamon, allspice, cloves, ginger, cumin, mint, parsley, bay leaves, garlic, and onions are used frequently. Skewer cooking and slow simmering are typical modes of preparation. All countries have rice and wheat dishes, stuffed vegetables, nut-filled pastries, and fritters soaked in syrup. Dishes are garnished with raisins, pine nuts, pistachios, and almonds.

Favorite fruits and vegetables include dates, figs, apricots, guava, mango, melon, papaya, bananas, citrus, carrots, tomatoes, cucumbers, parsley, mint, spinach, and grape leaves. Lamb and chicken are the most popular meats. Muslims are prohibited from eating pork and pork products (for example, lard). For Arab Christians, pork is not prohibited; however, pork consumption by Arab Christians is low. Similarly, because the consumption of blood is forbidden, Muslims are required to cook meats and poultry until well done. Bread accompanies every meal and is viewed as a gift from God. In many respects, the traditional Arab diet is representative of the U.S. Department of Agriculture's food pyramid. Bread is a mainstay, grains and legumes are often substituted for meats, fresh fruit and juices are especially popular, and olive oil is widely used. In addition, because foods are prepared "from scratch," consumption of preservatives and additives is limited.

Lunch is the main meal in Arab households. Encouraging guests to eat is the host's duty. Guests often begin with a ritual refusal and then succumb to the host's insistence. Food is eaten with the right hand because it is regarded as clean. Beverages may not be served until after the meal because some Arabs consider it unhealthy to eat and drink at the same time. Similar concerns may exist regarding mixing hot and cold foods.

Health-care providers should also understand *Ramadan*, the Muslim month of fasting. The fast, which is meant to remind Muslims of their dependence on God and the poor who experience involuntary fasting, involves abstinence from eating, drinking (including water), smoking, and marital intercourse during daylight hours. Although the sick are not required to fast, many pious Muslims insist on fasting while hospitalized, necessitating adjustments in meal times and medications, including medications given by nonoral routes. In outpatient settings, health-care providers need to be alert to potential "noncompliance." Patients may omit or adjust the timing of medications. Of particular concern are medications requiring constant blood levels, adequate hydration, or both (for example, antibiotics that may crystallize in the kidneys). Health-care providers may need to provide appointment times after sunset during Ramadan for individuals requiring injections (for example, allergy shots).

DIETARY PRACTICES FOR HEALTH PROMOTION

Arabs associate good health with eating properly, consuming nutritious foods, and fasting to cure disease. For some, concerns about amounts and balance among food types (hot, cold, dry, moist) may be traced to the **Prophet Mohammed**, who taught that "the stomach is the house of every disease, and abstinence is the head of every remedy" (Al-Akili, 1993: 7). Within this framework, illness is related to excessive eating, eating before a previously eaten meal is digested, eating nutritionally deficient food, mixing opposing types of foods, and consuming elaborately prepared foods. Conversely, abstinence allows the body to expel disease.

The condition of the alimentary tract has priority over all other body systems in the Arab perception of health (Meleis & La Fever, 1984). Gastrointestinal complaints are often the reason Arab Americans seek care (Lipson, Reizian, & Meleis, 1987; Reizian & Meleis, 1987). Obesity is a problem for second-generation Arab American women and children, most of whom report eating American snacks that are high in fat and calories. Most women try to lose weight by reducing caloric intake (Wayne County Health Department, 1994).

NUTRITIONAL DEFICIENCIES AND FOOD LIMITATIONS

In Arab countries, diet is influenced by income, government subsidies for certain foods (i.e., bread, sugar, oil), and seasonal availability. Arab Americans most at risk for nutritional deficiencies include newly arrived immigrants from Yemen and Iraq (Kurian, 1992) and Arab American households below the poverty level. Lactose intolerance sometimes occurs in this population. However, the practice of eating yogurt and cheese, rather than drinking milk, probably limits symptoms in sensitive people.

Many of the most common foods are available in American markets. Some Muslims may refuse to eat meat that is not **halal**, or slaughtered in an Islamic manner. *Halal* meat can be obtained in Arabic grocery stores and through Islamic centers or **mosques**.

Islamic prohibitions against the consumption of alcohol and pork have implications for American health-care providers. Conscientious Muslims are often wary of eating outside the home and may ask many questions about ingredients used in meal preparation: Are the beans vegetarian? Was wine used in the meat sauce or lard in the pastry crust? Muslims are equally concerned about the ingredients and origins of mouthwashes, toothpastes, and medicines (e.g., alcohol-based syrups and elixirs), as well as insulins and capsules (gelatin coating) derived from pigs. However, if no substitutes are available, Muslims are permitted to use these preparations.

Pregnancy and Childbearing Practices

FERTILITY PRACTICES AND VIEWS TOWARD PREGNANCY

Fertility rates in the countries from which most Arab Americans emigrate range from 2.5 in Tunisia and Lebanon to 6.5 in North Yemen (UNICEF, 2001). Fertility practices of Arabs are influenced by traditional Bedouin values supporting tribal dominance, popular beliefs that "God decides family size," "God provides," and Islamic rulings regarding birth control, treatment of infertility, and abortion.

High fertility rates are favored. Procreation is regarded

as the purpose of marriage and the means of enhancing family strength. Accordingly, Islamic jurists have ruled that the use of "reversible" forms of birth control is "undesirable but not forbidden." They should be employed only in certain situations, listed in decreasing order of legitimacy, such as threat to the mother's life, too frequent childbearing, risk of transmitting genetic disease, and financial hardship. Moreover, irreversible forms of birth control such as vasectomy and tubal ligation are **haram**, "absolutely unlawful." Muslims regard abortion as *haram* except when the mother's health is compromised by pregnancy-induced disease or her life is threatened (Ebrahim, 1989). Therefore, unwanted pregnancies are dealt with by hoping one miscarries "by an act of God" or by covertly arranging for an abortion. Recently, there has been great decline in fertility rates in Arab countries and among Arab Americans. According to Michigan's birth registration data, fertility rates among Arab Americans are highest (approximately 4) when compared to the total population (OMH, 2001).

Among Jordanian husbands, religion and the fatalistic belief that "God decides family size" were most often given as reasons why contraceptives were not used. Contraceptives were used by 27 percent of the husbands, typically urbanites of high socioeconomic status. Although the IUD and the pill were most widely favored, 4.9 percent of females used sterilization despite religious prohibitions (Hashemite Kingdom of Jordan, 1985). A survey of a random sample of 295 Arab American women in Michigan indicated that 29.1 percent of the surveyed women did not use any birth control methods because of their desire to have children, 4.3 percent did not use any form of contraceptives because of their husband's disapproval, and 6 percent did not use contraceptive methods because of religious reasons. The use of birth control pills was the highest (33.2 percent) among the users of contraceptive methods, followed by tubal ligation (12.9 percent) and IUD (10.7 percent) (Kulwicki, 2000).

Indeed, among Arab women, in particular, fertility may be more of a concern than contraception because sterility in a woman could lead to rejection and divorce. Islam condones treatment for infertility, as **Allah** provides progeny as well as a cure for every disease. However, approved methods for treating infertility are limited to artificial insemination using the husband's sperm and in vitro fertilization involving the fertilization of the wife's ovum by the husband's sperm.

PRESCRIPTIVE, RESTRICTIVE, AND TABOO PRACTICES IN THE CHILDBEARING FAMILY

Because of the emphasis on fertility and the bearing of sons, pregnancy traditionally occurred at a younger age and the fertility rate among Arab women was higher in the Arab world. However, as the educational and economic conditions for Arab women have improved both in the Arab world and in the United States, fertility patterns have also changed accordingly. The MDPH (1995) reported a median age of 25 for first pregnancies among Arab American women.

The pregnant woman is indulged and her cravings satisfied, least she develop a birthmark in the shape of the particular food she craves. Because of the preference for male offspring, the sex of the child can be a stressor for mothers without sons. Friends and family often note how the mother is "carrying" the baby as an indicator of the baby's sex (that is, high for a girl and low for a boy). Although pregnant women are excused from fasting during Ramadan, some Muslim women may be determined to fast and thus suffer potential consequences for glucose metabolism and hydration.

Labor and delivery are women's affairs. In Arab countries home delivery, with the assistance of **dayahs** (midwives) or neighbors was common because of limited access to hospitals, "shyness," and financial constraints. However, recently the practice of home delivery has decreased dramatically in Arab countries, and hospital deliveries have become common. During labor, women openly express pain through facial expressions, verbalizations, and body movements. Nurses and medical staff may mistakenly diagnose Arab women as needing medical intervention and administer pain medications more liberally to alleviate their pain.

Care for the infant includes wrapping the stomach at birth, or as soon thereafter as possible, to prevent cold or wind from entering the baby's body (Luna, 1994). The call to prayer is recited in the Muslim newborn's ear. Male circumcision is almost a universal practice, and for Muslims, it is a religious requirement.

Folk beliefs influence bathing and breast-feeding. Arab mothers may be reluctant to bathe postpartum because of beliefs that air gets into the mother and causes illness (Luna, 1994) and washing the breasts "thins the milk" (Cline, Abuirmeileh, & Roberts, 1986).

Breast-feeding is often delayed until the second or third day after birth because of beliefs that the mother requires rest, that nursing at birth causes "colic" pain for the mother, and that "colostrum makes the baby dumb" (Cline, Abuirmeileh, & Roberts, 1986). Postpartum care also includes special foods such as lentil soup to increase milk production and tea to flush and cleanse the body.

Statistics describing the pregnancy and birth experiences of Michigan mothers, including 2755 Arab Americans, depict the experiences of Arab American mothers and infants as fairly comparable to their white counterparts with regard to adequacy of prenatal care, maternal complications, infant mortality, and birth complications. In addition, fewer Arab American mothers smoke, drink alcohol, or gain too little weight. (MDPH, 1993). Although these statewide statistics are quite favorable, it is important to mention that earlier studies revealed an alarming rate of infant mortality among Arab American mothers in Dearborn, Michigan, a particularly disadvantaged community of new immigrants with high rates of unemployment. Factors contributing to poor pregnancy outcomes include poverty; lower levels of education; inability to communicate in English; personal, family, and cultural stressors; cigarette smoking; and early or closely spaced pregnancies. Fear of being ridiculed by American health-care providers and a limited number of bilingual providers limit access to health-care information.

Death Rituals

DEATH RITUALS AND EXPECTATIONS

Although Arabs insist on maintaining hope regardless of prognosis, death is accepted as God's will. According to Muslim beliefs, death is foreordained and worldly life is but a preparation for eternal life. Hence, from the Qur'an, Surrah III, v. 185:

Every soul will taste of death. And ye will be paid on the Day of Resurrection only that which ye have fairly earned. Whoso is removed from the Fire and is made to enter Paradise, he indeed is triumphant. The life of this world is but comfort of illusion. (Pickthall, 1977: 70)

Muslim death rituals include turning the patient's bed to face the holy city of Mecca and reading from the Qur'an, particularly verses stressing hope and acceptance. After death, the deceased is washed three times by a Muslim of the same sex. The body is then wrapped, preferably in white material, and buried as soon as possible in a brick- or cement-lined grave facing Mecca. Prayers for the deceased are recited at home, at the mosque, or at the cemetery. Women do not ordinarily attend the burial unless the deceased is a close relative or husband. Instead, they gather at the deceased's home and read the Qur'an. Cremation is not practiced.

Family members do not generally approve of autopsy because of respect for the dead and feelings that the body should not be mutilated. Islam allows forensic autopsy and autopsy for the sake of medical research and instruction.

Death rituals for Arab Christians are similar to Christian practices in the rest of the world. Arab American Christians may have a Bible next to the patient, expect a visit from the priest, and expect medical means to prolong life if possible. Organ donations and autopsies are acceptable. Wearing black during the mourning period is also common. For both Christians and Muslims, patients, especially children, are not told about terminal illness. The family spokesperson is usually the person who should be informed about death. The spokesperson will then communicate news to family members.

RESPONSES TO DEATH AND GRIEF

Mourning periods and practices may vary among Muslims and Christians emigrating from different Arab countries. Extended mourning periods may be practiced if the deceased is a young man, a woman, or a child. However, in some cases, Muslims may perceive extended periods of mourning as defiance of the will of God. Family members are asked to endure with patience and good faith in Allah what befalls them, including death. While friends and relatives are to restrict mourning to 3 days, a wife may mourn for 4 months, and in some special cases mourning can extend to one year. Although weeping is allowed, beating the cheeks or tearing garments is prohibited. For women, wearing black is considered appropriate for the entire period of mourning.

Spirituality

RELIGIOUS PRACTICES AND USE OF PRAYER

Most Arabs are Muslims. Prominent Christian groups include the Copts in Egypt, the Chaldeans in Iraq, and the Maronites in Lebanon (Kulwicki & Kridli, 2001). Despite their distinctive practices and liturgies, Christians and Muslims share certain beliefs because of Islam's origin in Judaism and Christianity. Muslims and Christians believe in the same God and many of the same prophets, the Day of Judgment, Satan, heaven, hell, and an afterlife. One major difference is that Islam has no priesthood. Islamic scholars or religious *sheikhs*, the most learned individuals in an Islamic community, assume the role of **imam**, or "leader of the prayer." The imam also performs marriage ceremonies and funeral prayers and acts as a spiritual counselor or reference on Islamic teachings. Obtaining the opinion of the local imam may be a helpful intervention for Arab American Muslims struggling with health-care decisions.

Observance of religious practices varies among Muslims. Patai (1958) makes a distinction between official Islam, as practiced by the educated, and popular beliefs and practices that influence the religious life of the "untutored folk." In addition, as with any other religion, there are nominal as well as practicing Muslims. However, because Islam is the state religion of most Arab countries, and in Islam there is no separation of church and state, a certain degree of religious participation is obligatory.

To illustrate, consider a few examples of Islam's impact on Jordanian life. Because of Islamic law, abortion is investigated as a crime and foster parenting is encouraged, whereas adoption is forbidden. The infertility treatments available are those approved by Islamic jurists. **Shariah**, Islamic law courts, rule on matters such as marriage, divorce, guardianship, and inheritance. Public schools have classes on Islam and prayer rooms. School and work schedules revolve around Islamic holidays and the weekly prayer. During Ramadan, restaurants remain closed during daylight hours and workdays are shortened to facilitate fasting. Because Muslims gather for communal prayer on Friday afternoons, the workweek runs from Saturday through Thursday. Finally, because of Islamic tradition that adherents of other monotheistic religions be accorded tolerance and protection, Jordan's Christians have separate religious courts and schools, and non-Muslims attending public schools are not required to participate in religious activities.

For Arab American Christians, church is an important part of everyday life. Most celebrate Catholic and Orthodox Christian holidays with fasting and ceremonial church services. They may display or wear Christian symbols such as a cross, a picture of the Virgin Mary, and so forth.

MEANING OF LIFE AND INDIVIDUAL SOURCES OF STRENGTH

For Muslims, adherents of the world's second largest religion, Islam means "submission to Allah." Life centers on worshipping Allah and preparing for one's afterlife by fulfilling religious duties as described in the Qur'an and the **hadith**. The five major pillars, or duties, of Islam are: (1) declaration of faith, (2) prayer five times daily, (3) almsgiving, (4) fasting during Ramadan, and (5) completion of a pilgrimage to Mecca.

Despite the dominance of familialism in Arab life, religious faith is often regarded as more important. Whether Muslim or Christian, Arabs identify strongly with their respective religious groups, and religious affiliation is as much a part of their identity as family name. God and his power are acknowledged in everyday life.

SPIRITUAL BELIEFS AND HEALTH-CARE PRACTICES

Many Muslims believe in combining spiritual medicine, performance of daily prayers, and reading or listening to the Qur'an with conventional medical treatment. The devout patient may request that his or her chair or bed be turned to face Mecca, and that a basin of water be provided for ritual washing or ablution before praying. Providing for cleanliness is particularly important because the Muslim's prayer is not acceptable unless the body, clothing, and place of prayer are clean.

Islamic teachings urge Muslims to eat wholesome food; abstain from pork, alcohol, and illicit drugs; practice moderation in all activities; be conscious of hygiene; and face adversity with faith in Allah's mercy and compassion, hope, and acceptance. Muslims are also advised to care for the needs of the community by visiting and assisting the sick and providing for needy Muslims.

Sometimes illness is considered punishment for one's sins. Correspondingly, by providing cures, Allah manifests mercy and compassion and supplies a vehicle for repentance and gratitude (Al-Akili, 1993). Others emphasize that sickness should not be viewed as punishment, but as a trial or ordeal that brings about expiation of sins and that may strengthen character (Ebrahim, 1989). Common responses to illness include patience and endurance of suffering because it has a purpose known only to Allah, unfailing hope that even "irreversible" conditions might be cured "if it be Allah's will," and acceptance of one's fate. Euthanasia and suicide are forbidden.

Spiritual beliefs and health-care practices for Arab American Christians are similar to those of Orthodox or Catholics. Caring for the body and burial practices are similar. A priest is always expected to visit the patient; if the patient is Catholic, a priest administers the sacrament of the sick.

Health-Care Practices

HEALTH-SEEKING BELIEFS AND BEHAVIORS

Good health is seen as the ability to fulfill one's roles. Diseases are attributed to a variety of factors such as inadequate diet, hot and cold shifts, exposure of one's stomach during sleep, emotional or spiritual distress, and envy or the evil eye. Arabs are expected to express and

acknowledge their ailments when ill. Muslims often mention that the Prophet urged physicians to perform research and the ill to seek treatment because "Allah has not created a disease without providing a cure for it," except for the problem of old age (Ebrahim, 1989: 5).

Despite beliefs that one should care for health and seek treatment when ill, Arab women are often reluctant to seek care. Because of the cultural emphasis placed on modesty, some women express shyness about disrobing for examination. Similarly, some families object to female family members being examined by male physicians. Because of the fear that a diagnosed illness, such as cancer or psychiatric illness, may bring shame and influence the marriageability of the woman and her female relatives, delays in seeking medical care may be common.

Evidence also suggests that the cultural preference for male offspring influences the health care that low-income parents provide for female children. In poor communities in Jordan, boys were better nourished, more likely to be immunized, and more apt to receive prompt medical attention for illnesses (West, 1987). Delay in seeking treatment was noted by a local health-care provider who diagnosed "failure to thrive" in a young Iraqi female infant when her refugee parents sought medical attention for a feverish male sibling.

While Arab Americans readily seek care for actual symptoms, preventive care is not generally sought (Kulwicki, 1996; Kulwicki, Miller, & Schim, 2000). Similarly, pediatric clinics are used primarily for illness and injury rather than for well-child visits (Lipson, Reizian, & Meleis, 1987). Laffrey and colleagues (1989) attributed these patterns to Arabs' present orientation and reluctance to plan, and to the meaning Arab Americans attach to preventive care. Whereas American health-care providers focus on screening and managing risks and complications, Arab Americans value information that aids in coping with stress, illness, or treatment protocols. Arab Americans' failure to use preventive care services may be related to other factors such as insurance coverage, the availability of female physicians who accept Medicaid patients, and the novelty of the concept of preventive care for immigrants from developing countries.

RESPONSIBILITY FOR HEALTH CARE

Dichotomous views regarding individual responsibility and one's control over life's events often cause misunderstanding between Arab Americans and health-care providers (Abu Gharbieh, 1993). For example, individualism and an activist approach to life are the underpinnings of the American health-care system. Accordingly, practices such as informed consent, self-care, advance directives, risk management, and preventive care are valued. Patients are expected to use information seeking and problem solving in preference to faith in God, patience, and acceptance of one's fate as primary coping mechanisms. Similarly, American health-care providers expect that the patient's hope be "realistic" in accordance with medical science.

However, in Arab culture, quite the opposite values—

familialism and fatalism—influence health care and responses to illness. For Arabs, the family is the context within which health care is delivered (Lipson, Reizian, & Meleis, 1987). Rather than engage in self-care and decision making, clients often allow family members to oversee care. Family members indulge the individual and assume the ill person's responsibilities. Although the patient may seem overly dependent and the family overly protective by American standards, family members' vigilance and "demanding behavior" should be interpreted as a measure of concern. For Muslims, care is a religious obligation associated with individual and collective meanings of honor (Luna, 1994). Individuals are seen as expressing care through the performance of gender-specific role responsibilities as delineated in the Qur'an.

Although most American health-care professionals consider full disclosure an ethical obligation, most Arab physicians do not believe that it is necessary for a client to know a serious diagnosis or full details of a surgical procedure. In fact, communicating a grave diagnosis is often viewed as cruel and tactless because it deprives clients of hope. Similarly, preoperative instructions are thought to cause needless anxiety, hypochondriasis, and complications. Apart from the educated, most clients are not interested in actively participating in decision making (Abu Gharbieh, 1993). They expect physicians, because of their expertise, to select treatments. The client's role is to cooperate. The authority of physicians is seldom challenged or questioned. When treatment is successful, the physician's skill is recognized; adverse outcomes are attributed to God's will unless there is evidence of blatant malpractice (Sullivan, 1993).

Not all Arabs may be familiar with the American concept of health insurance. Traditionally, the family unit, through its communal resources, provides insurance. Certain Arab countries, such as Saudi Arabia and Kuwait, provide free medical care, whereas in other countries many citizens are government employees and are entitled to low-cost care in government-sector facilities. Private physicians and hospitals are preferred because of the belief that the private sector offers the best care.

Because many medications requiring a prescription in the United States are available over the counter in Arab countries, Arabs are accustomed to seeking medical advice from pharmacists. In comparison with other Americans in Wayne County, Arab Americans were less likely to take prescription medications, but when they did, they were more likely to use medications as directed (Wayne County Health Department, 1994).

FOLK PRACTICES

Although Islam disapproves of superstition, witchcraft, and magic, concerns about the powers of jealous people, the evil eye, and certain supernatural agents such as the devil and **jinn** are part of the folk beliefs. Those who envy the wealth, success, or beauty of others are believed to cause adversity by a gaze, which brings misfortune to the victim. Beautiful women, healthy-looking babies, and the rich, are believed to be particularly susceptible to the evil eye, and expressions of congratu-

lations may be interpreted as envy. Protection from the evil eye is afforded by wearing amulets, such as blue beads or figures involving the number five, reciting the Qur'an, or invoking the name of Allah (Kulwicki, 1996). Barren women, the poor, and the unfortunate are usually suspects for casting the evil eye.

Mental or emotional illnesses may be attributed to possession by evil jinn. Some believe that insanity, or *jinaan* (meaning "possessed by the jinn"), may also be caused by the evil wishes of jealous individuals.

Traditional Islamic medicine is based on the theory of four humors and the spiritual and physical remedies prescribed by the Prophet. Because illness is viewed as an imbalance between the humors—black bile, blood, phlegm, and yellow bile—and the primary attributes of dryness, heat, cold, and moisture, therapy involves treating with the disease's opposite: hot disease, cold remedy. Although methods such as cupping, cautery, and phlebotomy may be employed, treating with special prayers or simple foods such as dates, honey, salt, and olive oil is preferred (Al-Akili, 1993). Yemeni or Saudi Arabian patients may apply heat (cupping, moxibustion) or use cautery in combination with modern medical technology.

BARRIERS TO HEALTH CARE

Newly arrived and unskilled refugees from poorer parts of the Arab world are at particular risk for both increased exposure to ill health and inadequate access to health care. Factors such as refugee status, recency of arrival, differences in cultural values and norms, inability to pay for health-care services, and inability to speak English add to the stresses of immigration (Kulwicki, 2000; Kulwicki, Miller, & Schim, 2000), affecting both health status and responses to health problems. Moreover, these immigrants are less likely to receive adequate health care because of cultural and language barriers, lack of transportation, limited health insurance, poverty, a lack of awareness of existing services, and poor coordination of services (Kulwicki, 1996, 2000).

Although a lack of insurance coverage affects a significant number of Wayne County Health Department respondents (Wayne County Health Department, 1994), other studies suggest that Arab Americans regard other barriers and services as more significant. For instance, language and communication remain serious barriers for recent Arab American immigrants (Kulwicki, 2000). Transportation to health-care facilities and culturally competent service providers also add to the problems of accessing health-care services.

CULTURAL RESPONSES TO HEALTH AND ILLNESS

Arabs regard pain as unpleasant and something to be controlled (Reizian & Meleis, 1986). Because of their confidence in medical science, Arabs anticipate immediate postoperative relief from their symptoms. This expectation, in combination with a belief in conserving energy for recovery, often contributes to a reluctance to comply with typical postoperative routines such as frequent ambulation. Although expressive, emotional, and vocal responses to pain are usually reserved for the immediate family, under certain circumstances, such as childbirth and illnesses accompanied by spasms, Arabs express pain more freely (Reizian & Meleis, 1986). The tendency of Arabs to be more expressive with their family and more restrained in the presence of health professionals may lead to conflicting perceptions regarding the adequacy of pain relief. Whereas the nurse may assess pain relief as adequate, family members may demand that their relative receive additional analgesia.

The attitude that mental illness is a major social stigma is particularly pervasive. Psychiatric symptoms may be denied, attributed to "bad nerves" (Hattar-Pollara, Meleis, & Nagib, 2001) or evil spirits (Kulwicki, 1996). Underrecognition of signs and symptoms may occur because of the somatic orientation of Arab patients and physicians, patients' tolerance of emotional suffering, and relatives' tolerance of behavioral disturbances (El-Islam, 1994). Indeed, home management with standard but crucial adjustments within the family may abort or control symptoms until remission occurs. For example, female family members manage postpartum depression by assuming care of the newborn, and/or by telling the mother she needs more help or more rest. Islamic legal prohibitions further confound attempts to estimate the incidence of problems such as alcoholism and suicide, resulting in underreporting of these conditions because of a potential for severe social stigma.

When individuals suffering from mental distress seek medical care, they are likely to present with a variety of vague complaints, such as abdominal pain, lassitude, anorexia, and shortness of breath. Patients often expect and may insist on somatic treatment, at least "vitamins and tonics" (El-Islam, 1994). When mental illness is accepted as a diagnosis, treatment by medications rather than by counseling is preferred. Hospitalization is resisted because such placement is viewed as abandonment (Budman, Lipson, & Meleis, 1992). Although Arab Americans report family and marital stress as well as various mental health symptoms, they often seek family counseling or social services rather than a psychiatrist (Aswad & Gray, 1996).

Yousef (1993) described the Arab public's attitude toward the disabled as generally negative, with low expectations for education and rehabilitation. Yousef also related misconceptions about mental retardation to the dearth of Arab literature about disability and the public's lack of experience with the disabled. Because of social stigma, the disabled are often kept from public view. Similarly, although there is a trend toward educating some children with mild mental retardation in regular schools, special education programs are generally institutionally based.

Reiter, Mar'i, and Rosenberg (1986) found that parents who were most intimately involved with the developmentally disabled held rather positive attitudes. More tolerant views were expressed among Israeli-Arab parents, Muslims, the less educated, and residents of smaller villages than among Christians, the educated, and residents of larger villages with mixed populations. Reiter, Mar'i, and Rosenberg linked the less positive attitudes of the latter groups to the process of modernization, which affects a drive toward status and a weakening of family structures and traditions. Traditions include regarding the handicapped as coming from God, accepting the disabled person's dependency, and providing care within the home.

Dependency is accepted. Family members assume the ill person's responsibilities. The ill person is cared for and indulged. From an American frame of reference, the patient may seem overly dependent and the family overly protective.

BLOOD TRANSFUSIONS AND ORGAN DONATION

Although blood transfusions and organ transplants are widely accepted, organ donation is a controversial issue among Arabs and Arab Americans. Practices of organ donation may vary among Arab Muslims and non-Muslims based on their religious beliefs about death and dying, reincarnation, or based on their personal feelings about helping others by donating their organs to others or for scientific purposes (Kulwicki, 2001). Health-care professionals should be sensitive to personal, family, or religious practices toward organ donation among Arab Americans and should not make any assumptions about organ donation unless family members are asked.

Health-Care Practitioners

TRADITIONAL VERSUS BIOMEDICAL PRACTITIONERS

Although Arab Americans combine traditional and biomedical care practices, they are very cognizant of the effective medical treatments in the West, and consider themselves privileged to be able to use the American health-care system, which would not have been accessible to them in their country of origin (Kulwicki, 1996). Because of their profound respect for medicine, Arab Americans seek treatments for physical disorders or ailments. Medical treatments that require surgery, removal of causative agents, or eradicating by intravenous treatments are valued more than therapies aimed at health promotion or disease prevention. Although most Arab Americans have high regard for medicine related to physical disorders, many do not have the same respect or trust for mental or psychological treatment. There is a pervasive feeling among many Arab Americans that psychiatric services or therapies related to mental disorders are not effective, and are only required for individuals who have severe mental disorders or who are considered "crazy." Psychiatric services are, therefore, underutilized among Arab Americans despite greater need for such services among distressed immigrant populations.

Gender and, to a lesser extent, age are considerations in matching Arab patients and health-care providers. In Arab societies, unrelated males and females are not accustomed to interacting. Shyness in women is appreciated, and Muslim men may ignore women out of politeness. Health-care settings, client units, and sometimes waiting rooms are segregated by sex. Male nurses never care for female patients.

Given this background, many Arab Americans may find interacting with a health-care professional of the opposite sex quite embarrassing and stressful. Discomfort may be expressed by refusal to discuss personal information and by a reluctance to disrobe for physical assessments and hygiene. Arab American women patients may refuse to be seen by male American health-care providers, excluding or denying them the opportunity to interact or appropriately diagnose health conditions for high-risk Arab Americans.

STATUS OF HEALTH-CARE PROVIDERS

Arab Americans have great respect for science and medicine. Most Arab Americans are aware of the historical contributions of Arabs in the field of medicine and are proud of their accomplishments. Knowledge held by a doctor is thought to convey authority and power. When ill, most Arab American clients who lack English communication skills prefer to see Arabic-speaking doctors because of their feelings of cultural and linguistic affinity toward Arab American doctors. Many Arabic-speaking clients also feel that Arab American doctors understand them better and feel more at ease speaking with someone from their own culture. However, clients who are able to communicate in English do not usually show preferences for seeing Arab doctors rather than American doctors. In some cases, these clients prefer to be seen by American doctors because they view American doctors as more professional and more respectful to clients than their Arab American counterparts.

Although medicine is perhaps the most respected profession in Arab society, nursing is viewed as a menial profession that conflicts with societal norms proscribing certain female behavior. In this conservative culture, where contact between unrelated males and females is often discouraged, nursing is considered particularly undesirable as an occupation since it requires close contact between the sexes and work during evening and night hours (Abu Gharbieh, 1993). American nurses are regarded more favorably because of their education, expertise, and performance of roles ascribed solely to Arab physicians (for example, performing physical examinations). However, younger immigrants, and especially immigrants who come from Lebanon, Iraq, and Jordan, have more favorable perceptions about nursing as a profession than the older generation of Arab American immigrants (Kulwicki & Kridli, 2001).

Perhaps because Arab physicians tend to be older males and Arab nurses are typically young females, the status and roles of physicians and nurses mirror the hierarchical family structure of Arab society. Physicians require that nurses "know their place" and leave the interpretation of data, decision making, and disclosure of information to them. Nurses conform to the role expectations of physicians and the public and function as medical assistants and housekeepers rather than as critical thinkers and health educators.

CASE STUDY Mrs. Ayesha Said is a 39-year-old Muslim Arab housewife and mother of six who immigrated to the United States from a rural town in southern Iraq 2 years ago. Her mother-in-law and her husband, Mr. Ahmed Said, accompanied her to the United States as participants in a post–Gulf War resettlement program, after spending some time in a Saudi Arabian refugee camp. Their relocation was coordinated by a local international institution that provided an array of services for finding employment and establishing a household, enrolling the children in public schools, and applying for federal aid programs.

Mr. Ahmed, who completed the equivalent of high school, works in a local plastics factory. He speaks some English. He plans to attend an English-language class held at the factory for its many Iraqi employees. Mrs. Ayesha, who has very little formal schooling, spends her day cooking and caring for her children and spouse with the assistance of her mother-in-law. She leaves their home, a three-bedroom upper flat in a poor area of the city, only when she accompanies her husband shopping or when they attend gatherings at the local Islamic center. These events are quite enjoyable because most of those using the center are also recently arrived Iraqi immigrants. She also socializes with other Iraqi women by telephone. Except for interactions with the American personnel at the institute, Mr. Ahmed and Mrs. Ayesha Said remain quite isolated from American society. They have discussed moving to Detroit because of its large Arab community.

Four of the Said children attend public elementary schools, participating in the English as a Second Language (ESL) program. Mr. Ahmed and Mrs. Ayesha are dismayed by their children's rapid acculturation. Although Muslims do not practice holidays such as Halloween, Christmas, Valentine's Day, and Easter, their children plead to participate in these school-related activities.

Mrs. Ayesha is being admitted to the surgical unit after a modified radical mastectomy. According to the physician's notes, she discovered a "lump that didn't go away" about 6 months ago while breast-feeding her youngest child. She delayed seeking care, hoping that *inshallah*, the lump would vanish. Access to care was also limited by Mrs. Ayesha's preference for a female physician and her family's financial constraints; that is, finding a female surgeon willing to treat a patient with limited financial means. Her past medical history includes measles, dental problems, headache, and a reproductive history of seven pregnancies. One child, born prematurely, died soon after birth.

As you enter the room, you see Mrs. Ayesha dozing. Her husband, mother-in-law, and a family friend who speaks English and Arabic and acts as the translator, are at her bedside.

STUDY QUESTIONS

1 Describe Arab Americans with respect to religion, education, occupation, income, and English-language skills. Compare the Said family with Arab Americans as a group.

2 Assess the Said family's risk for experiencing a stressful immigration by relating factors and personal characteristics discussed by Lipson and Meleis (1985).

3 Describe the steps you would take to develop rapport with Mrs. Ayesha and her family during your initial encounter. Include nonverbal behavior and social etiquette, as well as statements or questions that might block communication.

4 Identify interventions that you would employ to accommodate Mrs. Ayesha's "shyness" and modesty.

5 You notice that although Mrs. Ayesha is alert, her husband and sometimes her mother-in-law reply to your questions. Interpret this behavior within a cultural context.

6 Although Mrs. Ayesha is normothermic and states her pain is "little," Mr. Ahmed insists that his wife be covered with several additional blankets and receive an injection for pain. When you attempt to reassure him of his wife's satisfactory recovery, noting as evidence of her stable condition that you plan to "get her up" that evening, he demands to see the physician. Interpret his behavior within a cultural context.

7 Discuss Arab food preferences as well as the dietary restrictions of practicing Muslims. If you filled out Mrs. Ayesha's menu, what would you order?

8 When you give Mrs. Ayesha and her family members discharge instructions, what teaching methods would be most effective? What content regarding recovery from a mastectomy might most Arab Americans consider "too personal"?

9 Identify typical coping strategies of Arabs. What could you do to facilitate Mrs. Ayesha's use of these strategies?

10 Discuss predestination as it influences the Arab American's responses to death and bereavement.

11 Discuss Islamic rulings regarding the following health matters: contraception, abortion, infertility treatment, autopsy, and organ donation and transplant.

12 Describe the Arab American's culturally based role expectations for nurses and physicians. In what ways do the role responsibilities of Arab and American nurses differ?

13 What illnesses or conditions are Arab Americans unlikely to disclose because of Islamic prohibitions or an attached stigma?

14 Compile a health profile (strengths versus challenges) of Arab Americans by comparing beliefs, values, behaviors, and practices favoring health and those negatively influencing health.

REFERENCES

Abu Gharbieh, P. (1993). Culture shock. Cultural norms influencing nursing in Jordan. *Nursing and Health Care, 14*(10), 534–540.

Al-Akili, M. (1993). *Natural healing with the medicine of the prophet.* Philadelphia, PA: Pearl Publishing House.

Arab human development report. (2000). Retrieved October 30, 2002, from http://www.UNESCO.org/education.

Aswad, B. (1999). Arabs in America: Building a new future. In M. W. Suleiman (Ed.), *Attitudes of Arab immigrants toward welfare* (pp. 177–191). Philadelphia: Temple University Press.

Aswad, B. C., & Gray, N. (1996). Challenges to the Arab-American family and ACCESS (Arab Community Center for Economic and Social Services). In B. C. Aswad & B. Bilgé (Eds.), *Family and gender among American Muslims: Issues facing Middle Eastern immigrants and their descendants* (pp. 223–240). Philadelphia: Temple University Press.

Budman, C., Lipson, J., & Meleis, A. (1992). The cultural consultant in mental health care: The case of an Arab adolescent. *American Journal of Orthopsychiatry, 62*(3), 359–370.

Cainkar, L. (1996). Immigrant Palestinian women evaluate their lives. In B. C. Aswad & B. Bilgé (Eds.), *Family and gender among American Muslims: Issues facing Middle Eastern immigrants and their descendants* (pp. 41–58). Philadelphia: Temple University Press.

Cline, S., Abuirmeileh, N., & Roberts, A. (1986). *Woman's life cycle. Fundamentals of health education* (pp. 48–77). Yarmouk, Jordan: Yarmouk University.

Ebrahim, A. (1989). *Abortion, birth control and surrogate parenting. An Islamic perspective.* Indianapolis, IN: American Trust Publications.

El-Badry, S. (1994, January). The Arab-American market. *American Demographics*, pp. 22–31.

El-Islam, M. (1994). Cultural aspects of morbid fears in Qatari women. *Social Psychiatry Psychiatric Epidemiology, 29,* 137–140.

Eisonlohr, C. J. (1996). Adolescent Arab girls in an American high school. In B. C. Aswad & B. Bilgé (Eds.), *Family and gender among American Muslims: Issues facing Middle Eastern immigrants and their descendants* (pp. 250–270). Philadelphia: Temple University Press.

Global Gayz. (2002). http://www.globalgayz.com.

Hamamy, H., & Alwan, A. (1994). Hereditary disorders in the Eastern Mediterranean region. *Bulletin of the World Health Organization, 72*(1), 145–154.

Hashemite Kingdom of Jordan, Department of Statistics. (1985). *Jordan's husbands' fertility survey.* Amman, Jordan: Author, in collaboration with Division of Reproductive Health, Centers for Disease Control, Atlanta, GA.

Hattar-Pollara, M., Meleis, A. I., & Nagib, H. (2001). A study of spousal role of Egyptian women in clerical jobs. *Health Care for Women International, 21*(4), 305–517.

Kasem, C. (1994). *Arab Americans: Making a difference.* Washington, DC: Arab American Institute.

Kulwicki, A. (1996). Health issues among Arab Muslim families. In B. C. Aswad & B. Bilgé (Eds.), *Family and gender among American Muslims: Issues facing Middle Eastern immigrants and their descendants* (pp. 187–207). Philadelphia: Temple University Press.

Kulwicki, A. (2000). Arab women. In M. Julia (Ed.), *Constructing gender: Multicultural perspectives in working with women* (pp. 89–98). Canada: Brooks/Cole.

Kulwicki, A. (Ed.). (2001). *Ethnic resource guide.* Dearborn, MI: Henry Ford Hospital.

Kulwicki, A., & Cass, P. (1994). An assessment of Arab-American knowledge, attitudes, and beliefs about AIDS. *IMAGE: Journal of Nursing Scholarship, 26*(1), 13–17.

Kulwicki, A., & Kridli, S. (2001). Health-care perceptions and experiences of Chaldean, Arab Muslim, Arab Christian, and Armenian women in the metropolitan area of Detroit. Unpublished manuscript.

Kulwicki, A., & Miller, J. (1999). Domestic violence in the Arab American population: Transforming environmental conditions through community education. *Issues in Mental Health Nursing 20*(3) 199–215.

Kulwicki, A., Miller, J., & Schim, S. (2000). Collaborative partnership for culture care: Enhancing health services for the Arab community. *Journal of Transcultural Nursing, 11*(1), 31–39.

Kurian, G. (Ed.). (1992). *Encyclopedia of the third world.* New York: Facts on File.

Laffrey, S., Meleis, A., Lipson, J., Solomon, M., & Omidian, P. (1989). Assessing Arab-American health care needs. *Social Science and Medicine, 29*(7), 877–883.

Levy, R. (1993). Ethnic and racial differences in response to medicines: Preserving individualized therapy in managed pharmaceutical programmes. *Pharmaceutical Medicine, 7,* 139–165.

Lipson, J., & Meleis, A. (1985). Culturally appropriate care: The case of immigrants. *Topics in Clinical Nursing, 7*(3), 48–56.

Lipson, J., Reizian, A., & Meleis, A. (1987). Arab-American patients: A medical record review. *Social Science and Medicine, 24*(2), 101–107.

Luna, L. (1994). Care and cultural context of Lebanese Muslim immigrants: Using Leininger's theory. *Journal of Transcultural Nursing, 5*(2), 12–20.

Meleis, A., & La Fever, C. (1984). The Arab American and psychiatric care. *Perspectives in Psychiatric Care, 22,* 72–86.

Michigan Department of Public Health. (1993). *Health profiles of Michigan populations.* Lansing, MI: Author.

Michigan Department of Public Health. (1995). *Health profiles of Michigan populations.* Lansing, MI: Author.

Naff, A. (1980). *Arabs in America: A historical overview* (pp. 128–136), Boston, MA: Harvard Encyclopedia of American Ethnic Groups.

Nydell, M. (1987). *Understanding Arabs. A guide for Westerners.* Yarmouth, ME: Intercultural Press.

Office of Minority Health (OMH). (2001). *Health facts.* Retrieved October 21, 2001, from http://www.mdch.state.mi.us/pha/omh/aram-ch.htm.

Patai, R. (1958). *The kingdom of Jordan.* Princeton, NJ: Princeton University Press.

Pickthall, M. (1977). *The meaning of the glorious Qur'an.* Mecca, Saudi Arabia: Muslim World League.

Reiter, S., Mar'i, S., & Rosenberg, Y. (1986). Parental attitudes toward the developmentally disabled among Arab communities in Israel: A cross-cultural study. *International Journal of Rehabilitation Research, 9*(4), 335–362.

Reizian, A., & Meleis, A. (1986). Arab-Americans' perceptions of and responses to pain. *Critical Care Nurse, 6*(6), 30–37.

Reizian, A., & Meleis, A. (1987). Symptoms reported by Arab-American patients on the Cornell Medical Index (CMI). *Western Journal of Nursing Research, 9*(3), 368–384.

Rice, V., & Kulwicki, A. (1992). Cigarette use among Arab Americans in the Detroit metropolitan area. *Public Health Reports, 107*(5), 589–594.

Seikaly, M. (1999). Arabs in America: Building a new future. In M. W. Suleiman (Ed.), *Attachment and identity: the Palestinian community of Detroit* (pp. 25–38). Philadelphia: Temple University Press.

Sullivan, S. (1993) The patient behind the veil: Medical culture shock in Saudi Arabia. *Canadian Medical Association Journal, 148*(3), 444–446.

UNICEF. (2001). Life expectancy and infant mortality estimates from Population Division of the United Nations Secretariat. *World population prospects: The 2000 revision.* Supplemented by demographic yearbook 1998 and population vital statistics report, statistical papers, series A, vol. 53, no. 2. Geneva: UNICEF.

Vincent-Barwood, A. (1986). The Arab immigrants. *Aramco World Magazine, 37*(5), 10–13,15.

Wayne County Health Department. (1994). *Arab community in Wayne County, Michigan: Behavior risk factor survey (BRFS).* East Lansing, MI: Michigan State University, Institute for Public Policy and Social Research.

West, M. (1987, April 29). *Surveys indicate girls face discrimination in provision of nutrition and health care.* Jordan Times.

World Health Organization. (2001a). *AIDS update.* Retrieved October 21, 2001, from http://www.emro.who.int/aidnews/June1999/AIDSSupdate.

World Health Organization, (2001b). *EMR country profile-health status indicators.* Retrieved October 21, 2001, from http://www.emro.who.int/emrinfo/socioeconomic.inc.

Yousef, J. (1993). Education of children with mental retardation in Arab countries. *Mental Retardation, 31*(2), 117–121.

Zogby, J. (1990). Arab America today. A demographic profile of Arab Americans. Washington, DC: Arab American Institute.

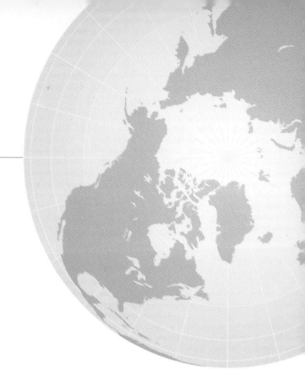

Chapter 7

People of Chinese Heritage

YAN WANG

Overview, Inhabited Localities, and Topography

OVERVIEW

Although some Western health-care providers categorize all Asians together in one group, each nationality is very different. Cultural values differ even among Chinese according to their geographic location within China—north, south, east, west; rural versus urban; interior versus port city—as well as other primary and secondary characteristics of culture (see Chapter 1). Chinese immigrants to Western countries are even more diverse, with a mixture of traditional and Western values and beliefs. These differences must be acknowledged and appreciated.

Most Chinese are **Han** (almost 92 percent); the remaining 8 percent are a mixture of 56 different nationalities, religions, and ethnic groups. Because of the complexity of their values, it is impossible to develop specific cultural interventions appropriate for all Chinese clients. Therefore, the information included in this chapter should serve simply as a beginning point for understanding Chinese people, not as a definitive profile.

Children born to Chinese parents in Western countries tend to adopt the Western culture easily. Their parents and grandparents tend to maintain their traditional Chinese culture in varying degrees. Chinese who live in the "Chinatowns" of North America maintain many of their cultural and social beliefs and values and insist that health-care providers respect these values and beliefs with their prescribed interventions.

HERITAGE AND RESIDENCE

The Chinese culture is one of the oldest recorded cultures in human history, beginning with the Xia dynasty, dating from 2200 B.C., to the present-day People's Republic of China (PRC). The Chinese name for their country is *Zhong guo*, which means "middle kingdom" or "center of the earth." Many of the current values and beliefs of the Chinese remain grounded in their history; many believe that Chinese culture is superior to other Asian cultures. Ideals based on the teachings of Confucius (551–479 B.C.) continue to play an important part in the values and beliefs of the Chinese. These ideals emphasize the importance of accountability to family and neighbors and reinforce the idea that all relationships embody power and rule.

During early Communist rule, an attempt was made to break down the values grounded in Confucianism and substitute values consistent with equal social responsibility. This was initially achieved, and rank in society was no longer seen as important. During the People's Revolution, feudal rank frequently meant loss of social importance, physical punishment, imprisonment, and even death. Later, during the Cultural Revolution, the young were held responsible for the deaths of many previously esteemed elderly and educated Chinese. Today, many of the Confucian values have reasserted themselves. Families, the elderly, and highly educated individuals are again considered important. Research completed by the Chinese Culture Connection (a group of Chinese sociologists) lists 40 important values in modern China, including filial piety, industry, patriotism, paying deference to those in hierarchal status positions, tolerance of others, loyalty to superiors, respect for rites and social rituals, knowledge, benevolent authority, thrift, patience, courtesy, and respect for tradition (Hu & Grove, 1991).

The population of China is 1.26 billion people, with 80 percent of the Chinese living in rural communities. The country is over 9.6 million square kilometers (3.7 million square miles), with 23 provinces, 5 regions, (including Tibet, Hong Kong, and Taiwan), and 3 municipalities. Each province, region, and municipality functions independently and in many different ways. The Chinese consider each region as part of greater China and predict that the day will come when all of China is reunited. Tibet has already been reassimilated, Hong Kong returned to Chinese control in 1997, and Macau in 1999.

Chinese Americans comprise the largest subgroup among Asians/Pacific Islanders (APIs), exceeding 1.6 million people, and they are the second largest immigrant group after Mexicans. Every year the quota for Chinese immigration to the United States has been filled, with more than 40,600 immigrants arriving from mainland China, Taiwan, and Hong Kong. It is estimated that at the current rate of immigration to the United States, the Chinese American population will double every 10 years (Wong, 1987). Chinese Americans reside in various regions of the country, but the largest communities are in California, New York, Hawaii, and Texas (Ma, 1999).

REASONS FOR MIGRATION AND ASSOCIATED ECONOMIC FACTORS

Chinese immigrated to the United States in three different waves: in the 1800s, in the 1950s, and in recent years. Chinese immigration was initially fueled by economic needs. Over 100,000 male peasants from Guangdong and Fujian came to the United States without their families in the early 1830s to make their fortune on the transcontinental railroad. This immigration continued through the Gold Rush of 1849. Many believed that they could make money in the United States to help their families and later return to China. Unfortunately, most found that opportunities were limited to hard labor and other vocations that were not desired by European Americans. Their culture and physical features made them readily identifiable in the predominantly white American society. They could not simply change their names and blend in with other primarily European immigrant populations. The Chinese had few rights. They were barred from becoming American citizens. Racial violence and prejudice against them were common, and the courts did not punish the violators. Compared with other ethnic groups, their immigration numbers were small until 1952, when the McCarran-Walters Bill relaxed immigration laws and permitted more Chinese to enter the country.

The most recent immigrants from Taiwan, Hong Kong, and mainland China are strikingly different from earlier Chinese immigrants in that they are more diverse. In addition, while many emigrated to reunite with families, there were also students, scholars, and professionals flocking to the United States to pursue higher education or research. For their safety and the maintenance of their cultural values, most Chinese settled in closed communities.

EDUCATIONAL STATUS AND OCCUPATIONS

Education is compulsory in China, and most children receive the equivalent of a ninth-grade education. Middle-school students must complete a state examination to determine their eligibility to enter a general high school, to go to a preparatory high school before entering technical school or college, or to begin their lives as workers. Those who complete either the general or preparatory high school experience compete academically to continue their education at college and university levels. The Chinese educational system is complex and is not presented here in its entirety; further study is encouraged.

A university education is highly valued; however, few have the opportunity to achieve this life goal because enrollments in better educational institutions are limited. Because competition for top universities is keen, many families select less-valued universities to ensure that their child is accepted into a university rather than slated for a technical school education. After their undergraduate or graduate programs, many young adults come to Western countries to attend universities to seek more advanced education or research. A foreign education is considered prestigious in China.

In the West, the Chinese tend to be either highly or poorly educated. This dichotomy may result in health-care providers categorizing clients in a similar manner, but usually assuming that clients have a poor education because they may not have attained positions of power or high economic levels. Many people believe that Chinese occupations are limited to restaurants, service employment, and the garment industry. However, this phenomenon has changed in the past decade. A significant number of Chinese students and scholars from the PRC and Taiwan come to the United States to study every year. Because of the competitive educational system in mainland China and Taiwan, where only the brightest students go to a university, Chinese immigrants with a college education are often very well educated. Student immigrants are expected to return to China or Taiwan when their education and research are completed. However, many do not return, but elect to remain in Western countries, having obtained graduate degrees in the United States and having found employment in high technology companies or in educational and research institutes.

Another group of Chinese immigrants are professionals from Hong Kong who moved to Canada, the United States, and other Western countries to avoid the repatriation in 1997. These immigrants usually have family connections or close friends in Western countries who are highly educated and skilled. A third group of immigrants consists of uneducated individuals with diverse manual labor skills. Finding employment opportunities for these Chinese people may be more difficult. They often settle with family members who are not skilled or highly educated. This arrangement drains family resources for many years until they obtain financial security, learn the language, and become acculturated in other ways.

Communication

DOMINANT LANGUAGE AND DIALECTS

The official language of China is Mandarin (**pu tong hua**), which is spoken by about 70 percent of the population, primarily in northern China, but there are 10 major, distinct dialects, including Cantonese, Fujianese, Shanghainese, Toishanese, and Hunanese. For example, *pu tong hua* is spoken in Beijing, the capital of China in the north, and Shanghainese is spoken in Shanghai. The two cities are only 1462 kilometers (about 665 miles) apart, but because the dialects are so different, the two groups cannot understand one another verbally. Even though people from one part of China cannot understand those from other regions, the written language is the same throughout the country. It consists of over 50,000 characters (about 5000 common ones); thus, most children are at least 10 to 12 years old before they can read the newspaper.

Although many times Chinese sound loud when talking with other Chinese, they generally speak in a moderate to low voice. Americans are considered loud to most Chinese, and health-care providers must be cautious about tone of voice when interacting with Chinese in English so that intentions are not misinterpreted.

When possible, health-care providers should use the Chinese language to communicate (see Table 7–1 for some common phrases), being careful to avoid jargon and use the simplest terms. Many times verbs can be omitted because the Chinese language has only a limited number of verbs. The Chinese appreciate any attempt to use their language. They do not mind mistakes and will correct speakers when they believe that it will not cause embarrassment. When asked whether they understand what was just said, the Chinese invariably answer yes, even when they do not understand. Such an admission causes loss of face; thus, it is better to have clients repeat the instructions they have been given.

Negative queries are difficult for Chinese people to understand. For example, do not say, "You know how to do that, don't you?" Instead say, "Do you know how to do that?" Also, it is easier for them to understand instructions placed in a specific order, such as "One, at nine o'clock every morning get the medicine bottle. Two, take two tablets out of the bottle. Three, get your hot water. Four, swallow the pills with the water." Do not use complex sentences with *ands* and *buts*. The Chinese have difficulty deciding what to respond to first when the speaker uses compound or complex sentences.

Table 7–1 Frequently Used Words and Phrases

English Word or Phrase	Chinese Pinyin	Phonetic Pronunciation
Hello	*Nǐ hǎo*	Nee how (note tones to be used*)
Goodbye	*Zài jiàn*	Dzai jee en
How are you?	*Nǐ hǎo mā*	Nee how mah
Please	*Qing*	Ching
Thank you	*Xǐe xie*	Shee eh shee eh
I don't understand	*Wo bù dǒng*	Wah boo doong
Yes	*Shì de* or *dui*	Shur da or doee (no real yes or no comparable saying—this means I agree or okay)
No	*Bú shì de* or *bu hǎo*	Boo shur or boo how
My name is	*Wo jiào*	Wah djeeow
Very good	*Hen hǎo*	Hun hao
Hurt	*Téng*	Tung
I, you, he/she/it	*Wo, nǐ, tā*	Wah, nee, tah
Hot	*Rè*	Ruh
Cold	*Lěng*	Lung
Happy	*Gāo xìngu*	Gow shing
Where	*Nǎ li*	Na lee
Not have	*Méi yǒu*	May yo
Doctor	*Yī shēng*	Yee shung
Nurse	*Hù shì*	Who shur

* *Note:* Each *pu tong hua* Chinese word is pronounced with five different tones:
1. First tone is high and even across the word (¯).
2. Second tone starts low and goes high (ˊ).
3. Third tone starts neutral, goes low, and then goes high (ˇ).
4. Fourth tone curt and goes low (ˋ).
5. Fifth tone is neutral and pronounced very lightly.

CULTURAL COMMUNICATION PATTERNS

Chinese have a reputation for not openly displaying emotion. Although this may be true among strangers, among family and friends they are open and demonstrative. The Chinese share information freely with health-care providers once a trusting relationship has developed. This is not always easy because Western health-care providers may not have the patience or time to develop such relationships. In situations where Chinese people perceive that health-care practitioners or other people of authority may lose face or be embarrassed, they may choose not to be totally truthful.

Touching between health-care providers and Chinese clients should be kept to a minimum. Most Chinese maintain a formal distance with each other, which is a form of respect. Many are uncomfortable with face-to-face communications, especially when there is direct eye contact. Because they prefer to sit next to others, the health-care practitioner may need to rearrange seating to promote positive communication. When touching is necessary, the practitioner should provide explanations to Chinese clients.

Facial expressions are used extensively among family and friends. The Chinese love to joke and laugh. They use and appreciate smiles when talking with others. However, if the situation is formal, smiles may be limited. Other body movements are used when communicating with family and friends or when they are angry. In formal business situations or greeting people with high rank, their use of body movements may be limited. It is best to watch them for cues of expression.

FORMAT FOR NAMES

Among Chinese people the manner of introductions, either by name card or verbally, is different from Western countries. For example, the family name is stated first and then the given name. Calling individuals by any name except their family name is impolite unless they are close friends or relatives. If a person's family name is Li and the given name is Ruiming, then the proper form of address is Li Ruiming. Men are addressed by their family name, such as *Ma*, and a title such as *Ma xian sheng* ("Mister Ma") or *lao Ma* ("respected elder Ma") or *xiao Ma* ("young Ma"). Titles are important to Chinese people, so when possible, identify the person's title and use it.

Women in China do not use their husband's name after they get married. Therefore, unless the woman is from Hong Kong or Taiwan, or has lived in a Western country for a long time, do not assume that her last name is the same as her husband's. Her family name comes first, followed by her given names and finally by her title. Many Chinese take an English name as an additional given name because their name is difficult for Westerners to pronounce. Their English name can be used in many settings. It is better to address them as "Miss Millie" or "Mr. Jonathan" rather than simply by their English name. Even though they have adopted an English name, some Chinese may give permission to use only the English name. In addition, some Chinese switch the order of their names to be the same as Westerners, with their family name last. This practice can be confusing; therefore, health-care providers should address Chinese clients by their whole name or by their family name and title, and then ask the person how they wish to be addressed.

Family Roles and Organization

HEAD OF HOUSEHOLD AND GENDER ROLES

Kinship traditionally has been organized around the male lines. Fathers, sons, and uncles are the important, recognized, relationships between and among families in politics and in business. Each family maintains a recognized head that has great authority and assumes all major responsibilities for the family.

Another traditional practice in many rural Chinese families is the submissive role of the daughter-in-law to the mother-in-law. Many times the mother-in-law is demanding and hostile to the daughter-in-law and may treat her worse than the servants. This relationship has changed significantly since modern culture was introduced to Chinese society. However, such relationships may continue to influence some Chinese families today to some extent, or mothers-in-law and daughters-in-law may simply not get along with each other.

The Chinese view of women is perpetuated to ensure male dominance in a society that has existed for centuries. Men still remain in control of the country largely because of stereotypical roles of men and women. However, since the founding of the People's Republic of China, this has been changing somewhat. In 1949, the Communist Party stated that "women hold up half the sky" and are legally equal to men. In China today, over 90 percent of the women work (Chin, 1988), and many hold professional positions or are prestigious leaders. Even though legally women are considered equal, they are frequently forced to accept more menial positions. The traditional gender roles of women are changing, but a sense remains that the woman's responsibility is to maintain a happy and efficient home life, especially in rural China. In recent times, some Chinese men include housework, cooking, and cleaning as their responsibilities when their spouses work. Most Chinese believe that the family is most important and, thus, each family member assumes changes in roles to achieve this harmony.

PRESCRIPTIVE, RESTRICTIVE, AND TABOO BEHAVIORS FOR CHILDREN AND ADOLESCENTS

Children are highly valued in China, especially now that China's one-child rule is in effect. Because of overpopulation in China, the government has mandated that each married couple may only have one child; however, in some rural areas if the first-born child is female, the couple may get permission to have a second child. Families often wait many years, until they are financially secure, to have a child. After the child is born, many family resources are lavished on the child. Families may only be able to afford to live with relatives in a two-room apartment, but if the family believes that the child will benefit by having a piano, then the resources will be found to provide a piano. Children are well dressed and kept clean and well fed.

In China, the child is protected from birth and independence is not fostered. The entire family makes decisions for the child even into young adulthood. Children usually depend on the family for everything. Few teens earn money because they are expected to study hard and to help the family with daily chores rather than to seek employment. Children feel a lot of pressure to succeed to help improve the future of the family and the country. Their common goal is to score well on the national examinations when they reach age 18 years. Most Chinese children and adolescents value studying over playing and peer relationships. They recognize that they are constantly evaluated on having healthy bodies and minds and achieving excellent marks in school.

In rural communities, male children are more valued than female children because they continue the family line and provide labor. In urban areas, female children are valued as highly as male children. Children in China are taught to curb their expression of feelings because individuals who do not stand out are successful. However, this is changing. The young in China today frequently think that their parents are too cautious. The children are becoming even more outspoken as they read more and watch more television and movies.

From elementary school to university, students take courses in Marxist politics and learn not to question the doctrine of the country. If they do, they may be interrogated and ridiculed for their radical thoughts. Nationalism is important to Chinese children, and they want to help their country continue to be the center of the world. Children are also expected to help their parents in the home. Many times in the cities when children get home from school before their parents, they are expected to do their homework immediately and then do their household chores. They exhibit their independence not so much by expressing their individual views but by performing chores on their own. However, since China's one-child rule, parents and grandparents spoil most children. They are expected to earn good grades and household chores are not encouraged. While it is acceptable for the children to perform chores on their own, it is not encouraged. If children wish to do chores on their own, it is acceptable.

Lin and Fu (1990) studied 138 children (44 Chinese, 46 Chinese Americans, and 48 white Americans) in kindergarten through second grade and found that both Chinese and Chinese American parents expected increased achievement and parental control over their children. One surprising finding was the high expectation for independence in Chinese and Chinese American children.

Boys and girls play together when they are young, but as they get older, this changes because their roles, and the corresponding expectations, are predetermined by Chinese society. Girls and boys both study hard. Boys are more active, and take pride in physical fitness. Girls are not nearly as interested in fitness as boys, and often enjoy reading, art, and music.

Adolescents are expected to determine who they are and where they want to end up in life. Adolescents maintain their respect for elders even when they disagree with them, and while they may argue with their parents and teachers, they have learned that it seldom does any good. Teens value a strong and happy family life, and seldom do things that jeopardize that unanimity. Adolescents question affairs of life and make great efforts to see at least two sides of every issue. They enjoy exploring different views with their peers and try to explore them with their parents.

Teenage pregnancy is not common among the Chinese, but it is increasing among Chinese Americans (Butterfield, 1990). Young men and women enter the workforce immediately after high school if they are unable to continue their education. Many continue to live with their parents and contribute to the family even after marriage (in their twenties) and the birth of a child (in their thirties).

FAMILY GOALS AND PRIORITIES

The Chinese perception of family is through the concept of relationships. Each person identifies himself or herself in relation to others in the family. The individual is not lost, just defined differently from individuals in Western cultures. Personal independence is not valued; rather, Confucian teachings state that true value is in the relationships a person has with others, especially the family.

Older children who experienced the Cultural Revolution may feel some discomfort with their traditional parents. During the Cultural Revolution, the young were encouraged to inform on elders and peers who did not espouse the doctrine of the time. Most of those who were reported were sent to "reeducation camps" where they did hard labor and were "taught the correct way to think." As a result, many families have been permanently separated.

Extended families are important to the Chinese and function by providing ways to get ahead. Often children live with their grandparents or aunts and uncles so individual family members can obtain a better education or reduce financial burdens. Relatives are expected to help each other through connections (**guan xi**), which are used by Chinese society in a manner similar to the use of money in other cultures. Such connections are perceived as obligations and are placed in a mental bank with deposits and withdrawals. These commitments may remain in the "bank" for years or generations until they are used to get jobs, housing, business contacts, gifts, medical care, or anything that demands a payback.

Filial loyalty to the family is extended to other Chinese. When Chinese immigrants need additional assistance, health-care providers may be able to call on local Chinese organizations to obtain help for clients.

Elderly people in China are venerated just as they were in earlier years. Chinese government leaders are often elderly and remain in power until they are in their seventies, eighties, and beyond. Traditional Chinese people view the elderly as very wise, a view that communism has not changed. Chinese children are expected to care for their parents, and in China this is mandated by law.

Younger Chinese who adopt Western ideas and values may find that the expectations of their elders are too demanding. Even though younger Chinese Americans do not live with their elders, they maintain respect and visit them frequently. Elderly Chinese mothers are viewed as central to family feelings, and elderly fathers retain their roles as leaders. As generations live in areas removed from China, families become more Westernized, and family relationships need to be assessed on an individual basis. An extended-family pattern is common and has existed for over 2000 years. The traditional marriage still remains nuclear. Historically in China, marriage was used to strengthen positions of families in society.

Kinship relationships are based on the concept of loyalty, and the young experience pressure to improve the family's standing. Many parents give up items of daily living to provide more for their children, thereby increasing opportunities for them to get ahead.

Maintaining reputation is very important to the Chinese and is accomplished by adhering to the rules of society. Because power and control are important to Chinese society, rank is very important. True equality does not exist in the Chinese mind; their history has demonstrated that equality cannot exist. If more than one person is in power, then consensus is important. If the person in power is not present at decision-making meetings, barriers are raised and any decisions made are negated unless the person in power agrees. Even after negotiations have been concluded and contracts signed, the Chinese continue to negotiate.

The Chinese concept of privacy is even more important than recognized social status, corresponding values, and beliefs. The Chinese word for privacy has a negative connotation and means something underhanded, secret, and furtive. People grow up in crowded conditions, they live and work in small areas, and their value of group support does not place a high value on privacy. The Chinese may ask many personal questions about salary, life at home, age, and children. Refusal to answer personal questions is accepted as long as it is done with care and feeling. The one subject that is taboo is sex and anything related to sex. This may create a barrier for a Western health-care provider who is trying to assess a Chinese client with sexual problems. They may feel uncomfortable discussing or answering questions about sex with honesty. Privacy is also limited by territorial boundaries. Some Chinese may enter rooms without knocking or invade privacy by not allowing a person to be alone. The need to be alone is viewed as "not good" to some Chinese, and they may not understand when a Westerner wants to be alone. A mutual understanding of these beliefs is necessary for harmonious working relationships.

ALTERNATIVE LIFESTYLES

Alternative lifestyles are not common and not encouraged by Chinese society. The Chinese do not condone same-sex relationships. In many provinces, they are illegal and punishable by death. The goals of all men and women are supposed to be marriage and the procreation of one child. Chinese women and men generally are not encouraged to marry until they are between the ages of 25 and 28 years because of the government's population control policy. There are few single-parent families unless a death has occurred. Divorce is legal, but not encouraged. For reasons such as tradition, consideration of children's feelings, and difficulty in remarrying, many Chinese families would rather stay in an unhealthy marriage than divorce. Remarriage is encouraged, but some difficult relationships may occur in this new family, especially remarriage with children from previous marriages.

Workforce Issues

CULTURE IN THE WORKPLACE

China is becoming more Westernized with high technology and increased knowledge. The Communist Party is responsible for establishing the **dan wei**, local Chinese work units that are responsible for jobs, homes, health, enforcing governmental regulations, and problem-solving for families. Although recent immigrants know that the culture in the workplace is different in the United States, they adapt to it quickly. The Chinese acculturate by learning as much as possible about their new culture in the workplace. They observe people from the culture and listen closely for nuances in language and interpersonal connections. They frequently call on other Chinese people to teach them and to discuss how to fit into the new culture more quickly. Chinese Americans support one another in new cultures and help each other find resources and learn to live effectively and efficiently in the new culture. They also watch television and go to movies to learn about Western ways of life. They read about the new culture in magazines, books, and newspapers. They love to travel, and when an opportunity arises to see different aspects of the new culture, they do not hesitate to do so.

The Chinese are accustomed to giving coworkers small gifts of appreciation for helping them acculturate and adapt to the American workforce. Often, Americans seek opportunities to reciprocate with a gift, such as at a birthday party, farewell party, or other occasion. Whereas a wide variety of gifts are appropriate, some gifts are not. For example, giving an umbrella means that you wish to have the recipient's family dispersed; giving a gift that is white in color or wrapped in white could be interpreted as meaning the giver wishes the recipient dead; and giving a clock or watch could be interpreted as never wanting to see the person again or wishing the person's life to end (Smith, 2002).

On the surface, Chinese Americans form classic external networks. These five traditional bases for Chinese networks include groupings by: (1) family surname, (2) locality of origin in China, (3) dialect or subdialect spoken, (4) craft practiced, and (5) trust from prior experience or recommendation. Therefore, Chinese Americans approximate external networks with some characteristic of internal networks (Haley, Tan, & Haley, 1998).

Guanxi is a Mandarin term with no exact English translation. This term includes the concept of trust and presenting uprightness to build close relationships. It definitely helps to build networks. This *Guanxi* network can be used in the work-related, decision-making process and is also used with family, friends, and community-related issues in the Chinese American community.

ISSUES RELATED TO AUTONOMY

Historically, the Chinese have been autonomous. They had to exhibit this characteristic to survive through difficult times. However, their autonomy is limited, and is based on functioning for the good of the group. When a new situation arises that requires independent decision making, many times the Chinese know what should be done but do not take action until the leader or superior gives permission. However, the Western workforce expects independence, and some Chinese may need to be taught that true autonomy is necessary to advance. Health-care providers should be aware, however, that the training might not be successful because it is foreign to Chinese cultural values. It is best to demonstrate alternatives, leaving it up to the individuals to determine if assertiveness can be a part of their lives. After acculturation takes place, Chinese Americans do not differ significantly in assertiveness.

Language may be a barrier for Chinese immigrants seeking assimilation into the Western workforce. Western languages and Chinese have many differences, among them sentence structure and the use of intonation. Chinese does not have verbs that denote tense, as in Western languages. While the ordering of the words in a sentence is basically the same, with the subject first and then the verb, the Chinese language places descriptive adjectives in different orders. Intonation in Chinese is in the words themselves, rather than in the sentence. Chinese people who have taken English lessons can usually read and write English competently, but they may have difficulty in understanding and speaking it.

Biocultural Ecology

SKIN COLOR AND OTHER BIOLOGIC VARIATIONS

The skin color of Chinese is varied. Many have skin color similar to Westerners with pink undertones. Some have a yellow tone, while others are very dark. Mongolian spots, dark bluish spots over the lower back and buttocks, are present in about 80 percent of infants. Bilirubin levels are usually higher in Chinese newborns, with the highest levels occurring on the fifth or sixth day after birth.

While the Chinese are distinctly Mongolian, their Asian characteristics have many variations. China is very large and includes people from many different backgrounds, including Mongols and Tibetans. Generally, men and women are shorter than Westerners, but some Chinese are over 6 feet tall. Differences in bone structure are evidenced in the ulna, which is longer than the radius. Hip measurements are significantly smaller: females are 4.14 centimeters smaller, and males 7.6 centimeters smaller than Westerners (Seidel et al., 1994). Not only is overall bone length shorter, but also bone

density is less. Chinese have a high hard palate, which may cause them problems with Western dentures. Their hair is generally black and straight, but some have naturally curly hair. Most Chinese men do not have much facial or chest hair. The Rh-negative blood group is rare, and twins are not common in Chinese families, but are greatly valued, especially since the emergence of China's one-child law.

DISEASES AND HEALTH CONDITIONS

Many Chinese who come to the United States settle in large cities like San Francisco and New York, so they are at risk for the same problems and diseases experienced by other inner-city populations. For example, crowding in large cities often results in poor sanitation and increases the incidence of infectious diseases, air pollution, and violence.

The three major causes of death in China are the same as in the United States: heart disease, other circulatory diseases, and cancers (Lawson & Lin, 1994). Life expectancy in China is 67 years for males and 71 years for females, an amazing increase from a longevity of 35 years in the 1970s. Life expectancy is roughly the same in the United States (Lawson & Lin, 1994). Disease incidence has decreased as well, but major problems still exist in rural China, where perinatal deaths and deaths from infectious diseases remain high. Tobacco use is a major problem and results in an increased incidence of lung disease. Health-care providers must screen newer immigrants from China for these health-related conditions and provide interventions in a culturally congruent manner.

Thalassemia, a genetic disease, affects Chinese people in one of two ways. One form (β-thalassemia) is evidenced by a smaller but increased number of red blood cells, and does not usually affect one's health status; the other form (α-thalassemia) is evidenced as anemia followed by an early death (Gaspard, 1994). A sex-linked genetic disease common in the Chinese is glucose-6-phosphate dehydrogenase deficiency (G-6-PD), an enzyme deficiency affecting the person's red blood cells, resulting in anemia (Gaspard, 1994). Finally, the Chinese have an increased incidence of lactose intolerance, resulting in diarrhea, indigestion, and bloating when milk and milk products are consumed.

Many Chinese immigrants have an increased incidence of hepatitis B and tuberculosis. Poor living conditions and overcrowding in some areas of China enhance the development of these diseases, which persist after immigrants settle in other countries.

Studies by the Office of Minority Health Resource Center in Washington, D.C., have found that Chinese American women have a 20 percent higher rate of pancreatic cancer and higher rates of suicide after the age of 45 years, and all Chinese have higher death rates due to diabetes. The incidence of different types of cancer, including cervical, liver, lung, stomach, multiple myeloma, esophageal, pancreatic, and nasopharyngeal cancers, is higher among Chinese Americans (Office of Minority Health Resource Center, 2001). Overall, the incidence of disease in this population has not been studied sufficiently, and continuing research is desperately needed.

VARIATIONS IN DRUG METABOLISM

Multiple studies outlining problems with drug metabolism and sensitivity have been conducted among the Chinese. Results suggest a poor metabolism of mephenytoin (for example, diazepam) in 15 to 20 percent of Chinese; sensitivity to beta-blockers, such as propranolol, as evidenced by a decrease in the overall blood levels accompanied by a seemingly more profound response; atropine sensitivity, as evidenced by an increased heart rate; and increased responses to antidepressants and neuroleptics given at lower doses. Analgesics have been found to cause increased gastrointestinal side effects, despite a decreased sensitivity to them. In addition, the Chinese have an increased sensitivity to the effects of alcohol (Levy, 1993).

Delineating specific variations in drug metabolism among the Chinese is difficult because various studies tend to group them in aggregate as Asians. Much more research needs to be completed to determine variations between Westerners and Asians as well as among Asians.

High-Risk Behaviors

High-risk behaviors are difficult to determine with accuracy among Chinese in the United States because most of the data on Chinese are included in the aggregate called Asian Americans. However, the Chinese are not without high-risk health behaviors. Smoking is a high-risk behavior for many Chinese men and teenagers. Most Chinese women do not smoke, but recently the numbers for women are increasing, especially after immigration to the United States. Travelers in China see more cigarette vendors in the streets than any other type of vendor. The decrease in smoking in the United States resulted in cigarette manufacturers' identifying China as a good market in which to sell their product.

Even though alcohol consumption among Chinese has been high at times, the level is currently low (Weatherspoon, Danko, & Johnson, 1994). Despite these findings, the use of alcohol contributes to a high incidence of vehicle accidents and related trauma. HIV, AIDS, and sexually transmitted diseases are lower among Chinese and other Asian Americans compared with other groups in the United States (Centers for Disease Control, 2001).

Nutrition

MEANING OF FOOD

Food habits are important to the Chinese, who offer food to their guests at any time of the day or night. Most celebrations with family and business events focus on food. Foods served at Chinese meals have a specific order, with the focus on a balance for a healthy body. The importance of food is demonstrated daily in its use to promote good health and to combat disease and injury. Traditional Chinese medicine frequently uses food and food derivatives to prevent and cure diseases and illnesses and increase the strength of weak and elderly people.

COMMON FOODS AND FOOD RITUALS

The typical Chinese diet is difficult to describe because each region in China has its own traditional diet. Peanuts and soybeans are popular. Common grains include wheat, sorghum, and maize (a type of corn). Rice is usually steamed but can be fried with eggs, vegetables, and meats as well. Many Chinese just eat beans or noodles instead of rice. The Chinese eat steamed and fried rice noodles, which are usually eaten with a broth base and include vegetables and meats. Meat choices include pork (the most common), chicken, beef, duck, shrimp, fish, scallops, and mussels. Tofu, an excellent source of protein, is a staple of the Chinese diet. It is prepared in many different ways, from fried to boiled, or cold like ice cream. Bean products are another source of protein, and many of the desserts or sweets in Chinese diets are prepared with red beans.

At celebrations, before-dinner toasts are usually made to family and business colleagues. The toasts may be interspersed with speeches, or the speeches may be incorporated in the toasts. Cold appetizers often include peanuts and seasonal fruits. Chopsticks, a chopstick holder, a small plate, and glass are part of the table setting. If the foods are messy, like Beijing duck, then a finger towel may be available. The Chinese use ceramic or porcelain spoons for soup. Knives are unnecessary because the food is usually served in bite-sized pieces. Chopsticks may be difficult for some at first, but the Chinese are good-natured and are pleased by any attempt to use them. Chopsticks should never be stuck in the food upright because that is considered bad luck (Smith, 2002). Westerners soon learn that slurping, burping, and other noises are not considered offensive, but are appreciated. The Chinese are very relaxed at meals and commonly rest their elbows on the table.

Fruits and vegetables may be peeled or eaten raw. Some vegetables commonly eaten raw by Westerners are usually cooked by the Chinese. Unpeeled raw fruits and vegetables are sources of contamination due to unsanitary conditions in China. The Chinese enjoy their vegetables lightly stir-fried in oil with salt and spice. Salt, oil, and oil products are important parts of the Chinese diet.

Drinks with dinner include tea, soft drinks, juice, or beer. Foreign-born Chinese and older Chinese may not like ice in their drinks. They may just not like cold while eating, or some may believe that it is damaging to their body and shocks the body systems out of balance. On the other hand, hot drinks are enjoyed and believed to be safe for the body. This "goodness" of hot drinks may stem from tradition when the only safe drinks were made from boiled water. All food is put in the center of the table. It may come all at one time, but usually multiple courses are served. The host either serves the most important guests firsts or signals everyone to start.

DIETARY PRACTICES FOR HEALTH PROMOTION

Food is important for the Chinese in maintaining their health. Foods that are considered yin and yang prevent sudden imbalances and indigestion. A balanced diet is considered essential for physical and emotional harmony. Health-care providers need to provide special instructions regarding risk factors associated with diets that are high in fats and salt. For example, the Chinese may need education regarding the use of salty fish and condiments, which increase the risk for nasopharyngeal, esophageal, and stomach cancers.

NUTRITIONAL DEFICIENCIES AND FOOD LIMITATIONS

The Chinese diet is generally vegetarian, although meat is often served. Little information is available about dietary deficiencies in the Chinese diet. The life span of the Chinese is long enough to suggest that severe dietary deficiencies are not common as long as food is available. Periodically, some deficiencies, such as rickets and goiters, have occurred. The Chinese government added iodine to water supplies, and fish, which is rich in iron, is encouraged to enhance the diets of people with goiters. Native Chinese generally do not drink milk or eat milk products because of a genetic tendency for lactose intolerance. Their healthy selection of green vegetables limits the incidence of calcium deficiencies. Health-care providers may need to screen newer Chinese immigrants for these deficiencies and assist them in planning an adequate diet.

Most Chinese do not eat desserts that are high in sugar content. Their desserts are usually peeled or sliced fruits or desserts made of bean and bean curd. The higher death rate from diabetes in Western countries mentioned earlier in this chapter may be due to a change from the typical Chinese diet with few sweets to a Western diet with many sweets.

Pregnancy and Childbearing Practices

FERTILITY PRACTICES AND VIEWS TOWARD PREGNANCY

China is attempting to slow the rate of population growth by enforcing a one-child law. The most popular form of birth control is the intrauterine device. Sterilization is common even though oral contraception is available. Contraception is free in China. Abortion is fairly common, but statistics are hard to find.

Most Chinese families see pregnancy as positive and important in the immediate and extended family. Many couples wait a long time to have their first and only child. If a woman does become pregnant before the couple is ready to start a family, she may have an abortion. When the pregnancy is desired, the nuclear and extended family rejoices in the new family member. Overall, pregnancy is seen as women's business, although the Chinese male is beginning to demonstrate an active interest in pregnancy and the welfare of the mother and baby. Health-care practitioners need to understand this traditional view. Because Chinese women are very modest, many women insist on a female midwife or obstetrician. Some agree to use a male physician only when an emergency arises.

PRESCRIPTIVE, RESTRICTIVE, AND TABOO PRACTICES IN THE CHILDBEARING FAMILY

Pregnant women usually add more meat to their diets because their blood needs to be stronger for the fetus. Many women increase the amount of organ meat in their diet, and even during times of severe food shortages, the Chinese government has tried to ensure that pregnant women receive adequate nutrition. These traditions are also reflected in Chinese families living in the West.

Other dietary restrictions and prescriptions may be practiced by pregnant women, such as avoiding shellfish during the first trimester because it causes allergies. Some mothers may be unwilling to take iron because they believe that it makes the delivery more difficult.

The Chinese government is proud of the fact that since the People's Revolution, in 1949, infant mortality has been significantly reduced (Ministry of Public Health, 1992). This has been accomplished by providing a three-level system of care for pregnant woman in rural and urban populations. Over 90 percent of childbirths take place under sterile conditions either by an obstetrician or a midwife. This has reduced the maternal mortality rate significantly (Ministry of Public Health, 1992). Therefore, most Chinese who have immigrated to Western countries are familiar with modern sterile deliveries.

In China, a woman stays in the hospital for 5 to 7 days after delivery to recover her strength and body balance. Traditional postpartum care includes 1 month of recovery, with the mother eating foods that decrease the **yin** (cold) energy. The Chinese government supports this 1-month recuperation period through labor laws that entitle the mother from 56 days to 6 months of maternity leave with full pay (Ministry of Public Health, 1992). Women who return to work are allowed time off for breast-feeding, and in many cases, factories provide a special lounge for the women to breast-feed. Families who come to Western societies expect the same importance to be placed on motherhood and may be surprised to find that many Western countries do not provide similar benefits.

Prescriptive and restrictive practices continue among many Chinese women during the postpartum period. Drinking and touching cold water are taboo for Chinese women in the postpartum period. Raw fruits and vegetables are avoided because they are considered "cold" foods. They must be cooked and be warm. Mothers eat five to six meals a day with high nutritional ingredients including rice, soups, and seven to eight eggs. Brown sugar is commonly used because it helps rebuild blood loss. Drinking rice wine is encouraged to increase the mother's breast milk production. But mothers need to be cautioned that it may also prolong the bleeding time. Many mothers do not expose themselves to the cold air and do not go outside or bathe for the first month postpartum because the cold air can enter the body and cause health problems, especially for older women. Some women wear many layers of clothes and are covered from head to toe, even in the summer, to keep the air away from their bodies.

Death Rituals

DEATH RITUALS AND EXPECTATIONS

Chinese death and bereavement traditions are centered on ancestor worship. Ancestor worship is frequently misunderstood; it is not a religion, but rather a form of paying respect. Many Chinese believe that their spirits can never rest unless living descendants provide care for the grave and worship the memory of the deceased. These practices were so important to the Chinese that early Chinese pioneers to the West had statements written into their work contract that their ashes or bones be returned to China (Halporn, 1992).

The belief that the Chinese greet death with stoicism and fatalism is a myth. In fact, most Chinese fear death and avoid references to it, and teach their children this avoidance. The number 4 is considered unlucky by many Chinese because it is pronounced like the Chinese word for death; this is similar to the bad luck associated with the number 13 in many Western societies. Huang (1992) writes:

> At a very young age, a child is taught to be very careful with words that are remotely associated with the "misfortune" of death. The word "death" and its synonyms are strictly forbidden on happy occasions, especially during holidays. People's uneasiness about death often is reflected in their emphasis on longevity and everlasting life. . . . In daily life, the character "Long Life" appears on almost everything: jewelry, clothing, furniture, and so forth. It would be a terrible mistake to give a clock as a gift, simply because the pronunciation of the word "clock" is the same as that of the word "ending." Recently, many people in Taiwan decided to avoid using the number "four" because the number has a similar pronunciation to the word "death." (p. 1)

The purchase of insurance may be avoided because of a fear that it is inviting death. The color white is associated with death and is considered bad luck. Black is also a bad-luck color. Red is the ultimate good-luck color.

Many Chinese believe in ghosts, and the fear of death is extended to the fear of ghosts. Some ghosts are good and some are bad, but all have great power. Communism discourages this thinking and sees it as a hindrance to future growth and development of the society, but the ever-pragmatic Chinese believe it is better not to invite trouble with ghosts just in case they might exist.

The dead may be viewed in the hospital or in the family home. Extended family members and friends come together to mourn. The dead are honored by placing objects around the coffin that signify the life of the dead: food, money designated for dead person's spirit, and other articles made of paper. In China, cremation is preferred by the state because of a lack of wood for coffins and a lack of space for burial. The ashes are placed in an urn and then in a vault. As cities grow, even the space for vaults is limited. In rural areas, many families prefer traditional burial and have family burial plots. It is preferable to bury an intact body in a coffin.

RESPONSES TO DEATH AND GRIEF

The Chinese react to death in various ways. Death is viewed as a part of the natural cycle of life, and some believe that something good happens to them after they die. These beliefs foster the impression that Chinese are stoic. In fact they feel similar emotions to Westerners but do not overtly express those emotions to strangers. During bereavement, a person does not have to go to work, but instead can use this mourning time for remembering the dead and planning for the future. Bereavement time in the larger cities is 1 day to 1 week, depending on the policy of the government agency and the relationship of family members to the dead. Mourners are recognized by black armbands on their left arm and white strips of cloth tied around their heads.

Spirituality

DOMINANT RELIGION AND USE OF PRAYER

In mainland China the practice of formal religious services is minimal. The ideals and values of the different religions are practiced alone rather than with people coming together to participate in a formal religious service. In recent years, in some parts of China, religion is becoming more popular. The main formal religions in China are Buddhism, Catholicism, Protestantism, Taoism, and Islam.

As immigration from China increases, Chinese people who practice Christian religions have become more visible on the American landscape. Chinese immigrants from the PRC may express different perspectives on religious beliefs than the Chinese from other countries, or from Hong Kong and Taiwan, where they have been permitted to practice Christianity. At first they may go to a church attended by other Chinese people. Some eventually are baptized, and some continue to attend Bible studies. In cities in the United States, churches are playing a very important role in the local Chinese community in terms of providing support and services to Chinese immigrants, students, scholars, and their families. An understanding of this concept is essential when the health-care provider attempts to obtain religious counseling services for Chinese clients.

Prayer is generally a source of comfort. Some Chinese do not acknowledge a religion such as Buddhism, but if they go to a shrine they burn incense and offer prayers.

MEANING OF LIFE AND INDIVIDUAL SOURCES OF STRENGTH

The Chinese view life in terms of cycles and interrelationships, believing that life gets meaning from the context in which it is lived. Life cannot be broken into simple parts and examined because the parts are interrelated. When the Chinese attempt to explain life and what it means, they speak about what happened to them, what happened to others, and the importance and interrelatedness of those events. They speak not only of the importance of the current phenomena, but also about the importance of what occurred many years ago, maybe even centuries, before their lives. They live and believe in a true systems framework.

"Life forces" are sources of strength to the Chinese. These forces come from within the individual, the environment, the past and future of the individual, and society. Chinese use these forces when they need strength. If one usual source of strength is unsuccessful, they try another. The individual may use many different techniques such as meditation, exercise, massage, and prayer. Drugs, herbs, food, good air, and artistic expression may also be used. Good-luck charms are cherished, and traditional and nontraditional medicines are used.

The family is usually one source of strength. Individuals draw on family resources and are expected to return resources to strengthen the family. Resources may be financial, emotional, physical, mental, or spiritual. Calling on ancestors to provide strength as a resource requires giving back to the ancestors when necessary. The interconnectedness of life provides a source of strength for individuals from before birth to death and beyond.

Health-care providers need to understand this multidimensional manner of thinking and believing. Assessments, goal setting, interventions, and evaluations may be different for Chinese clients than for American clients. The context of client problems is the emphasis, and the physical, mental, and spiritual aspects of the person's life are the focal points.

Health-Care Practices

HEALTH-SEEKING BELIEFS AND BEHAVIORS

Health care in China is provided for most citizens. Every work unit and neighborhood has its own clinic and

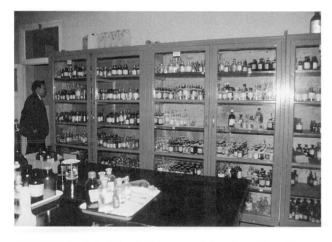

FIGURE 7–1 A traditional Chinese medicine shop. Many Chinese practice traditional Chinese medicine, either alone or in conjunction with Western medicine.

hospital. Traditional Chinese medicine shops abound (Fig. 7–1). Even department stores and supermarkets have Western medicines and traditional Chinese medicines and herbs.

The focus of health care has not changed over the centuries, and includes having a healthy body, a healthy mind, and a healthy spirit. Preventive health-care practices are a major focus in China today. An additional focus is placed on infectious diseases such as schistosomiasis, tuberculosis, childhood diseases, and malaria; cancer; heart diseases; and maternal-infant care. Reported human immunodeficiency virus remains at low levels in China, mostly because of the stigma associated with sexually transmitted diseases and drug use in the society.

While many Chinese have made the transition to Western medicine, others maintain their roots in traditional Chinese medicine, and still others practice both types of medicine. The Chinese are similar to other nationalities in seeking the most effective cure available. Younger Chinese people usually do not hesitate to seek health-care providers when necessary. They generally practice Western medicine unless they feel that it does not work for them; then they use traditional Chinese medicine. On the other hand, elderly people may try traditional Chinese medicine first, and only seek Western medicine when traditional medicine does not seem to work.

Among Chinese Americans, these health-seeking beliefs, practices, and patterns remain the same as the ones in China. This results in sicker elderly people seeking care from Western health-care providers. Even after seeking Western medical care elderly Chinese may continue to practice traditional Chinese medicine in some form. However, some Chinese clients may not tell health-care providers about other forms of treatment they have been using because they are conscious of saving face. Health-care providers need to understand this practice and include it in their care. Members of the health-care team need to develop a trusting relationship with Chinese clients so that all information can be disclosed. Health-care providers must impress upon clients the importance of disclosing all treatments because some may have antagonistic effects.

RESPONSIBILITY FOR HEALTH CARE

Chinese people often self-medicate when they think that they know what is wrong, or if they have been successfully treated by their traditional medicine or herbs in the past. They share their knowledge about treatments and their medicines with friends and family members. This often happens among Chinese Americans as well because of the belief that occasional illness can be ameliorated through the use of nonprescription drugs. Many consider seeing Western health-care providers as a waste of time and money. Health-care providers need to recognize that self-medication and sharing medications are an accepted practice among the Chinese. Thus, health-care providers should inquire about this practice when making assessments, setting goals, and evaluating the results of treatments. A trusting relationship between members of the health-care team and the client and family is necessary to enhance the disclosure of all treatments.

TRADITIONAL CHINESE MEDICINE PRACTICES

Traditional Chinese medicine is practiced widely, with concrete reasons for the preparation of medications, the taking of medicine, and the expected outcomes. Western medicine needs to be explained to Chinese people in equally concrete terms.

Traditional Chinese medicine has many facets, including the five basic substances (**qi**, energy; **xue**, blood; **jing**, essence; **shen**, spirit; and **jing ye**, body fluids); the pulses and vessels for the flow of energetic forces (**mai**); the energy pathways (**jing**); the channels and collaterals, including the 14 meridians for acupuncture, moxibustion, and massage (**jing luo**); the organ systems (**zang fu**); and the tissues of the bones, tendons, flesh, blood vessels, and skin. The scope of traditional Chinese medicine is vast and should be studied carefully by professionals who provide health-care to Chinese clients.

Acupuncture and moxibustion are used in many of the treatments. Acupuncture is the insertion of needles into precise points along the channel system of flow of the *qi* called the 14 meridians. (The system has over 400 points.) Many of the same points can be used in applying pressure and massage to achieve relief from imbalances in the system. The same systems approach is used to produce localized anesthesia.

Moxibustion is the application of heat from different sources to various points. For example, one source, such as garlic, is placed on the distal end of the needle after it is inserted through the skin, and the garlic is set on fire. Sometimes the substance is burned directly over the point without a needle insertion. Localized erythema occurs with the heat from the burning substance, and the medicine is absorbed through the skin. Cupping is another common practice. A heated cup or glass jar is put on the skin creating a vacuum, which causes the skin to be drawn into the cup. The heat that is generated is used to treat joint pain.

The Chinese believe that health and a happy life can be maintained if the two forces, the **yang** and **yin**, are balanced. This balance is called the **dao**. Heaven is yang, Earth is yin; man is yang, woman is yin; the sun is yang, and the moon is yin; the hollow organs (bladder, intestines, stomach, gallbladder), head, face, back, and lateral parts of the body are yang; and the solid viscera (heart, lung, liver, spleen, kidney, and pericardium), abdomen, chest, and the inner parts of the body are yin. The yang is hot and the yin is cold. Health-care providers need to be aware that the functions of life and the interplay of these functions, rather than the structures, are important to Chinese people.

Central to traditional medicine is the concept of the *qi*. It is considered the vital force of life; includes air, breath, or wind; and is present in all living organisms. Some of the *qi* is inherited, and other parts come from the environment, such as in food. The *qi* circulates through the 14 meridians and organs of the body to give the body nourishment. The channels of flow are also responsible for eliminating the bad *qi*. All channels (the meridians and organs) are interconnected. The results resemble a system where a change in one part of the system results in a change in other parts, and one part of the system can assist other parts in their total functioning.

Diagnosis is made through close inspection of the outward appearance of the body, the vitality of the person, the color of the person, the appearance of the tongue, and the person's senses. The practitioner uses listening, smelling, and questioning techniques in the assessment. Palpation is used by feeling the 12 pulses and different parts of the body. Treatments are based on the imbalances that occur. Many are directly related to the obvious problem, but many more are related through the interconnectedness of the body systems. Many of the treatments not only "cure" the problem but are also used to "strengthen" the entire human being. Traditional Chinese medicine cannot be learned quickly because of the interplay of symptoms and diagnoses. It takes many years for practitioners to become adept in all phases of diagnosis and treatment.

T'ai chi, practiced by many Chinese, has its roots in the 12th century. This type of exercise is suitable for all age groups, even the very old. Liu (1972) stated, "It relaxes the mind as well as the body. It helps digestion, quiets the nervous system, benefits the heart and blood circulation, makes joints loose, and refreshes the skin" (p. 1). T'ai chi involves different forms of exercise, and some can be used for self-defense. The major focus of the movements is mind and body control. The concepts of yin and yang are included in the movements, with a yin movement following a yang movement. Total concentration and controlled breathing are necessary to enable the smoothness and rhythmic quality of movement. The movements resemble a slow-motion battle, with the participant both attacking and retreating. Movements are practiced at least twice a day to bring the internal body, the external body, and the environment into balance.

Herbal therapy is integral to traditional Chinese medicine. It is even more difficult to learn than diagnosis, acupuncture, and moxibustion. Herbs fall into four categories of energy (cold, hot, warm, and cool), five categories of taste (sour, bitter, sweet, pungent, and salty), and a neutral category. Different methods are used to administer the herbs, including drinking and eating, applying topically, and wearing on the body. Each treatment is specific to the underlying problem or a desire to increase strength and resistance.

BARRIERS TO HEALTH CARE

In China the government is primarily responsible for providing basic health care within a multilevel system. Native Chinese are accustomed to the neighborhood work units called *dan wei*, where they get answers to their questions and health-care services are provided. After transition to the United States, Chinese clients face many of the same barriers to health care faced by Westerners, yet they have other special concerns and difficulties that prevent them from accessing health care services. Ma (2000) summarized these barriers as following:

1 *Language barriers:* This is one of the major reasons that Chinese Americans do not want to see Western health-care providers. They feel uncomfortable and frustrated with not being able to communicate with them freely and not being able to adequately express their pains, concerns, or health problems. Even highly educated Chinese Americans, who have limited knowledge in the medical field and are unfamiliar with medical terminology, have difficulty complying with recommended procedures and health prescriptions.

2 *Cultural barriers:* Lack of culturally appropriate and competent health-care services is another key obstacle to health-care service utilization. Many Chinese Americans have different cultural responses to health and illness. Although they respect and accept the Western health-care provider's prescription drugs, they tend to alternate between Western and traditional Chinese physicians.

3 *Socioeconomic barriers:* Being unable to afford medical expenses is another barrier to accessing health-care services for some Chinese Americans. However, having health insurance does not always assure the utilization of the health-care system or the benefits of health insurance. There may be a sense of distrust between patients and health-care providers or between patients and insurance companies. Additionally, many do not know the cost of the service when they enter a clinic or hospital. They are frustrated with being caught in the battle between health insurance companies and the clinic or hospital.

4 *Systemic barriers:* Not understanding the Western health-care system and feeling inconvenienced by managed care regulations deters many from seeking Western health-care providers unless they are seriously ill. The complexity of the rules and regulations of public agencies and medical assistance programs such as Medicaid and Medicare blocks their effective use.

Tan (1992), in a different perspective, summarized barriers for Chinese immigrants seeking health care.

1 Many Chinese Americans have great difficulty facing a diagnosis of cancer because families are the main source of support for patients, and many family members are still in China.

2 Because many Chinese Americans do not purchase medical insurance, any serious illness will lead to heavy financial burdens on the family.

3 Once the client responds to initial treatment, the family tends to stop treatment and the client does not receive follow-up care or becomes noncompliant.

4 Chinese American families may be reluctant to allow autopsies because of their fear of being "cut up."

5 The most difficult barrier is frequently the reluctance to disclose the diagnosis to the patient or the family.

CULTURAL RESPONSES TO HEALTH AND ILLNESS

Chinese people express their pain in ways similar to those of Americans, but their description of pain differs. A study by Moore (1990) includes not only the expression of pain but also common treatments used by Chinese. The Chinese tend to describe their pain in terms of more diverse body symptoms, whereas Westerners tend to describe pain locally. The Western description includes words like "stabbing" and "localized," whereas the Chinese describe pain as "dull" and more "diffuse." They tend to use explanations of pain from the traditional Chinese influence of imbalances in the yang and yin combined with location and cause. The study determined that the Chinese cope with pain by using externally applied methods, such as oils and massage. They also use warmth, sleeping on the area of pain, relaxation, and aspirin.

The balance between yin and yang is used to explain mental as well as physical health. This belief, coupled with the influence of Russian theorists such as Pavlov, influence the Chinese view of mental illness. Mental illness results more from metabolic imbalances and organic problems. The effect of social situations on a person's mental well being (such as stress and crises) is considered inconsequential, but physical imbalances from genetics are the important factors. Because a stigma is associated with having a family member who is mentally ill, many families initially seek the help of a folk healer. Many use a combination of traditional and Western medicine. Many mentally ill clients are treated as outpatients and remain in the home.

Although Chinese do not readily seek assistance for emotional and nervous disorders, a study of 143 Chinese Americans found that younger, lower socioeconomic, and married Chinese with better language ability seek help more frequently (Ying & Miller, 1992). The researchers recommended that new immigrants be taught that help is available when needed for mental disorders within the mental health-care system.

Chinese people in larger cities are becoming more supportive of the disabled but, for the most part, support services are rare. Because the focus has been on improving the overall economic growth of the country, the needs of the disabled have not had priority. The son of Deng Xiaoping was crippled in the Cultural Revolution and has been active in making the country more aware of the needs of the disabled. In the summer of 1994, games for the physically disabled were held in Beijing. Because most city households have televisions, the televised games increased the awareness of the Chinese people about the abilities of the disabled. Overall, the Chinese still view mental and physical disabilities as a part of life that should be hidden.

The expression of the sick role depends on the level of education of the client. More educated Chinese people, who have been exposed to Western ideas and culture, are more likely to assume a sick role similar to that of Westerners. However, the highly educated and acculturated may exhibit some of the traditional roles associated with illness. Each client needs to be assessed individually for responses to illness and for expectations of care. Traditionally, the Chinese ill person is viewed passive and accepting of illness. To the Chinese, illness is expected as a part of the life cycle. However, they do try to avoid danger and to live as healthy a life as possible. To the Chinese, all of life is interconnected; therefore, they seek explanations and connections for illness and injury in all aspects of life. Their explanations to health-care providers may not make sense, but the health-care provider should try to determine those connections so the connections can be incorporated into treatment regimens. The Chinese believe that because the illness or injury is caused from an imbalance, there should be a medicine or treatment that can restore the balance. If the medicine or treatment does not seem to do this, they may refuse to use it.

The Chinese respect their bodies but may not seem modest. Their bathrooms may have no doors, and they frequently go to communal showers. However, they are very modest when it comes to touch. They feel uncomfortable touching their own bodies, which may be problematic when they need to use touch to provide their own health care, for example, breast self-examinations. People of the same sex may use touch if they are close friends or family. Men and women do not touch each other, and even couples who have been married for a long time do not show physical affection in public. Most Chinese women feel uncomfortable being touched by male health-care providers and most seek female health-care providers.

Native Chinese and Chinese Americans like treatments that are comfortable and do not hurt. Treatments that hurt are physically stressful and drain their energy. Health-care providers who have been ill themselves can appreciate this way of thinking, because sometimes the cure seems worse than the illness. Treatments will be more successful if they are explained in ways that are consistent with the Chinese way of thinking. The Chinese depend on their families and sometimes on their friends to help them while they are sick. These people provide much of the direct care; health-care providers are expected to manage the care. The family may seem to take over the life of the sick person, and the sick person is very passive in allowing them the control. One or two primary people assume this responsibility, usually a spouse. Health-care providers need to include the family members in the plan of care and, in many instances, in the actual delivery of care.

BLOOD TRANSFUSIONS AND ORGAN DONATION

Modern-day Chinese accept blood transfusions, organ donations, and organ transplants when absolutely essential, as long as they are safe and effective. Chinese Americans have the same concerns as Americans about blood transfusion because of the perceived high incidence of HIV positive and hepatitis B. No overall ethnic or religious practices prohibit the use of blood transfusions, organ donations, or organ transplants. Of course, some individuals may have religious or personal reasons for denying their use.

Health-Care Practitioners

TRADITIONAL VERSUS BIOMEDICAL PRACTITIONERS

China uses two health-care systems. One is grounded in Western medical care, and the other is anchored in traditional Chinese medicine. The educational preparation of physicians, nurses, and pharmacists is similar to Western health-care education. Ancillary workers have responsibility in the health-care system, and the practice of midwifery is widely accepted by the Chinese. Physicians in Chinese medicine are trained in universities, and traditional Chinese pharmacies remain an integral part of health care.

STATUS OF HEALTH-CARE PROVIDERS

Traditional Chinese medicine practitioners are shown great respect by the Chinese. In many instances, they are shown equal, if not more, respect than Western practitioners. The Chinese may distrust Western practitioners because of the pain and invasiveness of their treatments. The hierarchy among Chinese health-care providers is similar to that of the Chinese society. Older health-care providers receive respect from the younger providers. Men usually receive more respect than women, but that is beginning to change. Physicians receive the highest respect, followed closely by nurses with a university education. Other nurses with limited education are next in the hierarchy, followed by ancillary personnel.

Health-care practitioners are usually given the same respect as elders in the family. Chinese children recognize them as authority figures. Physicians and nurses are viewed as individuals who can be trusted with the health of a family member. Nurses are generally perceived as caring individuals, but many times they do not provide much direct care for patients. The family is expected to oversee the direct care, while the physician makes the decisions about the type of treatment. Adult Chinese also respond to practitioners in the same way, but if they disagree with the health-care provider, they may not follow instructions. Moreover, they may not verbally confront the health-care provider because they fear that either they or the provider will suffer a loss of face.

CASE STUDY Mr. Chen, age 30, and his wife age 28, have three children, ages 7, 5, and 2 years. Many of their extended families also live in the United States near them. Mr. Chen and his parents own several Chinese restaurants. Mr. Chen, an extremely important member in this family, was diagnosed with end-stage renal disease (ESRD) in 1996. The entire family has been under stress for a variety of reasons: the uncertain outcomes of Mr. Chen's illness, three young children, living in a foreign country and in a different cultural environment, and barriers to accessing health care effectively.

Mr. Chen immigrated to the United States in the early part of 1988 to join his parents and work in their successful Chinese restaurant in New York City. His fiancé immigrated to the United States in late 1988, and they married in 1990. The Chen family and Mr. Chen's parents moved to Albany, New York, and eventually opened three new restaurants before he became ill. His wife cared for their children at home. Mrs. Chen's parents remained in New York City where her father is a minister in the Chinese Christian Church.

In December 1995, Mr. Chen felt extremely sick with fatigue, nausea, vomiting, and weight loss. At that time he did not have health insurance. Because of language barriers and the high cost of health care in the United States, he returned to China for medical care. In China, Mr. Chen was diagnosed with ESRD. His physician recommended a kidney transplant. Mr. Chen's parents also returned to China because of the seriousness of their son's health. Mr. Chen sold his three restaurants to obtain money for his medical expenses. In May 1996, Mr. Chen received a cadaver kidney transplant in China and recuperated without complications. In July 1996, he returned to the United States with a fully functioning kidney. Mr. Chen continued taking antirejection immunosuppressive agents prescribed by the Chinese physician until October 1996, a period of 5 months post-transplantation. At that time, he saw an American physician to obtain a prescription for refilling his antirejection medication. The physician told him that he did not need to continue the medication. He questioned the physician because the Chinese physician had told him that he needed to continue the medication for the rest of his life. Again, he was told that his condition was stable and he stopped taking the medication. After 20 days, kidney rejection occurred and he began the long-term hemodialysis under Medicare.

Hemodialysis left him feeling exhausted and unable to work outside his home. His diet was limited, and he suffered a number of complications, including hepatitis B and liver failure. In December 1997, he suffered a seizure while visiting friends. After Mr. Chen became ill, Mrs. Chen began working as a waitress in a friend's restaurant, and became the sole financial provider for the family. To reduce rent expenses and to be closer to his wife's work, they moved to a four-bedroom house, which they shared with two other Chinese families who were close friends. Also Mr. Chen initiated the extensive application process for disability and Medicaid and long-term hemodialysis. The language barrier made this process even more complicated. He felt frustrated because he was unable to care for his family. However, he is still hopeful, and plans to someday to return to China for another kidney transplant. His extended family is very supportive and they are saving money to support his second kidney transplant.

STUDY QUESTIONS

1 Initially, what were the main reasons why Chinese people immigrated to the United States? How does this differ from their current reasons for immigrating?

2 How did Americans treat the Chinese in the early 1800s?

3 How do Chinese Americans form networks to support one another?

4 What are some effective ways for Western health-care providers to communicate with Chinese clients who may have difficulty understanding English?

5 Compare and contrast the Chinese meaning of life and ways of thinking with the Western cultural perceptions of the meaning of life and ways of thinking.

6 Why did Mr. Chen initially not seek health-care providers in the United States?

7 What are some of the difficulties that Mr. Chen might have as a long-term hemodialysis patient with a Chinese cultural background?

8 If you were Mr. Chen's health-care provider, what might you do to improve the quality of life for the Chen family?

9 How might the Chen family go about seeking a kidney transplant in the United States?

10 How might the extended family be more involved with the Chen family?

11 Would you suggest to Mr. Chen that he ask his extended family to be tested for compatibility for being a kidney donor for him?

12 Explain the relationship of *yin* and *yang.*

REFERENCES

Butterfield, F. (1990). *China: Alive in the bitter sea* (rev. ed.). New York: Random House.
Centers for Disease Control. (2001). http://www.cdc.gov.
Chin, A. (1988). *Children of China: Voices from recent years.* New York: Alfred A. Knopf.
Gaspard, K. J. (1994). The red blood cell and alterations in oxygen transport. In C. M. Porth (Ed.), *Pathophysiology: Concepts of altered states* (4th ed., pp. 323–339). Philadelphia: J. B. Lippincott.
Haley, G., Tan, C., & Haley, U. (1998). *New Asian emperors: The overseas Chinese, their strategies and competitive advantages.* Woburn, MA: Butterworth-Heinemann.
Halporn, R. (1992). Introduction. In C. L. Chen, W. C. Lowe, D. Ryan, A. H. Kutscher, R. Halporn, & H. Wang (Eds.), *Chinese Americans in loss and separation* (pp. v–xii). New York: Foundation of Thanatology.
Hu, W., & Grove, C. L. (1991). *Encountering the Chinese.* Yarmouth, MA: Intercultural Press.
Huang, W. (1992). Attitudes toward death: Chinese perspectives from the past. In C. L. Chen, W. C. Lowe, D. Ryan, A. H. Kutscher, R. Halporn, & H. Wang (Eds.), *Chinese Americans in loss and separation* (pp. 1–5). New York: Foundation of Thanatology.
Lawson, J. S., & Lin, V. (1994). Health status differentials in the People's Republic of China. *American Journal of Public Health, 84*(5), 737–741.
Levy, R. A. (1993). Ethnic and racial differences in response to medicines: Preserving individualized therapy in managed pharmaceutical programmes. *Pharmaceutical Medicine, 7,* 139–165.
Lin, C. C., & Fu, V. R. (1990). A comparison of child-rearing practices among Chinese, immigrant Chinese, and Caucasian-American parents. *Child Development, 61,* 429–433.

Liu, D. (1972). *T'ai chi and I ching: A choreography of body and mind.* New York: Harper & Row.

Ma, G. X. (1999). *The Culture of health: Asian communities in the United States.* London: British Library Cataloguing in Publication Data.

Ma, G. X. (2000). Barriers to the use of health services by Chinese Americans. *Journal of Allied Health, 29*(2) 64–70.

Ministry of Public Health. (1992). *A brief introduction to China's medical and health services.* Beijing: People's Republic of China.

Moore, R. (1990). Ethnographic assessment of pain coping perceptions. *Psychosomatic Medicine, 52,* 171–181.

Office of Minority Health Resource Center. (2001). http://www. minority-health.gov.

Seidel, H., Ball, J., Dains, J., & Benedict, W. *Quick reference to cultural assessment.* (1994). St. Louis, MO: Mosby.

Smith, C. S. (2002, April 30). Beware of cross-cultural faux pas in China. *New York Times.* Retrieved April 30, 2002, from http://www.nytimes.com.

Tan, C. M. (1992). Treating life-threatening illness in children. In C. L. Chen, W. C. Lowe, D. Ryan, A. H. Kutscher, R. Halporn, & H. Wang (Eds.), *Chinese Americans in loss and separation* (pp. 26–33). New York: Foundation of Thanatology.

Weatherspoon, A. J., Danko, G. P., & Johnson, R. C. (1994). Alcohol consumption and use norms among Chinese Americans and Korean Americans. *Journal of Studies on Alcohol,* March: 203–206.

Wong, B. (1987). Economic survival: The case of Asian-Americans elderly. *Sociological Perspectives, 27*(2), 197–217.

Ying, Y., & Miller, L. S. (1992). Help-seeking behavior and attitude of Chinese Americans regarding psychological problems. *American Journal of Community Psychology 20*(4), 549–556.

Chapter 8

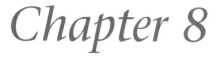

People of Cuban Heritage

LARRY D. PURNELL

Overview, Inhabited Localities, and Topography

OVERVIEW

The Republic of Cuba, with a population of over 11 million people, is located 90 miles south of Key West, Florida. Approximately the size of Pennsylvania, it is the largest island in the West Indies. The capital, Havana, is the largest city, with 2.5 million people, followed by Santiago de Cuba, with a population of 440,000, and Camaquey, with a population of 293,000. Fidel Castro has been president of this communist country since 1959. Major agricultural products and industries include sugar, petroleum, tobacco, textiles, nickel, copper, cement, and fertilizer. Cuba is a multiracial society, with a population of primarily Spanish and African origins, although other significant ethnic groups include Chinese, Haitians, and Eastern Europeans.

Although Cuban Americans are the smallest Hispanic group in the United States, they are the largest ethnic group in metropolitan Miami, Florida, and have been credited with the socioeconomic transformation of that city. Miami is in fact the dominant center of Cuban settlement. In this ethnic enclave, Cubans have created businesses and rejuvenated the economy, leading some to speak of the "great Cuban miracle." The distinctive Cuban culture is evidenced by their music, dance, and art. Cubans have made a number of dances popular, including the rumba, the cha-cha, the guaracha, the bolero, and the conga. Classical arts, such as the opera *Carmen* and the ballet *Alicia Alonso,* were created in Cuba. The film *Fresa y Chocolate (Strawberries and Chocolate)* won the Silver Bear Award at the Berlin Film Festival in February 1995 (Cultural Orientation Resource Center, 2002).

The experience of Cubans in their homeland and in the United States is distinct from that of other Hispanic groups. The history and culture of Cuba and the Cuban people have been heavily influenced by Spain, the United States, the Soviet Union, and, through the slave trade in Cuba's sugar industry, West African groups such as the Yoruba.

Cuba was under Spanish control from 1511 until 1898, making it one of Spain's last colonies in the New World. Control of the sugar industry by Spanish *peninsulares* (individuals born in Spain) was challenged by the growing class of *criollo* landowners (individuals of Spanish ancestry born in Cuba) and the *independentista* movement. This absentee ownership created political turmoil and social imbalances that gave rise to the Cuban national character. The mistrust of government reinforced a strong personalistic tradition, sense of national identity evolving from family and interpersonal relationships (Szapocznik & Hernandez, 1988).

Unlike most other immigrant groups, Cubans were welcomed by the U.S. government, provided with support (for example, the Cuban Refugee Program begun by the Kennedy administration), and met with relatively little prejudice (Portes & Zhou, 1994). Cubans engaged in a wide range of entrepreneurial activity, both in sales and services, within the shelter of the Cuban community. Consequently, newer Cuban immigrants found networks of support and were somewhat protected from the difficulties associated with a competitive labor market. Cubans in the United States are a strong pres-

The author wishes to acknowledge the contributions of Divina Grossman, who wrote this chapter in the first edition.

ence, not only economically but also politically. An exile ideology, a preoccupation with events in Cuba, and militant opposition to the regime of Fidel Castro characterize their predominant political stance. Overwhelmingly, Cuban Americans tend to be conservative, Republican, and anticommunist. They have demonstrated high voter turnout and tend to vote in blocks during local and national elections (National Council of la Raza, 2002).

Cubans have managed to adjust to mainstream American culture while remaining close to their Cuban roots. However, young adults and adolescents who were educated in Cuba with strict communist ideation and who emigrated with their parents may find the clash in values between Cuba and their new country confusing and negative. The bicultural Cuban American population can help in their adjustment. Many Cubans outside Cuba possess a strong ethnic identity, speak Spanish, and adhere to traditional Cuban values and practices at home while working in the dominant culture of their new homeland.

HERITAGE AND RESIDENCE

Racially, Cubans are 51 percent mulatto, 37 percent white, 11 percent black, and 1 percent Chinese. The Cuban culture is relatively new in terms of world cultures. The native Arawak Indian population that inhabited the island when Columbus landed in 1492 died from diseases brought by Spanish settlers.

Cubans have a rich historical heritage. Spain launched its conquest of Mexico from Cuba in 1519. During the Spanish colonial period (1511–1898), Spanish boats stopped in Havana on their way to Mexico and Central America. In the 19th century, the Monroe Doctrine led to a special relationship between Cuba and the United States. The United States military controlled the island from 1898 to 1902. In 1902, Cuba was a politically independent capitalist state. In 1959, Fidel Castro led a revolution to free Cuba of U.S. influence and subsequently established a socialist government, which still controls the country.

The highest concentration of Cuban Americans is in Florida, although significant numbers live in New Jersey, New York, Illinois, and California. The median age of Cubans in the United States is 34, compared with the overall Hispanic population in the United States whose median age is 26 (National Women's Health Information Center, 2002).

REASONS FOR MIGRATION AND ASSOCIATED ECONOMIC FACTORS

About 1 million Cubans immigrated to the United States between 1959 and 1980. Most arrived on the U.S. mainland after the 1959 revolution that brought Fidel Castro to power and changed the social, economic, and political landscape of Cuba. Although the American government has defined the exodus as a political rather than an economic migration, a combination of these factors provided the motivation for migration. The desire for personal freedom, the hope of refuge and political

exile, and the promise of economic opportunities have been the main reasons for Cuban immigration.

Portes and Bach (1985) identify six stages of Cuban immigration to the United States:

First stage: departures from January 1959 to October 1962. When Fidel Castro overthrew the government of Fulgencio Batista in January 1959, approximately 250,000 landowners, industrialists, professionals, and merchants left on commercial flights from Havana for the United States.

Second stage: departures from November 1962 to September 1965. The confrontation between Cuba and the United States over Russian missiles in Cuba ended all direct flights from Cuba to the United States. At this time, about 56,000 people left on small boats and rafts because no direct transportation was available.

Third stage: departures from October 1965 to April 1973. Cuba and the United States reached an understanding in which an airlift was allowed from Varadero Beach to Miami. These "freedom flights" or "family reunification flights" provided the opportunity for about 297,000 people to immigrate.

Fourth stage: departures from May 1973 to September 1978. The Cuban government unilaterally ended the airlift. Travel to Spain, Mexico, and Jamaica became the only means of leaving Cuba. About 39,000 people arrived in the United States on commercial flights by way of these countries.

Fifth stage: departures from October 1978 to March 1980. Fidel Castro allowed political prisoners from Cuban jails to leave with their families. About 10,000 people arrived in this manner on airplane flights, boats, and rafts.

Sixth stage: departures from April to September 1980. The Cuban government again allowed a massive boatlift from the Mariel Harbor to Key West, Florida. Approximately 125,000 people arrived, including people with criminal records, homosexuals, deaf-mutes, lepers, and patients from mental institutions. About 5000, or 4 percent, of these were hard-core criminals, causing an increase in the levels of violent crime in the metropolitan Miami and New York areas.

Since December 1960, the Cuban Refugee Program under the Department of Health, Education, and Welfare (now the Department of Health and Human Services) has been responsible for coordinating the processing and resettlement of Cubans in the United States. Between 1962 and 1971, the federal government spent over 730 million on Cuban immigrant assistance programs, which covered relocation costs, housing subsidies, job training, medical care, low-cost college loans, food distribution, and cash allotment (Boswell & Curtis, 1983; Olson & Olson, 1995; Portes & Bach, 1985).

In the two decades of Cuban immigration, significant change has been observed in the waves of immigrants, from the elite classes of the first stage, called the "golden exiles," to the **Marielitos** of the sixth stage. Each wave is distinct: the earliest immigrants had higher educational and economic status in Cuba than subsequent waves; the later groups were more representative of the Cuban population. The motivation for immigration also changed from the desire to escape political and religious persecution in the earlier waves to the hope for economic improvement in the later waves (Boswell & Curtis, 1983).

EDUCATIONAL STATUS AND OCCUPATIONS

The level of educational attainment of Cuban Americans is higher than that of other Hispanic groups, approximating that of the white non-Hispanic American population (Ginzberg, 1991). Cubans under age 35 also have the highest school enrollment rates of any population in the United States, including non-Hispanic whites. Even at the preschool level (children aged 3 and 4), about 42 percent of Cuban children are enrolled in school (Perez, 1984).

In comparison with other Hispanic groups, a higher proportion of Cubans are self-employed. Relatively high proportions of Cubans work in areas such as wholesale and retail trade, banking and credit agencies, insurance, real estate, and finance. A lower proportion of Cubans are employed in the extractive industries (oil, coal, and timbering); public administration; and the manufacture of durable goods (Perez, 1984). Cubans are found in larger percentages than other Hispanic groups and than the total U.S. population in nonclerical white-collar occupations such as executive, administrative, and managerial; professional and technical; and sales (57 percent of Cubans versus 38 percent of other Hispanics and 56 percent of total U.S. population) (Ginsberg, 1991). Cuban Americans report the highest income of the three main Hispanic groups and are more likely to report dual-income families (Smart & Smart, 1992). In 1987, the unemployment rate among Cubans was 5.5 percent—the lowest of any ethnic group in the United States—compared with 7 percent for the rest of the country (Olson & Olson, 1995).

Communication

DOMINANT LANGUAGE AND DIALECTS

Language is often used as an index of assimilation of an immigrant group into the dominant culture. Virtually all first-generation Cubans in the United States speak Spanish as their first language. A survey by Diaz (1980) found that most Cuban immigrants speak only Spanish at home, with slightly over 50 percent speaking only Spanish at work. In contrast, more than 50 percent who attend school speak English exclusively, and less than 20 percent of those speak mostly Spanish. For all age groups, Cubans with a higher level of education are more likely to speak English at home.

A study by the National Commission for Employment Policy (1982) revealed that only 18 percent of Cuban-born Americans consider English to be their dominant language, compared with 30 percent for the Mexican and Puerto Rican populations. Because Cubans live and transact business in Spanish-speaking ethnic enclaves, they have little need or motivation to learn English (Boswell & Curtis, 1983).

The large number and variety of Spanish-language media, including newspapers, magazines, and radio programs, also reflect Cuban immigrants' preference for Spanish rather than English. Research by Diaz (1980) indicated that about 60 percent of Cubans listen to mostly Spanish-language programs, and over 55 percent primarily read newspapers in Spanish. Taking a stroll through Little Havana in Miami or Little Havana North along New Jersey's Union City–west New York corridor, the preference for Spanish is reflected in billboard and poster advertisements. There signs announcing *joyeria* (jewelry store), *carniceria* (butcher shop), *muebleria* (furniture store), *farmacia* (drug store), or *zapateria* (shoe store) are quite commonplace (Boswell, 1991).

The inability to speak English has been identified as one of the most important problems faced by first-generation Cuban immigrants. According to a study by Portes and Clark (1980), three years after immigration, learning English was still identified as the foremost problem, with economic difficulties moving to second place, and transportation to third place.

Compared with their first-generation predecessors, second-generation Cubans speak Spanish, but frequently in a functional, elementary way. They may speak Spanish exclusively at home, but converse with friends or peers in "Spanglish," a mixture of Spanish and English. The smooth transition from Spanish to English and vice versa in the same sentence may be observed in such expressions as *Vamos de shopping* or *Tenga un nice day* (Boswell & Curtis, 1983). In addition, Cubans in the United States have incorporated into their everyday Spanish many English words, such as *futbol, rosbif, coctel, sueter, frigidaire,* and *bridge*. For Cuban Americans, Spanglish becomes a reflection of both their Cuban and American heritages.

CULTURAL COMMUNICATION PATTERNS

Like other Hispanic groups, Cubans value **simpatia** and **personalismo** in their interactions with others. *Simpatia* refers to the need for smooth interpersonal relationships, and is characterized by courtesy, respect, and the absence of harsh criticism or confrontation. *Personalismo* emphasizes intimate interpersonal relationships over impersonal bureaucratic relationships. **Choteo**, a lighthearted attitude with teasing, bantering, and exaggerating, may be observed often in the way Cubans communicate with one another (Bernal, 1994; Queralt, 1984).

Conversations among Cubans are characterized by animated facial expressions, direct eye contact, hand gestures, and gesticulations. Voices tend to be loud, and the rate of speech faster than may be observed with non-Cuban groups. Linguistically, the use of the second-person form *usted* to address older people and authority figures has fallen into disuse, replaced by the familiar form *tu* (Sandoval, 1979). The use of *tu* in interpersonal situations serves to reduce distance and promotes *personalismo* (Bernal, 1994). Touching, in the form of handshakes or hugs, is acceptable among family, friends, and acquaintances. In the health-care setting, clients and family members may hug or kiss the health-care provider to express gratitude and appreciation.

Cubans feel a sense of "specialness" about themselves and their culture that may be conveyed in communication with others. This sense of specialness arises from pride in their unique culture, a fusion of European and African, the geopolitical importance of Cuba in relation to powerful countries in history, and the exceptional success they have achieved in adapting to their new environment. This sense of specialness, combined with the fast rate and loud volume of speech, may sometimes be interpreted as arrogance or grandiosity in a non-Cuban cultural context (Bernal, 1994).

TEMPORAL RELATIONSHIPS

Cubans tend to be present-oriented compared with future-oriented European Americans. A greater emphasis is paid to current issues and problems rather than on projections into the future. In the clinical setting, health-care providers must realize that Cuban clients tend to be motivated to seek help in response to crisis situations. Hence, visits to health-care providers for resolution of a crisis must be used as opportunities for teaching and promotion of personal growth (Szapocznik et al., 1978; Queralt, 1984).

Hora cubana (Cuban time) refers to a flexible time period that stretches from 1 to 2 hours beyond the designated clock time. A Cuban understands that when a party starts at 8 P.M., the socially acceptable time to arrive is between 9 and 10 P.M. However, families who have acculturated to American values may adhere to a more rigid clock time. When setting up appointments for clinic visits, the health-care provider must determine the client's level of acculturation with respect to time, and make arrangements for flexible scheduling, if necessary.

FORMAT FOR NAMES

As in other Latin American societies, Cubans use two surnames, representing the mother's and the father's sides of the family. To illustrate: a woman may use the name Regina Morales Colon, indicating that her patrilineal surname is Morales and her matrilineal surname is Colon. When a Cuban woman marries, she adds *de* and her husband's name after her father's surname and drops her mother's surname. In the previous example, if Regina marries Mr. Ordonez, her name will be Regina Morales de Ordonez (Boswell & Curtis, 1983).

When addressing Cuban clients, especially the elderly, the health-care provider should use the formal rather than the familiar form, unless told otherwise. In the previous example, the appropriate appellation would be Señora Morales, or Mrs. Morales, instead of Regina.

Family Roles and Organization

HEAD OF HOUSEHOLD AND GENDER ROLES

Among Cubans, the family is the most important social unit (Bernal, 1994). The traditional Cuban family structure is patriarchal, characterized by a dominant and aggressive male and a passive, dependent female (Queralt, 1984). Fox (1979) found that the concepts of *la casa* (the

home) and *la calle* (the street) underscore the distinction between the roles of men and women. *La casa* is considered the province of the woman, and *la calle* the domain of the man. *La calle* includes everything outside the home, which is considered a proper testing ground for masculinity, but dangerous and inappropriate for women.

Traditionally, Cuban wives are expected to stay at home, manage the household, and care for the children. Husbands are expected to work, provide, and make major decisions for the family. Richmond's (1980) work on Cuban family structure demonstrated that Cuban husbands helped very little with household chores, but those whose wives worked helped more. In the same study, Cuban wives who contributed to the family income were more likely to receive help from their husbands with household chores and acquired greater decision-making power than women who did not work outside the home.

Cultural values acquired through four centuries of Spanish domination influence the behavior of Cuban men and women toward each other. The concept of **honor** is described as personal goodness or virtue, which can be lost or diminished by an immoral or unworthy act. Honor is maintained mainly by fulfilling family obligations and by treating others with *respeto* (respect). **Verguenza**, a consciousness of public opinion and the judgment of the entire community, is considered more important for women than men. **Machismo** dictates that men display physical strength, bravery, and virility (Fox, 1979).

Fox (1979) reported that the qualities Cuban men found most admirable in women were *puntuales a sus esposos*, *obediente*, and *atienda bien a sus esposos*, all indicating submissive and passive qualities. In women, being *moral* (virtuous), *aseada* (clean), and *decente* are desirable qualities. A double standard is often applied to male and female behavior (Fox, 1979). For example, it may be socially acceptable for men, but not for women, to engage in extramarital affairs. Chaperoning is expected for single, respectable women who go out on dates (Boswell & Curtis, 1983).

Since the massive migration from Cuba to the United States in 1959, the traditional Cuban family has undergone a transition to a less male-dominated, less segregated, and more egalitarian structure. Cuban women who arrived in the United States were frequently the first in the family to find jobs and contribute to the survival of the family. According to Gallagher (1980), Cuban immigrant women were more receptive to life in the United States, more flexible, and more readily hired for jobs than men. Eventually, as their contributions to the family's economic well-being increased, the women's power to make decisions was enhanced. Cuban American women have the highest rate of labor participation when compared with all other groups of women in the United States (Suarez, 1993). Thus, contemporary Cuban families from the 1980s to the present may demonstrate greater gender equality in decision making for the family (Szapocznik & Hernandez, 1988). Although customs are changing, the gender role distinctions are still greater among Cuban Americans than European Americans in the United States (Queralt, 1984).

PRESCRIPTIVE, RESTRICTIVE, AND TABOO PRACTICES FOR CHILDREN AND ADOLESCENTS

Cuban parents tend to pamper and overprotect their children, showering them with love and attention (Queralt, 1984). Fox (1979) reported that in Cuban families, the expectation is that children study, respect their parents, and follow *el buen camino* (the straight and narrow). Children are encouraged to acquire knowledge and learning *porque eso no te lo puede quitar nadie* (because no one can take that away from you) (Bernal, 1994).

Gender differences are evident in the differing expectations of boys and girls. A boy is expected to learn a trade or prepare himself for work, whereas a girl is expected "to keep herself honorable while single" and to prepare herself for marriage. Boys are enjoined to stay away from vices. Girls are instructed to avoid the opposite sex and not to go out without "ample protection" (Fox, 1979).

When a Cuban daughter reaches the age of 15 years, a *quince*, or 15th birthday party, is typically held to celebrate this rite of passage. Socially, the *quince* is indicative of the young woman's readiness for courting by a *novio* (boyfriend). In Cuba, the *quince* was celebrated with plenty of good food, music, and dancing with family and friends. In Miami's Cuban enclave, the *quince* is a major social event. Parents may save up for years to prepare for a daughter's *quince*, which has today evolved into a large, extravagant party (Mendez, 1994).

Evidence suggests that younger and second-generation Cubans are acculturating faster than older and first-generation Cubans (Bernal, 1994). Cuban adolescents may undergo an identity crisis, not knowing whether they are fully Cuban or American. During this time, they may reject traditional cultural values, and parents may feel threatened that their authority is being challenged. The opposing values and demands of their Cuban heritage and American society create a potential for tension and conflict between Cuban adolescents and their parents. Some examples are the Cuban practice of chaperoning unmarried couples when they go dating. The custom has persisted of protecting young unmarried daughters and expecting them to live at home with the family until they marry (Boswell & Curtis, 1983).

FAMILY GOALS AND PRIORITIES

Cubans have tightly knit nuclear families that allow for inclusion of relatives and *padrinos* (godparents). *La familia* (the family) is the most important source of emotional and physical support for its members. Multigenerational households are common, with grandparents often being part of the nuclear family.

In comparison with other Hispanic ethnic or cultural groups, Cubans have the lowest proportion of families with children. Cubans also have the highest proportion of people aged 65 and older who live with their relatives. The high proportion of elderly people living with family members has led to the typical three-generation Cuban family (Perez, 1984).

In Cuban families, hierarchical relationships are the norm, with husbands expecting obedience from their wives, and parents expecting the same from their children (Szapocznik & Hernandez, 1988). As is typical of many Latin American societies, Cubans tend to rely on family and personal relationships rather than on the government or organizations (Boswell & Curtis, 1983).

A system of personal relationships known as **compadrazgo** is also typical. A set of godparents, or *compadres*, is selected for each child who is baptized and confirmed. *Compadres* tend to be close friends or relatives of the child's natural parents, and may be counted on for moral or financial assistance. *Compadres* are usually considered part of the Cuban family whether or not a true blood relationship exists (Boswell & Curtis, 1983).

As Cubans become acculturated to American society, the traditional closely knit family may be disrupted. Intergenerational differences may occur, with highly Americanized children feeling alienated from their parents. The number of Cubans over the age of 65 years can be expected to double by the early part of the 21st century (Perez, 1994).

ALTERNATIVE LIFESTYLES

There is a high proportion of divorced women among Cuban Americans compared with other Hispanic and non-Hispanic groups in the United States. In spite of this, Cubans have the highest percentage of children under 18 years living with both parents, a low percentage of families headed by women with no husbands present, and the lowest rate of mothers and children living within a larger family. One explanation for these patterns may be that divorced Cuban women return to their parents' home, but because they typically have fewer children, they do not tend to be accompanied by children (Perez, 1994).

In dealing with some Cuban Americans, health-care providers may hear the term *Marielito* used in a derogatory manner to refer to the estimated 4 percent of the 125,000 Cubans who arrived during the Mariel boatlift. Because some of the *Marielitos* were hard-core criminals released from Cuban jails, the increased levels of crime in metropolitan Miami and New York have been attributed in part to their arrival. Although very few of them were criminals, unfortunately the negative attitudes toward them have been extended to Cuban Americans as a group. The *Marielitos* were predominantly single, black, working-class Cuban males, in contrast to the professional and managerial workers of earlier waves of migration (Boswell & Curtis, 1983). They experienced many difficulties in adjusting to life in the United States, had lower median incomes, and were more likely to be unemployed and receiving public assistance than earlier Cuban immigrants (Olson & Olson, 1995).

Little or no data are available on the occurrence of homosexuality among Cuban Americans, although the gay lifestyle would be contradictory to the prevailing machismo orientation of Cuban culture. Same-sex couples living together may be alienated from their families, especially among first-generation Cubans who adhere closely to traditional gender roles and family values. Given the stigma associated with homosexuality in this culture, a matter-of-fact, nonjudgmental approach must be used by health-care workers when questioning Cuban clients regarding sexual orientation or sexual practices.

Workforce Issues

CULTURE IN THE WORKPLACE

As stated previously, Cubans have enjoyed tremendous economic success in the United States. According to the U.S. Bureau of the Census (1989), 62 percent of Cubans have completed a high school education, a higher percentage than for other Hispanic groups. The relatively high educational achievement is reflected in the proportion of Cuban Americans (57 percent) who are employed in professional and technical jobs, the two highest paying occupational categories. Cuban families also have proportionately more people participating in the labor force and earning a higher median income than Mexican or Puerto Rican families (Suarez, 1993).

Cuban Americans exhibit strong entrepreneurial abilities, and many own their own businesses. These businesses tend to be concentrated in construction, transportation, textiles, wholesale, and retail trades. Cuban American businesses have the highest annual gross receipts when compared with those of other recent immigrant groups (Olson & Olson, 1995). The existence of several Cuban ethnic enclaves with a familiar language and culture has created numerous employment opportunities for recent Cuban immigrants.

Blank and Slipp (1994) discussed some of the workplace concerns of Hispanics, including Cubans. A major complaint is that regardless of different cultural heritages, Hispanics tend to be lumped together as a group. Although they share the same language with other Hispanic groups, Cubans prefer to be identified with their own group and appear to take greater pride in their heritage.

In a study of Cuban immigrants, Martinez (1984) found that one of the most frequently encountered workplace difficulties was in the area of interpersonal relationships. Cubans tend to be hierarchical in their relationships, recognizing supervisors or superiors as authority figures and treating them with respect and deference. In mainstream American culture, collegial relationships, where workers can exercise initiative, question the supervisor, and participate in decision making, may make Cubans uncomfortable. Cubans value a structure characterized by *personalismo*, that is, one that is oriented around people rather than around concepts or ideas. For Cubans, personal relationships at work are considered an extension of family relationships. Cuban workers may function best in a working environment that is warm, friendly, and fosters *personalismo*. Because of the emphasis on the job or task in the American workplace, many Cubans view this workplace as being too individualistic, businesslike, and detached.

A frequent source of tension in the workplace is the tendency of Cubans to speak Spanish with other Cuban or Hispanic coworkers. Speaking the same language allows them to form a common bond, relieve anxieties at work, and feel comfortable with one another. In Blank and Slipp's (1994) study, one Cuban supervisor asserted, "Others should know that we tend to go back and forth in language—Spanish when we're talking personally and English when it's professional."

ISSUES RELATED TO AUTONOMY

Diaz (1980) reported that the percentage of Cuban Americans who spoke Spanish exclusively at work was 34 percent in Miami and 39 percent in Union City, New Jersey. A small proportion spoke only English at work—23 percent in Miami and 17 percent in New Jersey. The existence of a Cuban ethnic enclave and the high labor force participation among Cuban Americans suggest that proficiency in English was not a requisite for employment for most individuals in this group (Boswell & Curtis, 1983). Nevertheless, for Cuban Americans as a whole, the slow progress of linguistic assimilation has created a political backlash from European Americans and African Americans, who fear further latinization of their community. In 1980, overwhelming support in Miami for an antibilingualism ordinance, stating that "the expenditure of county funds for the purpose of utilizing any language other than English, or promoting any culture other than that of the United States, is prohibited" is cited as a manifestation of the anti-Cuban sentiment (Portes & Stepick, 1993). To some degree, the language barrier may have also insulated Cuban Americans from the dominant culture, retarded acculturation, and fostered some interethnic tensions (Grenier & Stepick, 1992).

Biocultural Ecology

SKIN COLOR AND OTHER BIOLOGICAL VARIATIONS

During the period of Spanish colonization, the indigenous Arawak Indians were almost completely annihilated. Unlike people from Mexico and Central and South America, therefore, Cubans have no Indian ancestry (Queralt, 1984).

A higher proportion of Cuban Americans than Cubans are white: more than 80 percent. Only 5 percent of Cuban Americans are black (Olson & Olson, 1995). Because of their predominantly European ancestry, Cuban Americans have skin, hair, and eye colors that vary from light to dark. A minority, who are of African Cuban extraction are dark-skinned and may have physical features similar to African Americans.

DISEASES AND HEALTH CONDITIONS

Data from the Hispanic Health and Nutrition Examination (HHANE) survey indicate that 29 percent of Cuban American men, and 34 percent of Cuban American women are overweight, compared with 25 percent and 37 percent of Puerto Rican males and females, and 30 percent and 39 percent of Mexican American males and females (National Center for Health Statistics, 1989; Council on Scientific Affairs, 1991). The same study found that 16 percent of Cuban Americans aged 45 to 74 had diabetes mellitus, compared with 26 percent of Puerto Ricans and 24 percent of Mexican Americans (Council on Scientific Affairs, 1991).

Among Cuban Americans in Dade County, Florida, approximately 23 percent of the males and 16 percent of the females were hypertensive—rates that are significantly lower than those for whites and blacks nationally. Cuban American hypertensive men were more likely to be on medication than Puerto Rican and Mexican hypertensive men. With the hypertension threshold designated as 160/95, and the control threshold considered to be 140/90, the proportion of men with controlled hypertension was 26 percent for Cuban Americans, compared with 23 percent for Mexicans and 12 percent for Puerto Ricans (Pappas, Gergen, & Carroll, 1990). The Cuban population in Miami was found to have an inordinately high rate of nonalcoholic cirrhosis, but attempts to link this trend with the hepatitis B surface antigen have not proved successful (Diaz, 1980).

The HHANE survey revealed that the prevalence of self-reported bronchitis was lower among Cuban Americans (1.7 percent) and Mexican Americans (1.7 percent) than among Puerto Ricans (2.9 percent). The prevalence of chronic bronchitis was two times greater among smokers than nonsmokers among Cubans and Puerto Ricans but less for Mexican Americans (Bang, Gergen, & Carroll, 1990).

In the HHANE survey, Cubans had a significantly higher prevalence of total tooth loss than both Mexican Americans and Puerto Ricans. In adults, Cuban Americans had the highest mean number of filled teeth of the three Hispanic subgroups. Also, the prevalence of gingival inflammation and periodontitis in Cuban Americans is higher than that in the white non-Hispanic population (Ismail & Szpunar, 1990). The Cuban diet, which is high in sugar and starches, may explain the high prevalence of these conditions among Cuban Americans.

VARIATIONS IN DRUG METABOLISM

Although some studies have reported differences in drug metabolism among Hispanics, little or no data is available specific to Cuban Americans.

High-Risk Behaviors

The HHANE survey found that Hispanic men were twice as likely to smoke as Hispanic women, with a prevalence rate of 42 percent for Cuban American men. The prevalence rate of smoking among Cuban women was 24 percent, compared with 30 percent among Puerto Ricans and 24 percent among Mexicans. All three Hispanic groups showed higher smoking rates than the non-Hispanic white population in the National Health Interview Survey (Sandoval, 1994). The prevalence of smoking among Cuban American women in their thirties was higher than the national average, and they smoked significantly more cigarettes than Puerto Rican and Mexican American women in the same age group (Pletsch, 1991).

The HHANE survey also revealed that drinking alcohol was significantly more common among Cuban males than females, and among younger versus older Cuban groups, a pattern that was similar to that in Mexicans and Puerto Ricans. Among middle-aged and older Cuban males, who tend to be relatively well educated and have higher incomes, control of intoxication is important, compared with the younger, more recent Cuban immigrants. Among Cuban women, the proportion of lifelong abstainers increased significantly from the younger to the older groups (Black & Markides, 1994).

Violent deaths account for high mortality rates among adolescents and young adults of Cuban, Mexican American, and Puerto Rican origin. Cuban and Puerto Rican suicide rates also exceed those of the white non-Hispanic population (Council on Scientific Affairs, 1991).

HEALTH-CARE PRACTICES

An obstacle to good nutritional practice is the Cuban cultural perspective of the "healthy body." A healthy and beautiful Cuban infant is fat. Even among adults, a little heaviness is considered attractive. *Que gordo estas!* (How fat you are!) is considered a compliment. The traditional Cuban diet, high in calories, starches, and saturated fats, predisposes individuals to the development of obesity.

As shown in the HHANE survey, about one-third of Cuban men and women are overweight (National Center for Health Statistics, 1989). Lopez and Masse (1993) found that unmarried Cuban American women who had little recreational activity tended to have a higher mean weight. In addition, in contrast to Mexican American and Puerto Rican women, body fatness in Cuban American women was not significantly associated with income (Lopez & Masse, 1993).

In Cuba, health care is viewed as a basic human right and occupies a prominent place in the Cuban government's domestic and foreign policies. Polyclinics in communities are the basic unit of health care. Physician-nurse teams attend clients in these polyclinics as well as in the home, school, day-care center, and workplace. In the United States, Cubans exhibit high levels of preventive health behavior, as evidenced by routine physical examinations within the last 2 years. The utilization of preventive services was usually associated with accessibility, which, in turn, was significantly influenced, by education, annual income, and age (Solis et al., 1990).

Nutrition

MEANING OF FOOD

Food has a powerful social meaning among Cuban Americans, allowing families to reaffirm kinship ties, promote a sense of community, and perpetuate their customs and heritage (Boswell & Curtis, 1983). To grasp this fully, one needs only to observe multigenerational families assembled for dinner on a Saturday or Sunday evening in a Cuban restaurant in Miami's Little Havana, or Cuban friends sharing a cup of *cafe cubano* and *pastelitos* at a stand-up sidewalk counter. In Miami alone,

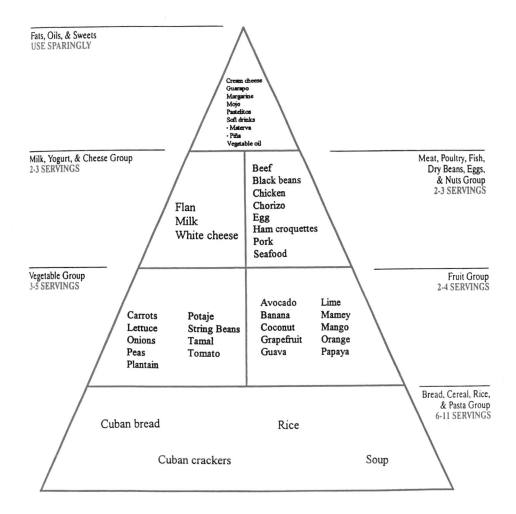

Fats, Oils, & Sweets
USE SPARINGLY

Cream cheese
Guarapo
Margarine
Mojo
Pastelitos
Soft drinks
• Materva
• Piña
Vegetable oil

Milk, Yogurt, & Cheese Group
2-3 SERVINGS

Flan
Milk
White cheese

Beef
Black beans
Chicken
Chorizo
Egg
Ham croquettes
Pork
Seafood

Meat, Poultry, Fish,
Dry Beans, Eggs,
& Nuts Group
2-3 SERVINGS

Vegetable Group
3-5 SERVINGS

Carrots
Lettuce
Onions
Peas
Plantain

Potaje
String Beans
Tamal
Tomato

Avocado   Lime
Banana   Mamey
Coconut   Mango
Grapefruit Orange
Guava   Papaya

Fruit Group
2-4 SERVINGS

Cuban bread

Rice

Bread, Cereal, Rice,
& Pasta Group
6-11 SERVINGS

Cuban crackers

Soup

FIGURE 8–1   The Food Guide Pyramid for Cubans. (From *Hispanic Americans in Florida: An overview of their food habits*, by A. Rodriguez, 1995.)

the demand for Cuban food and food products has resulted in the establishment of about 400 Latin restaurants, mostly Cuban, and some 700 *bodegas*, or grocery stores.

COMMON FOODS AND FOOD RITUALS

Cuban foods reflect the environmental influences of Cuba's tropical climate and agriculture, the historical influences of Spanish colonial rule, the African slave trade, and the Arawak Indians' cultivation methods. Figure 8–1 depicts the food pyramid for Cubans. Typical staple foods are root crops like yams, yucca, malanga, and boniato; plantains; and grains. Traditional Spanish dishes like *arroz con pollo* and *paella* are frequently served. Many dishes are prepared with olive oil, garlic, tomato sauce, vinegar, wine, lime juice, called *sofrito*, and spices. Meat is usually marinated in lemon, lime, sour orange, or grapefruit juice before cooking (Boswell & Curtis, 1983).

The main course in Cuban meals is meat, usually pork or chicken. Some popular entrees are roast pork (*lechon*),

fried pork chunks (*masas de puerco*), sirloin steak (*palomilla*), shredded beef (*ropa vieja*), pot roast (*boliche*), and roasted chicken (*pollo asado*). A roasted suckling pig is traditionally served on Christmas Eve and New Year's Day, and during other festive celebrations. Black beans are prepared with a sauce containing fat, pork, and other spices. Ripe plantains (*platanos maduros*) or green plantains (*platanos verdes*) are served fried. Fried green plantains (*tostones* or *mariquita*) may also be smashed between a brown paper bag and the fist (*un cartucho y el puno*), giving them the familiar name *platanos y punetazo*. Desserts are rich and very sweet, such as custard (*flan*), egg pudding (*natilla*), rice pudding (*arroz con leche*), coconut pudding (*pudin de coco*), or bread pudding (*pudin de pan*) (Boswell & Curtis, 1983).

Beverages may include sugar cane juice (*guarapo*), iced coconut milk (*coco frio*), milkshakes (*batidos*), Cuban soft drinks such as Iron Beer or Materva, sangria, or beer. The strong and bittersweet coffee called *cafe cubano* is a standard drink after meals and throughout the day, whether at home, in restaurants, or in other social situations. In the United States, Cubans may drink the *cafe cubano* as *cortadito* or with a dash of milk to cut the strength and bittersweet taste (Boswell & Curtis, 1983). A traditional Cuban meal includes a generous helping of white rice with black beans or black bean soup, fried plantains, roasted pork or fried chicken, a tuber such as malanga or yucca, followed by dessert and espresso. Thus, the typical diet is high in calories, starches, and saturated fats. As in Spain and other Hispanic countries, a leisurely noon meal (*almuerzo*) and a late evening dinner (*comida*), sometimes as late as 10 or 11 P.M., are customary.

NUTRITIONAL DEFICIENCIES AND FOOD LIMITATIONS

As seen in Figure 8–1, the major food groups are well represented in the Cuban diet; however, leafy green vegetables may be lacking in the average Cuban meal. Therefore, in assessing the nutritional adequacy of a Cuban client's diet, the health-care provider must ensure that there is sufficient fiber content.

Pregnancy and Childbearing Practices

FERTILITY PRACTICES AND VIEWS TOWARD PREGNANCY

The fertility rate of Cuban women is lower than that of Mexican American and Puerto Rican women (Smith & Weinman, 1995). The low rate of reproduction, which is consistent in every maternal age group, has been attributed to three factors (Perez, 1984):

1 Cuban American women have a high rate of labor force participation.

2 Before the revolution, Cuba had the lowest birth rate in Latin America.

3 Cuba's current reproductive rate is among the lowest in the developing world.

In an analysis of HHANE data, Stroup-Benham and Trevino (1991) found that Mexican American women were twice as likely to use oral contraceptives (16 percent) as Cuban American women (8 percent). Among Cuban American women who were considered at risk for pregnancy, only 9 percent took oral contraceptives, compared with 11 percent among Puerto Ricans and 20 percent among Mexican Americans.

In the same study, hysterectomies, oophorectomies, and tubal ligations were found to be less common among Cuban American women than among either Mexican American or Puerto Rican women. Based on these data, Cuban American women appear to be at greatest risk for unintended pregnancies. Paradoxically, they have the lowest birth rate among the three groups of Hispanic women (Stroup-Benham & Trevino, 1991). A possible explanation for this inconsistency may be the high divorce rate and the high labor force participation rate among Cuban American women.

The rate of prenatal care among Cuban mothers is 85 percent, compared with 80 percent in white non-Hispanics, 59 percent in Mexican Americans, and 65 percent in Puerto Ricans (U.S. Department of Health and Human Services, 1993). The prevalence of preterm births (infants born before 37 weeks of gestation) was found to be lowest (13 percent) among Cuban American women, followed by Mexican American women (14 percent), and Puerto Rican women (15 percent), compared with 11 percent for non-Hispanic white women (Mendoza et al., 1991).

In the Linked Birth and Infant Death data sets of 1983 and 1984, the neonatal mortality risk (the risk of death in infants less than 28 days after birth) was 1.0 among Cuban Americans and Mexican Americans, compared with 2.3 among Puerto Rican Islanders and 1.5 among continental Puerto Ricans. The post-neonatal mortality risk, the risk of death in infants between 28 to 364 days of life, was highest among Puerto Ricans (1.2) and lowest among Cuban Americans (0.6) (Becerra et al., 1991).

Many Cuban folk beliefs and practices surround pregnancy. For example, some Cuban women believe that they have to eat for two during the pregnancy and end up gaining excessive weight. Some believe that morning sickness is cured by eating coffee grounds; that eating a lot of fruit ensures that the baby will be born with a smooth complexion; and that wearing necklaces during pregnancy causes the umbilical cord to be wrapped around the baby's neck (Brewer, 1995).

Among Cuban Americans, childbirth is a time for celebration. Family members and friends congregate in the hospital, awaiting the delivery of the baby. Although traditionally it was not acceptable for Cuban men to attend the birth of their children, the younger and more acculturated Cuban fathers tend to be present to support their wives during labor and delivery. In the postpartum period, it is believed that ambulation, exposure to cold, and bare feet place the mother at risk for infection. Because of this, family members and relatives often care for the mother and baby for about 4 weeks postpartum (Brewer, 1995).

PRESCRIPTIVE, RESTRICTIVE, AND TABOO PRACTICES IN THE CHILDBEARING FAMILY

Thomas and DeSantis (1995) found that most Cuban women (77 percent) who migrated to the United States in the 1980s considered breast-feeding better than bottle feeding, but only 40 percent chose to breast-feed one or more of their infants. In the same study, Cuban mothers weaned infants from the breast and introduced solid foods at a median age of 3 months. Weaning from the bottle occurred in Cuban infants at a median age of 4, compared with 1 year of age recommended in the medical literature.

Thomas and DeSantis (1995) related the early introduction of solid foods and prolonged bottle feeding of Cuban children to the traditional Cuban beliefs that "a fat child is a healthy child," and that breast-feeding may contribute to a deformity or asymmetry of the breasts. In the same study, 97 percent of Cuban mothers indicated that they administer vitamin preparations to promote healthy development of their children. Cuban mothers also used advice about child health given by their spouses, mothers, mothers-in-law, and clerks and pharmacists who sold them over-the-counter drugs (Thomas & DeSantis, 1995).

Death Rituals

DEATH RITUALS AND EXPECTATIONS

In death, as in life, the support of the extended family network is important. Whether in the hospital or at home, the dying person is typically attended by a large gathering of relatives and friends. In Catholic families, individual and group prayers are held for the dying to provide a peaceful passage to the hereafter. Religious artifacts such as rosary beads, crucifixes, *estampitas* (little statues of saints) are placed in the dying person's room.

Depending on the dying person's religious beliefs, a Catholic priest, a Protestant minister, a rabbi, or a **santero** may be summoned to the deathbed to perform appropriate death rites. For adherents of **Santeria**, death rites may include animal sacrifice, chants, and ceremonial gestures. Health-care providers need to be open-minded and responsive to both the physical and psychosocial needs of the dying and the bereaved and, regardless of religious beliefs, accord them the utmost respect and privacy.

After a person's death, candles are lighted to illuminate the path of the spirit to the afterlife. A wake, or *velorio*, is usually held at a funeral parlor, where friends and relatives gather to support the bereaved family. The wake lasts for 2 to 3 days until the funeral. Burial in a cemetery is the common practice for Cuban Catholics, although others may choose cremation.

RESPONSES TO DEATH AND GRIEF

Bereavement is expressed openly among Cuban Americans, with loud crying and other physical manifestations of grief considered socially acceptable. Death is an occasion for relatives living far away to visit and commiserate with the bereaved family. Women from the immediate family usually dress in black during the period of mourning. Visitors make offerings of candles and floral wreaths (*coronas*), provide assistance with household chores, and attend to visitors or funeral arrangements. Cuban Americans customarily remember and honor the deceased on their birthdays or death anniversaries by lighting candles, offering prayers or masses, bringing flowers to the grave, or gathering with family members at the grave site.

Spirituality

DOMINANT RELIGION AND USE OF PRAYER

Approximately 85 percent of Cuban Americans are Roman Catholics, with the remaining 15 percent being Protestants, Jews, and believers in the African Cuban practice of *Santeria*. The Roman Catholic Church has been an important source of support, especially for first-generation Cuban immigrants. A number of predominantly Cuban parishes with Cuban clergy are located in Florida and New Jersey, where large Cuban populations reside. In south Florida, about 1 in 5 Cuban Catholics regularly attend mass (Jorge, Suchlicki, & Leyva de Varona, 1991). The Roman Catholic Church has exerted an important influence on Cuban families by providing educational opportunities at Catholic schools. Many Cuban parents, especially the upper middle class, prefer to have their children educated in private Catholic schools.

Roman Catholicism as practiced by Cubans is personalistic, rather than institutional, in nature. The religious practice of Cuban Catholics is characterized by devotion and intimate, confiding relationships with the Virgin Mary, Jesus, and the saints (Boswell & Curtis, 1983).

Some families may have shrines dedicated to *La Caridad del Cobre* (the patron saint of Cuba) or other saints at the entrance to their homes, in their yards, or in commercial establishments. The three favorite saints that are enshrined are Santa Barbara, San Lazaro, and *La Caridad del Cobre*. Inside the home, crucifixes and pictures or statues depicting images of saints may be found. When someone is ill, small pictures of saints, called *estampitas,* may be placed under the pillow or at the sick person's bedside.

Significant religious holidays for Cuban families include Christmas, *Los Tres Reyes Magos* (Three Kings Day), and the festivals of the *La Caridad del Cobre* and Santa Barbara (Boswell & Curtis, 1983). The Cuban community usually celebrates the feast of *La Caridad del Cobre* (September 8) by transporting the statue of the patron saint on a boat to a specific location, where a mass is held in her honor. Cuban families also celebrate Christmas Eve (*Noche Buena*) with a traditional Cuban meal. Typically a pig is cooked all day in a wooden box lined in metal (*una caja china*) and set in the backyard. The pig is placed at the bottom of the box and the charcoal on top. The meat is served with black beans and rice, yucca, and *turones* (Spanish dessert). The evening concludes with the family attending midnight mass (*Misa de Gallo*).

Santeria, or *Regla de Ocha*, is a 300-year-old African Cuban religious system that combines elements of Roman Catholicism with ancient Yoruba tribal beliefs and practices. Santeria originated among the Yoruba people of Nigeria, who brought their beliefs with them when they arrived in the New World as slaves. As a condition of their entry into the West Indies, slaves were required to be baptized as Roman Catholics (Murphy, 1988). In the process of adapting to their new non-African environment, the slaves altered their beliefs to incorporate those of their predominantly Catholic masters. Thus, Santeria became the product of a syncretism between "the gods of the slaves and the Catholic saints of their masters" (Sandoval, 1979: 138).

Santeria evolved from two main cultural antecedents: the worship of the **orishas** among the Yoruba tribe of Nigeria and the cult of saints from the Roman Catholicism of Spain. Through their exposure to the Catholic religion, the slaves came to associate their African gods, called *orishas*, with the Roman Catholic saints, or *santos*. The worship of the *orishas* and the asso-

Table 8–1 Seven African Powers or Main Orishas

Orisha	Christian Saint	Function/Power	Punishment	Propitiation
Eleggua	Holy Child of Atocha	Guardian of entrances, roads, and paths; Trickster		Blood of goats; black rooster; smoked fish; smoked junia; yams, sugar cane
Obatala	Our Lady of Mercy	Father of all human beings, gives advice, is source of energy, wisdom, purity, and peace	Blindness, paralysis, and birth deformities	White pigeons, white canaries; female goat; plums; yam puree
Chango	Saint Barbara	Warrior deity that controls thunder and violent storms, lightning and fire	Death, suicide by fire	Roosters, goats, lambs; apples, and bananas
Oshun	Our Lady of Charity	Deity that controls money and love, makes marriages, protects genitals	Abdominal distress, social and domestic strife	Female goat, white chickens, sheep; honey
Yemaya	Our Lady of Regla	Primary mother of the santos, protects womanhood, owns seas	Respiratory distress	Ducks, lambs, female goats; watermelons; black-eyed peas
Babaluaye	Saint Lazarus	Patron of the sick, especially diseases of the skin	Leprosy, gangrene, skin diseases	Spotted rooster; snakes; cigars; pennies; glasses of water
Ogun	Saint Peter	Warrior deity, owns all metals and weapons	Violent death (such as an automobile accident)	Blood and feathers; young bulls, roosters; steel knife; railroad tracks

Source: Adapted from Martinez, R., & Wetli, C. (1982). Santeria: A magicoreligious system of Afro-Cuban origin. *American Journal of Social Psychiatry, 2*(3), p 34, with permission.

ciated beliefs, rituals, incantations, magic, and spirit possession are central to Santeria.

Table 8–1 displays the seven African powers, or main *orishas* (Martinez & Wetli, 1982). The Yoruba deity of fire and thunder, called Chango, became identified with Santa Barbara, the patron saint of the Spanish artillery, who appeared in Catholic lithographs in red, the color of the *orisha* (Sandoval, 1979). Chango, the most popular god in Santeria, controls thunder, violent storms, lightning, and fire. The six other *orishas,* the Catholic saints with whom they are identified, and their corresponding functions and powers, are also shown in Table 8–1.

When people decide to practice Santeria, their *orishas* become known to them and must be worshipped throughout their lives. Followers of Santeria believe in the magical and medicinal properties of flowers, herbs, weeds, twigs, and leaves. Sweet herbs such as *manzanilla, verbena,* and *mejorana* are used for attracting good luck, love, money, and prosperity. Bitter herbs such as *apasote, zarzaparilla,* and *yerba bruja* are used to banish evil and negative energies.

Adherents of Santeria also believe in the power of consecrated objects such as stones (*otanes*) in which the *orishas* reside. Necklaces, bracelets, and charms may be given by *santeros* to their clients to protect them from evil and strengthen their well-being. The *orishas* must be propitiated for the person to avoid punishment. For example, white pigeons and plums must be offered to the god Obatala to avoid the punishments of blindness, paralysis, and birth deformities (Martinez & Wetli, 1982).

Sacrifice, or **ebo** (pronounced "egbo" or "igbo"), is a central ritual in Santeria. The main purpose of *ebo* is to

establish communication between the spirits and human beings. The initiation of a *santero* involves the sacrifice of a four-legged animal and a series of rites lasting 7 days (Murphy, 1988). Transition through major life events such as birth, death, and marriage require ritual sacrifices to appease the gods and solicit their support.

Sacrificial objects in Santeria include plants, foods, and animals. Plants and foods include plantains, malanga, yam, okra, flour, gourds, and ground black-eyed peas wrapped in plantain leaves. Animals used for sacrifice, such as hens, birds, lambs, or goats, are killed by wringing the head or severing the carotid arteries with a knife. The animal's blood is offered as a type of communion with the deities. In 1993, the Supreme Court struck down anti-animal sacrifice laws in Hialeah, Florida, and recognized the right of a Santeria sanctuary, the Church of Chango Eyife, to offer animal sacrifice as a religious sacrament (Gonzalez, 1995).

Santeria is viewed as a link to the past, and is used among Cubans and other Hispanic groups to cope with physical and emotional problems. When someone is sick, that person's physical complaints may be diagnosed and treated by a physician, but the *santero* may be summoned to assist in balancing and neutralizing the various aspects of the illness. Santeria is actively practiced by middle-class Cubans in Miami and in areas of New York, New Jersey, and California where Cubans reside (Sandoval, 1979).

In eliciting a complete history from clients, health-care providers must include information regarding the type of religion being practiced, if any. Clients' religious beliefs and practices must be viewed in an open, sincere, and nonjudgmental manner. In the hospital setting, maintenance of privacy is important if clients and families need to perform certain rituals or prayers. A visit from a priest, rabbi, or *santero* may provide a sense of psychological support and spiritual well-being. At times, *santeros* have been known to make sacrificial offerings at the client's hospital bedside. As long as standards of safety and sanitation are maintained, families must be allowed space and privacy to be able to engage in specific religious ceremonies.

MEANING OF LIFE AND INDIVIDUAL SOURCES OF STRENGTH

As in other Latin American communities, the family is the most important source of strength, identity, and emotional security. Cubans usually rely on a network of family members and relatives for assistance in times of need. The sense of specialness Cubans feel, stemming from pride in their culture and their remarkable success in adapting to their new country is, likewise, a source of self-esteem and self-identity. For many Cubans, deeply held religious beliefs have provided guidance and strength during the long and difficult process of migration and adaptation, and continue to play an important role in their day-to-day lives.

SPIRITUAL BELIEFS AND HEALTH-CARE PRACTICES

Research indicates that Cubans tend to be fatalistic, feeling that they lack control over circumstances influencing their lives (Szapocznik et al., 1978). The belief in a higher power is evident in a variety of practices Cubans may engage in for the purpose of maintaining health and well being or curing illness, such as using magical herbs, special prayers or chants, ritual cleansing, and sacrificial offerings.

When Cuban clients consult health-care providers, in all likelihood they have already tried some folk remedies advised by older women in their family or obtained from a botanica. Most folk remedies are harmless and do not interfere with biomedical treatment. In most cases, clients may be allowed to continue using these remedies, such as herbal teas.

Health-care providers should be alert to the frequent practice of sharing prescription medications in families and among relatives. A family member who found an antibiotic effective in curing an ailment may share the medication with another relative suffering from the same symptoms. The health history must always include assessment of past or present medication use, whether traditional, over-the-counter, or prescription. Appropriate explanations must be given regarding the actions and adverse effects of drugs and the reasons why they cannot be shared with other family members.

Health-Care Practices

HEALTH-SEEKING BELIEFS AND BEHAVIORS

As in other Latin American societies, Cubans rely on the family as the primary source of health advice. Typically, the older women in the family are sought out for information such as traditional home remedies for common ailments. Herbal teas or mixtures may be prepared to relieve mild or moderate symptoms. Concurrently or alternatively, a *santero* may be consulted or a trip to the botanica may be warranted to obtain treatment.

Socialized into a strong health ideology and successful primary care system in Cuba, Cubans are able to use biomedical services as primary or secondary sources of care. Cuba has a regionalized, hierarchically organized, national health system that provides universal coverage and standardization of services. An innovative family practice program assigns physicians and nurses to city blocks and remote communities to promote physical fitness, detect risk factors for disease, and cure disease. In the United States, many Cuban clinics have evolved into health maintenance organizations (HMOs).

RESPONSIBILITY FOR HEALTH CARE

Of the three Hispanic groups, Cuban Americans with the most education and the highest incomes are most likely to have private insurance (Council on Scientific Affairs, 1991). The Current Population Survey estimated that the rate of uninsured was 20 percent for Cuban Americans, compared with 37 percent for Mexican Americans, 16 percent for Puerto Ricans, and 10 percent for non-Hispanic whites (U.S. Bureau of the Census, 1989). In addition, Cuban Americans averaged more visits per year to a physician (6.2 visits) than Mexican Americans (3.7 visits) and white non-Hispanics (4.8 visits) (Trevino et al., 1991).

Research indicates that the utilization of preventive services by Cuban Americans was determined more by access to care than by acculturation. Among Cuban Americans without health insurance, 40 percent reported not having visited a physician for more than 1 year (Trevino et al., 1991). Moreover, among Cuban Americans, access to care was positively associated with higher education, greater annual income, and age (Solis et al., 1990).

FOLK PRACTICES

Cubans may use traditional medicinal plants in the form of teas, potions, salves, or poultices. In Cuban communities like Little Havana in Miami, stores called **botanicas** sell a variety of herbs, ointments, oils, powders, incenses, and religious figurines to relieve maladies, bring luck, drive away evil spirits, or break curses. In addition, Santeria necklaces and animals used for ritual sacrifice are available at botanicas. (See Fig. 8–2.)

According to Estape (1995) herbal teas that may be used to treat common ailments include:

Cosimiento de anis (anise): to relieve stomach aches, flatulence, and baby colic; also to calm nerves
Cosimiento de limon con miel de abeja (lemon and honey): to relieve cough and respiratory congestion
Cosimiento de apasote (pumpkin seed): to treat gastrointestinal worms
Cosimiento de canela (cinnamon): to relieve cough, respiratory congestion, and menstrual cramps
Cosimiento de manzanilla (chamomile): to relieve stomachaches

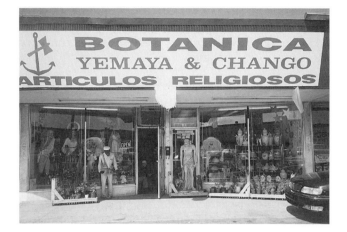

FIGURE 8–2   In Cuban communities, *botanicas* such as this one sell herbs, ointments, oils, powders, incenses, and religious figurines to relieve maladies, bring luck, or drive away evil spirits.

Cosimiento de naranja agria (sour orange): to relieve cough and respiratory congestion

Cosimiento de savila (aloe vera): to relieve stomachaches

Cosimiento de tilo (linden leaves): to calm nerves

Cosimiento de yerba buena (spearmint leaves): to relieve stomachaches and calm nerves

Fruits and vegetables, abundant in the natural tropical environment of Cuba, that may be used include:

Chayote (vegetable): to calm nerves

Zanaoria (carrots): to help problems with vision

Toronja y ajo (grapefruit and garlic): to lower blood pressure

Papaya y toronja y pina (papaya, grapefruit, and pineapple): to eliminate gastrointestinal parasites

Remolacha (beets): to treat influenza and anemia

Cascara de mandarina (fruit): to relieve cough

Other home remedies that may be used include:

Agua con sal (salt water): to relieve sore throat

Agua de coco (coconut water): to relieve kidney problems and infections

Agua raja (turpentine): applied to sore muscles and joints to relieve pain

Bicarbonato, limon y agua (baking soda, lemon, and water): to relieve stomach upset or heartburn

Cebo de carnero (fat of lamb): applied directly on the skin to treat contusions and swelling

Mantequilla (butter): applied directly on burns to soothe pain

Clara de huevos (egg white): applied directly over scalp to promote hair growth

Cuban families may use an *azabache, la manito de coral,* or *ojitos de Santa Lucia* for various protective purposes. The *azabache* is a black stone placed on infants and children as a bracelet or pin to protect them from the evil eye. *La manito de coral,* symbolic of the hand of God protecting a person, may also be worn as a necklace or bracelet. *Los ojitos de Santa Lucia,* or the eyes of Saint Lucy, may be hung on a bracelet or necklace for prevention of blindness and protection from the evil eye.

BARRIERS TO HEALTH CARE

Poverty may be a barrier to health care for only 14 percent of Cuban families, compared with 65 percent of Puerto Ricans, 47 percent of Mexicans, and 10 percent of non-Hispanic whites in the United States (Juarbe, 1995). In a study of Cuban households, Diaz (1980) examined difficulties encountered in the utilization of health-care services. Nearly half of those who used public clinics and public hospitals reported at least one or more types of difficulties. These included language, time lag, red tape, and transportation. For those who used private clinics and private health practitioners, the difficulties were cost of services, inconvenient hours, language, and red tape.

Moreover, Cuban families that used hospitals, both public and private, named language as a major difficulty in obtaining health services. Thus, hospitals may not be as accommodating to the bilingual needs of Cuban clients as are other types of health-care providers (Diaz, 1980).

CULTURAL RESPONSES TO HEALTH AND ILLNESS

Because of the many losses they experienced in leaving their homeland and the difficulties associated with adaptation to a new culture and environment, Cuban immigrants may suffer from loneliness, depression, anger, anxiety, insecurity, and health problems (Queralt, 1984). In evaluating Cuban families, Bernal (1994) suggested that health-care providers assess the following:

1   *Migration phase associated with the family.* It is important to know how long the family has lived in the United States and the reasons for migration. Information about political and social pressures that prompted the move should be elicited. Because family members acculturate at different rates, the level of acculturation should also be determined.

2   *Degree of connectedness to the culture of origin.* Conflicts in value orientations must be identified when assessing Cuban families. For example, the varying expectations between mainstream American and Cuban cultures with respect to dependence and independence may give rise to tension and conflict.

3   *Differentiation between the stresses of migration and differences in cultural values and family developmental conflicts.* In a clinical situation, health-care providers must be able to recognize whether the clients' responses are due to migration-related problems, value orientation conflicts, or dysfunctional family development.

Among Cuban Americans, dependency is a culturally acceptable sick role. Sick family members are showered with attention and support. Frequently, a hospitalized Cuban client will have a room full of flower arrangements and visitors. Favorite dishes may be brought to the hospital from home. The extended family network is relied on to temporarily assume the household chores and other tasks usually performed by the sick person. Family members are consulted and typically participate in decision making relative to the client's treatment.

Cuban Americans tend to seek help in response to crisis situations. The experience of pain constitutes a signal of a physical disturbance that warrants consultation with a traditional or biomedical healer. Similar to other Hispanic clients, Cuban Americans tend to express their pain and discomfort. Verbal complaints, moaning, crying, and groaning are culturally appropriate ways of dealing with pain. The expression of pain itself may serve a pain-relieving function and may not necessarily signify a need for administration of pain medication.

African Cubans may seek biomedical care for organic diseases but consult a *santero* for spiritual or emotional crises. Conditions such as **decensos** (fainting spells) or **barrenillos** (obsessions) may be treated solely by a *santero* or simultaneously with a physician. As pointed out by Sandoval (1979), the trance state achieved through Santeria enables the Cuban client to act out emotional problems in a manner that is nonthreatening to the person's self-esteem.

BLOOD TRANSFUSIONS AND ORGAN DONATION

Receiving blood transfusions and organ donations are usually acceptable for Cubans. This is probably due to their experience with the sophisticated, high-technology medical care system in Cuba.

Health-Care Practitioners

TRADITIONAL VERSUS BIOMEDICAL PRACTITIONERS

As with many other cultural groups, Cubans use both traditional and biomedical care. Initially, folk remedies may be used at home to treat an ailment or illness. If the condition persists, folk practitioners such as *santeros* and biomedical practitioners may be used either simultaneously or successively. When seeing Cuban clients, health-care providers must always ask about the use of folk remedies and consultations with folk practitioners to prevent conflicting therapeutic regimens.

Although Santeria was associated with the lower, uneducated classes in Cuba, it has emerged as a viable and dynamic religious and health system among middle-class Cubans in the United States. The *santero* may prescribe treatment or perform the appropriate rituals or ceremonies to enable ill people to recover. The *santero* may invoke various types of supernatural deities to intervene in their lives and make them well. Often, even if a physician is being consulted, clients may believe that the *santero* is needed to rally supernatural forces toward their recuperation (Sandoval, 1979).

Unlike most health-care agencies, which are open for only 8 or 9 hours a day, Santeria houses are open to help their adherents about 18 hours a day (Sandoval, 1979).

Many Cubans consult a family physician for primary care. Before the revolution, Cuba had an organized government-supported health program that provided medical care to most citizens. Since the 1959 revolution, the Cuban government has articulated a fundamental principle that health care is a right of all and a responsibility of the state. Thus, a national health-care system provides universal coverage, equitable geographic distribution of health-care facilities, and standardization of health services.

Cuban families in Miami gained access to primary health-care services predominantly through private health practitioners and private clinics, whereas in Union City the main sources of health care were private health practitioners. An extensive network of privately owned and operated health clinics exist in Dade County, mainly located in Miami's Cuban ethnic enclaves, Little Havana and Hialeah. The private health clinics are believed to be popular among the Cubans because they provide services that are culturally sensitive to Cuban needs, such as emphasis on the family, use of the Spanish language, focus on preventive health-care behaviors, and low cost.

In contrast to the high utilization rate of private clinics, very small proportions of Cuban families in Miami and Union City used public clinics for primary health-care services. Moreover, only 1 percent of Cuban households in both cities reported using a *santero* for health-care services, a surprisingly low proportion given the popular belief that the practice of Santeria is widespread. In contrast, 7 percent of the Miami respondents and 23 percent of the Union City respondents indicated they would approach a *santero* if needed. Diaz suspected some degree of underreporting in this survey because of the sensitive nature of the question; therefore, the true figures may actually be higher.

STATUS OF HEALTH-CARE PROVIDERS

Although Hispanics, including Cubans, will soon exceed 13 percent of the U.S. population, they are seriously underrepresented in the health occupations. Only 1 percent of registered nurses; 2 to 3 percent of dentists, pharmacists, and therapists; and 5 percent of physicians are of Hispanic origin (Ginzberg, 1991; Rojas, 1994). More effort needs to be directed toward increasing the number of Hispanic students in health professional schools as well as enhancing programs and resources to assist in successful retention and completion.

CASE STUDY Mrs. Demetilla Hernandez is a 63-year-old Cuban woman who seeks consultation at the Liberty HMO Clinic because of weakness, lethargy, and fatigue that she has experienced for the last 2 months. A week ago, while cooking dinner at her daughter Mariana's house, she momentarily lost her balance and slipped on the kitchen floor. Although Mrs. Hernandez sustained only a mild bruise on her leg, her daughter Mariana insisted on taking her to the clinic for a checkup because of her persistent symptoms.

Mrs. Hernandez, widowed 4 years ago when her husband died of a heart attack, lives with her daughter Mariana, age 40. Mariana is divorced and has three children: Luis, 15; Carolina, 10; and Sofia, 7. Since moving into Mariana's house, Mrs. Hernandez has been managing the household while Mariana is at work. Mrs. Hernandez prepares the family's meals, attends to the children when they come home from school, and performs light housekeeping chores. Mariana is employed full-time as a supervisor at the local telephone company. The family, originally from Cuba, has been living in Miami for 12 years. Carolina and Sofia were born in Miami, but Luis came from Cuba with his parents when he was 3 years old. Mrs. Hernandez, who does not speak English, converses with her daughter and grandchildren in Spanish. Although the children and their mother occasionally speak English among themselves, the family's language at home is Spanish.

At the Liberty HMO Clinic, Mrs. Hernandez was diagnosed with essential hypertension and non-insulin-dependent diabetes mellitus. The physician prescribed an oral hypoglycemic drug and advised Mrs. Hernandez to exercise daily and to limit her food intake to 1500 calories a day. Mrs. Hernandez was concerned because she usually prepares traditional Cuban meals at home and was not sure whether she could tolerate being on a diet. Besides, she explained to Mariana, she thought the dishes she prepares are very "healthy." Proof of that, she stated, is that her three grandchildren are plump and nice-looking. Mrs. Hernandez told her daughter that instead of buying the prescribed medicine, perhaps she should go to the *botanica* and obtain some herbs that would help lower her blood sugar.

STUDY QUESTIONS

1 As a health-care provider, what are the typical Cuban communication patterns you need to be aware of in dealing with Mrs. Hernandez?

2 Describe the traditional Cuban food patterns. How would you assist Mrs. Hernandez in developing a plan for a 1500-calorie diet and regular exercise?

3 Would you encourage Mrs. Hernandez to go to the *botanica* to purchase some herbs? How would you approach her desire to use herbs instead of the prescribed oral hypoglycemic agent?

4 Discuss some common folk practices that Cuban families may use to maintain health or cure common ailments.

5 Explain how time orientation may influence Mrs. Hernandez' compliance with follow-up clinic visits.

6 Formulate three important goals in teaching Mrs. Hernandez and her family about health care.

7 Identify the typical family and value structure among Cuban Americans.

8 List three major health problems among Cuban Americans.

9 If you were the health education specialist at the clinic, what would you teach the staff about Cuban culture to help them provide culturally comptent care?

10 Discuss traditional child-rearing practices among Cuban Americans.

REFERENCES

Bang, K., Gergen, P. J., & Carroll, M. (1990). Prevalence of chronic bronchitis among U.S. Hispanics from Hispanic Health and Nutrition Examination Survey 1982–84. *American Journal of Public Health, 80*(12), 1495–1497.

Becerra, J. E., Hogue, C. J., Altrash, H., & Perez, N. (1991). Infant mortality among Hispanics: A portrait of heterogeneity. *Journal of the American Medical Association, 265*(2), 217–221.

Bernal, G. (1994). Cuban families. In M. Uriarte-Gaston & J. Canas-Martinez (Eds.), *Cubans in the United States* (pp. 135–156). Boston: Center for the Study of the Cuban Community.

Black, S. A., & Markides, K. S. (1994). Aging and generational patterns of alcohol consumption among Mexican Americans, Cuban Americans and mainland Puerto Ricans. *International Aging and Human Development, 39*(2), 97–103.

Blank, R., & Slipp, S. (1994). *Voices of diversity* (pp. 63–64). New York: American Management Association.

Boswell, T. D. (Ed.). (1991). *South Florida: Winds of change.* Miami, FL: American Geographers Association.

Boswell, T. D., & Curtis, J. R. (1983). *The Cuban-American experience: Culture, images, and perspectives.* Totowa, NJ: Rowman & Allanheld.

Brewer, S. (1995). *Conception, pregnancy and childbirth rituals, taboos and beliefs within the Filipino and Cuban cultures.* Unpublished manuscript. Miami, FL: Florida International University.

Council on Scientific Affairs, American Medical Association. (1991). Hispanic health in the United States. *Journal of the American Medical Association, 265*(2), 248–252.

Cultural Orientation Resource Center. (2002). *The Cubans: Their history and culture.* Retrieved March 17, 2002, http://www.culturalorientation.net.cubans/index.htm.

Diaz, G. M. (1980). *Evaluation and identification of policy issues in the Cuban community.* Miami, FL: Cuban National Planning Council.

Estape, E. (1995). *The Cuban culture: Folk remedies and magicoreligious beliefs.* Unpublished manuscript. Miami, FL: Florida International University.

Fox, G. F. (1979). *Working-class émigrés from Cuba.* Palo Alto, CA: R & E Research Associates.

Gallagher, P. L. (1980). *The Cuban exile: A socio-political analysis.* New York: Arno Press.

Ginzberg, E. (1991). Access to health care for Hispanics. *Journal of the American Medical Association, 265*(2), 238–241.

Gonzalez, A. M. (1995, June 11). Santeria still shrouded in secrecy. *The Miami Herald*, pp. 1B–5B.

Grenier, G. J., & Stepick, A. (Eds.). (1992). *Miami now! Immigration, ethnicity, and social change.* Gainesville, FL: University Press of Florida.

National Women's Health Information Center. (2002). *Hispanics: Women of color.* Retrieved March 17, 2002, from http://www.4women.gov.

Ismail, A. I., & Szpunar, S. M. (1990). The prevalence of total tooth loss, dental caries, and periodontal disease among Mexican Americans, Cuban Americans, and Puerto Ricans: Findings from HHANES 1982–84. *American Journal of Public Health, 80*, 66–70.

Jorge, A., Suchlicki, J., & Leyva de Varona, A. (1991). *Cuban exiles in Florida: Their presence and contributions.* Miami, FL: University of Miami.

Juarbe, T. C. (1995). Access to health care for Hispanic women: A primary health care perspective. *Nursing Outlook, 43*, 23–28.

Lopez, L. M., & Masse, B. R. (1993). Income, body fatness, and fat patterns in Hispanic women from the Hispanic Health and Nutrition Examination Survey. *Health Care for Women International, 14*, 117–128.

Martinez, J. C. (1984). The Cuban immigrant of 1980: An exploration of psychosocial issues in the migration experience. In M. Uriarte-Gaston & J. Cana-Martinez (Eds.), *Cubans in the United States* (pp. 181–184). Boston: Center for the Study of the Cuban Community.

Martinez, R., & Wetli, C. (1982). Santeria: A magico-religious system of Afro-Cuban origin. *The American Journal of Social Psychiatry, 2*(3), 496–503.

Mendez, A. (1994). *Cubans in America.* Minneapolis, MN: Lerner Publications.

Mendoza, F. S., Ventura, S. J., Burciaga Valdez, R., Castillo, R., Saldivar, L., Baisden, K., & Martorell, R. (1991). Selected measures of health status for Mexican-American, mainland Puerto Rican, and Cuban-American children. *Journal of the American Medical Association, 265*(2), 227–232.

Murphy, J. M. (1988). *Santeria. An African religion in America*. Boston: Beacon Press.

National Center for Health Statistics. (1989). Anthropometric data and prevalence of overweight for Hispanics: 1982–84. DHHS Publication No. 89-1689. Hyattsville, MD: Department of Health and Human Services.

National Commission for Employment Policy. (1982). *Hispanics and jobs: Barriers to progress*. Report No. 14: Washington, DC: Author.

National Council of la Raza. (2002). http://www.nclr.org.

Olson, J. S., & Olson, J. E. (1995). *Cuban Americans: From trauma to triumph*. New York: Twayne Publishers.

Pappas, G., Gergen, P. J., & Carroll, M. (1990). Hypertension prevalence and the status of awareness, treatment, and control in the Hispanic Health and Nutrition Examination Survey (HHANES) 1982–84. *American Journal of Public Health, 80*(12), 1431–1436.

Perez, L. (1984). The Cuban population of the United States. The results of the 1980 U.S. census of population. Keynote address at meeting of the Institute of Cuban Studies, Miami, Florida.

Perez, L. (1994). Cuban families in the United States. In R. L. Taylor (Ed.), *Minority families in the United States: A multicultural perspective* (pp. 95–112). Englewood Cliffs, NJ: Prentice Hall.

Pletsch, P. K. (1991). Prevalence of cigarette smoking in Hispanic women of childbearing age. *Nursing Research, 40*(2), 103–106.

Portes, A., & Clark, J. (1980). *Cuban immigration to the United States, 1772–79. A preliminary report of findings*. Durham, NC: Duke University.

Portes, A., & Bach, R. L. (1985). *Latin journey: Cuban and Mexican immigrants in the United States*. Berkeley, CA: University of California Press.

Portes, A., & Stepick, A. (1993). *City on the edge. The transformation of Miami*. Berkeley, CA: University of California Press.

Portes, A., & Zhou, M. (1994). Should immigrants assimilate? *The Public Interest, 116*, 18–33.

Queralt, M. (1984). Understanding Cuban immigrants: A cultural perspective. *Social Work, 29*(2), 115–121.

Richmond, M. L. (1980). *Immigrant adaptation and family structure among Cubans in Miami, Florida*. New York: Arno Press.

Rojas, D. (1994). Leadership in a multicultural society: A case in role development. *Nursing and Health Care, 15*(5), 258–261.

Sandoval, V. A. (1979). Santeria as a mental health system: An historical overview. *Social Sciences and Medicine, 13B*, 137–151.

Sandoval, V. A. (1994). Smoking and Hispanics: Issues of identity, culture, economics, prevalence, and prevention. *Health Values, 18*(1), 44–53.

Smart, J., & Smart, D. (1992). Cultural issues in the rehabilitation of Hispanics. *Journal of Rehabilitation, 58*(2), 29–36.

Smith, P. B., & Weinman, M. L. (1995). Cultural implications for public health policy for pregnant Hispanic adolescents. *Health Values 19*(1), 3–9.

Solis, J. M., Marks, G., Garcia, M., & Shelton, D. (1990). Acculturation, access to care, and use of preventive services by Hispanics: Findings from HHANES 1982–84. *American Journal of Public Health, 80* (Suppl.), 11–19.

Stroup-Benham, C. A., & Trevino, F. M. (1991). Reproductive characteristics of Mexican-American, mainland Puerto Rican, and Cuban-American women. *Journal of the American Medical Association, 265*(2), 222–226.

Suarez, Z. E. (1993). Cuban Americans. From golden exiles to social undesirables. In H. P. McAdoo (Ed.), *Family ethnicity: Strength in diversity* (pp. 164–176). Newbury Park, CA: Sage Publications.

Szapocznik, J., Scopetta, M. A., Arandale, M., & Kurtines, W. (1978). Cuban value structure: Treatment implications. *Journal of Consulting and Clinical Psychology, 46*(5), 961–970.

Szapocznik, J., & Hernandez, R. (1988). The Cuban American family. In C. H. Mindel, R. W. Habenstein, & R. Wright (Eds.), *Ethnic families in America* (3rd ed, pp. 160–172). New York: Elsevier.

Thomas, J. T., & DeSantis, L. (1995). Feeding and weaning practices of Cuban and Haitian immigrant mothers. *Journal of Transcultural Nursing, 6*(2), 34–42.

Trevino, F. M., Moyer, E., Valdez, R. B., & Stroup-Benham, C. A. (1991). Health insurance coverage and utilization of health services by Mexican Americans, mainland Puerto Ricans, and Cuban Americans. *Journal of the American Medical Association, 265*(2), 233–237.

U.S. Bureau of the Census (1989). *Current population survey: March 1989*. Washington, DC: U.S. Government Printing Office.

U.S. Bureau of the Census (1993). *Statistical abstracts of the United States* (113th ed.). Washington, DC: U.S. Government Printing Office.

U.S. Department of Health and Human Services (1993). *Safe motherhood*. Retrieved from http://www.cdc.gov/nccdphp/drh/mh_diabet-preg.htm.

Chapter 9

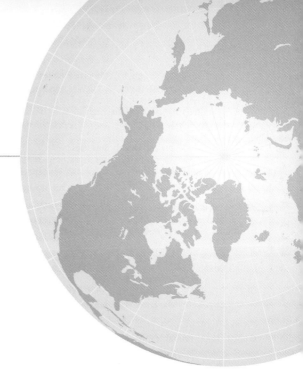

People of Filipino Heritage

DULA F. PACQUIAO

Overview, Inhabited Localities, and Topography

OVERVIEW

The Philippine archipelago consists of 7107 islands located in southeastern Asia, east of Vietnam and slightly north of the equator. With a landmass of 300,000 square kilometers, it is slightly larger than Arizona. The three major islands of Luzon, Visayas, and Mindanao have mostly mountainous terrain with narrow to extensive coastal lowlands. The western region is bound by the South China Sea, the east by the Pacific Ocean, the south by the Sulu and Celebes seas, and the north by the Bashi Channel. The tropical climate is suitable for year-round agriculture and fishing, but is affected by the seasonal northeast and southwest monsoons. In 2001, the total population was estimated at 82.84 million inhabitants, with a growth rate of 2.03 percent. Although the country is rich in natural resources and has a mixed economy of agriculture, light industry, and support services, 41 percent of the population lives below poverty level (World Factbook, 2001).

The Spaniards who colonized the country for over three centuries named the islands Las Islas Filipinas (the Philippine Islands). Following the Spanish-American War in 1898, Las Islas Filipinas was ceded to the United States and its name was anglicized to the Philippines. Filipinas (Pilipinas) and Philippines are used interchangeably today. Native speakers refer to the country as Filipinas or Pilipinas and use Philippines when speaking to outsiders or when writing in English.

The issue of whether to use *F* or *P* in referring to the country, its people, or its national language is a matter of debate among the country's scholars and historians. There is no letter *F* in the indigenous Tagalog language, which is spoken in central Luzon, including Manila, the nation's capital. When the country gained its independence from the United States in 1946, it adopted the Tagalog-based Pilipino as its national language. In 1959, Pilipino was officially declared as the national language. In 1986, however, the national assembly declared the national language as Filipino, based on existing Philippine and other languages (Gendrano, 1990). Usually, *Filipino* is used interchangeably with *Filipino American*. The term *Pilipino* is generally used to distinguish indigenous identity and nationalistic empowerment.

Filipino Americans are a diverse group because of regional variations in the Philippines, which influence the dialect spoken, food preferences, religion, and traditions (Fig. 9–1). Generational differences exist within families associated with age and time of migration from the Philippines. Other factors influencing diversity include pre- and post-migration level of education, occupation, and intermarriage. This chapter discusses the major characteristics of mainstream Filipino culture, offering some insights into some differences among groups. The reader should avoid using this information as a universal template for every Filipino.

The author wishes to acknowledge the contribution of Iluminada "Nini" Jurado in obtaining relevant literature from the Philippines for this chapter as well as the work of Beatriz F. Miranda, Magelende R. McBride, and Zen Spangler, authors of the chapter on Filipino Americans in the previous edition.

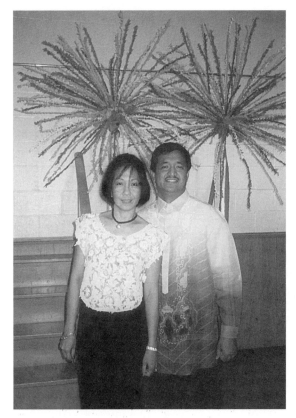

FIGURE 9–1   Traditional Filipino costumes.

HERITAGE AND RESIDENCE

The Filipino way of life is a tapestry of cultural influences superimposed on indigenous tribal origins. The people are predominantly of Malayan ancestry, influenced by the neighboring Chinese, Japanese, East Indian, Indonesian, Malaysian, and Islamic cultures. The Philippine culture is distinct from its Asian neighbors largely because of major influences from the Spanish and American colonizations. Spanish colonization spanned 350 years and was followed by 50 years of American domination. The Spaniards introduced Roman Catholicism, which has remained the dominant religion in the country; as much as 83 percent of the population is Catholic (World Factbook, 2001). The Americans, who emphasized English as the medium of instruction to give the Filipinos a common language, introduced free public education.

The Filipino way of life has evolved from the everyday situations that the people have to deal with living on scattered islands surrounded by large bodies of water and exposed to natural disasters such as volcanic eruptions, typhoons, floods, and droughts, as well as threats of foreign invasion. Gorospe (1977) traced the evolution of the Filipino sense of morality and justice from tribal times and the pre-Spanish era. *Barangays*, close-knit, kin-based, hierarchical communities emerged that placed emphasis on values instrumental to protecting communities from outside atrocities. These communal values stressed collective welfare and solidarity, significant values in harnessing individual energies for security in an unstable environment. Indeed, outsiders to the culture

may recognize these values expressed in the Filipino traits of collective loyalty, generosity, hospitality, and humility. These basic values are strong components of childhood socialization in the family. "Filipinos inculcate a strong sense of family loyalty which spreads beyond the nuclear family of parents and children. Family obligations extend to cousins several times removed, to in-laws, and to others who are made part of the family by such ceremonies as sponsors of marriage or a baptism" (Guthrie, 1968: 55).

Most Filipinos in North America were born in the Philippines. Between 1990 and 2000, Asian and Pacific Islanders (API) increased from 2.9 percent to 3.7 percent of the U.S. population. In 2000, there were approximately 1.85 million Filipinos in the United States concentrated in the states of California, Hawaii, Illinois, New Jersey, New York, Washington, and Texas. Filipinos comprised the second largest foreign-born population after Mexicans in the United States (The Philippine Diaspora in the United States, 2001; U.S. Bureau of Census, 2001). In 1996, of the total Canadian population of 28.5 million, Asians comprised 2.28 million, with Filipinos representing the third largest group after Chinese and East Indians. In the province of Manitoba, Filipinos constituted the largest Asian group (Statistics Canada, 1997).

REASONS FOR MIGRATION AND ASSOCIATED ECONOMIC FACTORS

The first Filipinos in North America were part of the labor force in Spanish galleons who settled in Louisiana as early as 1753, and introduced the dry shrimp industry to the United States (Espina, 1988). Filipino immigration to the United States began in 1902, when the Philippines became an American territory. Most of the first groups of migrants were U.S.-sponsored students who completed their college education and then returned to the Philippines. Nonsponsored students followed these groups; the majority were unable to complete their studies, but chose to remain in the United States and became unskilled laborers. From 1909 until the 1920s, male Filipino laborers were recruited to work on Hawaiian plantations and businesses on the West Coast (Tompar-Tiu & Sustento-Seneriches, 1994). These early migrants were ineligible for citizenship and were denied privileges such as types of employment that required citizenship, union membership, the right to own land, and the right to marry in states with antimiscegenation laws (McBride, Mariola, & Yeo, 1995). The Depression heightened racial animosity toward Filipino workers, and passage of the Tydings-McDuffie Act (Philippines Independence Act) in 1934 virtually ended immigration.

The United States eased immigration restrictions toward Filipinos in 1946 and granted Filipinos naturalization rights. Between 1946 and 1965, 33,000 immigrants entered the United States and contributed to a 44 percent increase in the Filipino population in America (Melendy, 1981). The Immigration Act of 1965 initiated a period of renewed mass immigration by promoting family reunification and recruitment of occupational immigrants. Since the passage of the 1965 act, the

Philippines has become the largest source of immigrants from Asia (Bouvier & Gardner, 1986). The post-1965 Filipino immigration has consisted of two distinct chains—one deriving from Filipinos who entered the United States before 1965 and the other from the flow of highly trained personnel who began immigration in the 1960s (Liu, Ong, & Rosenstein, 1991). Economic and educational opportunities and reunification with family members in the United States continue to be the primary motivating factors for emigration (McBride & Parreno, 1996). Working adults sponsored Filipino elders to come to the United States and care for their grandchildren. This in turn facilitated the subsequent emigration of other members of the nuclear families from the Philippines (Pacquiao, 1993).

Because the Philippine economy has been unable to provide jobs for college graduates, large numbers of Filipino professionals have emigrated in what has been dubbed a "brain drain." Export of professional and skilled labor is one of the biggest industries in the Philippines. Remittances sent home by émigrés has added billions of dollars annually to the Filipino economy. In 1995, Filipino nurses represented 75 percent of the foreign nurse labor force recruited and working in U.S. hospitals (Brush, 1995).

EDUCATIONAL STATUS AND OCCUPATIONS

The Americans introduced mass public education to the Philippines in the 1900s. English became the official medium of instruction in schools. Early training of schoolteachers was provided by the Thomasites, forerunners of the U.S. Peace Corps. The development of educational programs in the Philippines was highly influenced and patterned after the United States, as in the case of nursing and medicine. Early missionaries and philanthropic organizations such as the Daughters of the American Revolution, the Catholic Scholarship Fund, and the Rockefeller Foundation were instrumental in the Westernization of health-care education and practice in the Philippines (Brush, 1995). American nursing educators went to the Philippines, and Filipino nurses were sent to the United States for training. They subsequently returned to the Philippines and assumed pioneering leadership positions in nursing schools and hospitals in the Philippines. Since 1970, all educational programs in nursing in the Philippines have offered a 4-year degree in nursing (B.S.N.).

The Philippines has one of the highest literacy rates in Asia (96 percent). It is the third largest English-speaking country after the United States and the United Kingdom (Travel Information: The Philippines, 2002). Schools are either public (government) or private. Formal education starts at the age of 7, with 6 years of primary education. Pre-primary level (nursery school and kindergarten) is offered in most private schools. Students get 4 years of secondary education, either in a vocational-technical or an academic school. A high school graduate is 2 years younger than those graduating from U.S. high schools because of the omission of middle school years.

Filipinos view educational achievement as a pathway to economic success, status, and prestige for the individual and the family. A person's profession is always identified when introducing, addressing, or writing about the person (for example, Doctor Makalintal, Attorney Perez, or Engineer Sumulong). A family's status in the community is enhanced by the educational achievement of the children. Both male and female children are expected to do well in school, and parents do their best to provide for their full-time education. Adolescents' education is considered an investment of the whole family rather than an individual effort. Adolescents who closely identify with their families are usually concerned about how their scholastic achievement may affect the reputation of their families (Salazar et al., 2000). It is common to find family members and other relatives who contribute toward the financial support of kin. Among lower- and middle-class families, siblings take turns going to college in order to maximize resources for one member to finish school and then contribute to the education of the other siblings. One's choice of profession is generally a family decision, and is based on potential economic return to the group (Pacquiao, 1993).

A growing concern among Filipino leaders in the United States is the increasing dropout rate among members of the younger generation (Pilipino Mini-Health Forums Committee, 1993). Academic achievement of Filipinos in high school does not appear to match their academic performance in higher education. In two high schools in Vallejo, California, Filipinos were found to excel academically compared to other racial-ethnic groups. The dropout rate for Filipino students at the University of California at Davis between 1980 and 1989 was 33 percent. Some of the reasons cited included the following: intense parental pressure to succeed, predominance of parental wishes over children's voices and choices, differentiated parental expectations and attitudes toward their sons and daughters, fear of not meeting parental expectations, inability to seek support from parents for failures in school, and experienced tension between assimilation and racism in the outside society (Wolf, 1997).

Filipino immigrants since 1965 have had relatively high educational attainment (Kao, 1995), a high level of labor participation (particularly among women), a high percentage working as professionals (Cabezas, Shinagawa, & Kawaguchi, 1986), and the lowest rate of poverty in the United States (Oliver et al. 1995; Rumbaut, 1995). Filipinos appear to be assimilated and successful and tend to blend into American society, which gives them a reputation as a "model minority." In reality, high educational attainment of American-born and immigrant Filipinos does not guarantee their entry into well-paying or high-status jobs in the United States. The restricted labor market limits the match between their education and experience, resulting in many individuals competing for low-level jobs for which many are overqualified. Only those who are educated in health-care fields tend to find jobs that are consistent with their education. This is the same for all foreign graduates.

In contrast to nursing education in the United States, which stresses the process of thinking, mastery of facts, and rote learning have greater emphasis in the Philippines. A defined hierarchy, with the teacher as the expert authority, is congruent with the social organization of the broader society, where age and position are permanent markers of one's status. Students and younger generations are rewarded for accepting the ideas and counsel of elders and teachers. Thus, challenging authority and asserting one's creative ideas are unnatural predispositions, especially for the young, who are expected to acquiesce to those who are older and in positions of authority (Pacquiao, 1996a). In a study of Filipino nursing students in a school in New Jersey, faculty described them as taking things at face value, avoiding conflict, communicating nonassertively, and learning by rote memorization. In contrast to their faculty, students saw effort rather than ability as a key ingredient for success (Pacquiao, 1996b). Traditional values at home were in conflict with values in school and teacher expectations (Pacquiao, 1995). Hence, facilitating understanding of the dominant cultural values and norms in school, in addition to teaching the subject matter, is essential to facilitate academic success among Filipino students.

Communication

DOMINANT LANGUAGE AND DIALECTS

Between 87 and 111 languages and dialects are spoken in the Philippines, depending on how dialects are aggregated (Garrote-Trinidad, 2001). Distinct ethnic groups speak eight dialects: Tagalog (29.6 percent), Cebuano (24.2 percent), Ilocano (10.3 percent), Ilonggo (9.2 percent), Bicolano (3.5 percent), Waray (4 percent), Kapampangan (2.8 percent), and Pangasinenses (less than 1 percent) (Enriquez, 1994; Tompar-Tiu & Sustento-Seneriches, 1994). Most Filipinos speak the national language, Filipino. English is used for business and legal transactions, and is used in school instruction beyond the third grade. Business and social interactions commonly use a hybrid of both Tagalog and English (Tag-Lish) in the same sentence. Tag-Lish is often used in health education.

Many Spanish words are found in the Filipino language such as *sopa* (soup), *calle* (street), *hija/hijo* (daughter/son), and *respeto* (respect). The influence of indigenous Filipino and Spanish languages produces distinct characteristics when Filipinos speak English. Specific nouns are used to denote a person's age, gender, and position in the social hierarchy. For instance, *Manang* and *Manong* are used to refer to or address older woman and men, respectively. These nouns are used in lieu of the generic and gender-neutral pronouns *siya* (singular "he/she") and *sila* (plural "they/them"). Hence, it is customary for Filipinos to use "he" and "she" interchangeably in reference to the same individual.

Filipinos do not enunciate short *i*, long *a*, and long *o* sounds. Hence, *sit* may be sounded as *seat*, *fair* as *fir*, and *slow* as *slaw*. Many Filipinos are unable to differentiate *s* from *sh* (*physiology* as *fishiology*), *u* from short *o* or short *a* sounds (*fond* as *fund*; *church* as *charts*).

Although many Filipinos speak English, their ethnic language or dialect, their knowledge and use of the English language, and their age of migration to the United States often influence enunciation, pronunciation, and accentuation. Elderly Filipinos who originated from non-Tagalog-speaking regions may understand and speak better English than other Filipinos. In multigenerational Filipino American families, different languages may be used to communicate with family members and friends. Although many Filipinos speak and write fluently in English, they may have difficulty understanding American idiomatic expressions. For example, to a new immigrant, "How are you?" may be interpreted as a question about the person's well-being, requiring an elaboration of one's situation, rather than a mere greeting. Filipinos may have difficulty communicating their lack of understanding to others, and may use ritualistic language and euphemistic behavior that appears to be the opposite of how they actually perceive the situation. Saving face, a characteristic pattern of behavior employed to protect the integrity of both parties, is a consequence of the cultural value placed on maintaining smooth interpersonal relations with others. Desirous of group approval, the individual becomes sensitive to the feelings of others and, in turn, develops a high sense of sensitivity to personal insults.

Traditional Filipino communication is highly contextual. The individual is enculturated to attend to the context of the interaction and to adopt appropriate behaviors. Many Filipinos are observant, displaying an intuitive feeling about the other person and the contextual environment during interactions. Contextual variables include the presence of *ibang tao* (outsiders) versus *hindi ibang tao* (insiders), and the age, social position, and gender of the other individual. In the company of insiders, such as one's family, each member develops an intuitive knowledge of the other so that words are unnecessary to convey a message, and meanings are embedded in nonverbal communication. In the presence of outsiders, a child's emotional outburst may be met with adults' stern silence, indifference, or euphemistic grins. These behaviors imply to insiders that emotional outbursts are inappropriate in front of outsiders. An individual's interaction depends on the variable context of the situation. For example, one may not disagree, talk loudly, or look directly at a person who is older and who occupies a higher position in the social hierarchy. Honorific terms of address denoting an individual's status within the hierarchy exist in all dialects. In Tagalog, when communicating to an elder or a person in a position of higher authority than oneself, the person is addressed using gender and age-specific nouns such as "Grandpa" or "Grandma," "older sister" or "older brother," or prefixes such as Mr., Mrs., Miss, or Ms.

The emphasis on maintaining smooth interpersonal relationships brings a consequent ambiguity in communication to prevent the risk of offending others. Filipino interpersonal and social life operates by maintaining smooth interpersonal relationships. Filipinos may sacrifice clear communication to avoid stressful interpersonal conflicts and confrontations. Saying no to a superior may be considered disrespectful, which predisposes an ambiguous positive response. Filipinos are often puzzled, and sometimes offended, by the precision and exactness of American communication. Newly recruited Filipino nurses are stunned by their American coworkers' abrasiveness and open expressions of anger toward each other and their subsequent behavior of sitting down at coffee "as if nothing happened." To many traditional Filipinos, actions speak louder than words. They value respect and might find questions like "Do you understand?" or "Do you follow?" disrespectful. Health-care workers should ask indirectly whether the Filipino client understands and should have the person or family member do a return demonstration of a procedure or repeat an instruction, rather than question his or her comprehension. Allowing time for a Filipino to respond not only communicates respect but also gives time for translating the dialect into English. Speaking clearly and slowly facilitates appreciation of varying pronunciation and accentuation of the English language across cultures.

CULTURAL COMMUNICATION PATTERNS

Relational orientation has been suggested as the essence of Asian social psychology (Ho, 1993). Enriquez (1993) posited that the Filipino core values of shame, yielding to the leader or majority, gratitude, and sensitivity to personal affront emphasize a strong sense of human relatedness. These values originate from the central concept of *kapwa*, which arises from the awareness of shared identity with others. *Kapwa* embraces the insider-outsider categories of human relations, and prescribes different levels of interrelatedness or involvement with others. *Pakakikipagkapwa* ("being one with others") implies accepting and dealing with the other individual as a fellow human being (Enriquez, 1986). *Kapwa* is grounded in the fundamental value of shared inner perception or feeling for another, from which all other attributes for human relations are made possible (Enriquez, 1993).

The eight levels of social interactions identified by Enriquez within the core concept of *kapwa* follow. These levels demonstrate a hierarchy of human relatedness within the Filipino language and context of meanings. The contextual axis of interactions is conceptualized within a continuum of how the "other" is categorized— whether as an insider or outsider. The degree of sharing and involvement with outsiders may progress from level 1 to 5, while interactions at levels 6 to 8 are observed with insiders (Enriquez, 1986; McBride & Parreno, 1996). Enriquez (1993) describes these eight levels as civility, interacting, participating, conforming, adjusting, understanding and accepting, getting involved, and being one with.

Developing working relationships with Filipinos requires understanding of where one is likely to be perceived within the continuum of the insider-outsider category. Outsiders can move toward higher levels of interactions by observing cultural norms of communication, using trusted gatekeepers to mediate conflicts, seeking validation of perceptions of behaviors from more acculturated members of the group, and allowing opportunities to save face to prevent embarrassment and personal denigration. When confronting a Filipino coworker, provide privacy and point out positive attributes, as well as the problem. Observing nonverbal behaviors and interpreting them within the Filipino cultural context promotes culturally congruent interactions. Accommodating differential sharing and involvement between insiders and outsiders shows cultural understanding that enhances development of intercultural relationships. For example, speaking Filipino with others reinforces the value of being one with others. Learning and using some Filipino greetings and honorific terms of address facilitate movement of the relationship to higher levels of involvement. Developing an algorithm of work situations where English should be spoken in lieu of Filipino demonstrates cultural sensitivity and accommodation. The insider and outsider delineations may be less important to some Filipinos who are highly educated and take pride in their global outlook. Unlike other immigrants who settle in ethnic enclaves, more recent Filipino immigrants acculturate, finding it easy to relate with people from various cultures.

Smiling and giggling are often observed, especially among young Filipino women. The meanings of these spontaneous and highly unconscious behaviors are embedded in the context of the situation and may range from glee, genuine interest, and agreement all the way to discomfort, politeness, or indifference. It is helpful to point out how the behavior, if inappropriate to the situation, can be misinterpreted by patients and others. Behavior change can be expected if done in a timely, respectful, and sincere manner.

Having a heightened sensitivity to personal insults, Filipinos have a remarkable ability to maintain a proper front to protect their self-esteem when threatened. Conflict avoidance behaviors include euphemistic denial of anger, minimization of pain, and silence. Pent-up emotions and accumulated resentment may result in explosive anger, depression, and somatization. Practitioners should be sensitized to these behaviors and explore the underlying causes by establishing trust and maintaining respectful relationships. Offering pain medications and attending to nonverbal behaviors, rather than waiting for the patient to verbalize his or her needs, are culturally congruent approaches.

First-generation Filipinos in North America present themselves in therapy sessions as polite, cooperative, verbal, and engaging. Agreement with suggested interventions by health-care providers does not ensure that clients will follow through with the recommendations. Cimmarusti (1996) suggests that health-care providers should be comfortable with clients' deferential attitude without resorting to authoritarian approaches, which may be perceived as oppressive and may encourage euphemistic complaint behaviors. Filipinos who are accustomed to indirect communication may perceive focusing on action-oriented strategies and outcomes as coercive.

Direct eye contact varies among Filipinos depending on the degree of acculturation, length of time in America, age, and education. Some individuals may avoid prolonged eye contact with authority figures and older people as a form of respect. Older men may refrain from maintaining eye contact with young women because it may be interpreted as flirtation or a sexual advance. Filipinos are comfortable with silence, and may allow the other person to initiate verbal interaction as a sign of respect. During a teaching session, a Filipino client's nod may have several meanings, such as comprehension or agreement, "Yes, I hear you," "Yes, we are interacting," "Yes, I can see the instructions," or some other message that may be difficult for the client to disclose.

Touch is used freely especially with co-ethnics and insiders. Greater distance is observed when interacting with outsiders and people in positions of authority. Same-gender closeness and touching, which may be perceived as homosexual adult behavior in America, are considered normal behaviors among Filipinos. Young adults of the same gender may hold hands, put one arm over another's shoulder, or walk arm-in-arm. As they become more acculturated, many Filipinos become aware of the differences and adapt to the new culture.

TEMPORAL RELATIONSHIPS

Filipinos have a relaxed temporal outlook. They have a healthy respect for the past, the ability to enjoy the present, and hope for the future. Past orientation is evident in their respect for elders, strong sense of gratitude, obligation to older generations, and honoring the memories of dead ancestors. Future orientation is manifested in the strong sense of family commitment to provide for the education of the young, parental participation in the care of their children and grandchildren, and strong work ethic. Their firm present orientation is associated with the cultural emphasis on maintaining relationships with others. Permanent social bonds with kin and significant others outside of kin are nurtured. Filipinos enjoy their families, fiestas, and life and spend generously to make family events memorable and enjoyable. Although most Filipinos have adapted to American punctuality in the business sphere, promptness for social events is situationally determined. "Filipino time" means arriving much later than the scheduled appointment, which can be from one to several hours. The focus is on the gathering rather than on the schedule. It is common for a Filipino host to invite American guests at least one hour later than the Filipino guests in the hope that both will arrive at the same time.

Attending to the present situation to promote interpersonal relationships is inherent in Filipino time orientation. Many Filipino nurses have difficulty leaving a patient who is upset or in the middle of a procedure such as a bed bath. Addressing the present needs of patients, and ensuring smooth relationships with them, may be interpreted by their American coworkers as poor time management and an inability to determine work priorities. Newly recruited nurses are disturbed by their inability to complete the caretaking tasks that, in their assessment, would clearly please and ensure the comfort of their patients. Differential time orientation between Filipinos and Americans should be made part of job orientations. Defining expressions of these different time orientations can prevent conflicts at work and help provide culturally relevant mentoring.

FORMAT FOR NAMES

The Filipino kinship system is extended bilineally, and is reflected in the format for names. Kinship and family affinity can be legally and spiritually claimed equally from both sets of families, giving the child the identity and extended family. Children carry the surnames of both their father and their mother. For example, Jose Romagos Lopez and Leticia Romagos Lopez are the children of Maria Romagos and Eduardo Lopez. The middle name or initial is the mother's maiden name. After marriage, Eduardo keeps the same name, while his sister's name becomes Leticia Lopez Lukban (her husband being Ernesto Lukban). The middle name is generally abbreviated as an initial.

Many Filipino names are of Spanish origin. Filipino females may have a Ma. before their given names: for example, Ma. Luisa stands for Maria Luisa. Although the name Maria is often given to girls, some males may use the same name as a first or second name; hence, Ma. Jose Romagos Lopez and Jose Ma. Paredes Castro. As interracial marriages occur among Filipinos and the practice of adapting the male spouse's surname continues, one can expect more Filipino Americans with surnames reflecting the ethnic origins of the father. Few Filipino American women keep their own surname after marriage, although this may increase among second-generation and third-generation Filipinos.

Adults use first names to address young children. Nicknames symbolizing affectionate regard for the person are commonly used instead of the first name; hence, Nini, Baby, Bongbong. First names are avoided when addressing Filipino adults who are older or who occupy higher positions in the hierarchy than the speaker. Formal business transactions use English forms of addresses such as Mr., Mrs., Miss, or Ms., or the person's professional degree before their name (Dr. Abaya or Attorney Abaya).

Family Roles and Organization

HEAD OF HOUSEHOLD AND GENDER ROLES

Since the pre-Spanish era, Filipino women have been held in high regard, having rights equal to those of men (Agoncillo & Guerrero, 1987). In contemporary Filipino families, although the father is the acknowledged head of the household, authority in the family is considered egalitarian, as is evidenced in gender-neutral Filipino words. The mother plays an equal, and often major, role in decisions regarding health, children, and finances (Fig. 9–2).

Traditional female roles include caring for the sick and children, maintaining positive relationships with kin, and managing the home. Parents and older siblings are involved in the care and discipline of younger children. In extended family households, older relatives and grandparents share much authority and responsibility for the care and discipline of younger members. Traditional Filipino families may not expect female children to engage in activities that are considered appropriate for men, and may include driving, bicycling, and other func-

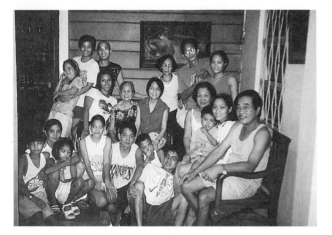

FIGURE 9–2   Members of a Filipino family that is bilaterally extended to three generations. (Photograph by Rowena Legaspi.)

tions requiring mechanical or technical skills. Blurring of roles between men and women occurs with increased education, urbanization, and emigration to a new culture, as in the United States.

In the United States, Filipinos are predominantly two-income families, with both spouses working. Family members and other Filipino friends or acquaintances are entrusted with the young children when parents are working. Elder parents, especially grandmothers, emigrate to the United States in time for the birth of their grandchildren and are expected to take care of them on behalf of their working adult children (Pacquiao, 1993). Filipino womanhood has evolved from the Spanish construct of modesty, demureness, and femininity to a contemporary image of a woman who is educated, working, and adept at balancing traditional roles and career demands. Since the 1950s, women represent close to 50 percent of university enrollments and pursue careers in law, medicine, and politics. Traditional Filipino parents expect their male and female children to pursue college education and economically productive careers and also have a family.

Studies of second-generation Filipino students in California high schools revealed greater parental control over daughters, with more latitude allowed for sons. For many Filipinas, high school achievement was met by parental control over their choice of colleges and pressure to remain close to home and family supervision (Wolf, 1997).

PRESCRIPTIVE, RESTRICTIVE, AND TABOO BEHAVIORS FOR CHILDREN AND ADOLESCENTS

Bulatao (1962) posited that the strong in-group consciousness of Filipinos is rooted in the centrality of family and kin to the exclusion of others in the socialization of individuals. "The family is the strongest unit of society, demanding the deepest loyalties of the individual and coloring all social activity with its own set of demands" (Grossholtz, 1964: 86). Ascriptive and particularistic personal ties with kin are significant in the allocation of rank, authority, and power to individuals.

Generational position conditions the status as well as the role performance of individuals. The family and one's family role define and order authority, rights, obligations, and modes of interaction. Younger generations are taught to be respectful and heed the authority of older siblings and relatives, parents, and grandparents. Respect is manifested in both speech and actions by using honorific terms of address, avoiding confrontation and offensive language, keeping a low tone of voice, greeting elders by kissing their forehead or back of the hand, avoiding direct eye contact when being admonished, offering food, touching, and so forth. Husbands and wives address each other using the honorific terms that they wish to model for their children. In front of the children, a husband will address his wife as *Inay* (mother) and the wife correspondingly refers to her husband as *Itay* (father). Under no circumstance are children permitted to call their parents by their first names. Friends of Filipino children are expected to show respect to adult members of the family when they visit.

Reciprocal obligations among kin are embodied in the value of *utang na loob*, a personal sense of indebtedness and loyalty to kin, which carries an obligation to repay or perform services for one another. Filial respect and obligation for caring for one's parents is the ultimate confluence of generational respect and reciprocal obligation. Childhood socialization to the mechanism of shame reinforces the value of *utang na loob* and generational respect. Failure to perform or recognize reciprocal obligations, as well as disrespect of elders or people of authority, results in the loss of one's self-esteem and status, as well as shame to one's family.

Children learn early to behave differently toward insiders and outsiders. Private affairs are reserved for close kin, and are well guarded from outsiders. High school students in California admitted that they were taught that all problems should be kept within the family, and that talking to outsiders such as friends, teachers, or counselors would bring shame to the family (Tompar-Tiu & Sustento-Seneriches, 1994; Wolf, 1997). Conditions such as mental illness, divorce, terminal illness, criminal offenses, unwanted pregnancy, and HIV/AIDS are not readily shared with outsiders until trust is established. The extent to which a Filipino client may disclose personal information is contextualized. Family presence may act as a barrier to full disclosure of conditions that may be perceived as putting the family at risk for shame.

Dating at an early age is discouraged for young daughters who are advised that a short courtship period may suggest that they are "easy to get." Young men with sincere intent must strive to get on the good side of the family and have patience with a long courtship. Open demonstrations of affection with sexual undertones are to be avoided by the young couple. Ideally, the groom's parents formally ask for the bride's parents' consent for the marriage of their children. Traditional families desire that their daughters remain chaste before marriage. Pregnancy out of wedlock brings shame to the whole family. Modernization and urbanization have changed the social mores in the Philippines, yet many Filipino American families are still perceived by younger family members as having an overly protective attitude toward children in matters of "hanging out" with friends, dating, and courtship.

FAMILY GOALS AND PRIORITIES

The Filipino family is extended to third cousins with a clear structure and network of relationships. In addition to blood relatives, it is possible to establish relationships through religious ceremonies, such as baptism and marriage, when friends and associates are invited to become godparents or surrogate parents. Fictive kinship is a significant support system for Filipino Americans who left families or relatives in the home country. In times of illness, the extended family provides support and assistance. Sometimes a family visit to the hospital takes on the semblance of a family reunion.

The family is the basic social and economic unit of Filipino kinship. Family relations strongly influence individual decisions and actions. Relatives and family constitute the reference group for individuals, determining their behavior as well as that of their relatives in any social exchange. Family loyalties and obligations supersede individual interests and residential migration. This is evident in migration patterns of adult children and aged parents, which are planned to maximize the economic welfare of the group.

Family emphasis on communal values and generational respect is highly institutionalized. Community activities generally center on the family. Fiestas, weddings, baptisms, illnesses, and funerals are occasions for reinvigorating relations with kin and rekindling local connections, where the presence and, more importantly, the absence of relatives are viewed as highly significant. Early childrearing practices are permissive, with emphasis on providing an emotionally secure environment for the child. Priority is placed on promoting the child's well-being and social acceptance The child is introduced early into various mechanisms designed to impose compliance with family values. A family's prestige is measured by the upbringing of their children, judged by their adherence to traditional cultural values.

The family emphasis on faithfulness to religious obligations is tied with the cultural values of generational respect and reciprocal obligation. Childrearing practices stress entire family participation in the religious education and adherence to rituals by the young members. Older generations share the responsibility in the reinforcement of these values. Religious sacraments, such as marriage, are embedded in the age-grading activities of the extended family (Fig. 9–3).

As the basic economic unit of society, the family defines the economic obligations of kin to each other. Interdependence within and across generations is fostered. Children are looked upon as economic assets and as sources of support for parents in old age. Thus, educating young members becomes a family priority. The socioeconomic status of the aged is closely linked with the family's wealth; if resources are limited, the elderly rely on children and relatives. Older parents and grandparents are integrated within the family, thus lessening the impact of advancing age. Traditional Filipinos

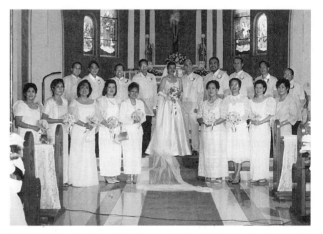

FIGURE 9–3 The Spanish influence in the Philippines is depicted in this Roman Catholic wedding featuring godparents as an important part of fictive kinship development for the couple and their families. (Photograph by Rowena Legaspi.)

consider institutionalization of aged parents tantamount to abandonment of filial obligation and respect for elders. Many elders aspire to returning to the Philippines and spending their remaining years with loving kin.

The development of *pakiramdam* (shared perception) and *kapwa* (shared identity) is the defining goal of the family. Group cohesiveness, loyalty, and faithfulness to shared obligation are expectations that transcend distant migration, marriage, and adulthood. There is significant evidence for the concept of shared perception and identity among Filipinos. Students who feel obligated to maintain their familys' reputations believe that effort and interest, rather than ability, can result in school success (Salazar et al., 2000). Older Filipinos in the United States have reported experiencing conflict between maintaining family obligations, such as babysitting for their grandchildren, and their desire to be more independent from their adult children. Family obligations may result in their inability to meet medical appointments, obtain needed medications, and make meaningful social connections because of lack of independent transportation. Depression has been associated with loneliness, feelings of isolation, and financial difficulty (McBride & Parreno, 1996; McBride, Mariola, & Yeo, 1995; Tompar-Tiu & Sustento-Seneriches, 1994). Elderly Filipinos identified integration in the family of their adult children, participation in community activities with family and close friends, and maintaining religious functions as highly important (Pacquiao, 1993).

The family provides primary support during illness. It is common to mobilize the extended family support system from the Philippines and in many parts of the United States to care for ailing family members. Many Filipinos believe that mental illness brings a stigma to the individual and the family; hence, support will likely come from family members. This is evident in the underutilization of mental health services and presentation of advanced symptoms by the patient on hospital admission (Weiner & Marvit, 1977). The first choice is caring by family members, rather than seeking health professionals (Tompar-Tiu & Sustento-Seneriches, 1994).

There is diversity in the degree to which Filipino

Americans adhere to the traditional cultural values. Superio (1993) reported that middle-aged immigrant Filipino parents raising families on the West Coast indicate that they do not expect to live with their children in their old age. In contrast, a younger group of immigrant and native-born Filipinos believe that children should take care of their elderly parents. Diversity in family member roles and priorities exists as a result of the financial resources of the family. Reciprocal obligations with kin are expressed differently based on the capacity of elders and adult children to meet them and may take economic, physical, emotional, or social support dimensions.

ALTERNATIVE LIFESTYLES

Traditional Filipino parents seldom provide sex education, and sex is not discussed openly at home. Homosexuality may be recognized and considered an aberrant behavior, but not openly practiced to save face and decrease stigmatization for the family. Younger gay, lesbian, bisexual, and transgender Filipinos in the Philippines and in the United States are taking a more active role in being recognized and expressing their rights (Tanikalang Ginto, 2002).

Although the tenets of the Catholic Church have a direct bearing on sexual mores for older generations of Filipinos, they have less influence on younger generations as is seen by the high incidence of teenage pregnancy reported by the San Francisco Health Commission. Filipino family values emphasizing shared identity and common shame may keep many Filipinos affected with AIDS from being open about their illness with kin. The family may not be the primary source of support for these individuals, who may be isolated to prevent stigma to the family. The nuclear family may protect the affected member from outsiders and intentionally remove themselves from contact with a network of friends and extended family. Providing an atmosphere that fosters the much-needed sense of belonging should be the goal of culturally congruent services.

Divorce can carry a stigma for older and more traditional Filipinos, especially those who are devout Catholics, although the stigma may be worse for Filipinos in the Philippines than for Filipino Americans. The more traditional see divorce resulting from failed marital duties, lack of mutual support between the partners, and marital infidelity (Asian Promise, 2002).

Workforce Issues

CULTURE IN THE WORKFORCE

Filipino ethnohistory with white colonizing powers may influence their perceptions of workplace experiences. Experience with racism is a continuing theme voiced by Filipino nurses working with white American nurses (Spangler, 1992). The recent business model used in recruiting nurses from the Philippines has removed some of the benevolent provisions for prolonged supportive training that were available to those nurses under the Exchange Visitors Program. The requirement

by the American Nurses Association for equal pay for the same job transformed foreign nurse recruitment into a competitive enterprise, where employers and existing staff expect recruited nurses to be functionally competent on the job as soon as they receive their American RN license because they will receive pay comparable to other RNs. In reality, providing transitional support for foreign nurses requires a significant time and financial investment and a prolonged acculturation process.

Filipino nurses have been recruited in large numbers to staff mostly evening and night shifts where acute shortages of American-trained nurses occur. This has reinforced the cultural tendency toward collective solidarity by defining the context of interactions within a continuum of insiders versus outsiders. Frequent entry of large numbers of new recruits into the same setting has reduced the number of cultural mentors who can help facilitate these nurses' acculturation to the organization and the cultural norms of the society at large. American nurses and administrators of health organizations with large contingents of Filipino nurses are becoming aware of the need for special knowledge and skills in understanding and managing a diverse workforce, and in developing culturally specific staff development programs.

Cultural conflicts in the workplace stem from different communication patterns: the dominant norm of assertiveness versus the highly contextual Filipino communication. The cultural concept of shared identity with other Filipinos creates a propensity among Filipino nurses to speak in their own dialect with each other to the exclusion of non-Filipino coworkers and patients. Lack of fluency in speaking and enunciating English words results in anxiety when interacting with outsiders. Nonsupportive reactions from others discourage further attempts to speak more English. Nonassertive communication becomes more difficult for those who lack fluency in speaking and have been conditioned to avoid conflict. Filipino nurses may consider it impolite and disrespectful for a subordinate to confront or challenge the authority of a superior. When a problem with a manager occurs, a Filipino nurse may communicate through a mediator, usually another Filipino nurse, who is in the same position within the hierarchy as her/his manager. Communicating disagreement with a physician is difficult for Filipino nurses. Conversely, Filipino registered nurses expect their subordinates to be deferential toward them.

Conflict can result from different cultural values about caring. Coming from a highly collective orientation, Filipinos define caring in terms of active caring for others. This perspective differs from the American value of self-care. Filipino nurses feel comfortable performing what they perceive as caring tasks for patients which American nurses expect patients to do for themselves. Initially they may not be inclined to teach and demonstrate procedures to patients, expecting them to be self-reliant about their care. Outsiders may misconstrue Filipino nurses' preoccupation with caring tasks as disorganization or lack of assertiveness.

Different views about a valued coworker may be another source of conflict. The Filipino values of shared perception and being one with others create a cooperative, rather than competitive, outlook. Valued Filipinos produce for the group and put the group above their own personal gain. Humility, hard work, loyalty, and generosity are admired. The businesslike and competitive perspectives of Americans, where behavior is internally motivated by individual gain, may be interpreted as selfish and uncaring. Self-proclamations of accomplishments are viewed as cocky and offensive. Instead, it is up to the group to recognize a member's achievement, which is assessed in terms of how this benefited the group.

Health-care organizations are cultural entities defined by norms that reflect the dominant values of the host society. Professional schools mirror these dominant societal norms, which are congruent with those of health-care organizations (Pacquiao, 1996a). For outsiders to the culture, the experience in American schools and health-care organizations is dissonant with previous life experiences, which require an understanding of both cultural and occupational role differences. Bicultural development of Filipino and non-Filipino staff should be the goal of occupational orientation and training. Biculturalism requires awareness of self and others and the ability to adapt behaviors that build positive relationships (Pacquiao, 2002). Understanding cultural differences and similarities allows for the development of intercultural understanding and skills that promote teamwork. Bicultural mentors who can teach cultural norms of the organization and work with diverse patients and staff will foster the individual health-care provider's ability to adapt behaviors. Staff development requires training in frame switching—using different frameworks to understand behaviors of others and commitment to the belief that other perspectives are equally sound in explaining our experiences (Pacquiao, in press). Impression management is a bicultural skill that is grounded in the ability to interpret behaviors of others within their own cultural context and manifest behaviors that promote relationship and intercultural understanding (Pacquiao, 2001).

ISSUES RELATED TO AUTONOMY

The Filipino cultural concept of *bahala na* is associated with trusting the hierarchy and the divine power to resolve conflicts and manage problems. *Bahala na* may be associated with avoiding taking an active role in controlling the situation or independently seeking a resolution to the problem. Outsiders may interpret this behavior as a lack of initiative or responsibility. Many Filipino nurses are hesitant to assume leadership roles and assert their points of view, especially with outsiders. After an initial effort, further attempts to resolve the problem are generally left to the leader or hierarchy. Providing support and role modeling helps these nurses assert themselves and feel confident in problem solving and conflict resolution. Filipinos are proud people, and it is important to maintain self-esteem and dignity by saving face and avoiding shame. Their sensitivity and attention to other people's feelings are often exhibited as indecisiveness, which many Americans interpret as lack of assertiveness.

Filipinos may achieve power and prestige by acquiring wealth, education, marriage, a distinguished position, or by age. Although this value has weakened among younger Filipinos, respect for the elderly and those in positions of power is firmly entrenched among most Filipinos, who are taught not to show open disagreement; loquacious Americans who uphold egalitarianism and candid expression of feelings and ideas are perplexed by the Filipino deference to authority. Less acculturated Filipinos may not understand the directness of Americans and, thus, may find it insulting. European American nurses saw the quiet, observant, tactful, patient, and slow-to-respond behaviors of Filipino nurses as unassertive (Spangler, 1992). The Filipino nurses saw outspoken, impatient, bold, and fast-moving behaviors of European American nurses as crass and insensitive. A Filipino may say yes to avoid hurting other people's feelings. A Filipino's response of yes must be examined in context to interpret its true meaning.

The Filipino hierarchy and emphasis on collectivity bring a consequent group-oriented sense of responsibility and accountability. The leader is respected, followed, and expected to make decisions on behalf of members. The leader is trusted to act in the best interests of the group. The concept of individual accountability and responsibility in a highly litigious society, such as the United States, may initially be difficult for Filipino nurses to understand. Supportive role modeling in assuming individual accountability is important for Filipino educated nurses.

Biocultural Ecology

SKIN COLOR AND OTHER BIOLOGICAL VARIATIONS

Variations in anthropomorphic, physical, and biophysiological characteristics of Filipinos exist as a result of ethnocultural and racial intermingling. One of the Filipino aboriginal tribes, the Aeta, is negroid and petite in stature. They are believed to have migrated from Africa through land bridges during the Ice Age (National Statistics Information Center, 1995). However, like other tribal groups in the Philippines, they are now a minority.

The typical native-born or immigrant Filipino may be of Malay stock (brown complexion) with a multiracial genetic background. It is important to note that intermarriage of Filipinos with other ethnic and racial groups occurs in many communities across the world. In clinical assessments, a family genogram identifying ethnic or racial blending is useful in tracking predisposition to genetic disorders.

The youthful features of Filipinos make it difficult to assess their age. Common Filipino physical features may include jet black to brunette or light brown hair, dark to light brown pupils with eyes set in almond-shaped eyelids, deep brown to very light tan skin tones, and mildly flared nostrils and slightly low to flat nose bridges. The eye structure may challenge health-care providers in assessment such as observing pupillary reactions for increased intracranial pressure, measuring ocular tension, and evaluating peripheral vision. The flat nose bridge may be overlooked by opticians when fitting and dispensing eyeglasses.

The high melanin content of the skin and mucosa may pose problems when assessing signs of jaundice, cyanosis, and pallor. This feature also poses difficulty in diagnosing retinal, gum-related, and oral tissue abnormalities. When performing skin assessments, practitioners should consider the complexion and skin tone of the Filipino client. The usual manifestations of anemia (pallor and jaundice) should be assessed in the conjunctiva. Newborns may have Mongolian spots (bluish green discolorations on their buttocks) that are physiological and eventually disappear.

Filipinos range in height from under 5 feet to the height of average Americans. Body weight varies according to nativity and other factors such as nutrition, physical activity, and heredity. Filipinos commonly gain weight when they come to the United States. There are no definitive studies relating nutrition with standard height and weight measures for this population; therefore, it is essential to assess for weight changes on an individual basis.

Filipinos have a small thoracic capacity. Approximately 40 percent have blood type B and a low incidence of the Rh-negative factor (Anderson, 1983). As more interracial families emerge in Filipino communities, changes in their serologic profile will likely occur.

DISEASES AND HEALTH CONDITIONS

Despite national efforts directed at health promotion and disease prevention, the Philippines is typical of any developing country. In 2001, the life expectancy at birth in the Philippines was estimated at 66.83 years for men and 71.88 years for women; APIs living in the United States have the highest life expectancy of all groups at 81.9 years (Demographics of Aging in America, 2002). In 1997, the infant mortality rate was 17 per 1000 live births, with a maternal mortality rate of 0.9 per 1000 live births. Infant mortality is associated with respiratory conditions, congenital anomalies, diarrhea, birth injury, septicemia, measles, meningitis, and nutritional deficiency. Leading causes of maternal mortality include complications of pregnancy, delivery, and puerperium such as hemorrhage and hypertension. In 1999, the 10 leading causes of morbidity among adults, in descending order, were diarrhea, bronchitis/bronchiolitis, pneumonia, influenza, hypertension, respiratory tuberculosis, malaria, heart disease, chickenpox, and typhoid/parathyroid fever. In 1997, the 10 leading mortality causes, in descending order, were heart disease, vascular system disease, pneumonia, accidents, malignancy, TB (all types), chronic obstructive pulmonary disease, other respiratory diseases, diabetes mellitus, and renal disease (Department of Health, Philippines, 2002a). Endemic diseases in the Philippines are related to the natural terrain and climate. The tropical climate increases risks for malaria, dengue fever, cholera, pneumonia, tuberculosis, and gastrointestinal diseases associated with bacteria and parasites. Injuries and physical disabilities occur during natural disasters such as tropical storms, volcanic eruptions, and coastal flooding.

Based on limited scientific literature on health risk factors specific to this group in the United States, Filipino immigrants are reported to be at high risk for developing coronary heart disease, hypertension, and diabetes at midlife and old age (Nora & McBride, 1996). This group is also reported to have a high predisposition to hypercholesterolemia, renal stones, hyperuricemia, gout (Guillermo, 1993), and arthritis (McBride, 1993). Compared to other Asians, Filipino men and women have the highest prevalence of hypertension (Garde, Spangler, & Miranda, 1994; Klatsky & Armstrong, 1991). High incidence of hyperuricemia is attributed to a shift from a Filipino diet to an American diet (McBride, Mariola, & Yeo, 1995).

Breast, cervical, prostate, thyroid, lung, and liver cancers are major threats to this population. A high incidence of late-stage breast and cervical cancers on diagnosis has been reported for Filipino women in the northern California region (Northern California Cancer Center, 1991). Liver cancer tends to be diagnosed in the late stages of the disease and appears to be associated with the presence of the hepatitis B virus. Silent carriers of the virus are common among Asians, and its presence is detected only when other problems are being evaluated. Health-care providers should routinely screen for hepatitis B virus, especially among recent immigrants. A high incidence of glucose-6-phosphate dehydrogenase (G-6-PD), thalassemias, and lactose intolerance and malabsorption exist among the Filipino population (Anderson, 1983).

VARIATIONS IN DRUG METABOLISM

Compared to the white American population, Asians require lower doses of central nervous system depressants such as haloperidol (Levy, 1993). Asians have a lower tolerance for alcohol, and are more sensitive to adverse effects of alcohol (Levy, 1993). Because of availability of over-the-counter antibiotics and lack of adequate medical monitoring of these drugs in the Philippines, Filipino immigrants may be insensitive to the effects of some anti-infectives. A positive reaction to tuberculin or Mantoux test is observed because of the practice of giving BCG vaccinations in childhood. Chest x-rays and sputum cultures are recommended for screening and diagnosis of TB. More research is needed to determine pharmacodynamics among Filipinos, including gender differences. Health-care providers need to assess Filipino clients individually when administering and monitoring medication effects.

High-Risk Behaviors

Gender differences are evident in the Filipino tolerance and acceptance of high-risk health behaviors related to alcohol, drugs, cigarettes, and sex, with higher incidences in men than women. A study of drinking patterns of Filipinos, Chinese, and Japanese in California reveals that men from all three ethnicities have approximately the same percentage of heavy drinkers (28 percent), whereas less than 4 percent of Filipino women are heavy drinkers (Chi & Kitano, 1989). Although Filipinos identified alcohol as a popular drink at social gatherings in a New Jersey study, 67 percent of the respondents reported that they did not drink alcohol. Only 1 percent reported having three or more drinks per day (Garde, Spangler, & Miranda, 1994). Because denial is closely associated with alcoholism, the frequency and amount of alcohol taken is generally underreported. Thus, the actual number of users may be slightly higher than reported, but probably still lower compared to the Western standard.

Cigarette smoking is more prevalent among Filipino men than women (Burns & Pierce, 1992). Smoking rates have been positively correlated with limited education and personal income (less than $15,000) (Garde, Spangler, & Miranda, 1994), a tendency to think or speak in a Filipino language (Asian American Health Forum, 2002), and for women, being born in the United States. In San Francisco, most Filipino youths reported living with an adult who smoked, and their first substance of choice was cigarettes, followed by alcohol and inhalants (Pilipino Mini-Health Forums Committee, 1993).

In 1996, the prenatal care rate among API women in the United States was 81.2 percent, with Filipinos at 82.5 percent. Filipinas have one of the highest incidences of low-birth-weight babies (8 percent) among APIs. Filipinas registered a rate of 3.5 percent for smoking during pregnancy compared to the overall rate of 3.3 percent for all APIs. Infant mortality rates among Filipinos rose from 5.1 per 1000 live births in 1991 to 5.6 per 1000 live births in 1995, in contrast to the overall decline in the total API population. Perinatal transmission of hepatitis B is common among APIs. Fifty percent of deliveries by women infected with the disease are Asian women. The combined hepatitis B rates for Chinese, Koreans, Filipinos, and southeast APIs range up to 15 percent versus 0.2 percent among the general U.S. population (Asian Pacific Islander American Health Forum, 2002).

Filipinos constitute the largest number of reported AIDS cases among APIs in the United States. Mortality data in the state of California for the period 1989–1991 showed that AIDS was the leading cause of death for American-born male Filipinos between the ages of 25 and 34, and the second leading cause of death for Filipino immigrants in the state. In 1998, Filipinos accounted for 37 percent of people with AIDS in San Francisco, and 32.4 percent of the people with AIDS among APIs living in California (Filipino Taskforce on AIDS, 2002). Culturally specific education programs on AIDS prevention has been a focus of the Filipino Task Force on AIDS. Low knowledge scores on information about HIV transmission and unprotected sex with multiple partners underscore the urgency of HIV and AIDS education and prevention.

HEALTH-CARE PRACTICES

Early Filipino immigrants reportedly do not seek health care in the United States until the illness is advanced (Anderson, 1983). Cultural, social, and economic factors have been implicated as reasons for their underutilization of health services. Lacking the rights and privileges of naturalized citizens, early Filipino immigrants remained in poverty and felt shunned and rejected as they grew older. Typical of the ethnically underserved elderly population in the United States, many were unaware of available services and were reluctant to access social and health services, particularly when culturally sensitive and bilingual providers were unavailable (McBride, 1993; Nora & McBride, 1996). Lack of transportation, fear of going to the area where services were located, and inappropriate program design were some of the other reasons for low utilization of services by this group (Pilipino Mini-Health Committee, 1993).

More recent Filipino immigrants differ significantly from their earlier counterparts in their access and utilization of health services. This group is highly educated and uses many of the socioeconomic opportunities in the United States. In a recent study in New Jersey, 78 percent of Filipinos had private or prepaid health insurance, 10 percent were on Medicare or Medicaid, and 7 percent had no insurance. Participants reported seeing a health-care provider at least every year, with only 2 percent not having seen a physician for more than 5 years (Garde, Spangler, & Miranda, 1994).

A group of older widows living in New York City compared their functional capacity with that of peers to determine their level of wellness and potential need for health-care services (Valencia-Go, 1989). Group differences may be attributed to variations in education, income, adjustment to the host culture, and acculturation experiences. Encouraging a Filipino American client to identify and describe the formal and informal resources that are used for health promotion can provide the health-care provider with a more realistic profile of the person's current health practices.

Nutrition

MEANING OF FOOD

To the Filipino, food is more than nourishment for the body; it is a fundamental form of socialization. Food and meal patterns are integral to the cultural emphasis on generosity, hospitality, and thoughtfulness that support group cohesiveness. No social gathering of Filipinos occurs without food. Food is offered as a token of gratitude and caring, to welcome others, to celebrate accomplishments and important events, to offer support in times of sickness or crisis, and to reinforce social bonds in everyday interactions. Younger family members are socialized into the closeness of the extended family, the community, and family values. Sharing food with others, or at the very least inviting others to share one's food, is expected of Filipinos and considered a sign of good upbringing. The insider versus outsider context influences the choice of food offered (Enriquez, 1993). Outsiders are served Westernized foods, while insiders are served native cuisines.

In the Philippines, traditional Filipino meals are labor-intensive, requiring participation of several family members. Meats are costly, so small amounts are cut in pieces and expanded using vegetables and starches to feed an entire family. It is common to offer refreshments and beverages or to invite guests to join in the family's meals. All family members, regardless of age, attend social gatherings where a variety of dishes are prepared to accommodate individual choices. The hosting family serves large amounts of food to accommodate guests of invitees who are expected to join if they happen to be around. It is customary for guests to linger for several meals as the focus is on the gathering. Latecomers are welcomed and expected to fully participate in the entire meal and the company of other guests. Dishes are served all at once from appetizers to desserts so guests are free to eat their courses without waiting for everyone to arrive. Guests are encouraged to return to the table to join arriving guests.

COMMON FOODS AND FOOD RITUALS

Indigenous Filipino cooking is characterized by simplicity of methods, such as boiling, steaming, roasting, broiling, marinating, or sour-stewing to preserve the fresh and natural taste of food. Spanish, Chinese, and American influences are integrated into contemporary Filipino cuisine. Foods may be sautéed, fried, or served with a sauce. Because of the tropical climate of the Philippines, many types of plants and animals flourish. Seafood forms the bulk of the Filipino diet. Animal sources of protein are chicken and pork because cows and water buffalo are primarily used for farming. Plants are the second most important food source and include a variety of seaweeds, edible roots, delicate leaves, tendrils, tropical fruits, seeds, and some flowers. Fruits and vegetables are consumed in large quantities in a variety of ways. Rice is a staple food and is eaten at every meal, either steamed, fried, or as a dessert.

Except for babies and young children, milk is almost absent in the Filipino diet. This may be partly due to lactose intolerance. However, milk in desserts such as egg custard and ice cream seems to be tolerated. In the Filipino food pyramid, milk and dairy products are incorporated in the major protein groups rather than as a separate category (Orbeta, 1998). Dietary calcium is derived from green leafy vegetables and seafood.

Regional variations in food preparation and use of spices exist in Filipino American households today. Nutrition counseling should take into account these variations when a Filipino needs to alter dietary patterns because of hypertension, diabetes, or other health problems. For instance, coconut milk is a common cooking additive among the Bicolanos of southern Luzon. Salty and spicy sauces complement meals. Less acculturated Filipinos tend to prepare and serve more traditional Filipino foods at home (De la Cruz, Padilla, & Agustin, 2000).

In the Philippines, breakfast consists of rice, meat or fish, and vegetable dishes or dinner leftovers. The breakfast beverage may be coffee, chocolate, or juice. In urban areas, Western-style meals are more common. For many Filipinos, breakfast, lunch, and dinner are not complete without steamed or fried rice served with fish, meat (especially pork), and vegetables. Snacks of bananas, yams, rice cake, and rice-flour cake are served as midday snacks, between meals, and before bedtime. The midday meal is the heaviest meal of the day, although this pattern is becoming more difficult among urban dwellers who cannot go home during lunchtime. Filipinos drink water with meals independently or in addition to another beverage of juice, soda, tea, or coffee.

DIETARY PRACTICES FOR HEALTH PROMOTION

Filipinos believe that health is maintained by moderation. Although Filipinos enjoy food and love to eat, they adhere to the wisdom that too much of a good thing can be harmful. In some parts of the Philippines, it is considered polite to leave food on one's plate. For many Filipino Americans, moderation in food intake is a special challenge because of the abundance and great variety of quality products at reasonable costs. Significant increases in weight are associated with changes in dietary patterns among new immigrants.

The abundance of plant life provides many medicinal plants and herbs for people in the Philippines. Filipino households may keep potted medicinal plants that are used for common colds, stomach upsets, urinary tract infections, and other minor ailments. Daily consumption of garlic to combat hypertension is common among Filipinos. Ginger root is boiled and served as a beverage to relieve sore throats and promote digestion. Bitter melon is prepared and eaten as a vegetable and believed to prevent diabetes. Greens such as *malunggay* and *ampalaya* leaves are used in stews to regain stamina for someone believed to be anemic or rundown.

NUTRITIONAL DEFICIENCIES AND FOOD LIMITATIONS

The nutrition of Filipinos, especially in the Philippines, is greatly affected by socioeconomic factors. Malnutrition persists in the country, especially among the poor and less educated, and remains as one of the 10 leading causes of infant mortality. In 1998, 9.2 percent of preschoolers were underweight, 5.4 percent had growth retardation, and 7.2 percent had wasting syndrome. Similar patterns were observed among school-aged children, with wasting syndrome reported more among boys and underweight reported more among girls (Department of Health, Philippines, 2002b).

In the United States, many Filipino immigrants may be at risk for nutritional deficiencies during their adjustment period, especially when they come with limited resources and without a support network of family and friends. Postmenopausal and pregnant women may be vulnerable to calcium deficiency owing to decreased intake of seafood and green leafy vegetables that were plentiful in the Philippines but limited in availability and variety in American food stores. Knowledge of indigenous food sources and meal patterns, nutritional content of Filipino foods and American food substitutes, and accessibility of traditional ingredients are important aspects of nutritional assessment and counseling for Filipinos in America.

Indigenous Filipino foods are often available in Asian American stores. Many cities have Filipino stores and restaurants that provide Filipino foods, although varieties may be limited.

Pregnancy and Childbearing Practices

FERTILITY PRACTICES AND VIEWS TOWARD PREGNANCY

The Roman Catholic Church and Filipino family values significantly influence childbearing and fertility practice. In marriage, the only acceptable method of contraception is the rhythm method. Abortion is considered a sin and is generally not acceptable. While these beliefs remain strong among many Filipinos, education, global communication, and modernization are causing changes, particularly in metropolitan cities such as Manila. Recent Filipino immigrants who come from large urban areas are more educated and less committed to the Church's position on birth control and premarital sex. Between 1993 and 1998, fertility rates of women in the Philippines decreased from 4.1 to 3.7 children. This decline is partly explained by an increase in contraceptive use among married women. Although there is a decline in female sterilization, it is still more common than the pill and other methods. There is a slight increase in the use of injectables and traditional methods such as rhythm and withdrawal. As many as 40 percent discontinue the use of contraception within 12 months of starting due to unwanted pregnancies (National Statistics Office, Philippines, 2002).

Although the median age for first birth is 23 years, the fertility rate is considerably higher than the rate of neighboring Southeast Asian countries. One reason is that many Filipino women want moderately large families consisting of 3 to 4 children. In 1998, 45 percent of pregnancies were unplanned, while 18 percent were unwanted (National Statistics Office, Philippines 2002). Filipino culture is child-centered, and abortion evokes strong reactions, even among liberal Filipinos. Though some may support the right to abortion, they may have moral qualms about obtaining one for themselves and feel guilty for considering this option.

Pregnancy is considered normal and is a time when a woman can demand attention and pampering from her husband and family members. Health-care providers who do not understand this special period for the pregnant Filipino woman may feel that their pregnant Filipino clients appear to be lazy (Stern, 1985). Pregnancy and childbirth are times for the family to draw closer together. Everyone assists in anticipation of the new baby, especially the pregnant woman's mother, who has a strong influence during this period. For mother and daughter, this is a special event in which the bond between them becomes closer. In the Filipino American community, women openly give advice to pregnant women, share their own birthing experiences, and ask personal questions that may be considered rather intrusive by outsiders.

PRESCRIPTIVE, RESTRICTIVE, AND TABOO PRACTICES IN THE CHILDBEARING FAMILY

Filipino practices surrounding pregnancy are influenced by indigenous beliefs, Western practices, and socioeconomic factors. A survey of birthing practices in the Philippines in 1999 showed that the practitioners most commonly sought during pregnancy and childbirth were nurses and midwives (49.4 percent), doctors (44.7 percent), and *hilots*, or traditional birth attendants (5.8 percent). Local *hilots* employed massage and were consulted for physical, spiritual, and psychological advice and guidance. Although more than 94 percent received prenatal care during their last pregnancy, only 80.6 percent completed three or more visits. In contrast to women from rural areas who saw nurses and midwives, urban dwellers sought doctors for prenatal care. Two-thirds of the infants were delivered at home (National Statistics Office, Philippines 2002).

After childbirth, the new mother continues to be pampered. Relatives help with the new baby and in running the household. Eighty percent of Filipino babies are breast-fed for some time, with a median duration of 13 months. More rural women breast-fed their infants, and for a much longer time (10 to 13 months) than their urban counterparts (1 to 3 months). Common reasons given for not breast-feeding were insufficient milk, mother working, nipple and breast problems, and mother's poor health. Supplementing breast-feeding with other liquids and foods occurs as early as 2 months (National Statistics Office, Philippines 2002). Lactating mothers are encouraged to take plenty of hot soups (chicken with papaya) to promote milk production. Only 64.5 percent of children between the ages of 12 and 23 months were fully immunized.

Stern (1985) reported that pregnant Filipino women in California refused to take vitamins because they were afraid that vitamins could deform the fetus. Some believe that when pregnant women crave certain foods, especially during the first trimester, the craving should be satisfied to avoid harm to the baby. Filipinos in America may continue to believe that the baby takes on the appearance of the craved food. Thus, if the mother craves dark-skinned fruit or dark-colored food, the infant's skin will be dark. Pregnant women are protected from sudden fright or stress because of the belief that this may harm the developing fetus. Table 9–1 provides a summary of traditional beliefs and practices observed among some Filipinos in Hawaii. Becoming aware of the pregnant Filipino woman's network of family and community health advisers, whose opinions she respects, is important for building trust and rapport in the client-provider relationship.

Some women prefer to have their mothers rather than their husbands in the delivery room. Mothers of pregnant women serve as coaches and teachers and are often respected over the health-care professional for their experience and knowledge. This may be puzzling to professionals who view pregnancy as an emancipating event. Conflicts are likely to occur if the coach and teacher believe in practices that are contrary to Western childbearing practices.

During postpartum, exposure to cold is avoided. Showers are prohibited because these may cause arthritis. However, the woman's mother gives a sponge bath with aromatic oils and herbs, or a *hilot* gives an aromatic herbal steam bath followed by full body massage, including the abdominal muscles, stimulating a physiological

Table 9–1 *Traditional Filipino Beliefs and Practices Surrounding Pregnancy and Childbirth*

Prenatal	Postpartum
Eating blackberries will make the baby have black spots.	Use warm water to drink and bathe for a month.
Eating black plums will give the baby dark skin.	Don't name the baby before it is born.
Eating twin bananas will result in twin births.	Don't name the baby after a dead person.
Eating apples will give the baby red lips.	Give money to charity or the needy when a baby comes to your house the first time.
When a woman's stomach is not round, the baby will be a boy.	Eating sour or ice cold foods may cause abdominal cramps.
If a woman's face is blemished, it will be a boy.	Wrap the baby's abdomen with a cloth until the umbilical cord falls off.
Going outside during a lunar eclipse is harmful to the baby.	The mother and baby should not go out for a month except to visit a doctor.
Going out in the morning dew is bad for the baby because evil spirits are present.	Putting garlic, salt, or a rosary near the baby's crib will keep evil spirits away.
Funerals are avoided because the spirit of the dead person may affect the baby.	Hanging the baby's placenta in a tree will make the baby a good climber.
Wearing necklaces may cause the umbilical cord to wrap around the baby's neck.	
Sitting by a doorway will make the delivery difficult.	
Sitting by a window when it is dark may let evil spirits come to the pregnant woman.	
Sweeping at night may sweep away the good spirits.	
Knitting might tangle the baby's intestines at birth.	

Source: Adapted from *http://www.hawcc.Hawaii.edu/nursing/RN/Filipino 2001.*

reaction that has both physical and psychological benefits.

Childbirth experience of Filipino women immigrants in a hospital in Brisbane, Australia, revealed the following (Asian Pacific Islander Maternity Coalition, 2001):

- Language and communication problems prevented some Filipino women from seeking antenatal care.
- They were embarrassed to have male doctors perform vaginal exams.
- Women who came from rural regions in the home country preferred the squatting position for birthing.
- They experienced conflict with practitioner expectation for their husbands' presence in the delivery room.
- They perceived discrimination by the hospital staff who did not consult them about their care.
- They preferred to deliver at home.

Death Rituals

DEATH RITUALS AND EXPECTATIONS

In the Filipino culture, death is a spiritual event. Illness and death may be attributed to supernatural and magicoreligious causes such as punishment from God, angry spirits, or sorcery. Religiosity and fatalism contribute to stoicism in the face of pain or distress as a way of accepting one's fate (Lipson, Dibble, & Minarik, 1996). Planning for one's death is taboo and may be considered tempting fate. Hence, many traditional Filipinos are averse to discussing advance directives or living wills (Pacquiao, 2001). When death is imminent, contacting a priest is important if the family is Catholic.

Religious medallions, rosary beads, a scapular, and religious figures may be found on the patient or at the bedside. Family members generally wish to provide the most intimate caregiving rituals to the patient regardless of the setting.

After death, a wake is planned. The wake may last from 3 days to 1 week (to wait for the arrival of kin from other states or countries). Although a wake is generally held in the home in the rural regions, funeral parlors are used in urban areas and in the United States. Families and friends gather to give support and recall the special traits of the deceased. Food is provided to all guests throughout the wake and after the burial.

The burial rites are consistent with the religious traditions of the family, which may be Judeo-Christian, Muslim, Buddhist, or other religions. Among Catholics, 9 days of novenas are held in the home or in the church. These special prayers ask God's blessing for the deceased. Depending upon the economic resources of the family, food and refreshments are served after each prayer day. Sometimes the last day of the novena takes on the atmosphere of a *fiesta* or a celebration. Filipino families in the United States follow variations of this ritual according to their social and economic circumstances. Funerals in the Philippines can be simple or elaborate, with a band accompaniment, several priests officiating, and a large throng of mourners. Reciprocal obligation continues in death through performance of rituals such as the wake, novenas, and establishing a burial site acceptable for the entire family.

On the first-year anniversary of death, family and friends are reunited in prayer to celebrate this memorable event. Most Filipino women wear black clothing for months or up to a year after the death. The one-year anniversary ends the ritual mourning. Before this period, family members postpone weddings and other celebrations in deference to the memory of the deceased. Memories and love for the deceased are shown on All Soul's Day, a Catholic feast day, when families visit and decorate the graves of their loved ones. Filipino American families may continue these traditions, particularly when strong kinship is present and the clan lives in close proximity. Many who die in the United States are buried in the Philippines and the family in that country continues the tradition.

Beliefs related to cremation vary according to individual preference. Ordinarily, bodies are buried, but cremation is acceptable to avoid the spread of disease. In America, some Filipinos who wish to return their deceased family members to the Philippines may choose cremation for practical and economic reasons.

RESPONSES TO DEATH AND GRIEF

Most Filipinos believe in life after death. Caring for the spiritual needs of the dying is one way of ensuring peaceful rest of the soul or one's spirit. Family presence around the dying and immediate period after death to pray for the soul of the departed is considered a priority. If the patient is Catholic, the priest anoints the patient and gives Holy Communion, if the patient is able to participate. Caring is shown by providing a peaceful environment, speaking in low tones, and praying with the ill person.

After death, grief reaction varies. Women generally show emotions openly by crying, fainting, or wailing. Men are expected to be more stoic and grieve silently. Young children are admonished for behaving inappropriately since this is considered disrespectful to the deceased. Family members gather together and provide physical and emotional support for each other. Praying for the deceased and following the implicit guidelines of behavior during mourning is a way of demonstrating grief appropriately. Wearing black or subdued colors (gray, white, navy, brown), avoiding parties and playing loud, distracting music, postponing weddings, or devoting time to one's studies to honor the dead are some of the acceptable ways of expressing grief. Honoring the memory of the deceased is a continuing obligation among close kin.

Spirituality

DOMINANT RELIGION AND USE OF PRAYER

The only predominantly Christian country in the Far East, the Philippines are 83 percent Catholic, 9 percent Protestant, 5 percent Muslim, and 3 percent Buddhist and other religions (World Factbook, 2001). Membership in the *Iglesia ni Christo, Aglipay,* Jehovah's Witness, and Seventh-Day Adventists is increasing. The spread of the fundamentalist movement within Roman Catholicism is becoming more evident. Christianity in the Philippines today is a blend of Spanish Catholicism, American Christianity, and surviving indigenous traditions (Russell, 2001) (Fig. 9–4).

Although Filipinos seek medical care, they believe that part of the efficacy of a cure is in God's hands or by some

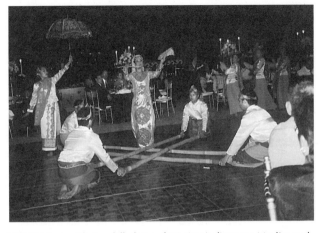

FIGURE 9–4 Filipino folk dance depicting indigenous Muslim and Malayan influences.

mystical power. Novenas and prayers are often said on behalf of the sick person. Families may bring religious items such as rosaries, medals, scapulars, and talismans for the sick person to wear. Talismans and amulets are believed to protect one from the forces of darkness, one's enemies, and sickness. Performance of religious obligations and sacraments and daily prayers are some of the ways many Filipinos believe health and peaceful death are achieved. Providing for spiritual needs of Filipino clients requires accommodation to their various ways of practicing beliefs.

MEANING OF LIFE AND INDIVIDUAL SOURCES OF STRENGTH

Filipinos consider a meaningful existence to be a healthy and appropriate relationship with nature, God, and kin. Indigenous Filipino beliefs are embedded in the relationship between humans within the cosmology of the universe. This concept is demonstrated by the integration of supernatural, magicoreligious, and natural phenomena in the belief system and practices toward health and illness. Filipinos do not see themselves as victims, but rather as part of the larger cosmos, subject to both the controllable and uncontrollable forces of nature. To the traditional Filipino, strength comes from an intimate relationship with God, family, friends, neighbors, and nature. The concept of self is formed from the relationship with a divine being and the social collective.

Many Filipinos find religion a source of strength in their daily lives. Some Filipinos are considered fatalistic in that they tend to accept fate easily, especially when they feel they cannot change a situation. However, acceptance of fate or destiny comes from their close relationship and healthy respect for nature. The acceptance of events they cannot change is tied to their religious faith. A common expression uttered by Filipinos is *bahala na*, originating from *bathala na*, (it is up to God). Enriquez (1994) explained that *bahala na* is often used when the person has used all resources to deal with a problem, and it is up to a higher power to take care of the rest. Nevertheless, there is an element of individualism among Filipinos, manifested by being confident that the situation is within their sphere of influence. An excellent example is the belief in the ability of education and hard work to change one's life.

SPIRITUAL BELIEFS AND HEALTH-CARE PRACTICES

Holism and integration characterize Filipino health-care beliefs and practices. Religious and spiritual dimensions are important components in health promotion. Belief in harmony between humans and nature, and the role of natural and supernatural forces in health and illness are found in their beliefs about causes of illness, and healing modalities. Prayers, religious offerings, appeasing natural spirits, and witchcraft may be simultaneously practiced along with biomedical interventions. Despite increasing notoriety and scandal associated with Filipino faith healers, this healing modality is widely sought in the Philippines. Many Filipinos seek biomedical and integrative ways of healing and do not subscribe to the competitive reductionism of the West. They believe in the synergistic relationship of differing modalities and have no problem subscribing to both ways of healing. Filipino Americans travel to Lourdes in France and to the shrine of Fatima in Portugal to pray for good health and healing.

Health-Care Practices

HEALTH-SEEKING BELIEFS AND BEHAVIORS

Filipinos seek out family and close kin first for help when they are ill. When illness is more defined, mobilization of support occurs within the family. Decisions about when, where, and from whom to seek help are largely influenced by the intimate circle of family. Among Filipino elders in the United States, choice of practitioners is based on accessibility and availability to their working adult children (Pacquiao, 1993). Linguistically and ethnically congruent practitioners are preferred. A dual system of personal health care exists for many Filipinos, including those who are established in American communities. Filipinos may accept and adhere to medical recommendations and may use alternative sources of care suggested by trusted friends and family members. Very often, they adhere to Western and indigenous medicine simultaneously, creating more choices to deal with their own or their family's health issues.

Many Filipinos consult an informal network of friends and family members who may be physicians, nurses, pharmacists, or neighbors who have had similar symptoms. Once the person finds the brand name of the "effective" medicine, the person can easily purchase the drug by asking family or friends to purchase medication in the Philippines. Hoarding prescription drugs and sharin medicine may be practiced by Filipinos in the United States (Pilipino Mini-Health Committee, 1993). Those who do not believe in wastefulness or those who believe that office visits are expensive may practice these behaviors.

When educating Filipino clients about medication, health-care professionals should stress that medications need to be taken as prescribed; medications are ordered specifically for each ailment; unused drugs should be discarded; and the use of medications by individuals other than the intended may have serious consequences. Assessing these behaviors and delivering the message in a respectful, courteous, and unhurried manner may enhance the client-provider relationship, especially for traditional Filipino clients.

Health-care practices stress balance and moderation for the Filipino. Health is the result of balance, and illness is the consequence of imbalance. Imbalances that threaten health are brought about by personal irresponsibility or immorality. Care of the body through adequate sleep, rest, nutrition, and exercise is essential for health. A high value is also placed on personal cleanliness. Keeping oneself clean and free of unpleasant body odors is viewed as good for one's health and face-saving. To be slovenly and disorderly is to be shamelessly irresponsible (Anderson, 1983). Aromatic baths are taken both for pleasure and to restore balance.

RESPONSIBILITY FOR HEALTH CARE

Parents may seek all possible assistance that they can personally generate from family, friends, the church, community, and the formal health-care system (often in that order) for a child who has cancer, eventually accepting the inevitability of death. From a Western perspective, the outcome may be slightly different than if formal services were accessed as early as possible. Adult children, especially those working in the United States, are responsible for the health care of their aged parents and extended kin. Responsibility may be in different forms such as decision making, financial responsibility, providing supportive presence, performing caretaking tasks, or negotiating with the health-care practitioner and the system.

In general, older adult women provide direct care for younger members. Older men participate in caring tasks like driving the patient to the clinic. Decisions and financial support are relegated to family members who are deemed qualified and able. The family acts as a unit and the individualistic paradigm commonly used by American caregivers is replaced by a social ethic of care. Before the decision is made to inform the patient about his or her terminal condition, a discussion among family members occurs, and they may request the doctor not to divulge the truth to protect the patient. The ethical principles of beneficence and nonmalfeasance take precedence over patient autonomy (Pacquiao, in press).

Filipino family hierarchy may require consulting with family members before decisions are made. This may pose a problem to Western practitioners who believe in adult patients' autonomy in making decisions about their own lives. The same perspective of Filipinos may result in their inability to question and assert ideas with the physician, who is regarded to be in a higher position of authority. Major decisions may be delegated to the physician rather than the patient or family taking an active collaborative role in decision making. Failure to develop a trusting relationship with the practitioner can lead to noncompliance with prescribed regimens because of a lack of participation in the decision-making process.

FOLK PRACTICES

Supernatural and magicoreligious beliefs about health and illness are integrated with scientific medicine. Mental illness may be attributed to an external cause such as witchcraft, soul loss, or spirit intrusion. Illness in infancy and childhood may be attributed to the evil eye. This belief system is consistent with the variety of Filipino folk healers. Healing rituals may involve religious (prayers and exorcism), sacrifices to appease the spirits, use of herbs, and massage.

Balance and moderation are embedded in the hot and cold theory of healing. The ideal environment is warm, moderate, and balanced. The underlying principle is that change should be introduced gradually. Sudden changes from hot to cold, from activity to inactivity, from fasting to overeating, and so forth, introduce undue bodily stresses, which can cause illness. After strenuous physical activity, a rest should precede a shower; otherwise the person could develop arthritis. Cold drinks or foods such as orange juice or fresh tomatoes are not served for breakfast to prevent stomach upset. Exposure to sudden cold drafts may induce colds, fever, rheumatism, pneumonia, or other respiratory ailments. Some Filipinos in the United States avoid hand-washing with cold water after ironing or heavy labor. Exposure to cold such as showers is avoided during menstruation and during the postpartum period.

The Department of Health in the Philippines has endorsed 10 herbal medicines as being scientifically proven and effective. These include bitter melon for diabetes, *sambong* as a diuretic, and guava leaves for cleaning wounds (National Statistics Office, Philippines, 2002). Some Filipinos in Hawaii use chives for cuts and bruises, garlic for hypertension, ginger for inflammation, and green bananas to treat fevers (Hawaii Community College, 2001).

BARRIERS TO HEALTH CARE

Studies of Filipinos in the United States show that, for many reasons, Filipinos generally do not seek care for illness until it is quite advanced. Some take minor ailments stoically and consider them natural imbalances that will run their normal course and disappear. Others claim to watch the progress of their illness so that the appropriate health-care provider can be consulted (Anderson, 1983). Still others may not seek help because of economic reasons, distrust of the health-care system, religious reasons, lack of knowledge, or an inability to articulate their needs (McBride, Mariola & Yeo, 1995; Pilipino Mini-Health Forums, 1993).

Some Filipinos may not have a primary health-care provider and may rely on emergency services instead. Many Filipinos are reluctant to participate in health-promotion programs such as cancer screening and health education. Aging Filipino veterans may be denied health services because of lack of insurance and consequently referred to various nonprofit community clinics (McBride, 1993). Older Filipino émigrés did not have adequate health benefits through their place of employment. Thus, they may have been used to postponing

seeking care until the illness was quite advanced. In contrast, recent immigrants have health insurance and behave differently, seeking preventive medical services regularly (Garde, Spangler, & Miranda, 1995).

Health-care providers should expect wide variations in health behaviors among Filipino American clients. Most important, nonjudgmental history taking should be well documented. Turning on the "multicultural ear" and listening with care to the context of these actions can provide insight for practitioners, particularly when the practitioner is under time pressure.

CULTURAL RESPONSES TO HEALTH AND ILLNESS

Filipinos view pain as part of living an honorable life. Some view this as an opportunity to reach a fuller spiritual life or to atone for past transgressions. Thus, they may appear stoic and tolerate a high degree of pain. Health-care providers may need to offer and, in fact, encourage pain relief interventions for Filipino clients who do not complain of pain despite physiological indicators. Others may have a strong sensitivity to the "busyness" of health-care providers, quietly diminishing their own need for attention so that others can receive care, or they may simply have little knowledge of how pain management can be maximized.

Minimal expressions of psychological and emotional discomfort may be observed. The discomfort in discussing negative emotions with outsiders may be manifested by somatic complaints or ritualistic behaviors, such as praying. Exploring the underlying meaning of somatization (loss of appetite, inability to sleep) and observing client interaction with others can provide valuable information. Filipino clients may display visible evidence of their religion such as religious medals, prayer cards, and rosary beads to manage anxiety and pain. These artifacts should be incorporated into their treatment regimen. Using cultural mediators or brokers to probe innermost feelings of patients may be helpful if used appropriately. Pain assessment can include the role of prayer by the patient and members of the support network. Questions such as "Do you have someone praying for you?" or "Is there a special prayer to help you deal with pain?" may provide vital information for individualizing care.

Most Filipinos believe that mental illness carries a certain amount of stigma, and some believe that mental illness is hereditary. Family members tend to take care of emotional problems to minimize exposing the problem to outsiders. Among rural residents and less-educated Filipinos in the Philippines, mental illness is generally attributed to external causes such as sorcery, soul loss, or spirit intrusion. Witch doctors, fortunetellers, and faith healers are often sought. Filipinos in the United States seek professional interventions when symptoms are advanced. Psychiatric symptoms are precipitated by a loss in self-esteem, loss of status, and shame related to the stresses of immigration. Separation from family, inability to find suitable employment, uncertainty, lack of money, and other relocation stressors, create serious psychological reactions among Filipinos. Talking to a trusted family member or friend, psychotherapy, staying involved, support and prayer groups, employment, and medication are the preferred treatment.

Using sociocultural behaviors learned early in life, Filipinos have a remarkable ability to maintain a proper front to protect their self-esteem and self-image. However, this front may be fragile, and chronic repression of resentment and anger may build up and erupt violently. Mental health providers should recognize that despite the possibility of a Filipino client's refusing professional mental health services, involving a trusted family member or friends, initiating contact with a Filipino mental health worker, especially a Filipino physician, or using both practices may increase the odds of getting the person into a culturally compatible treatment program (Nora & McBride, 1996). Deference to authority may successfully bring the Filipino client into treatment with the client's expectation that the authority figure will fix the problem. A family therapy framework can have a more beneficial outcome (McBride & Parreno, 1996).

The birth of a developmentally disabled child may be viewed as God's gift, an opportunity to become a better person or family, a curse from some unknown "angry spirit," negligence while pregnant, or a family matter that should be kept private (Tompar-Tiu & Sustento-Seneriches, 1994). Health-seeking behaviors are conditioned by the perceived cause. American-born Filipinos may be more inclined to accept rehabilitation services through a home-care program than through institutional placement, such as special schools and long-term-care facilities.

The cultural value of reciprocal obligation and the family as the main support exaggerate the burden of caring for a chronically ill family member. Institutionalization may not be readily accepted, causing considerable strains on the family relationships and resources. Self-sacrifice is believed to be virtuous and rewarded spiritually and in future life. Verbalization of care-taking hardships may not be tolerated and may cause guilt feelings on the individual caregiver. Practitioners should be sensitive to the needs of the family caregiver and work with the family unit in finding alternative ways of providing care for the chronically ill members. Reluctance to join support groups comprised of outsiders and non-Filipinos can be offset by involving other family members or friends.

BLOOD TRANSFUSIONS AND ORGAN DONATION

The value of blood transfusion is recognized and accepted by Filipinos. However, organ donation may be less acceptable, except perhaps in cases where a close family member is involved. Many Filipinos who follow Catholic traditions believe that keeping the body intact as much as possible until death is a reasonable preparation for the afterlife. A survey of Filipinos in New Jersey showed that most did not carry an organ donor card or know about the program. When asked if they would be willing to sign an organ donor card, only 29 percent agreed. Explanations offered were related to the rarity of organ donation and transplantation, and limited technological support for the procedures in the Philippine health-care system (Garde, Spangler, & Miranda, 1994).

Health-Care Practitioners

TRADITIONAL VERSUS BIOMEDICAL PRACTITIONERS

Western medicine is familiar and acceptable to most Filipinos. Many recent Filipino immigrants are educated in the health-care field. Some Filipinos accept the efficacy of folk medicine and may consult both Western-trained and indigenous healers. Traditional healers are sought more in the rural areas of the Philippines. Folk healers are less common in the United States, with the exceptions of the West Coast and Hawaii. When available, they contribute by facilitating cultural rapport between health-care providers and the client, and by increasing utilization of needed health-care services. For example, the *hilot* is often willing to be included in the counseling session and provide support for the patient's compliance with the medical treatment. The *hilot* may provide a special prayer to be incorporated into the medically prescribed treatment plan to increase the client's sense that all available resources are being used. In some areas on the West Coast, the *hilot* has a distinct role and function in the Filipino community. A few Filipino health professionals have learned the *hilot*'s art, skills, and spiritual approach, which they blend into their professional practice (McBride, 1993).

A practitioner of the same gender and the same culture may encourage more Filipinos to take advantage of disease prevention services. The availability of Filipino primary-care providers and, whenever possible, a bilingual person are critical to improving health care for elderly Filipino people.

STATUS OF HEALTH-CARE PROVIDERS

Filipinos generally consider the physician as the primary leader of the health-care team and other providers are expected to defer to the physician. As Filipino families become more acculturated and aware of how health-care services are accessed in the United States, changes in attitude and behavior may be expected.

When ill, Filipinos may first consult a family member or a friend who is a physician or other professional before arranging a medical appointment. Some prefer physicians from their own region, when possible, whereas others indicate preference for physicians who are knowledgeable and competent and have good bedside manners regardless of culture or ethnic background (Spangler, 1985). In San Francisco, a group of middle-aged immigrant Filipino women identified some of the criteria they used for choosing a health-care provider, such as their concern for privacy, feelings of modesty, approval from family members (especially the spouse), and most important, the overall caring environment in the system (McBride & Parreno, 1996).

CASE STUDY Sixty-eight-year-old Ramona Mag-pantay from the Philippines is visiting her daughter in New Jersey. She has been alternating with her husband in coming to the United States for 6 weeks at a time to keep their immigrant status in good standing. Although neither she nor her husband plan to reside in the United States permanently, they applied for immigration through the sponsorship of their daughter so they can facilitate immigration of their youngest child.

Ramona and her husband are both retired and live comfortably in the Philippines. She was an elementary school teacher and her husband maintains an accounting office with one of his sons, who is also an accountant. They have six children, three of whom reside in North America (two in New Jersey and one in Toronto). In the United States, they stay with their married daughter, Virginia, who lives with her husband and three children. Ramona's son Roberto lives with his wife and two children (a 3-year-old boy and a 1-year-old girl). Because her daughter Virginia is a full-time homemaker, Ramona stays with her son on the weekdays to help look after her grandchildren while the couple are working. She goes home to Virginia's family on weekends.

One Friday evening, Virginia phoned her friend, Rowena, a Filipino nurse residing in the same neighborhood. She asked Rowena to come and check her mother, who was not feeling well. Rowena sensed the urgency in Virginia's tone of voice and quickly drove to her home. She found Ramona in bed, fully covered with a comforter, with visible chest heaves and lifts. After examining Ramona and taking her vital signs, Rowena spoke with Virginia alone in the kitchen so Ramona would not hear their conversation. Rowena told Virginia that her mother should be taken to the hospital.

Virginia explained that her mother does not have medical insurance since she only stays for six weeks at a time and has a medical exam before her trips. She also told Rowena that her mother has diabetes, hypertension, and an irregular heartbeat. When Ramona's heart medications (Digoxin and Inderal) ran out, she did not inform Virginia. She did not want her to purchase her medications because she is not "working and earning." She also thought that since she would be going home in 2 weeks, she could wait until then. Before calling Rowena, Virginia already consulted her cousin Leticia, a physician who lives in Long Island, New York.

Rowena called her cousin's husband, who is a cardiologist, to get his recommendation. Upon hearing Ramona's symptoms, the cardiologist insisted that she be taken to the emergency room at once. When she heard his recommendation, Virginia agreed to call for an ambulance and accompanied her mother in the ambulance to the local hospital.

The ER physician determined that Ramona should be admitted to the cardiac care unit (CCU). Virginia requested that her cousin Leticia speak to the doctor before any decision was made. Leticia explained to the doctor the financial ramifications of Ramona's admission and explored the possibility of her discharge on medications. The ER physician vehemently disagreed with Leticia and explained the seriousness of Ramona's condition as well as her need for close medical supervision. Leticia then spoke with Virginia and apologized for her inability to convince the ER physician. She warned her to anticipate the high cost of CCU care.

Virginia's husband was called to sign the promissory note of payment for Ramona's hospitalization. He was resigned to the idea that Ramona's life was in danger and money should not be a barrier to her well-being. He was also confident that Virginia's two brothers in North America would share the cost. Ramona was never made aware of all these discussions. In her presence, Virginia and her husband did their best to present a calm, reassuring presence. She was told that she would be given a thorough examination, which is advantageous as it is done in a U.S. facility, far superior than health care in the Philippines.

Ramona spent 3 days in CCU, followed by 4 days in a medical unit. When visited by her daughter's friend, Rowena, she verbalized her concern for her daughter's family paying the cost of her hospitalization. What she tried hard to accomplish (not to burden her daughter) turned out to be a very expensive mistake. She had always wanted her daughter to go back to work as a medical technologist to help her husband. She said that with two incomes, her three grandchildren would be assured of a better future. Virginia admitted to Rowena that her mother had tried many times to convince her to return to work, but her previous experience with babysitters was traumatic and she decided to stay home and live economically to compensate for the loss of income. She said that she would consider returning to work when the children were much older.

Two weeks after her discharge, Ramona returned to the Philippines. She decided not to return to the United States, but assured her family that her husband would travel every year to maintain their immigration status. Her children made every effort to visit her regularly in the Philippines and speak with her frequently by phone.

STUDY QUESTIONS

1 Describe how these Filipino cultural values are manifested in this family.
- *Utang na loob:* reciprocal obligation to kin
- *Pakkipagkawa:* shared identity
- *Pakiramdam:* shared perception with others
- *Bahala na:* fatalism

2 Discuss how these values may have contributed to the crisis in the family.

3 | Identify potential problems that can arise from these values in a different cultural context such as in the United States.

4 | Explore culture-specific assessments and communication approaches for the patient and the family.

5 | Identify culturally competent care strategies for health promotion.

REFERENCES

Agoncillo, T., & Guerrero, M. (1987). *History of the Filipino people* (7th ed.). Manila, Philippines: Garcia Publishing.

Anderson, J. N. (1983). Health and illness in Pilipino immigrants. *Western Journal of Medicine, 139*(6), 811–819.

Asian American Health Forum. (2002). http://www.apiahf.org.

Asian Pacific Islander American Health Forum. (2002). *MCH facts.* Retrieved January 6, 2002, from http://www.apiahf.org.

Asian Pacific Islander Maternity Coalition. (2001). http://www.maternity-coalition.org.au.

Asian Promise. (2002). *Filipino divorce.* Retrieved April 14, 2002, from http://www.asianpromise.com.

Bouvier, L. F., & Gardner, R. W. (1986). Immigration to the United States: The unfinished story. *Population Bulletin, 41*(4), 1–50.

Brush, B. L. (1995). The Rockefeller agenda for American/Philippines nursing relations. *Western Journal of Nursing Research, 17*(5), 540–556.

Bulatao, J. (1962). Changing social values. *Philippine Studies, 10,* 206–214.

Burns, O., & Pierce, J. (1992). *Tobacco use in California 1990–1991.* Sacramento, CA: California Department of Health Services.

Cabezas, A., Shinagawa, L. H., & Kawaguchi, G. (1986). New inquiries into the socioeconomic status of Pilipino Americans in California. *Amerasia, 13,* 1–21.

Chi, I., & Kitano, H. H. L. (1989). Asian Americans and alcohol: The Chinese, Japanese, Koreans, and Filipinos in Los Angeles. *Alcohol use among U.S. ethnic minorities.* Research Monograph No. 18. Bethesda, MD: National Institute on Alcohol Abuse and Alcoholism.

Cimmarusti, R. A. (1996). Exploring aspects of Filipino-American families. *Journal of Marriage and Family Therapy, 22*(2), 205–218.

De la Cruz, F. A., Padilla, G. V., & Agustin, E. O. (2000). Adapting a measure of acculturation for cross-cultural research. *Journal of Transcultural Nursing, 11*(3), 191–198.

Demographics of Aging in America. (2002). Available at http://www.prcdc.org/summaries/aging/aging.html.

Department of Health, Philippines. (2002a). *Health indicators.* Retrieved January 4, 2002, from http://www.doh.gov.ph.

Department of Health, Philippines. (2002b). *Initial results of the fifth national nutrition survey.* Retrieved January 4, 2002, from http://www.doh.gov.ph.

Enriquez, V. G. (1985). Filipino psychology: Perspective and direction. In L. F. Antonio, E. R. Reyes, R. E. Pe, & N. R. Almonte (Eds.), Proceedings of the first national conference on Filipino psychology. Quezon City, Philippines: Pambansang Samahan sa Sikolohiyang Pilipino.

Enriquez, V. G. (1986). Kapwa: A core concept in Filipino social psychology. In V. G. Enriquez (Ed.), *Philippine worldview* (pp. 6–19). Singapore: Institute of Southeast Asian Study.

Enriquez, V. G. (1993). Developing a Filipino psychology. In U. Kim & J. W. Berry (Eds.), *Indigenous psychologies: Research and experience in cultural context* (pp. 162–169). Newbury Park, CA: Sage.

Enriquez, V. G. (1994). *From colonial to liberation psychology: The Philippine experience.* Manila, Philippines: De La Salle University Press.

Espina, M. E. (1988). *Filipinos in New Orleans.* New Orleans, LA: Laborde & Sons.

Filipino Task Force on AIDS. (2002). *Filipinos and AIDS.* Available at http://www.ftfa.org.

Garde, P., Spangler, Z., & Miranda, B. (1994). *Filipino-Americans in New Jersey: A health study.* Final Report of the Philippine Nurses' Association of America to the State of New Jersey Department of Health, Office of Minority Health.

Garrote-Trinidad, L. (2001). *Understanding the Filipinos and their culture.* Retrieved November 2, 2001, from http://www.fasgi.org/cultural.

Gendrano, V. P. (1990). The romance of Filipino language. *Heritage, 4*(3), 6–7.

Gorospe, V. R. (1977). Sources of Filipino moral consciousness. *Philippine Studies, 25,* 278–301.

Grossholtz, J. (1964). *Politics in the Philippines.* Boston: Little Brown.

Guillermo, T. (1993). Health care needs and service delivery for Asian and Pacific Islander Americans: Health policy. *LEAP: The state of Asian Pacific America—Policy issues to the year 2020.* Los Angeles, CA: University of California Los Angeles Press.

Guthrie, G. M. (1968). *Six perspectives on the Philippines.* Manila, Philippines: Bookmark.

Hawaii Community College. (2001). *Traditional Filipino beliefs surrounding pregnancy and childbirth. Filipino culture: Pregnancy and childbirth beliefs and superstitions. Traditional Filipino health practices.* Retrieved November 6, 2001, from http://www.web.hawcc.hawaii.edu/nursing/RNFilipino.

Ho, D. Y. (1993). Relational orientation in Asian social psychology. In U. Kim & J. W. Berry (Eds.), *Indigenous psychologies: Research and experience in cultural context* (pp. 240–259). Newbury Park, CA: Sage.

Kao, G. (1995). Asian Americans as model minorities? A look at the academic performance of immigrant youth. *Social Science Quarterly, 76,* 1–19.

Klastky, A. L., & Armstrong, M. A. (1991). Cardiovascular risk factors among Asian Americans living in Northern California. *American Journal of Public Health, 8*(11), 1423–1428.

Levy, R. (1993). Ethnic and racial differences in response to medicines: Preserving individualized therapy in managed pharmaceutical programmes. *Pharmaceutical Medicine, 7,* 139–165.

Lipson, J. G., Dibble, S. L., & Minarik, P. A. (1996). *Culture and nursing care: A pocket guide.* San Francisco: UCSF Nursing Press.

Liu, J. M., Ong, P. M., & Rosenstein, C. (1991). Dual chain migration: Post 1965 Filipino immigration to the United States. *International Migration Review, 25*(3), 487–513.

McBride, M. (1993). Health status of recently naturalized Filipino WWII Veterans. Paper presented at the annual conference of the American Society on Aging, Chicago, IL.

McBride, M., & Parreno, H. (1996). Filipino American families and caregiving. In G. Yeo & D. Gallagher-Thompson (Eds.), *Ethnicity and the dementias.* Washington, DC: Taylor & Francis.

McBride, M., Mariola, D., & Yeo, G. (1995). *Aging and health: Asian Pacific Islander American elders.* Stanford, CA: Stanford Geriatric Education Center.

Melendy, H. B. (1981). *Asians in America: Filipinos, Koreans and East Indians.* New York: Hippocrene Books.

National Statistics Information Center. (1995). *Philippine statistical yearbook.* (1995). Makati, Philippines: Author.

National Statistics Office, Philippines. (2002). *Philippine statistics.* Available at http://www.census.gov.ph.

Nora, R., & McBride, M. (1996). Health needs of Filipino Americans. *Asian Pacific Islander American Journal of Health, 3*(2), 13–23.

Northern California Cancer Center. (1991). Cervical cancer incidence among women in the San Francisco and Monterey Bay Area. *Bay Area Cancer Registry Report, 3*(3).

Oliver, J. E., Gey, F., Stiles, J., & Brady, H. (1995). *Pacific rim states demographic data book.* Oakland, CA: University of California, Office of the President.

One World. (2001). *Religion—Philippines: Holy week of folk rituals, gory spectacle.* Retrieved November 6, 2001, from http://www.oneworld.org.

Orbeta, S. S. (1998). The Filipino food pyramid. *Nutrition Today, 33*(5), 210–216.

Pacquiao, D. F. (1993). Cultural influences in old age: An ethnographic comparison of Anglo and Filipino elders. Doctoral dissertation, Graduate School of Education, Rutgers University, New Brunswick, NJ. Ann Arbor, MI: UMI.

Pacquiao, D. F. (1995). Multicultural issues in nursing education and practice. *Issues in Health Care, 16*(2)1, 4–5, 11.

Pacquiao, D. F. (1996a). Infusing philosophical thought into transcultural nursing. In V. M. Fitzsimons & M. L. Kelley (Eds.), *The culture of learning: Access, retention, understanding and mobility of minority students in nursing* (pp. 23–32). New York: National League for Nursing Press.

Pacquiao, D. F. (1996b). Educating faculty in the concept of educational biculturalism: A comparative study of sociocultural influences in nursing students' experience in school. In V. M. Fitzsimons & M. L. Kelley (Eds.), *The culture of learning: Access, retention, understanding and mobility of minority students in nursing* (pp. 129–162). New York: National League for Nursing Press.

Pacquiao, D. F. (2000). Editorial. Impression management: An alternative to assertiveness in intercultural communication. *Journal of Transcultural Nursing, 11*(1), 5–6.

Pacquiao, D. F. (2001). Cultural incongruities of advance directives. *Bioethics Forum, 17*(1), 27–31.

Pacquiao, D. F. (2002). Editorial. Foreign nurses recruitment and workforce diversity. *Journal of Transcultural Nursing, 13*(2), 89.

Pacquiao, D. F. (in press). Cultural competence in ethical decision-making. In M. M. Andrews & J. S. Boyle (Eds.), *Transcultural concepts in nursing care* (4th ed.). Philadelphia: Lippincott.

Philippine Department of Tourism. (2001). *General profile of the Philippines*. Retrieved November 2, 2001, from http://www.tourism.gov.ph.

The Philippine Diaspora in the United States. (2001). http://www.boondocksnet.com/centennial/sctexts/esj_94a.html.

Pilipino Mini-Health Forums Committee. (1993). *Executive report: Pilipino health assessment report to the San Francisco health commission.* San Francisco: Author.

Rumbaut, R. G. (1995). The new Californians: Comparative research findings on the educational progress of immigrant children. In R. G. Rumbaut & W. A. Cornelius (Eds.), *California's immigrant children* (pp. 17–70). La Jolla, CA: Center for Mexican Studies, University of CA, San Diego.

Russell, S. (2001). *Christianity in the Philippines.* Retrieved November 6, 2001, from http://www.seasite.niu.edu.

Salazar, L. P., Schuldermann, S. M., Schuldermann, E. H., & Hunyh, C. (2000). The Filipino adolescents' parental socialization for academic achievement in the United States. *Journal of Adolescent Research, 15*(5), 564–587.

Spangler, Z. (1985). Coping with cancer: Comparison of Philippine and American cancer patients. Unpublished qualitative interviews.

Spangler, Z. (1992). Transcultural nursing care values and caregiving practices of Philippine-American nurses. *Journal of Transcultural Nursing, 4*(2), 28–37.

Statistics Canada. (1997). *Nation series package no. 4: Ethnic origins.* Ottawa, Canada: Ministry of Industry.

Stern, P. N. (1985). A comparison of culturally approved behaviors and beliefs between Pilipina immigrant women, U.S.-born dominant culture women, and Western female nurses of the San Francisco Bay Area: Religiosity of health care. *Issues in Health Care, 6*(1), 123–133.

Superio, E. (1993). Beliefs held by Pilipinos regarding filial responsibility. Unpublished master's thesis, California State University, San Jose, CA.

Tanikalang Ginto. (2002). Available at http://www.filipinolinks.com/sexuality/gay_lesbian_bi_transgendered.

Tompar-Tiu, A., & Sustento-Seneriches, J. (1994), *Depression and other mental health issues: The Filipino American experience.* San Francisco: Jossey-Bass.

Travel Information: The Philippines (2002). Available at http://www.worldbex.com/travel_info.htm.

U.S. Bureau of Census. (2001). *2000 Census: Ethnic origin of population.* Washington, DC: U.S. Government Printing Office.

Valencia-Go, G. (1989). Integrative aging in widowed immigrant Filipinos. Unpublished dissertation, Adelphi University, Garden City, NY.

Weiner, B. P., & Marvit, R. C. (1977). Schizophrenia in Hawaii: Analysis of cohort mortality risk in a multi-ethnic population. *British Journal of Psychiatry, 131*, 497–503.

Wolf, D. L. (1997). Family secrets: Transnational struggles among children of Filipino immigrants. *Sociological Perspectives, 40*(3), 457–483.

World Factbook. (2001). *The world factbook—Philippines.* Retrieved November 10, 2001, from http://www.cia.gov/cia/publications/factbook.

Chapter 10

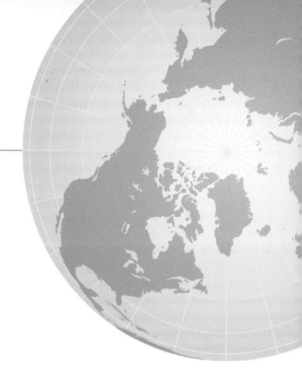

People of French Canadian Heritage

GINETTE COUTU-WAKULCZYK, DENISE MOREAU,
and ANN C. BECKINGHAM

Overview, Inhabited Localities, and Topography

OVERVIEW

Canada, with over 3,800,000 square miles and a population of 31,080,900 million, is larger than the entire United States, but has only one-ninth the population (Statistics Canada, 2001). The land mass covers six time zones and has fertile agricultural land, vast tundra, dense forests, and mountain ranges. The country is rich in minerals, coal, oil, and gas. Only 20 percent of the land is habitable.

Canada, a member of the Commonwealth of Nations, is a federation of 10 provinces, the Northwest and Yukon Territories, and, since April 1999, the Nunavut. The Constitution Act of 1981 transferred the Parliament from Britain to Canada. Even though the queen of England is also the queen of Canada, the Canadian constitution is entirely in the hands of the Canadians. People in each province elect their own premier and provincial legislative government. A lieutenant governor is symbolically appointed by the federal government in every province. The 10 provinces in descending order of population are Ontario, Quebec, British Columbia, Alberta, Manitoba, Saskatchewan, Nova Scotia, New Brunswick, Newfoundland, and Prince Edward Island. The Northwest Territories have been divided to form the Nunavut and Yukon Territories. Canada's largest cities are Toronto (4,881,400 people), Montreal (3,511.8 million), Vancouver (2,078.800 million), and the capital, Ottawa (1,106,900 people). The Francophone (French-speaking) population is over 6.6 million (Statistics Canada, 2001).

Before the latter half of the 18th century, most French people emigrating to Canada were Catholics, whereas French Protestants tended to come directly to the United States. After the French Revolution, an increased number of Catholics sought shelter in the United States. The bulk of those coming via Canada settled in the New England states and dispersed throughout the United States from there. Peaks of emigration occurred between the latter part of the 19th century and just prior to the Great Depression. Most of this latter migration was directly related to economic opportunities, and was part of an apparently contagious groundswell of immigration to the United States from Europe via Canada. As of 2000, it is estimated that more than 2.2 million people of French Canadian descent reside in the United States.

Because French Canadians vary according to the primary and secondary characteristics of culture (see Chapter 1), assessments must be carefully completed to avoid generalizations based on language and physical or racial traits. Additionally, the Multiculturalism Canada Act of 1988 provides guidelines for implementing policies regarding multicultural diversity.

HERITAGE AND RESIDENCE

Before the 1960s, people with French as their mother tongue were identified as French Canadians, referring to France as their country of origin. The ancestors of most French Canadians were the French "colons" who established themselves in the St. Lawrence Valley during the 17th and 18th centuries. They brought with them their native language and culture, their customs, songs, stories, and games, which have been enriched over the centuries by contact with indigenous peoples and other immigrant cultures to the region: the Basques, the Scots, and the Irish. The **Métis**, descendants of Native Americans and Europeans, are mainly, though not entirely, French-speaking. Some regard the Métis as a historically and culturally distinct people in their own right. Another major portion of Canada's French-speaking population are the **Acadians**. They are the descendants of the early French colonists, mainly people from west central France, who settled in the Maritime region of modern-day Nova Scotia and New Brunswick.

Today, the French-speaking population of Canada is far from homogeneous. In many homes English and French may be used equally. Canadians whose first language is French are called **Francophones**, a designation that broadly encompasses the multiethnic and cultural mosaic of the Canadian population. More recently, Francophones from former colonies under French rule such as Haiti, Lebanon, and Vietnam, have added to the French population of Canada. Also, during the last 20 years, many families in Quebec have adopted young children from Latin America and the Middle East. This practice has contributed to the development of an ethnic mosaic within the younger adult population. Although most French-speaking Canadians live in the province of Quebec, the French language is used daily for communication within families and communities from coast to coast, and as far north as the Yukon.

New France (Nouvelle France) was the name given to Canada when it was first settled in the 17th century, a period in which Portugal, Spain, Holland, France, and England all vied for territory. Although religious influences played a part in colonial policies, it was the mercantile system that stimulated exploration of the North American wilderness and the development of trading companies. One of the first permanent colonies in Canada was Quebec City. Soon after settling there in 1608, French explorers and traders moved up the St. Lawrence River, established a settlement at Ville-Marie (Montreal) in 1642, explored the Great Lakes (from which the St. Lawrence flows), opened fur-trading centers, and converted the natives to Christianity. In 1718, the French settled at the opposite end of the continent, in New Orleans. In 1750, approximately 80,000 French colonials lived within the vast area between the mouths of the St. Lawrence and Mississippi rivers. The French influence is still visible in large parts of Canada, and in cities such as St. Louis and New Orleans in the United States.

Around 1603, other groups of settlers established themselves in **Acadia**, north of what Giovanni da Verrazano, in 1534, referred to as Arcadia (note the *r*). This region is known today as Delaware, Maryland, and Virginia (Daigle, 1995). After a devastating experience during the winter of 1604–1605, the settlers moved to the Bay of Fundy and founded Port-Royal, which was to become the first coastal settlement and capital of Acadia (Cormier, 1994). By the middle of the 1700s, Acadians were caught in the crossfire of the imperial rivalries of England, France, and inhabitants of the American colonies, finally being absorbed into the British Empire.

With the Treaty of Utrecht in 1713, England secured Newfoundland, Acadia (renamed Nova Scotia), and the extensive region drained by the rivers flowing into the Hudson Bay. With the Treaty of Paris in 1763, France relinquished all its North American possessions east of the Mississippi River to England. Spain ceded Florida to England in exchange for the French territories west of the Mississippi River. Thus, as a geographic area, New France became only a memory. Yet, the French culture, language, and religious institutions remain as an everlasting tribute to the past. The heritage and early French architecture is well preserved through concentrated efforts and pride in restoration. Publication of information about monuments, houses, churches, and ramparts around Quebec City keep the public informed about the area's rich French heritage.

As a result of unresolved controversy over several highly contentious oaths of allegiance to the English between 1755 and 1762, a massive deportation occurred. Referred to as *le grand dérangement*, French-speaking Catholic Acadians were removed from their homes in Nova Scotia and New Brunswick. Some fled to Quebec, others took refuge in the woods, and many died. Still others dispersed to the south: Massachusetts, New York, Pennsylvania, Maryland, Virginia, the Carolinas, Georgia, and Louisiana. In 1774, some exiled Acadians returned to the Maritimes and attempted to recreate their lives. Unable to secure their former lands because of British occupation, they directed their energies to settling new areas, and gradually explored new activities such as fishing and forestry (Daigle, 1995). Today, 90 percent of the Acadians reside in northern and eastern New Brunswick, southern Nova Scotia, the Acadian region of Cape Breton, and the Evangeline region of Prince Edward Island (Beaudin & Leclerc, 1995).

Throughout Canada, important regional differences exist among the French-speaking population. Outside Quebec, the French-speaking population within each province or territory has its own association, which is organized nationally under the Fédération des Communautés Francophones et Acadiennes du Canada (FCFA).

An important consideration when health-care providers assess a family's cultural background is the number of mixed marriages leading to the adoption of English as the language spoken in the home and by the majority. French-speaking Canada has become an increasingly diverse society composed of various ethno-cultural groups. In the 1991 census, 31 percent of the population reported ethnic origins other than British or French (Ministry of Industry, Science and Technology, 1993).

REASONS FOR MIGRATION AND ASSOCIATED ECONOMIC FACTORS

Economic reasons, including the desire to cultivate the land and exploit fisheries, were the most frequent motivations for early French Canadian settlers in the 17th century. Most of these settlers originated from the French regions of Normandy, Perche, Poitou, and some from Aunis, Brittany, Ile de France, and Saintonge. During the 17th century in France, many nobles lost their fortune because of France's feudal system; thus, colonization of New France offered possibilities for regaining their prestige and land for their vassals. The richness and the quality of pelts available in the New World promoted fur trading with the Native Americans, and attracted merchants and their employees. In addition, missionaries and religious orders were among the earlier settlers. Today, French-speaking Canadians are represented in all trades and professions.

EDUCATIONAL STATUS AND OCCUPATIONS

Although the overall official literacy rate in Canada approaches 99 percent, the functional literacy rate is lower, and the educational levels of French Canadians represent a broad spectrum, depending on age group and geographic location. Fifty percent of Francophone students do not complete high school, and illiteracy reaches as high as 50 percent in some regions, especially among the elderly (Office of Francophone Affairs of Ontario, 1994). The postsecondary education rate for Francophones is approximately half the provincial rate for Ontarians. More recently, educational opportunities at all levels have become available in the French language in Ontario. Although a student dropout rate of 50 percent could reflect a phenomenon of the era rather than a provincial problem, the rate reaches 40 percent in some areas of Quebec. Nevertheless, the lack of professionals prepared for the delivery of services in French, as prescribed by the 1989 Ontario government, jeopardizes the development of a full network of services in some regions.

At the beginning of colonization, major occupations such as agriculture, fur trading, and fisheries were important for survival. In the latter part of the 19th century, French-speaking Canadians joined the developing industrial labor force. Factories, mining, forestry, and fisheries took advantage of the numerous hands available among the fertile Canadian families of French ancestry. Despite language barriers, this was a time when the borders of Quebec did not stop young families from moving across Canada for work. Throughout Canada, even in the Yukon, the origins of early French-speaking Canadian settlements can be traced to these years. Today, French-speaking Canadians are represented in all trades and professions. However, the elderly population may have a different life history, depending on their region of origin: Gaspésie, Abitibi, Beauce, Acadia, or the cities of Montreal and Quebec.

Communication

DOMINANT LANGUAGE AND DIALECTS

Canada has two official languages, French and English. Regional differences exist in accent, vocabulary, and degree of anglicization. However, French Canadians do not have difficulty understanding one another because the original French spoken in Canada includes some old 17th-century French words and expressions that are no longer used in France. Oral communication, in particular, has undergone assimilation. Indian words have been added and English words are incorporated into a syntax and grammar that is essentially French, resulting in a dialect, **joual**, which is spoken primarily by lower socioeconomic and undereducated groups. Age and location in Canada frequently determine language use and ability.

A population trend analysis in 1983 showed that despite the improved legal status of Francophones in Ontario, sociological conditions, particularly urbanization and economic pressures, are contributing to a decline in French-speaking Ontarians. This decrease is more noticeable in southern Ontario, with a lesser decline in the north and eastern counties bordering Quebec. As a result of urbanization, the distribution of Francophones in Ontario has become fragmented, although regional cohesion of French-speaking Ontario has remained strongly supported by active networks at the local and provincial levels.

Since 1969, the Official Languages Act of New Brunswick guaranteed the availability of government services and education in French and English at all educational levels. Although the act has increased the political and social utility of French, it has not reversed Acadians' use of English or the decline in the proportion of Francophones in the province. In an effort to prevent linguistic assimilation, a new policy for language teaching is used in the French schools of heavily anglicized regions. English as a second language is only taught beginning in grade 5. In all provinces except New Brunswick, where the French are the minority, a disproportionate number of young French Canadians are assimilated into the majority English-speaking society. In contrast, on Prince Edward Island the struggle to obtain education in French remains an ongoing issue.

A recent report prepared by the Official Language Community Development Bureau on behalf of the Consultative Committee for French-Speaking Minority Communities (CCFSMC) states that services in the user's language have benefits that extend far beyond simple respect for the user's culture (Public Works and Government Services Canada, 2001). They are indispensable for improving the health status of individuals, and for community empowerment in matters of health. Studies have shown that the health status of minority Francophones is generally poorer than that of their fellow citizens in any given province. In fact, between 50 and 55 percent of French-speaking minority communities often have little or no access to health services in their mother tongue. Of foremost importance, one of the recommendations is to increase the number of French-speaking health professionals who practice in minority communities and to support the establishment of a pan-Canadian Francophone consortium for the training of French-speaking health professionals.

From a health perspective, cultural heritage remains present long after words of the French language have been forgotten. Maintaining the use of French depends mostly on the strength of the local French community. As for other culturally diverse clients, health-care providers must respect the client's preference in choice of language by seeking interpreters when possible; gearing health teaching to the educational level of the client; and supplementing written directions with verbal instructions, demonstrations, and pictures.

CULTURAL COMMUNICATIONS PATTERNS

Conversation is very important to the French people. Among French Canadians, a conversation may be conducted with high voice crescendos, which do not necessarily mean anger or violence. Volume can increase with the importance and the emotional charge invested in the content of the message. Nonverbal communication patterns for French Canadians resemble those of their Latin and Mediterranean ancestors, which encourage sharing thoughts and feelings. Acadians are more reserved, quieter, shy, even self-effacing, and are less likely to share their thoughts and feelings than people from Quebec, using hand gestures for emphasis when speaking is common. Facial expressions for men and women of all ages are a part of communication, often replacing words. Health-care providers working with French-speaking Canadians need be attentive to nonverbal and paraverbal communication. These observations provide much of the information on affect, emotion, and mutual understanding between health-care providers and clients.

Spatial distancing for French-speaking Canadians differs among family members, close friends, and the public. When in the intimacy zone, people may touch frequently and converse in close physical space; however, they tend to avoid physical contact in public. When greeting another person, men usually shake hands, which is recommended for health-care providers. Close female friends and family members may greet each other with an embrace. However, in public and more formal situations such as the health-care environment, this is not a recommended practice.

Before radio and television reached the Port au Port Peninsula of Newfoundland, there was a public tradition of storytelling. Narrators were invited to a home where several families had gathered and an entire evening of storytelling took place. These public performances were time-consuming, followed stylistic conventions and formulas, and made dramatic use of gesturing. Since the 1960s, private storytelling has substantially replaced the public tradition. Stories are told within the confines of a single family or small group, and usually last less than an hour, about the length of a television episode. Narrators no longer use stylistic devices, literary formulas, or dramatic gesturing.

TEMPORAL RELATIONSHIPS

For the French Canadian people, relationships take a long time to develop, but once in place, the relationship becomes very important and enduring. Langelier (1996) states that once one enters the inner sanctum of close friendship, commitment and responsibility ensue. French-speaking Canadians from Quebec have a past, present, and future orientation in their worldview. Balancing the three dimensions depends on traditionalism, generation, religiosity, and urbanization (Pronovost, 1989). More traditional people, and many from rural

backgrounds, attach primary importance to living in the present and accepting day-to-day occurrences in a context of fatalism. Many elderly, with a strong religious background, maintain a future worldview regarding life after death, and a past orientation celebrating death anniversaries of family members and other events. However, many of the younger generation reject past traditions and attempt to balance enjoying the present, working, and planning for their future.

FORMAT FOR NAMES

Traditionally, until the late 1970s, women and children took the father's surname. Today, under Quebec law, a woman keeps her maiden name throughout her lifetime, although in other parts of Canada this practice is decided between the spouses. This situation has created tension and self-identity difficulties for some elderly. As for children, a Québécois family of two spouses and two children may well include four different surname combinations: one child may have the father's surname or the mother's surname alone or a hyphenated or nonhyphenated surname composed of those of the father and mother. For a second child, the surnames are the same, but in reverse order. The decision for using surnames rests entirely with the parents and must appear on the birth certificate. Today very few parents adhere to the official use of multiple surnames for children. Women married for several years before the new law often added their maiden name hyphenated with that of their husbands.

Many French-speaking Canadians have dropped the custom of naming the oldest son after the father or the grandfather. Also declining is the custom of adding Joseph to male infants' and Mary to female infants' names. Until 10 to 15 years ago, the custom was to use only one name without initials, except on legal documents, which used all three or four names as they appeared on the birth certificate. Another recent change is using names other than those of saints. All of these factors should alert the health-care practitioner to the potential for confusion in the name format for client cultural identification.

Family Roles and Organization

HEAD OF HOUSEHOLD AND GENDER ROLES

The profound social changes encountered after the "Quiet Revolution" of the late 1960s and early 1970s brought important modifications in education and industrialization and increased the role of women in economic activity. Women not only became producers of domestic goods in the household, but they also became productive outside the home environment. Traditionally, in French-speaking Canadian families, the man was seen as the moral authority and responsible for material well-being, such as economic provider and purveyor of affection and security. The woman served as the family mediator and social director, as well as being responsible for household activities, child care, and health care

(Langelier, 1996). French Canadians have always attributed great value to family relationships and obligations.

Using the husband's income as an index for comparing the family communication and relative independence on marital adjustment among 180 French-speaking couples, Aube and Linden (1991) found that the degree of marital discord was similar across different socioeconomic levels. However, quality of communication accounted for 16 percent of the variance in marital satisfaction among men, and only 13 percent of the variance among women. From a socioanthropological perspective, a national survey with 5614 females and 10,965 males demonstrated income differences between genders. Inequality, attributable to career interruptions by women, was estimated along with the importance of factors such as education, occupation, socioeconomic status, and number of hours worked per year. The income difference by gender among native and linguistic minorities in Canada showed that the inequality between sexes was smaller among French-speaking Canadians than other groups (Goyder, 1981).

By the end of the Quiet Revolution, marriages changed fundamentally, moving toward equality of husbands and wives, but not necessarily of children and parents. Wu and Baer (1996) found that Francophones are less committed than Anglophones to traditional values concerning marriage and relationships. Those results are consistent with Fong and Guilia's (1990) study showing that French Canadians had more permissive attitudes than English Canadians with respect to marriage, sexual activity, and nonmarried parenthood. On the other hand, French Canadians are more traditional than English Canadians when it comes to rating the importance of having children. Additionally, Catholicism is positively related to attitudes toward childbearing and difference in these attitudes among French and English Canadians.

Recent studies provide clear evidence of a profound transformation in attitudes toward family-related behaviors and gender roles in much of the Western world over the past three decades: increased acceptance of divorce, nonmarital cohabitation, unmarried parenthood, permanent nonmarriage, and voluntary childlessness. Norms for gender roles are also changing, with shifts toward gender egalitarianism with respect to the appropriate roles of women and men in the family and workplace.

PRESCRIPTIVE, RESTRICTIVE, AND TABOO BEHAVIORS FOR CHILDREN AND ADOLESCENTS

The greatest source of pride for French Canadian families is to see their children well established with a good education. On this issue, most of the present political elite, educated at religious colleges, shared the values and beliefs of their religious professors, not the prescribed behavior for their offspring.

FAMILY GOALS AND PRIORITIES

Traditional French Canadian intergenerational relationships are rapidly disappearing (Fig. 10-1). Urbani-

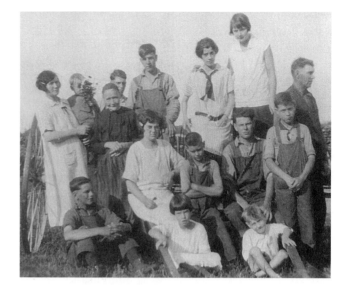

FIGURE 10–1   Traditional family returning from the fields.

zation, particularly without adequate social security measures, results in social dislocation of the young and old. Strategies for maintaining cohesion among the generations are required to avoid intergenerational conflict related to competition for scarce resources when survival challenges are real.

In Canada, many of the social policies are under provincial jurisdiction. Today, French Canadian families follow the same pattern of declining birth rates as other Canadians. Quebec has done the most in formulating a family policy and stimulating a widespread popular debate on the issue. Family policy, when geared toward protecting and fostering a particular type of family, contributes to the detriment of other types of families and becomes a prescribed structure for acceptance. For example, because children who were born out-of-wedlock were being penalized on the basis of their parents' relationship, the legal category of illegitimacy has been abolished in most Canadian provinces. The French Canadian family is more nuclear and autonomous than its counterpart in France. Historically, French Canadian women appear to have higher status and authority than their French counterparts (Hillstrom, 1995).

French-speaking Canadian family membership is known for its closeness, and some families are a "closed" family system. Urbanization and smaller families, along with the Quiet Revolution in Quebec, have encouraged people to open their borders and expand their circle to include others by broadening their family perspective. Nevertheless, within the microcosm of the French Canadian population, the physical and social quality of the microenvironment is more essential to health and survival than wealth and a physical connection (Evans & Stoddart, 1994). House, Landis, and Umberson (1988) reported widespread and strong correlations between mortality and social support networks—friends and family keep French Canadians alive! The sheer number of contacts one has is protective, regardless of the nature of the interaction (Evans, 1994).

Lambert and colleagues (1986), using the 1984 national election study of 3377 Quebec inhabitants, explored cognitive differences from a class perspective. English-speaking and French-speaking residents of Quebec were surveyed regarding their perceptions of social class, the importance of using characteristics to describe people from diverse social classes, and differentiation of the most important characteristics of social class. Approximately 45 percent stated that the idea of social class had no meaning to them, or that they were unsure of its meaning, with English-speaking Canadians being more likely to give this response. Generally, people who said they understood the concept believed that social classes differed materially, whereas those who did not understand the concept preferred to evaluate people on individual characteristics. French-speaking respondents defined social class in the materialistic sense of income and wealth, whereas English-speaking Canadians emphasized individuals in terms of character and ambition, and used ascriptive criteria such as country of origin, birth, or ancestry.

ALTERNATIVE LIFESTYLES

Traditionally, the Catholic Church dictated the parameters of sexual behavior, with high priority placed on marriage and the begetting and raising of children. In the years before 1960 abstinence from premarital sex was encouraged, and a sexual double standard existed, while the 1970s and 1980s witnessed a liberalization of sexual norms and the establishment of more egalitarian relationships between young men and women. At present, there is a growing trend for couples to live together without marrying. Many young couples answer that they cannot financially afford to get married. Yet, many of these same couples insist on having their children baptized and raise them according to Catholic Church principles.

Hobart (1992) studied sexual behaviors and attitudes toward sex, sexually transmitted diseases, and HIV/AIDS among 1775 Anglophone and 493 Francophone Canadian postsecondary students, surveying their expectations about condom use with different sexual partners. Results imply that women's patterns of sexual behaviors were more predictive than men's, but the relationships among variables were neither consistent nor strong. The most powerful predictors of safe-sex practices were the size of the home community and romantic love beliefs among Francophone women. A shift toward greater sexual permissiveness and recognition of female sexuality is apparent. There has been an increase in the percentage of sexually active adolescents, from less than 50 percent in the early 1980s to 76 percent in the mid-1990s, with an average age at the time of the first sexual relations of approximately 16 years in the mid-1990s (Samson, Otis, & Levy 1996).

An Internet search on gays and lesbians in Canada resulted in numerous Websites devoted to alternative life styles. Some Websites were hosted by universities, while others were hosted by gay and lesbian organizations (see, for example, *http://www.er.uqam.ca, http://www.clga.ca,* and *http://www.teleport.com*). In 1996, the Canadian government extended health, relocation, and other job benefits to same-sex partners of federal employees. During the same year, the Ontario Court of Appeals ruled that same-sex couples must be treated as common-law couples under the Family Leave Act. In 1999, a poll conducted by the Canadian federal government revealed that 53 percent of the Canadian public, across provincial and demographic lines, supported gay people's freedom to marry (International Recognition of Same-Sex Relationships, 2002).

Workforce Issues

CULTURE IN THE WORKPLACE

Among Canadians, workforce issues often correspond to educational background. In this respect, one must not forget the effects of the Durham Report and Law Number 17, which eliminated public schools' rights to teach in the French language, with the consequence of a high level of illiteracy among French Canadians. This situation was finally reversed with full rights to education in the French language in 1982, based on the Canadian Charter of Rights, article 23 (Denault & Cardinal, 1999). Hence, the overall educational level of French-speaking Canadians is lower than that of their English-speaking counterparts. In addition, the proportion of part-time and casual workers among French-speaking Canadians is higher, especially in Quebec hospitals. Labor unions support part-time and casual work as being shared work. However, many male workers are beginning to resent this approach, calling it "shared poverty." The strong laws to protect the French language in Quebec may have created another problem for its population. While promoting a pseudo sense of security by maintaining the dominance of the French language, a large portion of Quebec's French-speaking population lack sufficient knowledge of the English language to access the workforce outside their province and have difficulty in higher-education programs where readings are mostly in English.

Hofstede (as cited in Punnett, 1991) examined the preferred leadership styles within 113 Anglophone and 77 Francophone managers in Ottawa from the perspective of language and cultural values. The two groups were similar on their preferred style of leadership, but differed significantly in terms of individualism. Differences between this group and an earlier Canadian sample suggest that organizational influences may have more impact on expressed cultural values than language differences. To a large extent, outside the province of Quebec, French-speaking Canadians' patterns of acculturation are intermeshed with educational and work opportunities. From an educational perspective, in the 1970s a vast movement for French-immersion classes across Canada started changing the views of the younger generation. Also, the long battle for the administrative French school board system has reduced the acculturation process in many areas of Canada without stopping it. The availability of French-language higher education outside Quebec completes the realm of factors necessary to reverse acculturation and assure health services for French-speaking Canadians wherever they live.

In 1987, Ontario adopted legislation requiring equity in public services and recognized the necessity to look closely into the principles of equality and equivalence. The designation of a certain number of positions identified as Francophone, may have opened the door to a new phenomenon, that of ghettos (Denault & Cardinal, 1999). Most of these Francophone positions were created within the areas of essential population services and in the senior positions in the public services. Another aspect of the Francophone positions turns out be more task elasticity and work overload in the sense that the regular job must be completed in addition to the translation of whatever material is to be produced for the service to be delivered.

ISSUES RELATED TO AUTONOMY

Bilingualism, multiculturalism, and a focus on open-mindedness are the dominant themes in the Canadian workplace. With the exception of the Quebec province's position regarding French as the official language, very few places of employment want to identify an official language. However, geographic and regional aggregates shape the language of services offered.

Nurses' roles and activities remain consistent across Canada; however, changes in the mode of care and the language used in delivering services are apparent. Opportunities for Francophone nurses to function successfully outside Quebec are limited if they have not mastered the English language. Frustration occurs among Francophone nurses when the time and effort put into mastering and delivering services in both official languages are not recognized. In addition, the number of Francophone nurses academically prepared to serve in decision-making positions is limited outside the province of Quebec. This hinders the type and mode of services offered when decisions become public health policies.

Biocultural Ecology

SKIN COLOR AND OTHER BIOLOGICAL VARIATIONS

Canadians of French descent are white; however, Francophones, as a linguistic group, represent a mosaic of ethnocultural characteristics, including racial differences. Thus, individuals must be assessed individually according to their racial heritage.

DISEASES AND HEALTH CONDITIONS

Given the limited population density, multiculturalism, and regionalism factors affecting Canadian society, specific risk factors for Canadians of French ancestry are the same as those of other minority groups, except for those in Quebec. The primary causes of death among the Quebec population are cardiac diseases, lung cancer in men, breast cancer in women (Office of Francophone Affairs, 1988), premature birth rates (Coté, 1992), and trauma for those under age 30. In this assessment,

however, Quebec is not different from Ontario and the rest of Canada. Recently, a study conducted by Emard and colleagues (2001) reported a higher level of prostate cancer among the Francophone population of Quebec. Genetic susceptibility to breast cancer in French Canadians has been reported by Krajinovic and colleagues (2001), who associate the increase to the role of carcinogen-metabolizing enzymes and gene-environment interactions. In addition, Godar (1998) identified major influencing factors of risks for familial and sporadic ovarian cancer among French Canadians; these factors include a family history of breast or ovarian cancer, beginning use of oral contraceptives at a late age, and last childbirth at a late age.

In addition, suicide rates in Quebec are greater than in the United States, Japan, and Sweden (Office of Francophone Affairs, 1988). In 1978, approximately four times more Canadian men than women committed suicide (Health Canada, 1994). The suicide rate for men increased fivefold between 1950 and 1990, moving suicide from the ninth to the first place in Canada for all causes of death. A study in Quebec by Cormier and Klerman (1985) showed a correlation between unemployment and suicide rates among men between the years 1950 and 1981, and among women between the years 1966 and 1981. Platt (1984) concluded that there is a potential link between unemployment and suicide. However, in practice, this situation is not observed in other regions where prevalence of unemployment is chronically high. The high rate of suicide and suicidal ideation, particularly among adolescent and young adult males, is one aspect of mental health that health-care practitioners have yet to address adequately.

Today's French Canadian population suffers from the same endemic conditions and sensitivities to environmental diseases as the Canadian population as a whole. The harsh topography and low winter temperatures are responsible for 19 percent of the population's osteoarthritic disorders; and 13 percent of the allergies are related to urban air pollution, smog, and poor air circulation in public buildings (Pampalon et al., 1990). Distinctive features of idiopathic inflammatory myopathies in French Canadians were also reported by Uthman, Vazquez-Abad, and Sénécal (1996). Pausova and colleagues (2000) found an association in pedigrees of French Canadian origin. The TNF-α gene locus contributes to obesity and obesity-hypertension, and gender modifies the effect of the regional distribution of body fat.

A number of hereditary and genetic diseases more common among Québécois can be traced to early colonists. Familial chylomicronemia resulting from the lipoprotein lipase (LPL) deficiency, hyperlipoproteinemia type I, is an autosomal recessive disorder with a prevalence of 1 in 1 million individuals (Brunzell, 1989). Through genealogical research, this hereditary disorder has been traced to migrants from the Perche region of France (DeBraekeleer & Dao, 1994a, 1994b). The distribution of LPL deficiency among French Canadians of Quebec is the highest frequency worldwide (Ma et al., 1991). Within the French Canadian population of Quebec, its prevalence is especially high in the eastern part of the province (Gagné et al., 1989). Two separate mutations in the LPL gene introduced by French immigrants in the 17th century have been identified. Although the birthplaces of the obligate carriers were scattered throughout the province, three geographic clusters were identified: the Trois-Rivières-Mauricie region, the Saguenay-Lac-St.-Jean-Charlevoix region, and Beauce region (Dionne et al., 1993). The carrier rate of LPL deficiency is estimated to be 1 in 139 individuals in the province as a whole, but 1 in 85 individuals in eastern Quebec, with a peak of 1 in 47 individuals in Saguenay-Lac-St.-Jean (Dionne et al., 1993). With the discovery of a mutation in the human LPL gene, scientists have identified the most common cause of familial chylomicronemia in the French Canadian population (Ma et al., 1991). Furthermore, a single mutation of the fumarylacetoacetate hydrolase gene can lead to hereditary tyrosinemia type I (Grompe et al., 1994).

Familial hypercholesterolemia, leading to coronary thrombosis, supports the French origin of the French Canadian deletion. One century after settlement in North America, the founders originating from Perche had a large number of descendants. Among the 50 or more fertile couples, 14 came from Perche (Charbonneau et al., 1987). However, it is suggested that the high frequency of this mutation among French Canadian clients with hypercholesterolemia is due to a founder effect rather than to a high frequency within the population (Fumeron et al., 1992). Familial hypercholesterolemia (FH) is one of the most common autosomal codominant diseases. The frequency of FH among French Canadians in northern Quebec is higher than in most other populations (1 in 154 versus 1 in 500) due to high prevalence of few recurrent mutations in the LDL receptor gene (Levy et al., 1997).

A provincewide, long-term longitudinal study on all newborns identified a rare genetic disease among French Canadians. Profiles of phenylketonuria (PKU) in Quebec populations show evidence of stratification and novel mutations (Rozen et al., 1994). To date, five mutations account for almost 90 percent of PKU diagnoses among French Canadians from eastern Quebec (National PKU Index, 1992). Time and space clusters of the PKU mutation can be traced to France (Lyonnet et al., 1992). Studies by Vohl et al. (2000) and St-Pierre et al. (2001) on genetic mutation in the population of French Canadian origin are currently being conducted.

In addition, an increased incidence of cystic fibrosis occurs among French-speaking Canadians (Rozen et al., 1992). Muscular dystrophy, with a worldwide frequency of 1 in 25,000 individuals, occurs in 1 in 154 French Canadians of the Saguenay region (DeBraekeleer, 1991). Health-care providers working with this specialized population of Quebecers must screen for these genetic diseases and provide genetic counseling for clients expressing an interest.

VARIATIONS IN DRUG METABOLISM

Research supporting differences in drug metabolism related to race and ethnicity is beginning to identify genetic mutations among descendants of French Canadian settlers from specific areas of France. Although these findings may produce data related to drug metabolism, thus far, little has been published.

High-Risk Behaviors

Risk factors affecting French-speaking Canadians tend to be related to type of work, geographic region, communication, education, and age groups. In view of these risk factors, special attention must be given to Francophone elders living outside Quebec. Abuse of alcohol, tobacco, and psychotropic drugs are major health problems among Francophone Quebecers. Although the number of people who use tobacco is decreasing, 35 percent of men and 31 percent of women continue to smoke (Office of Francophone Affairs, 1988). The highest worldwide incidence of adult females who smoke is found in Quebec (Wharry, 1997). Smoking rates run a constant 5 to 10 percent higher for French Canadians than for English Canadians.

The French people have a long-standing appreciation of alcohol, with wine being their beverage of choice. Both French and French Canadians continue to view drinking favorably (Abbott, 2001). Two types of alcoholics have been identified. Delta alcohol users are associated with sociocultural and economic factors, whereas gamma alcohol users are frequently intoxicated and use alcohol to escape underlying psychological problems. Canadian drinkers tend to fall in between these two categories. French Canadians are more delta alcohol consumers, which is more socially acceptable in this culture, whereas English Canadians are more gamma alcohol users (Abbott, 2001). Disapproval of women drinking heavily is evident, and depression is higher among female alcoholics than among male alcoholics (Abbott, 2001). Francophone youth start drinking at younger ages than do Anglophones (DeWit & Beneteau, 1998).

Alcohol dependency is highest among the 20- to 24-year-old age group (Coté, 1992). Lapp's (1984) study on 132 female and 84 male college students in Montreal found that the use of psychotropic drugs is primarily among females. However, drug use is not associated with personality factors or depression when measured by Rotter's Internal-External Locus of Control Scale Depression Inventory. Tobacco and alcohol use is highest among French-speaking males, and is associated with masculine sex roles, higher self-esteem, and an external locus of control. Nonmedical drug use, primarily marijuana and hashish, most frequently involved men and was related to an internal locus of control.

HEALTH-CARE PRACTICES

Beliefs about methods for improving one's health are seen as influential factors in health-seeking behaviors. Edwards and Rootman's (1993) analysis of data from Canada's health promotion survey in 1990, on Canadians aged 15 and older, identified the following practices for improving health: smoking cessation (81 percent), increased relaxation (69 percent), increased exercise (65 percent), income security (45 percent), quantity of time spent with family (45 percent), weight loss (42 percent), better dental care (27 percent), job changes (22 percent), reduced drinking (16 percent), moving (14 percent), and reduced drug use (9 percent). According to Wharry (1997), Québécois probably give tobacco its strongest bulwark in the country; in health communication, one has to tailor the message. A communication method that works among the English does not mean it will automatically work among the French. Yet very little has been developed specifically for the French community.

Feather and Green's (1993) study on health behaviors found that good health practices were more prevalent among Canadian men under the age of 25 years and over the age of 65 than among men in their middle adult years. In contrast to men, the prevalence of good health practices among Canadian women increases until the age of 65 and then decreases. In addition, these practices were positively correlated with levels of education in both sexes, adequate income for women, and managerial or professional occupations for men.

Responses of French-speaking Canadians throughout Canada correlated more with the province in which they lived than with the selected cultural group. This correlation could be due to the method of data collection, which is less accurate with a small response rate. The higher proportion of respondents from Quebec and New Brunswick may have skewed the statistical outcome. Overall, age was a factor associated with beliefs about one's ability to achieve an improved health status. Results imply that elderly people focus more on personal well being than on health practices.

Nutrition

MEANING OF FOOD

The strong influence of nutritional status on health prompted the inclusion of questions on nutritional behaviors and diet changes in the 1990 health promotion survey to identify data among high-risk groups. In this survey, body mass index was used to calculate the ratio of weight relative to height and determine the potential for health risk. Age, gender, and education, rather than culture, were identified as positive influences on the practice of reading labels for nutritional value of food. Regardless of the reason, this practice demonstrates the importance individuals attribute to food in relation to health.

COMMON FOODS AND FOOD RITUALS

Common vegetables enjoyed by French Canadians include potatoes, turnips, carrots, asparagus, cabbage, lettuce, and tomatoes. Apart from citrus fruits, all other edible fruits and berries grown in gardens or the wild are prepared and preserved by French Canadians for the winter. Meat choices are mainly beef, pork, and poultry. Until the late 1960s, fish was often perceived as a Friday food. However, for the younger generation, this belief is no longer practiced. Increased immigration and fast-food availability have influenced food choices and customs to the point of transforming French Canadians' customs and food practices.

In Acadia, due to the proximity of the coastal areas, fresh fish and seafood are part of the diet. Common foods include *fricot* (stew made with a special spice called summer savory). Traditional foods such as *poutine réfrapées* (balls of dough made from grated potatoes) and *réfrapure* (grated potato) are not part of the regular diet, but are still enjoyed during special events. The equivalent to the French Canadian pea soup is named **fayots** soup in Acadia.

DIETARY PRACTICES FOR HEALTH PROMOTION

Most men and women report reading nutritional labels on food packages. This behavior is a good predictor of diet changes during the preceding year. As a whole, more Quebecers than other Canadians report eating breakfast. Only 10 percent of the French-speaking Canadians report skipping breakfast, which is significantly lower than among respondents from the rest of Canada (Craig, 1993). A similar study conducted with children of grades 1 to 3 yielded similar results in the northern part of Ontario (McIntyre & Doyle, 1992).

NUTRITIONAL DEFICIENCIES AND FOOD LIMITATIONS

In an industrialized country like Canada, six times as many women as men are underweight, yet half as many women as men rated themselves as underweight (Craig, 1993). However, one-third of all Canadians are trying to lose weight. The 1990 health promotion study demonstrates that being overweight is inversely proportionate to education and income for both men and women. For men, there was no association between being underweight and education and income, whereas for women, with the exception of the very poor, there was a positive correlation between being underweight and increased income (Craig, 1993).

Pregnancy and Childbearing Practices

FERTILITY PRACTICES AND VIEWS TOWARD PREGNANCY

Until the middle of the 20th century, French Canadians maintained high fertility rates, which is uncommon for a population living in an industrialized country. This phenomenon, called the "revenge of the cradles," has never been explained. Classic interpretations based on the economy, religion, or education do not hold up to scientific examination. The historical co-occurrence of the power of the Church and high birth rates do not prove a causal link. Instead, the "overfertility" of French Canadians appears to be a response to socialization that is distinguished by the prevalence of extended family ties (Fournier, 1989). Yet, Ansen (2000) found that the more education increases, the lower the fertility rate within the Francophone group, whereas the contrary is observed within the English group, meaning that as education level increases, so does the fertility rate.

For many years, French Canadian fertility practices have been closely tied to the Catholic religion. Before the 1960s, the only acceptable birth control method was abstinence, resulting in a high fecundity rate. From 1851 until the 1960s, Quebec families had a mean of 6.84 children per family. The number of children per family started to decline from 3.1 in 1965 to 1.5 in 1990 (Henripin & Martin, 1991), with a current record of 1.2 (Statistics Canada, 2001).

Effective contraception and family planning methods such as the pill, intrauterine devices, and tubal ligation have become available to all women. The pill remains the primary reversible method for birth control (Health and Welfare Canada, 1989). On the basis of relative frequency, tubal ligation and vasectomy follow the pill as nonreversible methods of fertility control. Diaphragms, foams, and creams are not commonly used for birth control, partially because perceptions imply that women are not supposed to, or do not like to, touch their genitals. Men are still reluctant to use condoms because they associate their use with prostitution. The beliefs that condoms reduce the level of sexual feeling during intercourse, or that contraception is not a man's responsibility, are inversely proportionate to the age of men. Many French-speaking Canadians believe that abortion is morally wrong, but it is legally available. The number of annual abortions by language or cultural subdivision is unavailable. However, figures published by province under the obstetric or gynecologic classification other than birth show that the frequency of abortion is greater than the frequency of rape and incest. Finally, new reproductive technologies are available but are used by a small number of French-speaking Canadians, more because of scarcity than cultural denial or restriction.

Although pregnancy is considered a normal life event, fear of labor and delivery prevails. This learned fear is transmitted to women from childhood and often reinforced by the health-care system. Midwives have officially been accepted by the government, but the use of midwives and maternity centers (*maisons des naissances*) are far from being the custom.

PRESCRIPTIVE, RESTRICTIVE, AND TABOO PRACTICES IN THE CHILDBEARING FAMILY

From a clinical perspective, prenatal medical visits are recommended once a month until the end of the seventh month, twice during the eighth month, and weekly during the last month. Since the mid-1970s, prenatal classes are well attended by both the mother and father-to-be. These classes are generally free of charge and focus on information regarding health and hygiene during pregnancy and on preparation and exercises for labor and delivery.

Alcohol and tobacco use are discouraged for the duration of pregnancy and the breast-feeding period. Intercourse restrictions are not commonly applied during pregnancy unless required for medical reasons. For the last 30 years, fathers have been encouraged to be present in the delivery room. They are invited to assume an active role by assisting the mother and the physician, receiving the baby, and cutting the cord. Most Canadian women of French descent still deliver in a dorsal position, even though lying on the back has been shown to be antiphysiological. However, with the advent of birthing rooms, more women are delivering their babies in half-sitting or side-lying positions.

More women are talking about the desire to deliver at home, but the number who actually use a midwife throughout labor and delivery at home is quite low. The use of analgesics, local anesthetics such as epidural for delivery, or both remain high. Very few French Canadians practice natural childbirth. During hospitalization, rooming-in of the mother and child is a relatively new practice. Many hospitals have made cohabitation a generalized practice, unless the child or mother must receive special treatment. Breast-feeding has regained importance after years of bottle-feeding. The mother's general hesitation to breast-feed relates to not having sufficient milk, experiencing sore nipples, losing breast firmness, and muscle wasting after the breast-feeding period. In practice, once the mother has made a decision regarding breast-feeding, the father's support and encouragement are key for a successful outcome.

Differences exist between English-speaking and French-speaking women with respect to breast-feeding. During the Health Survey of 1990, 44 percent of Canadian mothers reported breast-feeding their last child. Of these, 48 percent were Anglophones and 26 percent were Francophones. Craig (1993) found significant regional differences. Approximately one-quarter of women from the Maritimes, one-third from Quebec, and one-half from Ontario and the western provinces breast-feed their babies.

Women who breast-feed their babies to please the fathers or their families, or those who find it more comfortable to hide and isolate themselves to breast-feed the babies, are bound to fail. Mothers should not be made to feel guilty if they do not breast-feed. Bottle-feeding in these circumstances may be the best choice. Maternity and paternity leaves are available and range from 6 to 20 weeks. In practice, however, fathers often take only a few days to a few weeks of leave to help the mother care for the new baby and other children.

In general, French Canadians are particularly distinctive in terms of taboo behaviors. Some taboo practices related to pregnancy have persisted throughout the years. Although the movement used in washing a floor resembles that of an exercise aimed at strengthening the perineal muscles, this activity in the past was associated with the onset of labor and early or preterm deliveries. Another belief, which is shared by some nurses, is that the full moon plays a role in the onset of labor once the full-term period has been reached. This belief applies to pregnant women who are 2 weeks preterm or postterm. A much less common belief is that pregnant women who experience hyperglycemia give birth to boys and that lack of salt announces the birth of girls.

Death Rituals

DEATH RITUALS AND EXPECTATIONS

French Canadians do not differ from Canadians of other origins on issues related to death and death rituals. Expectations are closely related to Christian religious practices, in particular, those of the Roman Catholic Church, of which most French Canadians are members. Whether one is an active church-goer or not, religious funerals are the norm. Values and beliefs related to life after death, the soul, and God vary dramatically across the age span among French Canadians and, even more so, among Francophones. Thus, it is essential to assess each family individually when it comes to death rituals and expectations. For many years, cremation was seen by the Catholic Church as a ritual left for specific circumstances. Currently, the Catholic Church advocates cremation as an acceptable practice.

RESPONSES TO DEATH AND GRIEF

During the second half of the 20th century, long grief and mourning rituals imposed by social norms have been adapted to modern lifestyles. One aspect that has shaped the traditional responses to death and mourning periods is influenced by the place women hold in the workforce. Currently, the expression of grief among French Canadians is similar to the stages described by Kübler-Ross (1977). Supports for those who have lost a family member include openly acknowledging the family's right to express grief, being physically present, making referrals to appropriate religious leaders, and encouraging interpersonal relationships.

Spirituality

DOMINANT RELIGION AND USE OF PRAYER

Eighty-five percent of French Canadians identify themselves as Roman Catholic, and most are baptized at birth, though they may or may not remain active church members; fewer than 15 percent report active participation in their religion (Gannon et al., 1994). A growing number of births are registered through civil channels rather than through the traditional Catholic registry and baptism. Despite the sharp decline in actively practicing Catholics, most people from all socioeconomic levels turn to their church for important life events such as marriage and funerals. In some cases, even in a civil ceremony involving previously divorced spouses, the couple may ask a priest to say mass and bless the union. The Catholic Church does not allow a religious marriage and exchange of solemn vows for divorcees.

Religious holidays honored as civic holidays are New Year's Day, Good Friday, Easter Sunday and Easter Monday, and Christmas. In the province of Quebec, St. John the Baptist Day (June 24) is a civic holiday, and in most Acadian institutions, the national Acadian holiday feast of the Assumption is celebrated on August 15. All Saints Day, November 1, and the Epiphany, January 6, were dropped in the 1970s.

Older adults are more inclined to use prayers for finding strength and adapting to difficult physical, psychological, and social health problems. In times of illness and tragedy, French-speaking Canadians use prayer to help recovery. Many of the younger generation are not strongly influenced by religious values, beliefs, and faith practices. Many French Acadians still request the sacrament of the sick and a visit from the priest.

MEANING OF LIFE AND INDIVIDUAL SOURCES OF STRENGTH

Traditional French Canadians, who view themselves as the core (*gyron*) of the family, and who believe that the well-being of their children is more precious than their own life, have faded proportionally with the prevalence of divorce. For hard-working men and women of previous generations, leisure activity was a trivial expression. The little time that could be spared on holidays was dedicated to visiting distant relatives.

SPIRITUAL BELIEFS AND HEALTH-CARE PRACTICES

Although modern health promotion theories suggest that spiritual needs are a critical factor in comprehensive client care, this aspect of family needs has received little attention among French-speaking Canadians. Many health-care providers still equate spirituality with religion, which is often reflected in the patient's history at the time of admission. According to Rukholm and colleagues (1991), the most important issues are knowing that the patient is valued, recognizing the family, and respecting the client's values and spirituality. Their study of French and English cultural differences in family needs and anxiety in an intensive-care unit in three hospitals of northeastern Ontario found that spiritual needs and anxiety explained 33 percent of the variations in family needs.

Health-Care Practices

HEALTH-SEEKING BELIEFS AND BEHAVIORS

In the 19th century and early 20th century, sick people did not readily enter hospitals because mortality rates were high and care was often inhumane. Before Confederation, resources and preventive health care rested in the hands of religious sisterhoods, United Empire Loyalists, church groups, and local authorities (Allemag, 1995). As pioneers in health services, the Gray Nuns visited the sick and opened hospitals such as Bytown in Ontario in 1845 and St. Boniface in Manitoba in 1847. In 1860, they extended their services to an Indian settlement 400 miles north of Saskatoon, and in 1867 to Fort Providence on Great Slave Lake.

Beckingham, Coutu-Wakulczyk, and Lubin's (1993) study of rural elderly Francophones and Anglophones living in Ontario and Quebec showed that 71 percent of Ontarians rated their health as good or excellent, compared with 62.9 percent for Quebecers. Bourque and colleagues (1991) found that among elderly New

Brunswick Francophones, 58.5 percent rated their health as good or excellent. Using the same scales, Bellehumeur (1994) found similar results on a randomized sample of elderly French Canadian adults living in northeastern Ontario.

St.-Amant and Vuong (1994) surveyed 57 elderly former psychiatric clients from 14 organizations in New Brunswick on the relation between cultural affiliation, gender, and satisfaction with health-care services. The findings revealed that women's mental health was more fragile than men's. A positive correlation, and higher satisfaction with services, was found among those with longer institutionalization. The authors concluded that Francophones in New Brunswick rely more on an informal family support network, whereas Anglophones rely more on professional services.

Results of a 1990 Canadian health survey show that residents of British Colombia and Ontario reported the most favorable assessments of their health, with almost 3 out of 10 reporting excellent health. Lower levels of health were reported in eastern Canada, where 1 in 5 Nova Scotians reported excellent health. Canadians from New Brunswick, followed by those from Quebec, were more likely to report fair or poor health, with only 17 percent and 16 percent, respectively, reporting excellent health (Stephens & Fowler Graham, 1993). Good health was related to education and income, occupation, or both. However, lifestyle showed an inconsistent relationship with income. Among younger adults and older men, social class had little effect on income, whereas among women, the effect of income dominated over social class. Rather than attempting to identify risk factors for specific diseases, it may be more meaningful to identify those factors that affect general susceptibility to risk factors.

RESPONSIBILITY FOR HEALTH CARE

Canada's government-administered health system ensures free, universal health coverage at any point of entry into the system. A survey conducted by Renaud, Jutras, and Bouchard (1987) showed user satisfaction reaching 80 percent. However, many people in the upper socioeconomic classes call on their family physicians instead of the local community service centers. Among the lower socioeconomic classes of Quebec and the Maritimes, many do not seek health care until their health becomes a crisis situation.

Evans and Stoddart's 1994 White Paper, "Producing Health, Consuming Health Care," proposed that the determinants of health status are lifestyle, environment, human biology, and health-care organizations. According to this paper, lifestyle and, to a lesser extent, living environments are chosen by the individual. Corin (1994) offers a matrix of stressors for identifying high-risk behaviors within a perspective that avoids victim blaming. Lifestyle behaviors are readily perceived as being under the control of the individual. The broad set of relationships encompassed under the label of "stress," and predictive factors against stress, have demonstrated the importance of social relationships for preventing disease and mortality (Sapolsky, 1990).

In 1980, New Brunswick set up a novel program at the Extra-Mural Hospital to provide acute and chronic home-care services to a largely rural province with a small population density and limited financial resources. Because the willingness of clients and family members to participate actively in a plan of care is critical to the success of community-based services, the Extra-Mural Hospital program strongly encouraged self-care with family involvement. Unlike other community initiatives in Canada such as the Ontario home-care program, the Extra-Mural Hospital does not restrict services within specific boundaries, and offers a comprehensive, provincewide delivery system via a single-agency approach (Cormier-Daigle et al., 1995).

Hagan, O'Neill, and Dallaire (1995) raised the association between health promotion and community health nursing with conceptual and practical issues. In Quebec, the infrastructure for public health is different from that in other provinces. The community service centers, or CLSCs emerged from the Castonguay-Nepveu reform of health and welfare services in the early 1970s. The mission of the Fédération des CLSCs du Québec is to provide health and social services for primary and secondary prevention and rehabilitation. In a survey of health education roles and activities of 631 nurses, Hagan (1991) found that 89 percent of nurses have a humanistic vision of health education. This vision was defined as "teaching and establishing a helping relationship aimed at facilitating individuals' choices of strategies for improving or maintaining their global health" (p. 278).

French-speaking Canadians have joined the current trend toward over-the-counter drug use. However, from the health survey of 1990, their use of analgesics and tranquilizers shows strong provincial differences (Adlaf, 1993). As compared with the national average for the use of narcotic analgesics (11 percent), Quebec residents' use is only 5 percent. Residents of Quebec (67 percent) are less likely to use aspirin than the average Canadian (76 percent). However, the use of tranquilizers among Quebecers is slightly higher than the Canadian average (8 percent versus 5 percent). Drug use followed a pattern similar to that found in the healthy lifestyle practice. Despite the move toward healthy lifestyles, elderly French Canadian adults have not changed dramatically in comparison with younger age groups. In addition, in the 1990 health survey, the leisure time physical activity (LTPA) index reported a positive relation between adoption of healthy lifestyles and socioeconomic status, although not a smooth, linear one. In particular, the daily LTPA index decreased with increasing education.

FOLK PRACTICES

Saillant (1992) analyzed the importance, characteristics, and mechanics of women's knowledge of folk medicine in Quebec Francophone families at the beginning of the 20th century. This anthropological study focused on domestic activities. The ethnographic data were drawn from 4000 medical receipts dealing with the knowledge of women in folk-healing practices in Quebec and abroad to enhance the understanding of the roles played by women in rural society folk-healing tradition. The numerous connections between the culinary and therapeutic realms of activities bring one to rethink the link between nutrition and health practiced in the early years of the colony.

BARRIERS TO HEALTH CARE

Language differences may have an important impact on the patient, providers, and administrative interactions, and may become a barrier to continuity of care. However, language may also be a proxy for issues that can affect access to care. Language is closely related to culture, and language differences may signal variations in values about behaviors or use of health care. Current views toward multiculturalism include removing barriers so that all citizens have equal access and opportunities and cultural diversity needs are considered in decision making and resource allocation. For many elderly French Canadian adults raised outside the province of Quebec, French was the language used in daily living within their cultural environment, except for educational services. In their childhood, they attended English-speaking schools because the public school system was all that was available outside Quebec. This situation, and other issues, present challenges in organizing transcultural health-care delivery: the spoken language is French, yet reading skills (or what is left of them) are often English. Thus, the health-care team may need to supplement written messages and instructions with verbal instructions to ensure understanding.

CULTURAL RESPONSES TO HEALTH AND ILLNESS

Choinière and Melzack (1987), using the McGill Pain Questionnaire and a visual-analog intensity scale, assessed acute and chronic pain differences between 68 French-speaking and English-speaking people with hemophilia. The results showed a similarity in the sensory, affective, and evaluative properties between the two types of pain. French-speaking subjects rated their acute pain as more intense than chronic pain, and more affectively laden than the English-speaking group. From a different perspective, Rukholm, Bailey, and Coutu-Wakulczyk (1991), studying French and English cultural differences in family needs and anxiety in an ICU, found that English-speaking subjects rated their distress at seeing a relative in pain more highly than French-speaking subjects. Though puzzling, this finding deserves attention and additional research to better understand and plan health-care interventions and to assist family members involved with ICU services.

Adam (1989), as part of a broader package of health promotion, developed, implemented, and evaluated a 15-hour community program for French-speaking women living in minority situations, many of whom were socially and economically disadvantaged. The program was designed to increase the participants' ability to take charge of their lives and better manage their physical and mental health. After presenting the program to 29 groups, evaluations showed that women generally reported satisfaction as the program progressed. Most subjects were satisfied with their broader understanding of stress and relaxation techniques for controlling daily stress.

The deinstitutionalized physically and mentally disabled are protected from discrimination and abuse by federal and provincial laws in Canada. Physically disabled people, regardless of their ethnicity, benefit from equal-opportunity regulations. Throughout Canada, official general acceptance and an increased awareness have lead to the physical adaptation of the environment to facilitate access for the disabled. However, the homeless mentally disabled raise different concerns in regard to the cost of maintaining this segment of the population in the community for lack of adequate organized services.

Saillant (1990) studied the sick role among a French Canadian sample from a clinical anthropological perspective. This author (Coutu-Wakulczyk) explored the relation between discourse, knowledge, and the experience of cancer within the life story of a patient suffering from cancer. The underlying theoretical model drew on a cultural hermeneutic approach. The client's discourse was analyzed for cognitive and symbolic models used to understand the experience of cancer. The results of this study highlighted the gap between the client's actual medical knowledge and the health profession's perception of the client's experiences and discourse about cancer.

BLOOD TRANSFUSIONS AND ORGAN DONATION

As a cultural group, French Canadians have no official proscriptions against receiving blood or blood products. Those who are members of a religious group that prohibits the acceptance of a blood transfusion are rare in Canada. Organ donation and transplantation are relatively new treatments in Canada. The decision to donate or receive an organ is an individual decision without any cultural influence for French Canadians.

Health-Care Practitioners

TRADITIONAL VERSUS BIOMEDICAL PRACTITIONERS

French Canadians have discarded the idea that one goes to the hospital to die. With a publicly administered health-care system in place since the 1960s, the population has benefited from increased accessibility to health care. However, financing this "welfare state" (état providence) has imposed a tremendous burden on taxpayers. Although the overall impact on health-care services is minimal, alternative therapies are gaining popularity, which may reflect disillusionment with the biomedical model in Quebec.

Men have been members of the nursing profession since the early 1970s. Although male nurses receive the same training as female nurses, they still account for less than 10 percent of professional nurses in Canada. While bedside nursing is gaining in popularity for men, most still hold administrative or teaching positions.

STATUS OF HEALTH-CARE PROVIDERS

In Canada as a whole, health-care practitioners cover a broad realm of specialties and disciplines, each working within an interdisciplinary and intersectoral approach to well-being. However, the system is not ideal, and tension occurs within and among disciplines. Health-care providers hold a favorable status in the eyes of French Canadians, especially among elderly people. The prevalence study in three home-care community agencies in southern Ontario has shown the implications for cultural sensitivity training (Majumdar, Browne, & Roberts, 1995). To enhance staff knowledge and skills, in spite of their general assimilation, remnants of French cultural heritage must be recognized as both contributing to behavior and influencing the course of clinical intervention.

At the beginning of the century, parents and grandparents were pragmatic and practical people, sharing views about God's power over everyday life. For example, a mother would pray to have at least a priest and a nun among her children, and a physician or a nurse was next in her wish to God. Today, folk and traditional practitioners are almost nonexistent. The current universal health insurance system makes the folk practitioners less appealing. Professionals throughout Canada are vigilant in trying to avoid exploitation by traditional and folk healers, who are viewed as practicing outside the law.

CASE STUDY Mr. Tremblay, a retired 63-year-old car dealer, lives with his wife Aline, age 58, in a nice suburban bungalow. The couple has five children, each of whom have their own family now and no one is living close to them. Mrs. Tremblay has been a housewife since she married 40 years ago; she is not self-confident and is very dependent on her husband. Mr. Tremblay has always been the decision maker, but now he is not healthy and is tired of taking all the responsibilities.

Mrs. Tremblay comes into the emergency room complaining of chest pain for 2 weeks. She describes the pain as burning and squeezing; it is steady and ends gradually. The pain started while she was raking the lawn. She didn't say anything to her husband because he is an anxious man and she didn't want to worry him. When her daughter, a nurse, came to visit them a week ago, she talked about her symptoms. Her daughter said she should see her family doctor as soon as possible because her maternal grandfather died of an acute MI at the age of 59.

Although Mr. Tremblay is completely bilingual, Mrs. Tremblay never mastered the English language further than for the everyday needs of shopping. Mrs. Tremblay is hesitant to consult her family physician because he does not speak much French. She prefers to wait and see . . . until a stronger pain forces her to seek help.

STUDY QUESTIONS

1 What are the major obstacles to health and well-being for this elderly couple?

2 Which of the transcultural domains are in the most jeopardy?

3 What are the major obstacles to the Tremblays' independence and health? How do these differ from those that interfere with health and well-being?

4 How do the meanings people attach to health and well-being, the control they assume or wish to assume over their health, and the objective features of health reflect cultural differences in later life?

5 Discuss the role of the nurse and the implications for culturally competent care for this couple.

6 What types of assistance and relationships between generations are important in maintaining this family unit?

7 How important are kinship ties in minority settings with regard to the adjustment and morale of older adults?

8 Do cultural factors have a stronger impact on older adults than for other age groups?

REFERENCES

Abbott, D. (2001, Winter). *Alcohol, tobacco, and other drugs*. Retrieved April 17, 2002, from http://www.socialwork.rudgers.edu/pdf/highlights.

Adam, D. (1989). Women and stress: A community prevention and health promotion program. *Canada Mental Health, 37*(4), 5–8.

Adlaf, E. (1993). Alcohol and other drug use. *Health and welfare Canada: Canada's health promotion survey 1990. Technical report*. Cat. No. H39-263/2-1990E. Ottawa, Canada: Ministry of Supply and Services.

Allemag, M. M. (1995). Development of community health nursing in Canada. In M. J. Stewart (Ed.), *Community nursing: Promoting Canadians' health* (pp. 2–36). Toronto, Canada: W. B. Saunders Canada.

Ansen, J. (2000). Nationalism and fertility in Francophone Montreal: The majority as a minority. *Canadian Studies in Population, 27*(2), 377–400.

Aube, N., & Linden, W. (1991). Marital disturbance, quality of communication and socioeconomic status. *Canadian Journal of Behavioral Science, 23*(2), 125–132.

Beaudin, M., & Leclerc, A. (1995). The contemporary Acadian economy. In J. Daigle (Ed.), *Acadia of the Maritimes: Thematic studies from the beginning to the present* (pp. 1–44). Moncton, NB: Université de Moncton: Chaire d'études acadiennes.

Beckingham, A. C., Coutu-Wakulczyk, G., & Lubin, B. (1993). French-language validation of the DACL and MAACL-R. *Journal of Clinical Psychology, 49*(5), 685–695.

Bellehumeur, N. (1994). Influence de l'auto-évaluation de la santé et de l'humeur dépressive sur l'observance du régime thérapeutique auprès de personnes âgées à domicile. Unpublished master's thesis, Faculté des Lettres et Sciences Humaines, Université de Sherbrooke, Quebec.

Bourque, P., Blanchard, L., Sadeghi, M. R., & Arseneault, A. M. (1991). Etat de santé, consommation de médicaments et symptômes de la dépression chez les personnes âgées. *Canadian Journal on Aging, 10*(4), 309–319.

Brunzell, J. T. (1989). Familial lipoprotein lipase deficiency and other causes of the chylomicronemia syndrome. In C. R. Scriver, A. L. Beaudet, W. S. Sly, & D. Valle (Eds.), *The metabolic basis of inherited disease* (pp. 1165–1180). New York: McGraw-Hill.

Charbonneau, H., Desjardins, B., Guillemette, A., Landry, Y., Légaré, J., & Nault, F. (1987). *Naissance d'une population: Les Français établis au Canada au XVII siècle*. Paris: Institut National d'Études Démographiques.

Choinière, M., & Melzack, R. (1987). Acute and chronic pain in hemophilia. *Pain, 31*(3), 317–331.

Corin, E. (1994). The social and cultural matrix of health and disease. In R. G. Evans, M. L. Barer, & T. R. Marmor (Eds.), *Why are some people healthy and others not? The determinants of health of populations* (pp. 93–132). New York: Aldine De Gruyter.

Cormier, H. J., & Klerman, G. L. (1985). Unemployment and male-female labor force participation as determinants of changing suicide rates of males and females in Quebec. *Social Psychiatry, 20,* 109–114.

Cormier, Y. (1994). L'Acadie d'aujourd'hui: Guide des provinces maritimes Francophones. Moncton, NB: Editions d'Acadie.

Cormier-Daigle, M., Baker, C., Arseneault, A.M., & MacDonald, M. (1995). The Extra-Mural hospital: A home health-care initiative in New Brunswick. In M. J. Stewart (Ed.), *Community nursing: Promoting Canadians' health* (pp. 163–179). Toronto, Canada: W. B. Saunders.

Coté, M. (1992). *Health and welfare policy.* Québec, Canada: Le Ministère

Coutu-Wakulczyk, G., Larochelle, C., & Black, R. (1992). Perception de soi des étudiants de premier cycle: étude transculturelle. Ottawa, Canada: Université d'Ottawa. Rapport de Recherche.

Craig, C. L. (1993). Nutrition. In T. Stephens & D. Fowler Graham (Eds.), *Canada's health promotion survey 1990. Technical report.* Cat. No. H39-263/2-1990E. Ottawa: Health and Welfare Canada, Ministry of Supply and Services.

Daigle, J. (1995). Acadia from 1604 to 1763: An historical synthesis. In J. Daigle (Ed.), *Acadia of the Maritimes: Thematic studies from the beginning to the present* (pp. 1–44). Moncton, NB: Université de Moncton: Chaire d'Etudes Acadiennes.

DeBraekeleer, M. (1991). Deleterious genes. In G. Bouchard & M. DeBrackeleer (Eds.), *History of a genome: Population and genetics in Eastern Québec* (pp. 343–363). Québec, Canada: Presses de l'Université du Québec.

DeBraekeleer, M., & Dao, T. N. (1994a). In search of founders. I: Hereditary disorders in the French-Canadian population of Québec. *Human Biology, 66*(2), 205–224.

DeBraekeleer, M., & Dao, T. N. (1994b). Contribution of Perche (migrants from Perche, France). II: Hereditary disorders in the French-Canadian population of Québec. *Human Biology, 66*(2), 225–250.

Denault, A. A., & Cardinal, L. (1999). L'équité en matière d'emploi en Ontario et les Francophones, de 1986 à 1995. *Recherches Sociologiques, 40*(1), 83–101.

DeWit, D. J., & Beneteau, B. (1998). Predictors of the prevalence of alcohol use related problems among Francophones and Anglophones in the province of Ontario, Canada. *Journal of Studies on Alcohol, 59*(1), 78–88.

Dionne, C., Gagné, C., Julien, P., Murthy, M., Roederer, G., Davignon, J., Lambert, M., Chitayat, D., Ma, R., Henderson, H., Lupien, P. J., Hayden, M. R., & DeBraekeleer, M. (1993). Genealogy and regional distribution of lipoprotein lipase deficiency in French-Canadians of Québec. *Human Biology, 65*(1), 29–40.

Edwards, P., & Rootman, I. (1993). Supports for health. In T. Stephens & D. Fowler Graham (Eds.), *Canada's health promotion survey 1990. Technical report.* Cat. No. H39-263/2-1990E. Ottawa, Canada: Ministry of Supply and Services.

Emard, J., Drouin, G., Thouez, J., & Ghardirian, P. (2001). Vasectomy and prostate cancer in Québec, Canada. *Health & Place, 7*(2), 131–139.

Evans, R. G. (1994). Introduction. In R. G. Evans, M. L. Barer, & T. R. Marmor (Eds.), *Why are some people healthy and others not? The determinants of health of populations* (pp. 3–26). New York: Aldine De Gruyter.

Evans, R. G., & Stoddart, G. L. (1994). Producing health, consuming health care. In R. G. Evans, M. L. Barer & T. R. Marmor (Eds.), *Why are some people healthy and others not? The determinants of health of populations* (pp. 27–66). New York: Aldine De Gruyter.

Feather, J., & Green, K. L. (1993). Health behaviours and intentions. In T. Stephens & D. Fowler Graham (Eds.), *Canada's health promotion survey 1990. Technical report.* Cat. No. H39-263/2-1990E. Ottawa, Canada: Ministry of Supply and Services.

Fédération des CLSCs du Québec. (1992). *Les services infirmiers en CLSC: Document de réflexion.* Montreal: Author.

Fong, E., & Guilia, M. (1990). *Neighborhood changes within the Canadian ethnic mosaic.* University of Ontario, Canada: Author.

Fournier, D. (1989). Pourquoi la revanche des berceaux? L'hypothèse de sociabilité. *Recherches Sociographiques, 30*(2), 171–198.

Fumeron, F., Grandchamp, B., Fricker, J., Krempt, M. Wolf, L. M., Khayat, M. C., Boiffard, O., & Apfelbaum, M. (1992). Presence of the Canadian deletion in a French patient with familial hypercholesterolemia. *New England Journal Medicine, 326*(1), 69.

Gagné, C., Brun, L. D., Moorjani, S., & Lupien, P. J. (1989). Primary lipoprotein-lipase-activity deficiency: Clinical investigation of a French-Canadian population. *Canadian Medical Association Journal, 140*(4), 405–411.

Gannon, M. J. & Associates. (1994). *Understanding global cultures: Metaphorical journeys through 17 countries.* Thousand Oaks, CA: Sage.

Godar, C. (1998). Health Canada: Ovarian cancer in Canada. Retrieved April 17, 2002, from http://www.hc-sc.gc.ca.

Goyder, J. C. (1981). Income differences between the sexes: Findings from a national Canadian survey. *Canadian Review of Sociology and Anthropology, 18,* 321–342.

Grompe, M., St-Louis, M., Demers, S. I., Al-Dhalimy, M., Leclerc, B., & Tanguay, R. M. (1994). A single mutation of the fumarylacetoacetate hydrolase gene in French-Canadians with hereditary tyrosinemia type I. *New England Journal of Medicine, 331*(6), 353–358.

Hagan, L. (1991). Analyse de l'exercice de la fonction éducative des infirmiers et des infirmières des centres locaux de services communautaires du Québec. Unpublished doctoral dissertation, Faculty of Education Sciences, Université de Montréal.

Hagan, L., O'Neill, M., & Dallaire, C. (1995). Linking health promotion and community health nursing: Conceptual and practical issues. In M. J. Stewart (Ed.), *Community nursing: Promoting Canadians' health* (pp. 413–429). Toronto: W. B. Saunders.

Health and Welfare Canada (1989). Charting Canada's future: A report of the demographic review. Ottawa, Canada: Ministry of Supplies and Services.

Health Canada (1994). *Suicide in Canada: Update of the report of the task force on suicide in Canada.* Cat. No. H39-107/1995E. Ottawa, Canada: Ministry of Supply and Services.

Henripin, J., & Martin, Y. (1991). *La population du Québec d'hier à demain.* Montréal, Québec: Presses de l'Université de Montréal.

Hillstrom, L.C. (1995). French Americans. In J. Galens, A. Sheets, & R. V. Young (Eds.), & R. J. Vecoli (Cont. Ed.), *Gale encyclopedia of multicultural America,* vol. 1 (pp. 533–545). Detroit, MI: Gale Research.

Hobart, C. (1992). How they handle it: Young Canadians, sex and AIDS. *Youth and Society, 23*(4), 411–433.

House, J. S., Landis, K. R., & Umberson, D. (1988). Social relationships and health. *Science, 241,* 540–545.

International Recognition of Same-Sex Relationships. (2002). http://www.hrusa.org.

Krajinovic, M., Ghadirian, P., Richer, C., Sinnett, H., Gandini, S., Perret, C., Lacroix, A., Labuda, D., & Sinnett, D. (2001). Genetic susceptibility to breast cancer in French-Canadians: role of carcinogen-metabolizing enzymes and gene-environment interactions. *American Journal of Human Genetics, 59*(3), 633–643.

Kübler-Ross, E. (1977). *Death: The final stage of growth.* Englewood Cliffs, NJ: Prentice-Hall.

Lambert, R. D., Brown, S. D., Curtis, J. E., & Kay, B. J. (1986). Canadians' beliefs about differences between social classes. *Canadian Journal of Sociology/Cahiers Canadiens de Sociologie, 11*(4), 379–399.

Langelier, R. (1996). French-Canadian families. In M. McGoldrick, J. K. Pearce, & J. Giorano (Eds.). *Ethnicity and family therapy* (2nd ed.) (pp. 477–495). New York: Guilford Press.

Lapp, J. E. (1984). Psychotropic drug and alcohol use by Montreal college students: Sex, ethnic and personality correlates. *Journal of Alcohol Drug Education, 30*(1), 18–26.

Levy, E., Minnich, A., Cacan, S.L., Thibaut, L., Giroux, L.-M., Davignon, J., & Lambert, M. (1997). Association of an exon 3 mutation (Trp66→Gly) of the LDL receptor with variable expression of familial hypercholesterolemia in a French-Canadian Family. *Biochemical & Molecular Medicine, 60*(1), 59–69.

Lyonnet, S., De Braekelee, M., Labramboise, R., Rey, F., John, S. W., Berthelon, M., Berthelot, J., Journel, H., & Le Marec, B. (1992). Time and space clusters of the French-Canadian MIV phenylketonuria mutation in France. *American Journal of Human Genetics, 51*(1), 191–196.

Ma, Y., Henderson, H., Ven Marthy, M. R., Roederer, G., Monsalve, M. V., Clarke, L. A., Normand, T., Julien, P., Gagné, C., Lambert, M., Davignon, J., Lupien, P. Jé, Brunzell, J., & Hayden, M. R. (1991). A mutation in the human lipoprotein lipase gene as the most common cause of familial chylomicronemia in French-Canadians. *New England Journal of Medicine, 324*(25), 176–182.

Majumdar, B., Browne, G., & Roberts, J. (1995). The prevalence of multicultural groups receiving in-home service from three community agencies in Southern Ontario: Implications for cultural sensitivity training. *Canadian Journal of Public Health, 86*(3), 206–211.

McIntyre, L., & Doyle, J. B. (1992). Exploratory analysis of children's nutritional program in Canada. *Social Science Medicine, 35*(9), 1123–1129.

Office of Francophone Affairs of Ontario. (1994). *French language services: A historical overview.* Retrieved April 17, 2002, from http://www.ofa.gov.on.ca.

Pampalon, R., Gauthier, D., Raymond, G., & Beaudry, E. (1990). *Health map: A geographical distribution of the Québec Health Survey.* Québec, Canada: Ministere de la Santé et des Services Sociaux.

Pausova, Z., Deslauriers, B., Gaudet, D., Tremblay J., Koetchen, T. A., Larochelle, P. Cowley, A. W., & Hamet, P. (2000). Role of tumor necrosis factor-α gene locus in obesity and obesity-associated hypertension in French-Canadians. *Hypertension, 36*(1), 14–19.

Platt, S. (1984). Unemployment and suicidal behavior: A review of the literature. *Social Science and Medicine, 12*(2), 93–115.

Pronovost, G. (1989). Transformation in work time and leisure time. In G. Pronovost & D. Mercere (Eds.), *Time and societies* (pp. 37–61). Québec, Canada: Institut Québecois de Recherche sur la Culture.

Public Works and Government Services Canada. (2001). Available at http://www.pwgsc.gc.ca.

Punnett, B. J. (1991). Language, cultural values and preferred leadership style: A comparison of Anglophones and Francophones in Ottawa. *Canadian Journal of Behavioural Science, 23*(2), 241–244.

Rapport de la Commission d'Enquête sur les Services de Santé Sociaux. (1988). Retrieved April 17, 2002, from http://www.ofa.gov.on.ca.

Renaud, M., Jutras, S., & Bouchard, P. (1987). Solutions brought forth by Quebecers concerning social and health problems. Paper presented at the Inquiry Commission on health and social services. Québec, Canada: Les Publications du Québec.

Rozen, R., De Braekeleer, M., Daigneault, J., Ferrire-Rajabi, L., Gerdes, M., Lamoureux, L., Aubin, G., Simard, F., Fujiwara, T. M., & Morgan, K. (1992). Cystic fibrosis mutations in French-Canadians: Three CFTR mutations are relatively frequent in a Quebec population with elevated incidence of cystic fibrosis. *American Journal of Medical Genetics, 42*(3), 360–364.

Rozen, R., Mascisch, A., Lambert, M., Laframboise, R., & Scriver, C. R. (1994). Mutation profiles of phenylketonuria in Quebec populations: Evidence of stratification and novel mutations. *American Journal of Human Genetics, 55*(2), 321–326.

Rukholm, E., Bailey, P., & Coutu-Wakulczyk, G. (1991). Needs and anxiety in ICU: Cultural differences in northeastern Ontario. *Canadian Journal of Nursing Research, 23*(3), 67–81.

Rukholm, E., Bailey, P., Coutu-Wakulczyk, G., & Bailey, W. (1991). Needs and anxiety levels in relatives of intensive care unit patients. *Journal of Advanced Nursing, 16,* 920–928.

Saillant, F. (1990). Discourse, knowledge, and experience of cancer: A life story. *Cultural Medicine and Psychiatry, 14*(1), 47–72.

Saillant, F. (1992). Savoir et pratiques des femmes dans l'univers ethnomedical québécois. *Canadian Folklore (Canada), 14*(1), 47–72.

St.-Amant, N., & Vuong, D. (1994). Quand la language fait une difference: Ce que des "beneficiares" pensent du système de santé mentale. *Sociologie et Societes, 261*(1), 179–196.

St-Pierre, J., Vohl, M. C., Brisson, D., Perron, P., Despres, J. P., Hudson, T. J., & Gaudet, D. (2001). A sequence variation in the mitochondrial glycerol-3-phosphate dehydrogenase gene is associated with increased plasma glycerol and free fatty acid concentrations among French-Canadians. *Molecular Genetics & Metabolism, 72*(3), 209–217.

Samson, J. M., Otis, J., & Levy, J. J. (1996). Risques face au sida, relations de pouvoir et styles de communication sexuelle chez les étudiants des cégeps Francophones du Québec. Rapport de recherché. Département de sexology, Université du Québec à Montréal.

Sapolsky, R. M. (1990). Stress in the wild. Ottawa: Policy, Analysis and Research Directorate Multiculturalism. *Scientific American, 262*(1), 116–123.

Statistics Canada. (2001). Available at http://www.statcan.com.

Stephens, T., & Fowler Graham, D. (1993). Overview. In T. Stephens & D. Fowler Graham (Eds.), *Canada's health promotion survey 1990. Technical report.* Cat. No. H39-263/2-1990E. Ottawa, Canada: Ministry of Supply and Services.

Uthman, I., Vasquez-Abad, D., & Sénécal, J. L. (1996). Distinctive features of idiopathic inflammatory myopathies in French-Canadians. *Seminars in Arthritis & Rheumatism, 26*(1), 447–458.

Vohl, M. C., Lepage, P., Gaudet, D., Brewe, C. G., Betard, C., Perron, P., Houde, G., Cellier, C., Faith, J. M., Despres, J. P., Morgan, K., & Hudson, T. J. (2000). Molecular scanning of the human PPAR-α gene: Association of the L162V mutation with hyperapobetalipoproteinemia. *Journal of Lipid Research, 41*(6), 945–952.

Wharry, S. (1997). Canada: a country of two solitudes when smoking rates among Anglophones, Francophones compared. *Canadian Medical Association Journal, 156*(2), 244–245.

Wu, Z., & Baer, D. E. (1996). Attitudes toward family life and gender roles: A comparison of English and French-Canadian women. *Journal of Comparative Family Studies, 27*(3), 437–452.

Chapter 11

People of Iranian Heritage

HOMEYRA HAFIZI and JULIENE G. LIPSON

Overview, Inhabited Localities, and Topography

OVERVIEW

Estimates of the number of Iranians in the United States range from about 400,000 to over 1 million. Nearly half live in California. Over 64,000 live in Canada, mostly in Toronto. Remarkably little literature is published on the health of the North American Iranian population other than older clinical descriptions and research on health, health concepts, and adjustment (Lipson, 1992; Hafizi, 1990). Lack of literature necessitates using some information from Iran, not all of which is accurate for people in the United States.

Despite our focus on commonalities, Iranians vary enormously, from highly traditional to highly acculturated, in their reasons for leaving Iran, as well as their social class, education, religion, and ethnic background. In addition, the transition state of the U.S. Iranian immigrant population creates generational differences. For example, Iranian women in Los Angeles who left Iran at a young age have more liberal attitudes toward sex and intimate relationships and more conflicts about their Iranian and American identities (Hanassab, 1998).

Iran is about 636,000 square miles in area, and is bordered by Turkey, Iraq, Armenia, Azerbaijan, Turkmenistan, Afghanistan, and Pakistan. Most of the country is a mountainous plateau about 4000 feet above sea level and surrounded by mountain ranges, with the highest peak at 18,000 feet. Large salt deserts cover much of the area, but there are also many oases and forest areas. The climate varies from hot and dry summers to cold winters with snow in the higher altitudes.

Most of Iran's 70 million people live in the north and northwest. The capital, Tehran, has nearly 12 million residents, and a large proportion of the population lives in the cities. The United Nations estimates that with the current population growth rate of 1.4 percent per year, Iran's population will reach 99 million in 2025. Currently, 37 percent of the population is under the age of 15, and 5 percent are over 65.

The terms *Persian* and *Iranian* are used interchangeably in this chapter because some people call themselves Persian for historical and political reasons. In 1935, the country's name was changed from Persia to Iran (from the word *aryana*) to present an image of progress and in an attempt to unify into one nation the enormous diversity of urban dwellers and rural tribes, ethnic groups, and social classes.

HERITAGE AND RESIDENCE

Persian culture is very old and rich. Iranians are proud of their heritage, which includes the Zoroastrian religion and some of the world's greatest poets and leaders in medieval philosophy, astronomy, and medicine; for example, the physician Ibn Sina (Avicenna). The original Persians were an Indo-European group related to the Aryans of India who invaded the Middle East around 1500 BC. The Persian empire, founded by Cyrus the Great in 559 BC, covered an area from the Hindu Kush (now in Afghanistan) to Egypt, Palestine, Syria, and parts of Asia Minor.

Throughout its history, Persia was subjected to foreign rulers with customs, languages, and religions vastly different from its own; Persians managed to regain independence after centuries while maintaining their heritage. For example, Alexander the Great conquered Persia in 333 BC. Arabs brought Islam to Persia in the seventh century, and most Zoroastrian inhabitants were converted to Islam in the next two centuries. After Persia regained political and cultural autonomy, Turks and Mongols ruled Persia from the 11th century to 1502. In the 19th century, the British and Russian empires vied for influence.

In the past 70 years, Iran has seen the rise and fall of the Qajar dynasty; the Pahlavi dynasty (supported by the British); the short-lived National Front (social democratic organization led by Mossadeq, who rejected the British and returned the oil fields to the Iranians); the return of the Pahlavi dynasty led by Mohammed Reza Shah (supported by the United States); and finally, the current Islamic regime.

Reza Shah Pahlavi and his son instituted powerful social and economic reforms from the mid-1930s to the 1979 revolution, including national public health and education programs and a more secular society with decreased power for tribal chiefs, clergy, and landed aristocracy. During this period women were allowed to go unveiled, gained access to university education, and were fully enfranchised in 1963. By the late 1970s, women had become senators, cabinet ministers, physicians, and professors. However, despite these economic and social changes, Mohammed Reza Shah showed the same disrespect for democracy as did his father before him; for example, he reinstituted the secret police and had no tolerance for political opposition.

After conservative Moslem protests that led to the 1978 violence, martial law was declared and a military government was appointed to deal with striking oil workers. Early in 1979, the Shah fled Iran for the United States. The "reform" instituted by the new Islamic government was deeply colored by the traditional religious ideology of Shi'ia Islam. Since then, Iran has once again come to externally resemble the more conservative Muslim countries. However, some of the past radical social changes were simply forced underground. Urban women, for example, are covered and dress conservatively in public but dress stylishly indoors. The diversity created by these changes is reflected in the diversity of Iranian immigrants to the United States.

Iranian immigrants have faced considerable ethnic bias because of events in Iran. Anger and prejudice toward Iranians reached a peak during the 14-month occupation of the U.S. Embassy in Tehran beginning in November 1979. Americans were barraged daily with such television commentary as "Day 414 of the hostage crisis," which promoted hostility toward Iranians in the United States. This hostility was manifested by harassment of students of all ages and threats painted on store windows owned by Iranians immigrants. In the worst cases, Iranians were assaulted or received threatening telephone calls. Some immigrants were afraid to admit that they came from Iran, such as a Turkish-speaking Iranian woman who told people she was Turkish.

Los Angeles has the largest concentration of Iranians outside Iran, with hotly disputed estimates ranging from 74,000 to 300,000 in the mid-1980s (Kelly, Friedlander, & Colby, 1993); 1990 U.S. Census and Immigration and Naturalization figures through 1997 suggest there are nearly 400,000 Iranians in the United States. The Los Angeles population is ethnically and religiously diverse. While Muslims are still the majority, the Armenian, Jewish, and Baha'i communities are far larger than they were in Iran (Bozorgmehr, Sabagh, & Der-Martirosian, 1993). In other areas of the United States, Iranians do not live in ethnic enclaves that can assist newcomers to adjust. While many small and cohesive social networks exist, much of the Iranian population is divided by distrust based on political, religious, and social class differences.

REASONS FOR MIGRATION AND ASSOCIATED ECONOMIC FACTORS

Of the three waves of Iranian immigration to the United States, the first (1950 to 1970) consisted mostly of students from the social and professional elite class, many of whom remained in the United States after completing their education. The second wave (1970 to 1978) comprised immigrants who were more varied in social class background but were predominantly urban and affluent. They came mainly to pursue higher education, professional or economic opportunities, or to join family members. The 1975 to 1980 cohort included a higher proportion of minorities, such as Baha'is and Jews escaping religious persecution, as well as more women and elderly.

The third wave began with the Islamic revolution and included a large number of political exiles and forced migrants, who came mainly for personal or economic security. They are more heterogeneous in education, age, social class, religiosity, and exposure to Western culture. Many consider themselves exiles rather than voluntary immigrants and are ambivalent about having left Iran. While free of the social and political limitations imposed by the Islamic Republic, most still feel guilt and sorrow about leaving their families behind and live in an atmosphere of instability and uncertainty.

Length of time in the United States and the resources immigrants bring with them influence ease of transition and the issues with which they struggle. Relatively new immigrants frequently experience culture shock, problems associated with poor mastery of English, perceived loss of status, and difficulty finding work comparable to what they left behind, as well as the loss of their culture, habits, and identity. Financial problems are a source of considerable stress. Some wealthy people lost considerable money when they left Iran; other new arrivals have run out of savings, and income sources from Iran have dried up. Despite many having fled from Iran after the revolution because of fear for their safety, few were admitted as refugees. Thus they lack access to refugee social and financial programs. Some are undocumented and live in constant fear of discovery and deportation.

Some Iranians who have lived in the United States longer are concerned with occupational, financial, and academic functioning, and they may also experience more family problems. Although they have adjusted to life in the United States, many have become discouraged about their own achievements and consider their exodus as having been "for the sake of the children." Despite relative stability, upper middle-class and upper-class immigrants rarely recover the status they had in Iran.

Prerevolution immigrants experience stressors related to close family and cultural ties with Iran, such as fear of never seeing family members again or, during the Iran-Iraq war, fear of receiving the dreaded news that a relative had been killed. Despite their permanent status in the United States, some grieve the loss of their country. Iranians who are relatively financially secure experience more subtle stressors, such as perceptions of hostility and ethnic bias.

Elderly immigrants often express their ambivalence about being in the United States and may strongly believe they immigrated to care for their children with emotional and financial support, similar to elderly immigrants in Sweden (Emami et al., 2000). The elderly often feel isolated and do not learn English or participate in American culture; their desire to return home keeps them from making permanent commitments and cementing emotional ties. They are also concerned about their inability to keep their children from becoming too Americanized. They perceive American children as lacking respect for the elderly and having loose family ties.

Many younger Iranians lack social support in the United States. In Iran, friendships and relationships with extended family members are established from birth, and these relationships are sorely missed in the United States. Because most Iranians are highly social and dislike being alone, many "befriend" each other, despite having little in common but their national heritage and language. Because being Iranian becomes the basis on which a support network is formed, rather than on personal rapport or shared characteristics, the network may create undue stress and an underlying tension.

EDUCATIONAL STATUS AND OCCUPATIONS

Iranians are among the most highly educated immigrant group in the United States. Education is greatly valued and advanced degrees are highly respected; for example, those with doctorates are often consulted for their advice. In Iran, even poor villagers sacrifice their personal comfort to send their children to school. The children of immigrants in the United States are expected to do well in school and to attend college.

Occupational opportunities depend on the education and skills that immigrants brought from Iran, as well as the era and their age when they arrived in the United States. Those who immigrated before the 1979 revolution often chose to study medicine and engineering. American-educated Iranians represent the range of occupations available through higher education and other means. Many middle-aged physicians, engineers, professors, army generals, and government officials who were unable to find comparable work in the United States have gone into business for themselves. Some began with pizza parlors or gas stations, using their business acumen to maintain a middle-class or better lifestyle in the United States. In Los Angeles, 61 percent of Iranian heads of households claimed to be self-employed in 1987 and 1988 (Dallalfar, 1994), with Iranian Jews having a self-employment rate of 82 percent. Only 10 percent reported employment in blue-collar jobs (Bozorgmehr, Sabagh, & Der-Martirosian, 1993). Because health-care providers may encounter a jewelry store owner who is a former judge, they should not assume education and social class from occupation alone.

Iranian women are quite active in Los Angeles as owners and employees in such small businesses as travel agencies, accounting, and retail businesses; a number have home-based businesses; for example, seamstress, pastry maker, or make-up specialist. Very few are waitresses, and none were observed working in gas stations or as taxi drivers, an occupation in which Iranian men are quite visible (Dallalfar, 1994).

However, occupation remains a major concern for some immigrants, particularly for men from the Iran's upper social strata, who cannot get recognition through employment or status in their new country. Jobs that require manual labor are not respected, and some Iranian-Americans cannot accept that they have to take such menial jobs because of their limited skills in English. One study found a strong correlation between satisfactory employment and emotional well-being; discrepancy between social status in Canada and Iran was key in the development of psychiatric problems, particularly among middle-aged men (Bagheri, 1982).

Communication

DOMINANT LANGUAGE AND DIALECTS

Farsi (Persian) is the national language of Iran, and all school children are taught in Persian. An indication of modern Iran's Indo-European heritage is found in words similar to English words; for example, the English word "mother" is a cognate to the Persian word *madar*. However, nearly half the country's population speak different languages; for example, Turkish, Kurdish, Armenian, Baluchi, or other Iranian dialects. Well-educated and well-traveled immigrants may speak three or more languages, often using French as a cultural language or English in business settings.

CULTURAL COMMUNICATION PATTERNS

Communication among Iranians must be understood within the context of Iranian history, the personality style valued in the culture, and the structure of social relationships. The many foreign invasions of Persia and strict control by each ensuing government have influenced Iranians' interaction with outsiders, and have led them to be suspicious of foreigners. People adapted and assimilated without losing their own identity. The disclosure of personal thoughts to strangers is generally perceived to have detrimental consequences. Not verbalizing one's thoughts is viewed as a customary and useful defense; overt expressions of emotions to strangers may be culturally stigmatized.

Iranians engage in social conversation to build rapport before involving themselves in business. Their tone of voice depends greatly on their rural or urban background and the influence of traditionalism. Among women, patterns of speech may appear restrained or refined to avoid too much self-disclosure or to prevent loss of face, but overall, the situation guides the degree of expressiveness. Iranians give considerable detail rather than use blunt and succinct messages.

Bagheri (1992) described highly valued personality characteristics such as indirectness, subdued assertiveness, modesty, and politeness. Iranians are very concerned with respectability, a good appearance of the home, and a good reputation. They are embarrassed by financial troubles and even conceal such problems from relatives. **Zeranghi** (cleverness) is valued, but only among nonintimates; it means knowing how to manipulate bureaucratic structures and is used because government organizations were not trusted to function for the good of the people in Iran. The ability to bargain well is an example of *zeranghi*. In the public sphere, bargaining is how things get done in Iran; one never accepts the first price quoted or believes that a stated rule cannot be changed. However, it is very important to distinguish between "valued" or common cultural characteristics and individual personality characteristics.

In addition, Iranian communication patterns are influenced by a hierarchy of relationships, as well as the social status of the other person in relation to oneself. For example, communication may demonstrate support of lower-status individuals or competition with those of equal status. The influence of intimate versus public spheres and hierarchical social relationships is seen clearly in the practice of **ta'arof** (ritual expressed courtesy), which is not practiced with intimates. *Ta'arof* expresses the public face, with its respectful forms of speech and behavior, and is used when dealing with individuals whose status is unequal to one's own. In this system, there is a constant flow of offers of hospitality and compliments, which may sound very insincere to non-Iranians, particularly when they learn that taking these seriously is a social gaffe. However, such offers are sincere because they depend on the restraint of the respondent. The host has the pleasure of saying, "My house is your house" to a guest who enjoys this welcome but knows when to go home.

Social behavior is influenced by the constant awareness of the external judgment of others regarding whether a person is conforming to the ideal of "selflessness." It limits spontaneity and creates rules for approaching people of different ages and members of the opposite gender. What one says or feels is held back if it is believed to be outside the prescribed social script. An example of *ta'arof* occurs when a guest is offered tea; the guest initially refuses it, so as not to put the host to any trouble. The host offers again, and the guest again declines; the host offers again, and the guest finally accepts. The whole interaction is a ritual: the guest knows from the beginning that to refuse the tea or food would be an insult, but immediate acceptance would be seen as an act of egoism.

Communication in personal relationships in the public sphere, which is structured by social hierarchy, varies according to **baten** and **zaher**, and occurs on a continuum anchored at one end by the *baten* (inner self) in personal and intimate relationships, and at the other end by the *zaher* (public persona). A strong boundary exists between the internal world of family and close friends and the external world of acquaintances and everyone else. The *baten* is the true vulnerable self, a collection of freely expressed personal feelings. In contrast, *zaher* is proper and controlled behavior—a public face to protect and buffer the vulnerable world of the *baten* within. At the beginning of a new interaction, an Iranian is neither totally "outside" or "inside." If the exchange is oriented toward the *zaher* (outside), it is a sign of an unequal relationship where expressions become restricted or restrained. The Persian language, and its nonverbal accompaniments, has evolved to express and structure this exchange. Neither participant discloses the world of the *baten*; thus the relationship appears superficial, refined, and flawless, with social distance or aloofness being used to protect one's private self. Silence is used to guard confidential matters and to manage impressions.

In contrast to hierarchical public relationships, in communication among intimate friends and family—the *baten* or **andarun**—is shared. Overwhelmingly emotional or intense feelings can be expressed freely, are understood, and are not judged. Privacy is important in family affairs; family matters remain within the family and are not for others' ears. However, anger directed at people of higher status, like parents or superiors, is condemned. In addition, most Iranians refrain from showing anger or other strong emotions to outsiders. In Iranian society, where self-control is valued, showing anger can produce embarrassment, shame the family, or damage someone's reputation. To avoid embarrassment and to save face, Iranians may agree or say that they understand an outsider, whether they do or not.

In other words, a distinction exists between expressed emotion and felt emotion; a non-Iranian may view Iranians as highly emotional, but expressed emotion is based on the context of the situation in which it is appropriate to show emotions; for example, weeping and crying loudly in a public context such as a funeral. Inner feelings may not match the outer expression because of the importance placed on being polite, pleasant, and keeping social relationships smooth.

Health-care providers should be aware of the manner in which Iranians handle potentially disturbing information. In general, at the beginning of any health-care encounter, the provider should take time to "warm up" with social conversation before "getting down to business." Any kind of bad news must be handled carefully by revealing it gently and gradually, in several meetings if possible, or only to the family spokesperson. A person should never be given bad news alone, for example, being informed of a death or serious diagnosis.

Among more traditional Iranians, men and women do not hold hands or show affection toward each other in public. However, women often show affection for women and men for men, by walking hand in hand or greeting each other with a kiss on each cheek. In greeting acquaintances, some Iranians place the right hand on the chest and make a slight bow or extend a handshake. Strangers and health-care providers are greeted with both arms held at the sides or with a handshake. A slight bow or nod while shaking hands shows respect. Iranians generally stand when someone enters a room for the first time or when someone leaves. It is appropriate to offer something with both hands, which shows respect. Crossing one's legs when sitting is acceptable, but slouching in a chair or stretching one's legs toward another is considered offensive; it is considered rude to show the sole of one's foot. Beckoning is done by waving the fingers with the palm down. Tilting the head up quickly means "no." Tilting the head to the side means "what?" and tilting it down means "yes." Extending the thumb (like "thumbs up") is considered a vulgar sign. Health-care providers should refrain from using nonverbal behaviors that may be offensive to Iranians. Nonverbal communication among acculturated immigrants resembles that of Americans.

As in Mediterranean cultures, personal distance is generally closer than that of Americans or northern Europeans. The strength of the relationship does not alter communication distance, but it does affect how freely participants touch each other. For example, frequently touching one's sister and expressing emotions in conversation is acceptable, but this would not be done with a stranger. However, the greater the degree of acculturation, the more Iranians' behavior resembles that of Americans; although with health-care providers, respect for role and education might be demonstrated by keeping a wide distance.

Iranians maintain intense eye contact between intimates and equals of the same gender, but traditional Iranians tend to avoid eye contact with each other. Younger people and those of lower status do not sustain eye contact with those they perceive as being older or of higher status. When Iranians speak, smiling and using the arms and hands help to convey the message and to increase the expressiveness.

TEMPORAL RELATIONSHIPS

Temporal relationships are a combination of present and future orientations. The ideal is to maintain a balance between enjoying life to the fullest on a daily basis while saving enough money to ensure a comfortable future. Signs of daily gratification include intense family relationships and frequent visits, small trips, fashionable clothing, and proper meals. Financial planning, savings, and the importance of education demonstrate looking ahead.

With respect to health promotion, the future orientation enhances the effectiveness of health education. At the same time, a fatalistic theme in many Iranians' beliefs may hinder their understanding of teaching about risk reduction and health promotion.

Economic and social factors in Iran, especially scarce resources and virtually nonexistent competition,

make the theme of "time is money" meaningless in business. Iranians are not clock-watchers; rather, they are mood and feeling oriented. However, acculturation to American society brings with it timeliness and intense competition to sell goods and services.

Guests may arrive one to several hours after a social engagement begins. Thus, a party may last far into the night with guests arriving throughout the evening. While social time is flexible, Iranians meet the social expectations for timeliness in work and appointments.

FORMAT FOR NAMES

Iranians refrain from calling older people by their first names. In highly traditional families, privacy demands that husbands do not mention their wives' first names to other men. Close friends and children may be called by their first names by family members, but others should not do so. Shaking hands with a child shows respect to the parents, but a man should wait for a woman to extend her hand first. One is expected to greet every member of the family with a handshake. Health-care providers should heed nonverbal cues and greet Iranians in culturally congruent ways.

Family Roles and Organization

HEAD OF HOUSEHOLD AND GENDER ROLES

Iranian culture is patriarchal and hierarchical. The father rules the family and expects obedience and submission from family members. In the father's absence, the oldest son has authority. Families were traditionally large in Iran, with male children being highly desirable. Today, more Iranian families resemble the American norm. As a father ages, he may give property, the business, and control to the oldest son. In more traditional families, older male siblings have the authority to make decisions about younger siblings, even in the father's presence. However, this hierarchy is more flexible in cosmopolitan families. Siblings are taught from an early age to rely on each other for support, and sibling relationships are deep, trusting, and lively. Health-care providers should never underestimate the power of this hierarchy, or the family in general, in decision making. Individuals usually cannot or will not make decisions.

Iranian men see their role as protecting and providing for the family, managing the finances, and dealing with matters outside the home. Women are expected to maintain the home; even working women may place their priorities on the family and home and do the cooking, cleaning, and laundry. Until the social reforms of the 1960s in Iran, women were legally expected to be obedient and submissive to their husbands, who had the right to correct them and used this right frequently.

Women were traditionally expected to marry and bear sons as quickly as possible, although this is now changing. In traditional families, both daughters and sons stay at home until married, and in rural areas marriages are often arranged. In urban families in Iran and the United States, young people are free to select their own marriage partners, but families usually want to approve because of the importance of marriage alliances between families. Husbands are often five or more years older than their wives.

In the United States, stress occurs in Iranian families when men perceive that they have lost their power, particularly when they cannot regain their former social status. Many men complain that because of retirement, unemployment, or low-prestige jobs, their families no longer respect or obey them.

PRESCRIPTIVE, RESTRICTIVE, AND TABOO BEHAVIORS FOR CHILDREN AND ADOLESCENTS

In Iran, children in rural areas are just as responsible for the family economy as adults, but their rights as children are not well delineated. In urban families, Iranian children have the same rights as children in the Western world.

In general, immigrant Iranian families are child oriented. Parents pay a lot of attention to their children and are willing to sacrifice for their welfare, especially for their higher education. Children are expected to be loyal to their families and behave respectfully toward their elders. Manners are considered important even outside the home, where children are expected to be clean and well behaved and to refrain from rowdiness. Children are taught from an early age to avoid eating if no one else has yet been served at a meal, and never to speak rudely to elders. Girls are expected to behave and dress more modestly than boys, especially as they approach adolescence. Children and teens are usually included in adult gatherings. Young children are rarely left with babysitters.

Taboo behaviors for teens in Iran and in the United States differ only in degree and intensity. In Iran, parents are concerned about smoking, drugs, alcohol, and sex in that order. Young women are expected to remain virgins until they marry, but sexual activity by men outside marriage is tolerated. Dating is not allowed in the most traditional families, but this varies depending on ethnic group, length of time in the United States, and location.

While many adolescents in the United States resemble their non-Iranian peers in dress and outward behavior, they often behave more respectfully toward family members, particularly the elderly and other highly respected individuals. The fear of shaming the family and losing face in public acts as strong social constraints. For example, adolescents are unlikely to express their anger to parents or teachers, preferring instead to be silent, because showing respect is more important than acting on the aggressive impulse; however, it is acceptable to express anger toward peers.

Adolescents are often caught in a dilemma, pulled between their parents' attempts to maintain control and instill Iranian heritage and values, and their own desire to be like their American peers. Some who came to the United States at younger ages tend to become more American than American teens, retaining only faint remnants of popular Iranian culture, whereas those who

came at older ages—and are, therefore, likely to have developed a well-formed ego and personality—adjust more effectively to a bicultural identity.

FAMILY GOALS AND PRIORITIES

The family is the most important institution in Iranian culture. Family members often live close to each other so they can visit whenever possible. Most do not like to be isolated and, therefore, maintain strong intergenerational involvement with grandmothers, mothers, and children in the domestic sphere, and with male family members who are often employed in the family business. Families are child oriented, and a childless couple is considered incomplete. Iranians share their daily life difficulties; the elderly often function as counselors, because many Iranians are uncomfortable discussing their problems with someone outside the family circle.

The primary goal of family life is to ensure the well being and continuation of the family. Upholding the family's name is of great importance. Families desire good and well-educated children, safe and secure jobs, economic security, and social acceptance. If they are able, parents help to support their children financially throughout their lives by providing assistance with educational expenses, home buying, or starting businesses.

Iranians who live far from the support of their extended family members may experience a great deal of stress. Some Iranians complain about lack of close social ties in the United States, stating that they miss their families and old friends. Some socialize mainly or only with family members, stating that they have no "real" friends in the United States. They complain that Americans do not relate to and care for each other as Iranians do, giving as examples the "lack of closeness in families" and "lack of respect for old people" in American families. In other cases where many family members remain in Iran, relationships other than blood relationships, such as a network of friends, may define the extended family. Families gather for important events such as visiting a sick person, funerals, mourning days, **Norooz**, births, weddings, or **Eid** (celebration or commemoration of one of several religious holidays). The power of the family is based on supportive relationships among its members. Relationships among kin and kinlike friends are more important than any other social alignment.

Some Iranians have clothing that is only worn inside the home, and they change into these clothes when they get home. Often, they remove their shoes at the door and wear slippers. Outside the home, they tend to dress conservatively, but more traditional or religious women in the United States may choose to avoid bright colors, cover their arms and legs, and conceal their heads with head covers or scarves (**hejab**). In Iran, these coverings are mandatory, not a matter of choice. However, there is great variety in dress, depending on age and tradition. Many Iranians dress stylishly, valuing a good personal appearance in clothing, household furnishings, and decorations.

Age is a sign of experience, worldliness, and knowledge. Thus, regardless of kinship or relationship, an elder is treated with respect. When grandparents reach an age where they can no longer care for themselves, they live with and are cared for by the family. There are few nursing homes in Iran, and they are viewed negatively. Caring for the elderly is an obligation.

Respect for the elderly may be shown in various ways, including giving them attention, asking for their advice, or even agreeing (or being silent) when elders voice an opinion with which younger people disagree. In essence, although one may not appreciate the older person's wisdom, one is bound to respect them because of their age. Respect for age is shown not only to grandparents but also to aunts, uncles, older siblings, and neighbors.

Despite their esteemed role within the Iranian family, elders in the United States who do not speak English may feel lonely and isolated when adult children work and grandchildren are in school. Loneliness and isolation among elderly people are particularly common in neighborhoods where transportation is unavailable or walking is unsafe.

While social status in Iran is inherited, there is no caste system. One is usually born into the upper class, but one can ascend the class hierarchy through higher education and attainment of professional status. In addition, such valued individual characteristics as nobility, generosity, and courage are sources of social status. Parents often try to arrange marriages for their children with children of families of higher status. Sometimes marriages are arranged within the kin group (cousins) to maintain marital harmony or to cement family relationships.

While growth of the middle class in Iran was rapid in the 1970s, the enormous expense of getting out of Iran since the revolution prohibited all but the wealthy or professional middle class from immigrating to the United States. Rural people and those with limited financial resources could not afford plane tickets or lacked money to bribe officials.

ALTERNATIVE LIFESTYLES

Iranians are conservative about male-female relationships and may discourage dating. Older and more traditional Iranians may be uncomfortable with unrelated members of the opposite sex. Most Iranians strongly disapprove of the American practice of living together before marriage. While divorce is viewed negatively, its rate has been increasing among Iranians in the United States, partly as a result of the increase in intercultural marriages. Rezaian (1989) found that intraculturally married Iranians reported more marital satisfaction than Iranians married to Americans or intraculturally married Americans. This may be due to Iranians' greater emotional expressiveness and shared frame of reference, which can improve communication. Cultural mores also advocate ignoring or denying minor marital discord and acceptance of suffering for the sake of maintaining family stability.

In Iran, out-of-wedlock teen pregnancy is neither talked about nor prevalent, although it can have a devastating outcome. If it happens in the United States, it may be taken care of quietly to preserve the face of the family.

While homosexuality undoubtedly occurs in Iranians as frequently as in any other group, it is highly stigmatized and not discussed; gays or lesbians remain in the closet. Since 1979, when the legal and religious systems became synonymous, homosexuality, which is considered unnatural and sacrilegious, has been a capital offense punishable by death (Clark, 1995). Members of an Iranian gay support group in the San Francisco Bay area use anonymity and pseudonyms to protect themselves from potential physical harm by fundamentalist groups. However, in certain areas of the United States, younger Iranians are increasingly tolerant of alternative lifestyles. While there is considerable social and family pressure to marry, more people feel free to remain single, celibate, or both.

Workforce Issues

CULTURE IN THE WORKPLACE

The greatest difficulty faced by Iranian immigrant health-care providers is acquiring legal residency. This is followed by finding a position that is not too damaging to the person's self-esteem. Often, to satisfy the need for financial stability, employment of any sort may be accepted, which can lead to the person experiencing continual bitterness or sadness.

Iranians perceive ethnic bias toward them from many people in the United States, including clients and coworkers. This varies with location; for example, bias is much less evident in such highly multicultural areas as the San Francisco Bay area and is more evident in culturally homogenous areas. Common reactions include overt or subtle hostility, condescension, total lack of acknowledgment, or sarcasm. For example, one of the authors (Hafizi) encountered a physician who asked about her national origin, then responded, "Is this one of those countries that we like these days?" More acculturated immigrant professionals respond flexibly in the workplace. For example, when this same author perceives that a client is uncomfortable with her background or overtly expresses dislike, she uses ta'arof and becomes "super efficient." Her speech becomes polite and formal; she enters the room only to do clinically necessary tasks, and performs them so carefully that the client cannot complain that she is a "bad" or "rude" nurse. However, while her technical care is excellent, she is not satisfied because this approach lacks interpersonal rapport.

Iranian health-care workers strive for a balance of work, family, and leisure. If one spouse has to work, the wife is always the one who stays home. In some immigrant families, when the wife finds a job before the husband this creates problems for the entire family, despite the understanding that her employment is vital to the family's financial stability.

ISSUES RELATED TO AUTONOMY

In the workplace, Iranians are competitive and strive for a sense of personal accomplishment. They appreciate the importance of punctuality. Graduates of Iranian high schools are well educated in a broad curriculum with a sound science base. In contrast to the practical applications emphasized in American professional schools, professional education in Iran is formal, theory based, and rigid in nature, with an emphasis on memorization. Practice is obtained through on-the-job training.

Most Iranian health-care providers speak English, but newcomers may not be familiar with American slang. An ongoing stressor is the condescending attitudes directed at anyone who speaks English with a strong accent. For example, a nurse with a master's degree described her first year in the United States as follows:

I was seen as an ignorant nurse's aide who couldn't even speak English. One nurse used to follow me around, checking everything I did. I resented being treated that way, and my own self-esteem suffered (Lipson, 1992: 16).

Biocultural Ecology

SKIN COLOR AND OTHER BIOLOGICAL VARIATIONS

Iranians are a mixture of foreigners who invaded the area throughout Persian history and the ethnic groups who currently inhabit Iran. As white Indo-Europeans, their skin tones and facial features resemble those of other Mediterranean and Southern European groups. Their coloring ranges from blue or green eyes, light brown hair, and fair skin to nearly black eyes, black hair, and brown skin. Because of the variations in skin color, health-care professionals may need to assess jaundice and anemia in Iranians by examining the sclera and oral mucosa rather than by relying solely on skin assessments.

DISEASES AND HEALTH CONDITIONS

In Iran, the 2001 birth rate was 30 per 1000 people, and the infant mortality rate was 18 per 1000 infants, although some sources estimate that the infant mortality rate is 42 per 1000. Heat and humidity in some provinces provide fertile ground for the spread of cholera, including new and mutant strains. Malaria is widespread in Baluchistan (Southeast), with serological test results sometimes showing more than one strain in a single client. In rural areas that lack standardized sanitary systems, viral and bacterial meningitis, hookworm, and gastrointestinal dysenteries caused by parasites, are prevalent. Hypertension is widespread, with 2 million cases reported in Tehran, or one-sixth of its population. Ischemic heart disease is rising, and the rise is generally perceived as being related to the stress of living with daily uncertainties. Health-care providers should screen newer immigrants for diseases and illnesses common in their home country (Iranian Health Department, personal communication, April 14, 2001).

The most common health problems in Iran are linked to underdevelopment, the recent economic downturn, and lack of coordination of scarce but available funds and resources. For example, malnutrition (caused by protein and vitamin deficiencies), hepatitis A and B (caused by poor sanitary conditions, such as poor aseptic technique, or public health measures), rising rates of tuberculosis and syphilis, genetic problems (due to interfamily marriages), and blood dyscrasias. Interfamily marriage used to be common; however, increasing urbanization and scientific data has increased awareness of potential genetic diseases or birth defects resulting from these marriages, and has decreased the prevalence of this practice. Diseases and birth defects associated with marriages between cousins include epilepsy, blindness, several forms of anemia, and hemophilia.

The head of Iran's Institute of Mental Health estimates that 1.2 million people in Iran suffer from acute psychological illnesses. Forty to sixty percent of all Iranians suffer from an episode of mental illness that requires specialized medical intervention. The prevalence of diabetes is 1.5 percent, but about 50 percent of those diagnosed are unaware of having this disease, despite clear symptoms. Thalassemias, prevalent in northern and eastern provinces, are now being addressed through premarital screening for carriers and through genetic counseling. Individuals are also tested for vitamin B_{12} or folic acid deficiencies linked to an enzyme deficiency (Iranian Health Department, personal communication, April 14, 2001). Mediterranean glucose-6-phosphate dehydrogenase (G-6-PD) deficiency is also common among people of Iranian heritage, and can precipitate a hemolytic crisis when fava beans are eaten; it affects drug metabolism, such as increasing sensitivity to primaquine.

Allergies to plant pollens and air pollution induce pulmonary distress and exacerbate ischemic heart disease. Iranians in the United States also experience these problems. In the United States, many Iranians experience stress-related health problems from culture conflict and loss, homesickness for family and relatives, and the previous conditions of war. Although northern California Iranians in Lipson's (1992) study were generally healthy, many expressed their ongoing stress somatically, through intermittent general symptoms or physical discomfort. Several articulated a direct connection between their worries and illness; for example, three of the first seven people interviewed had suffered from ulcers, and attributed their "stomach problems" to their "worries" and "troubles." Others complained of headaches, backaches, a racing heart, or other manifestations of anxiety or depression. Iranians often focus their acute generalized stress on the alimentary system, attributing illness or its severity to something that has been eaten.

High-Risk Behaviors

Iranians' high-risk behaviors are similar to those in the general American population; however, they may occur less frequently in more traditional groups. Smoking is more prevalent in Iran than in the United States among both men and women. In general, health education, through the media and the influence of their children, encourages many Iranian immigrants to quit smoking.

Some alcohol and street-drug abuse occurs in the Iranian immigrant population, but the rate is no higher than that of the population at large. Alcohol is prohibited by the **Qur'an** (Holy Book), although many Iranians are not religious and drink socially, a few to excess. In Iran, the most popular street drug among the older generation is opium, traditionally used for medicinal purposes. In some people, years of opium use can create both psychological and physical addiction. Younger Iranians, who prefer heroin in Iran, take drugs for the same variety of reasons that American young people do, with availability and felt need determining continuation of use. Family responses to drug use range from complete support of the family member to disownment.

In the United States, alcohol is more generally accepted than in Iran. In some immigrants, abuse is related to a low level of acculturation and a sense of helplessness often experienced by displaced people. In other cases, Iranian men demonstrate their "masculinity" by being able to "hold" their liquor. This need to assert masculinity, combined with poor self-esteem, increases the risk of alcohol addiction.

HEALTH-CARE PRACTICES

Iranian children and young adults are more physically active than their elders, and exercise as frequently as their peers in nonimmigrant groups. Soccer remains popular in Iran; some men continue to play soccer in the United States and encourage their children to play. Soccer promotes family fun and closeness, and helps counteract the negative effects of peer pressure on children. Depending on their traditionalism, women may confine their exercise to housework or walking, or they may jog, swim, or do aerobics.

In Iran, seat belts were previously of lower priority than road conditions, but legislation was passed requiring seat belt use on intercity highways. However, the law was enforced only for a short period of time until recently, when a media campaign for wearing seat belts has encouraged enforcement of the legislation. In the United States, Iranians generally comply with seat belt and child restraint laws, valuing the safety of their children.

Diet is an important part of maintaining health and is described in the next section. Health-care providers need to encourage positive health-seeking behaviors among their Iranian clients by using culturally congruent approaches, and by carefully explaining the detrimental physical and psychological effects of smoking, recreational drug use, and excessive consumption of alcohol.

Nutrition

MEANING OF FOOD

Food is a symbol of hospitality for Iranians. They prepare their best food for guests and insist that guests eat several servings. More food is prepared and presented than is needed to actually feed guests to demonstrate lavish hospitality. Iranian hosts go all out to make guests comfortable, serving them first or giving them the most comfortable seats. If guests arrive at times other than mealtime, tea is offered, usually with such snacks as fruits and nuts. The courteous guest, however, should refuse "to trouble" the host by politely refusing tea or food at least once; when accepting food, guests should first offer it to other guests before taking any themselves.

COMMON FOODS AND FOOD RITUALS

Iranian food is flavorful and takes hours to prepare. Presentation is important. At any given table, there is usually a pleasing mixture of foods of different colors and ingredients, composed of a balance of **garm** (hot) and **sard** (cold) (see following section on Dietary Practices for Health Promotion). Tea and fruit are served for dessert after each meal. Iranians prefer to use only the freshest foods, although in some cases, cost is a factor in their using some dried herbs. Canned, frozen, and fast foods are perceived to have less nutritional value and contain preservatives that can affect health. Eating fast food may be less common because of concerns related to nutritional value and cost.

Hot tea is the most popular drink among Iranians. The most common starchy foods are rice and wheat bread. The art of preparing rice is the measuring stick against which teens and young women are judged as they complete their training in the kitchen. Long-grained, fluffy, and white rice is preferred. Bread is usually baked flat like **lavash** or pita. Corn and potatoes are used, but less favored. Beans and legumes, for example, lentils, pinto, mung, kidney, lima and green beans, and split and black-eyed peas, make up a fairly high proportion of the dietary intake and are commonly used in rice mixtures.

Dairy products are dietary staples, particularly eggs, milk, yogurt, and feta cheese, as well as dairy by-products, such as **doog** (yogurt soda) and **kashk** (milk by-product). Favorite meats are beef, chicken, fish, and lamb. Shellfish is sometimes eaten. Fresh fruit is always found in Iranian houses. Green leafy vegetables are used in cooking, and herbs such as parsley, cilantro (coriander), dill, fenugreek, tarragon, mint, savory, and green onions are served fresh at a meal.

Islam has a strict set of dietary prescriptions, **halal**, and proscriptions, **haram**. Slaughter of poultry, beef, and lamb must be done ritually to make the meat **halal**. Strict Muslims avoid pork and alcoholic beverages; a few avoid shellfish. Historically, pork was prohibited for hygienic reasons. As food habits are passed down through the generations, avoidance of pork and alcohol has become a mixture of cultural and religious traditions.

Generally, food is eaten with the right hand, and food or objects are passed with the right hand alone or with both hands. Traditional or older people may be most comfortable sitting on the floor with food on large platters in the center of a large tablecloth. Health-care providers may need to make adjustments to accommodate traditional food practices of Iranians, making provisions for the family to bring food from home if the client prefers. Having familiar food is much appreciated and assists in recovery.

DIETARY PRACTICES FOR HEALTH PROMOTION

Based on humoral theory, Iranians classify foods into one of two categories, **garm**, hot, and **sard**, cold, which sometimes correspond to high-calorie and low-calorie foods. The key is balance. The belief is that too much of one category can cause symptoms of being "overheated" or "chilled." Such symptoms are treated by eating food from the opposite group. For example, becoming overheated, sweating, itching, and rashes may result from eating too many hot foods, such as walnuts, onions, garlic, spices, honey, or candy. Or the stomach may become chilled, causing dizziness, weakness, and vomiting, after eating too many cold foods, such as grapes, rhubarb, plums, cucumbers, or yogurt or from drinking beer. One of the authors was served fish and green salad at a meal, after which her hosts strongly recommended that she eat some dates with tea to offset the possibility of developing **sardie**, a digestive problem from ingesting too much cold food. She was perceived to be susceptible because of her light complexion. Women are believed to be more susceptible to **sardie** than **garmie**, a digestive problem from too much hot food. Health-care providers may need to incorporate Iranian foods and dietary practices into health teaching to improve compliance with special dietary restrictions.

NUTRITIONAL DEFICIENCIES AND FOOD LIMITATIONS

Today, because of economic problems in Iran, certain foods are unavailable, with a corresponding increased incidence of protein and vitamin deficiencies. The emphasis of food has slightly changed from socializing around food to satisfying hunger. Because the Iranian immigrant diet is balanced and healthy, nutritional deficiencies are not usually a problem for those who have been in the United States for some time.

Almost all ingredients used in Iranian cooking can be found in the United States. When the cost of certain vegetables and herbs is too high, some families grow them in their backyards. Most commonly used medicinal herbs are available in Iranian or other middle eastern grocery stores. Iranians are not restricted from any foods whose absence might cause nutritional problems.

Pregnancy And Childbearing Practices

FERTILITY PRACTICES AND VIEWS TOWARD PREGNANCY

In rural areas of Iran, traditional beliefs and practices are influenced by Galenic or humoral medicine, particularly with regard to hot and cold temperament and the conditions of pregnancy and birth. Conception is explained as "the man contributes the seed and the woman provides the vessel in which the seed grows" (Good, 1980: 149). Menstrual blood is believed to be ritually unclean and physically polluting to the body and must be discharged monthly. Menstruating women are not allowed to touch holy objects or to have intercourse. Menstruation is also considered a time of great fragility when a woman should not exercise or shower exces-

sively, because these activities might cause a hemorrhage. At the end of the menses, the woman must wash and purify herself thoroughly before partaking in any religious rituals.

Before the 1979 revolution, birth control was rarely used in rural areas of Iran because having many children assured the continued financial success of the family. Women were concerned about the health of their uteri; thus, home remedies for infertility are often focused on improving the state of the uterus as a "vessel" of conception. Infertility was blamed on the woman. Baluch, Al-Shawaf, and Craft (1992) found that reasons for seeking infertility treatment differed for men and women: whereas men sought reproduction to ensure future support, women were fulfilling the social expectation to have babies at an early stage in the marriage.

Contraception is still rarely used in rural areas, but the rationale has changed from "many children assure family financial stability" to the Islamic emphasis on children as the symbol of God's blessing. With the recent population explosion and associated public health and welfare problems, birth control has again been cautiously encouraged. The annual growth rate remains at 3.8 percent, with higher fertility in the rural areas among tribal groups who marry young and have large families. Traditionally, prolonged breast-feeding was often used as a method of contraception.

In cosmopolitan and educated Iranian families, fewer children are the norm; a desirable family size is often three or four children. In the United States, young couples limit families to fewer children, the desirable number being two or three. Current methods used by Iranians to limit conception include the pill, intrauterine devices, and natural methods. Vasectomies are just beginning to gain acceptance.

Pregnancy after marriage is desirable among Iranian women for several reasons. Women believe that their bodies are in a less healthy state and are polluted with excess menstrual blood until they have given birth to a child. A women's prestige is at its height when she delivers her first child, particularly if it is a boy. Delivering the first child relieves anxiety and gives the young wife a more respected and cherished position with her in-laws. Health-care providers should consider these traditional beliefs of some Iranians in health teaching. Providing factual information regarding family planning is one area where health-care professionals can improve family care.

PRESCRIPTIVE, RESTRICTIVE, AND TABOO PRACTICES IN THE CHILDBEARING FAMILY

Food cravings during pregnancy are believed to result from the needs of the fetus for particular foods; thus cravings must be satisfied lest a miscarriage occur from not meeting the fetus's needs. Women avoid fried foods and foods that cause gas; fruits and vegetables are recommended, with special attention to the balance of hot and cold foods. Heavy work is thought to cause a miscarriage. Sexual intercourse is allowed until the last month. The pregnant woman receives considerable support from female kin including relieving the pregnant and postpartum woman of household tasks. This assistance begins in the sixth month and continues until after the birth.

During the birthing process, the woman receives support from her mother, sister, or aunt. In more traditional Iranian families, the father is not usually present at the birth. In the United States, delivery is typical of the dominant society, with some women choosing natural childbirth and involving their husbands fully in the process. However, some women do request analgesia for pain.

The postpartum period for Iranian women is 30 to 40 days. In rural Iran, female kin take primary responsibility for supporting the mother during the postpartum period. Because of the belief in the polluting nature of blood, postpartum women are required to take a ritual bath after they stop bleeding, so they can resume normal religious activities. To strengthen the postpartum woman, a **ghorse kamar** (a brown, flat disk of dried herbs) is mixed with eggs and placed on her lower back a few hours before bathing.

In rural Iran, postpartum diet and care are influenced by the need to balance hot and cold. Such hot foods as pistachio nuts and eggs are given to postpartum women to strengthen their bodies and combat **sardie**. New mothers avoid cold water for bathing, ablutions, or cleaning, although they now bathe sooner than the traditional first 30 days. Baby boys are considered "hotter" than baby girls, and mothers of sons are considered to have hotter bodies, hotter milk, and hotter temperaments than mothers of girls. Mothers of girls are given a mixture of honey and other nutrients, an herbal extract called **taranjebin**, to raise their bodily heat to ensure that the next child is a boy. Some families keep an infant home for the first 40 days; by that time, it is believed that the baby is strong enough to fight off environmental pathogens. The baby is given a ritual bath between the 10th and 40th days. Health-care providers should ask the childbearing family about prescriptive, restrictive, and taboo cultural practices that they customarily follow, and incorporate these practices in the care.

Death Rituals

DEATH RITUALS AND EXPECTATIONS

In discussing the withdrawal of life support of a terminal client, some families may demand that strenuous efforts be made to prolong life, so it is important to assess each family individually. To discuss termination of life support with a practicing Muslim, the health-care provider can begin the conversation by noting God's will for human beings and His power over our destiny. This discussion can be followed by a dialogue about life and death as necessary steps toward immortal life in heaven. Muslims may only need a gentle reminder that death is not a termination of life, but rather the beginning of a new and better life. However, Iranians may oppose stopping life support, viewing it as "playing God," even though they may have no objection to beginning life support, viewing it as the "gift" of medical technology (Klessig, 1992).

When an Iranian person is dying, family members and friends come to be with the patient and family. Among religious Muslims, the deathbed should be turned to face Mecca, so family members can read prayers from the Qur'an to assure that the dying person hears this at the time of death. Because few traditional Muslim cemeteries exist in the United States, some terminally ill traditional Muslims request to return to Iran either to die or be buried.

After death, another Muslim should wash the body in a ritual manner, using soap and water and proceeding from head to toe and front to back. All body orifices must be closed and slightly packed with cotton to prevent leakage of bodily fluids (considered unclean). The final rinse is performed with water. The body is then wrapped in a special white cotton shroud. Prayers and verses from the **Qur'an** are read during the procedure. A non-Muslim health-care provider should wear gloves when touching the body (Klessig, 1992).

There are no specific religious rules against autopsy. However, the body of the dead is to be respected; therefore, the reason for the autopsy must be made clear, and some may still refuse. In Iran, embalming of the dead is not practiced; rather, they are buried directly into the earth to facilitate the transition, from "dust to dust." The shroud is removed from the face, and one side of the face is turned to be in contact with the earth. Cremation is not practiced in Iran.

RESPONSES TO DEATH AND GRIEF

Iranians may express their grief over the death of a loved one by crying, wailing loudly, or even striking themselves or an object. While loss of a loved one is met with expressive and strong grieving and support from family and friends, death is seen as a beginning, not an end, in which the mortal life gives way to the spiritual existence, a cherished state of solidifying one's relationship with God. This "fatalistic" belief, and the belief in the power of God over all His creation, makes "letting go" easier for some families. In general, it seems that Iranians let their loved ones go more easily but grieve longer and more expressively than Americans, who let go less easily but grieve for a shorter period and more privately.

After a Muslim's death, relatives, friends, and acquaintances gather on the 3rd, 7th, and 40th days after the death. Clergy, family, relatives, and friends read prayers. Special foods are served, and grieving may be expressed loudly. Attending a funeral is essential for paying respect to the dead and for offering support to survivors. All Iranians wear black, and women relatives wear little or no makeup. Some believe that the family must pay the deceased's debts, or life after death will be less favorable. If the deceased is young, a more extensive ceremony is held. On the anniversary of the death, the family gathers again to pay respect to the dead. In Iran, money may be set aside to help the needy instead of holding an anniversary ceremony, but relatives still visit to pay their respects, especially on the first anniversary. Spouses or parents visit the grave of their loved ones weekly, generally on a Thursday or Friday.

Spirituality

DOMINANT RELIGION AND USE OF PRAYER

Islam exerted its influence on Iran and its culture in five domains: (1) the domain of temporal focus, (2) the fate of an individual, (3) humoral medicine, (4) dietary laws, and (5) family loyalty (Pliskin, 1987). However, certain norms embedded in Iranian culture transcend religious and ethnic boundaries, such as family loyalty and respect for elderly people.

Specific Muslim practices include prayers, read in the name of one of the 12 **Imams** (predecessors of the Prophet Mohammed), to provide peace of mind or to plead for a miracle. Sometimes, when an important asset needs protection, for example, a house, a child, or a life, a healer is sought to help with a sacrifice to keep the evil eye away. Although most Iranian Muslims in the United States are not ritually strict, devout religious Muslims pray five times daily and need privacy and water for ritual washing. They may fast from sunrise to sundown during Ramadan, although pregnant women and the ill are exempt from fasting. Jewish, Christian, and Baha'i Iranians have religious beliefs and practices similar to those of other ethnic groups. Health-care providers may need to make environmental adjustments that allow Iranian immigrant clients to practice their religious beliefs.

MEANING OF LIFE AND INDIVIDUAL SOURCES OF STRENGTH

An Iranian's understanding of, and outlook on, the world is influenced by national history and social expectations, which give every experience a rich context in which everything and everyone has significance. For religious Iranians of all faiths, belief in and acceptance of God's will is a source of strength and comfort, particularly in times of illness or crisis.

Family relationships and friendships are sources of strength and meaning in life for many individuals. Iranians are highly affiliative, and thrive on social relationships. Close and regular contact with family and friends is both a pleasure and a necessity. Given the importance of the family for providing meaning and strength for Iranians, health-care providers may need to adjust visiting policies in health-care settings to accommodate family and friends.

Family rules and societal norms are another source of strength for Iranians; they provide internal control over behavior, rather than the external control of law enforcement. Religious beliefs are also a source of strength for many Iranians, particularly for the elderly, who might consult a spiritual advisor and become more in tune with God as they come closer to death.

Iran has been called a "grief society," in which sadness, often associated with death, is a strong theme. This theme emerges in Iranian culture; expressions of the tragedies in life are depicted in poetry, art, music, and mythology. A sad person is considered deep, thoughtful, and sensitive, which are valued personality characteristics. Despite a cultural emphasis on sadness and political oppression, people still anticipate a better future and demonstrate drive, hope, and determination.

SPIRITUAL BELIEFS AND HEALTH-CARE PRACTICES

Tagdir, God's will and power over one's fate in life and death, is a common belief among Iranians. This belief fosters a sense of passivity and dependence on a superior force, which may be weaker or less prevalent among better-educated Iranians. Religious beliefs affect health-care beliefs, and are described more fully in the next section. Hafizi's (1990) research also clearly illustrates the integration of religion and health concepts. In the words of this highly educated, devout Muslim man:

> To ask me what health means is to ask me what my worldly outlook is. How I see myself in relation to God, my family, the society as a whole and my relation to my material body. Man is the embodiment of the unworldly spiritual being whereby the body and the spirit work in such a close connection that the two work as one unit. Life then becomes a passage through time. The mortal life represents only one stage of this passage. Death is not a finalization, rather a graduation to a higher level of being. I believe in God and *His* plan for the future. For example, being sick is not having a cold; rather it is not having the vision to deal with the cold (Hafizi, 1990).

Health-Care Practices

HEALTH-SEEKING BELIEFS AND BEHAVIORS

Traditional Iranian health beliefs and therapeutic processes are a combination of three traditions of medicine: Galenic (humoral), Islamic (sacred), and modern biomedicine. In classic humoral theory, illness arises from an imbalance (excess or deficiency) in the basic qualities, for example, of hot and cold or wet and dry. The purpose of treatment is to restore balance. The Galenic-Islamic tradition of humoral medicine is widely practiced throughout Iran, and influences the beliefs of the immigrant population. In Galenic thought, every individual has a distinctive balance of four humors, or **mezaj**, resulting in a unique temperament, or **tabi'at**. Physical and emotional illnesses are caused by an imbalance in humors of the body and mind that may coexist; thus, an emotional upset can cause physical illness and vice versa. Even among immigrants, practices related to the qualities of hot and cold and moist and dry in relation to food and climate are believed to significantly affect health. For example, wetness and wind are avoided; thus, a child's ears are covered on a windy day because cool wind is believed to cause earache or infection. Sacred medicine is from the **Qur'an** and **hadith**, and holy men are considered able to heal. The sacred tradition includes beliefs in the evil eye and **jinns** as disease agents, as well as healing by means of manipulating impurity. For those who believe strongly in God's control over their fate, a holy man can heal by writing prayers on a piece of paper, which can be placed in water and drunk or burned and the smoke inhaled to incorporate the prayers.

Health is a diffuse concept deeply rooted in Iranian culture, an idea central to the governing of daily chores and the routines of one's social and personal life. Illness is discussed and challenged, with advice solicited to remedy the ailment. For example, a balanced intake of hot and cold foods to maintain health is a daily consideration, although it may be practiced subconsciously and not articulated (Hafizi, 1990).

Among Iranians, **narahati** is a general term used to express a wide range of undifferentiated, unpleasant emotional or physical feelings, such as feeling depressed, uneasy, nervous, disappointed, or not fully well. **Narahati** is often expressed by silence, sullenness, crying, or avoidance of food. Iranians often somatize in a subconscious effort to communicate **narahati** or distress that cannot be otherwise expressed verbally. By somatizing, they construct an illness that is culturally sanctioned and socially understood. The source can be personal, social, spiritual, or psychological. Somatization also allows the individuals to distance themselves from the actual problem, while putting the responsibility and focus on the metaphoric body. Because Iranians generally shy away from overt expressions of "personal self" and the "somatic self" becomes a focal point in the health-care encounter. When **narahati** is seen as being caused by fright, the evil eye, or **jinns**, it may be treated with religious cures. If it is seen as caused by problems of blood, nerves, or humoral imbalance, it is treated with herbs or biomedicine.

Another cultural syndrome is **ghalbam gerefteh** (**narahatiye qalb**, or distress of the heart). Heart distress may be expressed as a feeling that the heart is being squeezed and can range in severity from mild excitation of the heart or palpitations to fainting and heart attack (Good, 1977). Good's (1977) classic study in rural Iran found that women of all ages represented two-thirds of those who reported experiencing heart distress, the same proportion found in Lipson's (1992) study of immigrants to the United States. Heart distress was attributed to great sadness, being homesick, or having problems that are overwhelming or seem insoluble. One woman stated, "I get it when I read Persian newspapers about the situation in Iran."

A widespread belief among Iranians is that fright or being startled by bad news negatively affects health. Symptoms caused by fright include extreme fatigue with chills and fever, as well as more severe symptoms. A client might be given salt or a mixture of hard sugar candy and water, taken to a physician, or be given herbal medicines or a religious cure. In other instances, a sudden ailment or symptom of puzzling origin may be attributed to the evil eye, or **cheshm-i-bad**, which is the belief that the eyes of another person can cause illness. **Cheshm-i-bad** can be unintentional (enthusiastically complimenting someone without saying "In the name of God") or intentional (cast out of jealousy or enmity). Some Iranians burn **esfand** (wild rue) in the fireplace to prevent it; more acculturated and younger people state that only their grandparents or rural people believe in "the evil eye."

Cheshm-i-bad and other folk syndromes are better understood by viewing the body in the context of its social and supernatural environment. Similar to somatizing, which distances an individual from the actual problem, **cheshm-i-bad** attributes illness to an outside person or force. In reality, the evil eye gives meaning to an occurrence of puzzling origin. It puts the blame on someone or something other than the client.

Hafizi's research (1990) found that Iranians' concepts of health represented two of Smith's (1983) four domains: the clinical view (health as absence of disease) and the adaptive view (health as the ability to cope successfully). These are integrated in a view of healthy human beings as physiochemical and sociopsychological systems able to cope successfully with the changing world. This health-illness paradigm is characterized by a dynamic relationship between the individual and the environment, a harmonious exchange between nature's available resources, and a person's capability to use these sources. Thus, health is not achieved through a preplanned, regimented schedule of diet, exercise, and therapy, but is a daily way of life marked by new demands and adaptations (Hafizi, 1990). Similar health concepts were found in elderly Iranian immigrants in Sweden (Emami et al., 2000).

Iranians accept both biomedical diagnoses and cultural illness categories. The concept of the body is viewed in relation to its total environment—society, God, and the supernatural. When someone has a discomforting symptom, often they are first asked whether they ate something that did not agree with their **mezaj** (humoral temperament). If the answer is no, then other causes are explored.

RESPONSIBILITY FOR HEALTH CARE

Iranians often seek relatively immediate relief or cures from the health-care system and may "shop around" until they find a provider they like. At the same time, they may seek advice from those who can suggest herbal remedies. Herbal remedies are used primarily to relieve symptoms. For example, mint tea and cilantro seeds are used to promote relaxation and sleep. Thus, Iranians' conceptions of illness are a combination of Western biomedical categories and culturally shaped explanatory models and syndromes.

To promote health, many Iranians watch their diets, particularly food choices and preparation; for example, including fruit and avoiding excessive fat and canned, frozen, or otherwise processed foods. They may be careful not to eat incompatible foods at the same meal, with an emphasis on balancing hot and cold. Iranians also protect their health by getting enough rest and exercise, by taking vitamins, and by keeping warm or dressing adequately. To introduce preventive education, Iranians can be reminded that prevention has always been and still remains a focal part of humoral medicine in Iran, and that Iranians have always unconsciously practiced prevention.

Iranians practice self-medication and use prescription and over-the-counter medications, as well as homemade herbal remedies. Antibiotics, codeine-based analgesics, mood-altering drugs in the benzodiazepine family (e.g., diazepam [Valium]), and intramuscular vitamins are available over the counter in Iran, and immigrants often bring these medications with them to the United States. Thus they are less cautious with these medications than Americans, who live under Food and Drug Administration regulations. Self-adjusting their dosage of prescribed medications is not uncommon in the United States, particularly when finances are a problem. American health-care providers should carefully consider the dosage and type of medication prescribed based on these self-medicating practices; for example, because of previous overuse, a first-generation antibiotic may not be strong enough for some Iranians.

When Iranians are ill, they are more inclined to be passive and taken care of by health-care providers and family members. When Iranians are hospitalized, family members are expected to visit frequently or to be present continuously until the client is discharged from the hospital or fully functioning again. Self-care is a less familiar concept to Iranians because, in Iran, the authoritative doctor describes the course of treatment. Even among acculturated immigrants in the United States, there is potential for misunderstanding because people rely on their cultural styles of coping in threatening situations like illness and hospitalization. For example, nurses on a neurosurgery unit requested consultation regarding an older male Iranian client because his wife and adult children were in constant attendance and demanded that the nurses take care of his every need immediately. The nurses did not understand that the family's unceasing attention to the client and their constant demands on staff were culturally appropriate ways of showing their care and concern. If the family did not insist on immediate care or left the patient alone, they would have been considered neglectful and unloving. Many Iranian clients do not seem motivated to practice self-care. This does not mean, however, that they do not care about their recovery. Rather, because of strong family values, self-care should be implemented by encouraging family members to assist with care of the sick person.

FOLK PRACTICES

Herbal remedies are used in a complementary manner with medications. Iranians often take herbal remedies recommended by relatives or friends to prevent illness or to treat symptoms. These remedies became increasingly popular in postrevolutionary Iran because of the economic embargo and scarcity of biomedical supplies; pharmacies and *atary* (herb shops) stock packaged herbal medications in tea bags, capsules, and creams. With the increasing popularity of herbal remedies, farm areas have been dedicated to the cultivation of plants for medicinal use.

Depending on the person's orientation, both in the United States and Iran, herbal remedies are used as either adjuncts to Western biomedicine or the first line of treatment for an illness. Therefore, American health-care providers should ask if herbal therapies are being used in addition to prescribed medications. Many Iranians believe that complementary treatments are more effective than a single treatment. The literature does not report any research data that contraindicate combining Iranian herbal and Western medications.

Common herbal remedies include dried flowers, seeds, leaves, and berries, steeped in hot or cold water and drunk for a variety of purposes, such as digestive problems, "cleaning the blood or kidneys," coughs, aches and pains, fevers, nerves or fear. Some common herbal medications include **gol-i-gov zabon** (dried foxglove flowers) for an imbalance in the digestive system or nervous upsets, which is sometimes taken with **nabat**, a concentrated sugar (Lipson, 1992). **Khakshir** (flat, brown rocket seed) is used for stomach problems and "dirty blood"; **razianeh** is used for halitosis; quince seeds are sucked for sore throats; and **sedr** prevents and treats dandruff. **Neshasteh** (wheat starch) is combined with boiling water and drunk for sore throats or coughs and also used to stop diarrhea. Mint extracts are used to relieve excess stomach gas. Plant extracts are popular both in Iran and the United States; for example, a plant called **shatareh** is thought to cure fever.

BARRIERS TO HEALTH CARE

Language and financial problems for some of the newest Iranian immigrants limit access to health care. For example, when a man with severely bleeding hemorrhoids telephoned a doctor and attempted to describe his problem as "pain in my back," he was told to come in the next day (Lipson, 1992). Lack of health insurance is a major barrier to health care. In Iran, health care is governmentally and privately financed, and the concept of health insurance does not hold the same significance as it holds in the United States.

CULTURAL RESPONSES TO HEALTH AND ILLNESS

On the whole, Iranians are more expressive about their pain than are Americans. Some justify suffering in light of later rewards. For example, the grandmother of a young women with a slow-growing brain tumor consoled herself and her granddaughter with the statement that suffering in this world assures her a place in heaven after death.

Mental illness is highly stigmatized among Iranians and is thought to be genetic. If a family member has a mental illness it is likely to be called a "neurological disorder" to avoid stigmatizing the family. Psychotherapeutic help may be avoided either because of stigma or because it is perceived as irrelevant. Bagheri (1992) stated that Iranians tend to pay more attention to somatic symptoms when under emotional stress, and consider psychopharmacological treatment most effective; such treatment also results in a higher rate of compliance.

Other than major mental illness, Iranian immigrants experience numerous stressors related to resettlement in a foreign culture. Health-care providers often do not recognize the subtle and not-so-subtle stressors their immigrant clients experience, such as daily necessities made difficult by financial strain or by accented or inadequate English. As measured by the Health Opinion Survey, 44 percent of Lipson's (1992) newer immigrant interviewees experienced medium or high stress compared with 14 percent of the longer-settled group. With reference to mood, about 35 percent of the informants answered "yes" when asked if they considered themselves to be "nervous," and about the same percentage stated that they did not have "peace of mind." The reasons given were mainly problems with life in the United States, missing family members, or concerns about relatives back home.

Despite these problems, most Iranian immigrants, like other middle eastern immigrants (Lipson & Meleis, 1983), stated that they were not likely to seek counseling or psychiatric help, preferring to discuss their problems with family members or to solve their problems by themselves. However, psychotherapy and counseling are becoming more accepted and perceived as helpful, particularly in dealing with children.

While mental disability is less tangible and understood, physical disability has received recent attention in Iran. Before 1979, the disabled were hidden at home because they brought stigma on the family and because few treatment options were available. The World Health Organization's Year of the Disabled stimulated Iran to institute civil rights for the disabled, guaranteeing access to health-care services and facilities. Today rehabilitation such as physical therapy and music therapy is embraced as the way to bring the disabled into the mainstream. Attitudes toward the disabled among Iranian immigrants depend partly on when they left Iran and vary from negative and embarrassed to open and helpful.

BLOOD TRANSFUSIONS AND ORGAN DONATION

Blood transfusions, organ donations, and organ transplants are widely practiced among Iranians. In Iran, donation of organs is often a business transaction—if a kidney is needed, it is purchased (Zargooshi, 2001).

Health-Care Practitioners

TRADITIONAL VERSUS BIOMEDICAL PRACTITIONERS

When asked to compare American medical care with that offered in Iran, most Iranian immigrants consider it to be very good, although they may shop around before finding a doctor they like. They most appreciate good facilities and equipment and the lack of corruption in the medical system. On the other hand, they complain about the expense of health care and health insurance. Others dislike waiting for appointments; as one woman noted, "The patient could die while waiting" (Lipson, 1992).

A frequent source of difficulties, even for immigrants with good English skills, is differing expectations regarding the proper roles of health-care providers and clients, and the differences in diagnostic styles between Iranian and American physicians. According to one woman, "Doctors here are horrible. They don't listen to you, they are always careful of malpractice, they don't want to be specific" (Lipson, 1992). Many Iranian clients request medication and expect quick results, visiting a new doctor if a cure is not imminent. In comparing American physicians with their counterparts in Iran, immigrants think that Iranian doctors make more authoritative and quicker diagnoses, using minimal technology, even if they may be uncertain or wrong. Sometimes, American physicians who are tentative, ask the client to describe the problem, or order too many tests are viewed as incompetent.

Their acculturation level influences whether a patient/family accepts a health provider of the opposite gender although, in general, Iranians prefer to be cared for by health-care providers of the same sex. Iranian women are modest in front of men so, if possible, male health-care providers should not ask women to undress fully for an examination or procedure. Some very traditional families may consider taking a woman client elsewhere or avoid care until the situation is acute, if only male health providers are available.

STATUS OF HEALTH-CARE PROVIDERS

Traditional religious and folk practitioners may be sought by extremely religious individuals or those who are superstitious, but not by most Iranian immigrants. If a magicoreligious healer's services are sought, it is generally for **narahatis** of unexplainable origin or nonmedical concerns.

The most respected health-care provider is an experienced, middle-aged to elderly male physician, with several degrees, and preferably with a high position in the hospital or university. He is considered the authority and is expected to act like one, making diagnoses quickly and prescribing remedies that cure the client. In Iran, physicians rely more on physiological cues than technology. Equipment such as computed tomography scanners is scarce, and the waiting lists are long for such equipment. Recently, the government of Iran has supported medical school admissions based on influential kin; therefore, graduates are of mixed quality.

The least respected health-care providers are students; immigrant families sometimes refuse student caregivers. Nurses are accorded little respect compared with physicians; male nurses or women who have gray hair and positions of authority are accorded more respect than young, single, female nurses. Nurses who encourage self-care may be perceived as uncaring or even incompetent.

CASE STUDY Hamid moved his family to the United States within five years of the revolution (1984). The restrictions of the Islamic government were increasingly affecting everyone's social, economic and private lives. With two young daughters and a third child on the way he "didn't want to take any chances by remaining in Iran." He thought that leaving while he was "fairly young" would allow him and his family to adjust better and more easily.

The family fled Iran with great hardship and settled in Pakistan until they could obtain their visa to enter the United States. A friend from high school was helping him. The friend had left Iran many years ago and had a successful accounting firm in a southeastern state. Hamid was promised a job and a company to sponsor him so he could get a green card. The year the family spent in Pakistan was filled with frustration, anger, and illness. Eventually, they managed to obtain tourist visas and entered the United States in 1985. By now the two daughters were 10 and 11 years old and the baby was 9 months old. Jaleh, Hamid's wife, was exhausted and weak. The pregnancy was problematic and without the support of her sisters and mother, her recovery had been slow and rocky.

Hamid and Jaleh began a constant stream of arguments because of her mental and physical state. She felt that their situation in the United States was no better than they had had in Pakistan. They could not afford housing in a good neighborhood; the girls and Jaleh were scared at night since Hamid had to work long hours at the accounting firm. Leaving Iran was a desire but never a priority for Jaleh, especially while she was pregnant.

Hamid's hours became longer and the work became more involved. He had to improve his English and increase his technical skills and knowledge of U.S. tax rules and regulations. His friend told him that to succeed in the United States he was expected to perform. "No time to feel sorry for yourself. What better place to be than here."

Jaleh had a probable genetic predisposition to mental illness. She had always heard rumors about different aunts, uncles, and cousins who had suffered from different forms of anxiety and depressive disorders. She was always told that they had a "nervous problem." But Jaleh had always thought that she was strong willed and would not succumb to the pressures. Unfortunately, as Hamid worked harder and longer, Jaleh became more and more depressed and nonattentive to the children.

Three years passed. The only easy task was changing from their tourist visa to permanent residency. Hamid's desire to excel had also been financially rewarding. They moved to a better house. Jaleh remained at home, didn't try to improve her English, and felt she should keep the baby at home. Neither she nor Hamid trusted leaving the baby in daycare.

The two girls were adjusting a little differently; the older was active and outgoing. She was befriended by classmates and neighbors and was enjoying her teenage years. The second daughter was now 13, reclusive and slightly overweight. Hamid constantly commented on her looks, and Jaleh attempted to protect her against his words. Jaleh thought of her as her soul mate. As the sisters drifted apart, the bond between Jaleh and her second daughter became stronger. The baby was often sick but Jaleh was increasingly too tired to care. One night, as the baby's fever spiked, he began to have difficulties breathing. Hamid rushed him and the family to the hospital. By this time, Jaleh's weight had dropped to 98 lbs. Even though she was small statured, the weight loss made her appear weak and unhealthy.

In the Emergency Department (ED), the family was assessed and evaluated by the triage nurse. She was attentive and noticed the strained family dynamics. In reporting the case to the ED physician, she stressed that the physician should consider the family's circumstances.

STUDY QUESTIONS

1 If you were the nurse or physician, what areas would you focus on first?

2 What initial interventions would you suggest?

3 How would you develop a relationship that would allow you to ask private and personal questions?

4 Would you talk to the family as a unit or separately? Why?

5 As a health-care provider, what might you do to help the two girls adjust in the United States?

6 Describe how Jaleh might perceive her changing behaviors and mood. Describe her perception of any effects the change might have on family dynamics.

7 How would you approach this family for mental health counseling?

8 Describe culturally congruent dietary counseling for Jaleh.

9 Why do Hamid and Jaleh not trust leaving the baby in daycare?

10 Why did the entire family accompany the baby to the Emergency Department?

11 Describe traditional Iranian health beliefs and practices.

REFERENCES

Bagheri, A. (1992). Psychiatric problems among Iranian immigrants in Canada. *Canadian Journal of Psychiatry, 37,* 7–11.

Baluch, B., Al-Shawaf, T., & Craft, I. (1992). Prime factors for seeking infertility treatments amongst Iranian patients. *Psychological Reports, 71,* 265–266.

Bozorgmehr, M., Sabagh, G., & Der-Martirosian, C. (1993). Beyond nationality: Religio-ethnic diversity. In R. Kelly (Ed.), *Irangeles: Iranians in Los Angeles* (pp. 59–79). Berkeley: University of California Press.

Clark, D. (1995, January 27). Small Iranian group maintains anonymity. *The Washington Blade,* p. 14.

Dallalfar, A. (1994). Iranian women as immigrant entrepreneurs. *Gender and Society, 8*(4), 541–561.

Emami, A., Torres, S., Lipson, J., & Ekman, S-L. (2000). An ethnographic study of a day care center for Iranian immigrant seniors. *Western Journal of Nursing Research, 22,* 169–88.

Good, B. J. (1977). The heart of what's the matter. *Culture, Medicine and Psychiatry, 1,* 25–58.

Good, M. D. (1980). Of blood and babies: The relationship of popular Islamic physiology to fertility. *Social Science & Medicine, 14b,* 147–156.

Hafizi, H. (1990). *Health and wellness: An Iranian outlook.* Unpublished master's thesis, University of California, San Francisco.

Hanassab, S. (1998). Sexuality, dating and double standards: Young Iranian immigrants in Los Angeles. *Iranian Studies, 31,* 65–76.

Kelly, R., Friedlander, J., & Colby, A. (1993). *Irangeles: Iranians in Los Angeles.* Berkeley: University of California Press.

Klessig, J. (1992). The effect of values and culture on life-support decisions. *Western Journal of Medicine, 157*(3), 316–322.

Lipson, J. (1992). Iranian immigrants: Health and adjustment. *Western Journal of Nursing Research, 14,* 10–29.

Lipson, J., & Meleis, A. (1983). Issues in health care of Middle Eastern patients. *Western Journal of Medicine, 139,* 854–861.

Pliskin, K. (1987). *Silent boundaries: Cultural constraints on sickness and diagnosis of Iranians in Israel.* New Haven, CT: Yale University Press.

Rezaian, F. (1989). A study of intra- and inter-cultural marriages between Iranians and Americans. Unpublished doctoral dissertation, California Institute of Integral Studies, San Francisco.

Smith, J. A. (1983). *The idea of health: Implications for the nursing profession.* New York: Teachers College.

Zargooshi, J. (2001). Iranian kidney donors: Motivations and relations with recipients, *Journal of Urology, 165,* 386–392.

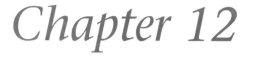

Chapter 12

People of Irish Heritage

SARAH A. WILSON

Overview, Inhabited Localities, and Topography

OVERVIEW

The Republic of Ireland, whose capital city is Dublin, is also known as **Eire** and the Emerald Isle, and covers most of the island bearing its name. The remainder of the island, Northern Ireland, is part of Great Britain. Ireland is the land of practical-joking, red-haired leprechauns with pots of gold at the end of the rainbow, fairy tales, queens of the underworld, banshees, and a land of superstitions.

With a population of 3.6 million, Ireland has a landmass of 32,500 square miles, slightly larger than the state of West Virginia (McDonald, 1999). The Irish Sea and St. George's Channel separate Ireland from Great Britain. Ireland is divided politically into 26 counties that make up the Republic of Ireland, and six counties that are part of Northern Ireland. Northern Ireland has a landmass of 5400 square miles and a population of 1.5 million (McDonald, 1999).

Ireland is bowl shaped with a central plain and low mountains. An agricultural country, its principal product is potatoes. Mining has become an important economic activity with the discovery of lead, copper, silver, and zinc. Surrounded by water, Ireland has a cool maritime climate with an average annual rainfall of 118 inches. Both winters and summers are mild, with average temperatures of 40°F in January, and temperatures of 60°F common in July. With this type of climate, the island cannot support a large variety of plant and animal species.

The history of Ireland is a chronicle of bloodshed, spirit, and pride. The Irish people have wit and a sense of humor and can laugh at themselves in the best possible way. More people of Irish descent live in the United States than Ireland itself (Byron, 1999). Irish was the second largest ancestry group reported in the 1990 U.S. census (U.S. Census, 2001). As a result of their influence, the United States celebrates St. Patrick's Day on March 17. St Patrick, the patron saint of Ireland, introduced Christianity in Ireland in 432 BC, and the country developed into a center of Gaelic and Latin learning.

The history of the Irish in America has not been harmonious. Early immigrants in America were subjected to religious persecution and economic discrimination. The Irish in America are a diverse group, and health-care providers must be careful to avoid generalizations or assumptions, such as the Irish being superstitious, heavy drinkers, and practical jokers, because these do not apply to all Irish. Factors that influence cultural beliefs of the Irish in America include primary and secondary characteristics of culture (see Chapter 1).

HERITAGE AND RESIDENCE

Historically, Ireland has been a melting pot. The Celts came to Ireland from Europe approximately 10,000 years ago. The Gales, a subgroup of **Celtic** people, gave Ireland the name Eire. The ancient Gaelic stock mixed with English, Scots, Welsh, French, Flemish, Norse, and German colonists. England dominated Ireland in the 16th century, creating a division between English Protestants and Irish Catholics.

The Irish immigrated to America in large numbers for almost three centuries beginning in the 1600s. The earliest settlements of Irish Catholics in America were in the colonies of Virginia and Maryland, with the Irish Catholics being the first Catholics to arrive in the United States in large numbers (Byron, 1999). The Irish ship, *St. Patrick*, arrived in Boston harbor in 1636. Irish Catholics experienced legal, social, and political discrimination in the early American colonies, and by 1699, Irish Catholic immigration was restricted in Virginia, Maryland, and South Carolina. For most of the 18th century, immigration from Ireland was dominated by Presbyterians. In the 19th and 20th century, most of the Irish immigrants were Catholic (Griffin, 1981).

Over 4 million Irish settled in the United States in the 19th century (Byron, 1999). Over a million arrived in just 7 years, from 1847 to 1854, nearly twice as many as had immigrated in the previous half century (Byron, 1999). The Irish heritage has been characterized as one of continuity and change. From initial experiences of bigotry and prejudice, the Irish in America brought their values of education, a strong work ethic, and the importance of children. They have made significant contributions to their new homeland in politics, the labor movement, the Catholic Church, the arts, and service to their country (Fig. 12–1).

Most Irish immigrants settled in industrial areas in the northeastern United States along the Atlantic coast. The cities of Philadelphia, New York, and Boston have the largest Irish settlements, followed by the commercial centers in Ohio, Illinois, and Michigan. By 1800, Philadelphia was the most Irish city in the United States (Boatman, 1992). After 1820, only German immigration into the United States exceeded the Irish. Irish settlements continued to concentrate in urban areas. Early Irish towns have been described as models for latter-day ghettos occupied by other groups whose race, religion, and nationality set them apart (Griffin, 1981). The Irish had the highest proportion of poor of any European American ethnic group by the early 20th century.

In 1920, 90 percent of all Irish in America resided in urban areas. However, second- and third-generation Irish families began leaving these areas around that time and moving to the suburbs. Suburban Irish became known as **lace-curtain Irish**, and those left in the city became known as **shanty Irish**.

REASONS FOR MIGRATION AND ASSOCIATED ECONOMIC FACTORS

The threat of famine was almost constant in early Ireland. Ireland had a population of 8.5 million until the **great potato famine** of 1846 to 1848, when the population decreased to 3.4 million, where it has remained relatively stable since. During the potato famine, thousands of Irish died from malnutrition, typhus, dysentery, and scurvy, and millions immigrated to America. Mass burials were organized because the demand for coffins could not be met.

Religious persecution and deplorable economic conditions were primary reasons for early immigration to America. The first Irish immigrants to arrive in America in the 1600s were Catholics. They came because of discrimination from Protestant English and Scots moving into Ireland. Oliver Cromwell, a Protestant leader in the English Parliament, ordered English armies into Ireland; Irish Catholics were forbidden to acquire land from Protestants or lease land for more than 31 years; they were forced to learn English; and they were not permitted to send their children to schools outside Ireland. Thus, early Irish immigrants who came to the United States had a history of oppression, violence, suffering, and misery (Greeley, 1972).

Most of the experiences of the Irish in America were similar to other immigrant groups, except for three features. First, the period of immigration lasted for well over a century. Many first-generation Irish in America saved money so other family members could come to America. Second, Irish women immigrated as single women rather than as part of a family group. This was in contrast to other immigrant groups, and was without parallel in the history of European immigration (Dezell, 2001). At the beginning of the twentieth century, over 60 percent of the Irish who came to the United States were single women (Dezell, 2001). Third, the established Catholic churches fulfilled a cultural and religious role for the Irish in America, became the center of their lives, and a symbol of identity. The Catholic parish was the cornerstone of the Irish community in America.

The Irish attained success in America because they spoke the same language, had the same physical appearance as other European Americans, and mastered the political system. They may have assimilated *less* than other ethnic groups because it was easier for them to blend in with the rest of society (Dezell, 2001). One-third of U.S. presidents trace their lineage to Irish descent. Three early presidents, Andrew Jackson, James Buchanan, and Chester Arthur were sons of Irish immigrants.

EDUCATIONAL STATUS AND OCCUPATIONS

Many Irish children in America went to work at a young age, often at the expense of their education, because they were needed to help provide for the family

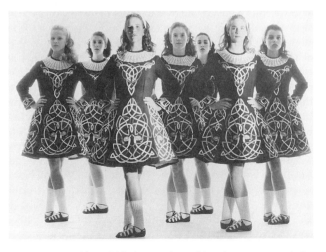

FIGURE 12–1 These Irish dancers in traditional costumes are helping to preserve and promote Irish culture in America. (Courtesy of Trinity Dance Company, Chicago, IL. Photo by Dan Harris.)

and to send money to Ireland for other family members. Educational attainment increased for each generation, with the descendants of Irish Catholic immigrants surpassing the general population in overall educational achievement (Blessing, 1980). According to the 1994 *Statistical Abstract of the United States* (U.S. Department of Commerce, 1994), 63.9 percent of the Irish in America are high school graduates, and 14.6 percent are college graduates.

Early Irish immigrants were primarily unskilled laborers from the agricultural regions of Ireland. On arrival in America, conditions were not what they expected. These rural farmers were not well prepared for life in large urban areas, and this lack of preparation was reflected by their failure to secure employment in their prescribed occupational roles. They were the only group in the late 19th century whose occupational mobility was limited almost as much as black Americans (Blessing, 1980).

Early Irish male immigrants contributed to the growth of America by helping build the Erie Canal, the transcontinental railroad, and skyscrapers. They served their new country by fighting in major military conflicts. By the turn of the century, the Irish made up 11 percent of policemen and 18 percent of the country's coachmen. The priesthood was the leading career choice for second-generation Irish men in the early 1900s (Blessing, 1980).

Communication

DOMINANT LANGUAGE AND DIALECTS

The major languages spoken in Ireland are English and Irish (Gaelic); the latter is the official language and is primarily spoken in the West of Ireland. The Celts developed a written language late and relied on oral transmission of traditions, laws, customs, philosophy, and religion (Greeley, 1981). Language used in oral tradition is more descriptive and flexible than the written form, and poetry is a useful mnemonic device for oral tradition. Ancient Irish folk heroes, such as Finn MacCool and Cuchulin, were in love with their own voices and enjoyed telling long complicated tales. Greeley (1981) suggested that modern-day Irish priests, politicians, and others share the love of using many words and playing with language not only for communication but also for enjoyment and entertainment. The Irish enjoy puns, riddles, **limericks**, and other storytelling. When one becomes accustomed to hearing the Irish-accented English used by the newer immigrants, there is little difficulty in understanding the speaker. This Irish accent has a nasal quality and is spoken with a strong inflection on the first syllable of a word, resulting in a loss of weak syllables. Words ending in a vowel weaken the consonants following them.

The Irish, in love with their own voices, use low-context English, using many words to express a thought. This low contextual use of the English language has its roots in the Celtic folk tradition of storytelling. The writings of famous Irish authors such as Jonathan Swift (although of English heritage, he was educated and wrote in Ireland), who wrote *Gulliver's Travels;* Lady Morgan, who wrote *The Wild Irish Girl;* Joseph Sheridan Le Fanu, who wrote *Uncle Silas* and *In A Glass Darkly;* and James Joyce, who wrote *Dubliners, Ulysses,* and *Finnegans Wake,* illustrate the low contextual use of the language. Some common Gaelic words and their meanings are *shamrock* for "emblem," *limer* for "folklore character," *colleen* or *lassie* for "girl," *sonsie* or *sonsy* for "handsome," *cess* for "luck," *brogue* for "shoe," *dudeen* for "pipe tobacco," and *paddy* for "Irishman."

CULTURAL COMMUNICATION PATTERNS

Even though most Irish delight in telling long stories, when discussing personal matters they are much less expressive unless they are talking with close friends and family. Even then, many are still reluctant to express their innermost thoughts and feelings. Humility and emotional reserve are considered virtues. Displays of emotion and affection in public are avoided, and are often difficult in private. Family members are expected to know that they are loved without being told. To many, caring actions are more important than verbal expressions. The Irish are unusual compared to other ethnic groups in not passing on family histories or cultural traditions to their children (Dezell, 2001).

The Irish use direct eye contact when speaking with each other. Not maintaining eye contact may be interpreted as a sign of disrespect, guilt, or evidence that the other person cannot be trusted.

Personal space is important to the Irish in America, who may require greater distance in spatial relationships. When speaking, they stand farther apart than other European Americans (Greeley, 1981). Although the Irish may be less physically expressive with hand and body gesturing, facial expressions are readily displayed, with frequent smiling even during times of adversity. However, health-care providers must remember that responses vary from person to person and are influenced by personality features and acculturation.

TEMPORAL RELATIONSHIPS

The Irish in America, with their strong sense of tradition, are typically past oriented. They have an allegiance to the past, their ancestors, and their history. The past is often the focus of Irish stories. However, many are past, present, and future oriented. While respecting the past, they balance "being" with "doing," and plan for the future by investing in education and saving money. Many Irish Americas see time as being elastic and flexible. Therefore, Irish Americas may have to be encouraged to arrive early for appointments.

FORMAT FOR NAMES

Mac before a family name means "son of," whereas the letter *O* in front of a name means "descended from." Gaelic names such as Brian, Maureen, Sheila, Sean, and Moira have become popular first names for American children. Otherwise, names are written with the surname, and the person is called by his or her first name in informal situations.

Family Roles and Organization

HEAD OF HOUSEHOLD AND GENDER ROLES

The family life of the Irish in America reveals its strong continuity over generations (Griffin, 1981). Families in western and southern Ireland were farmers who married young and had large families. The family structure was patrilineal, with land divided among the sons. The father ruled the family, but the mother had a significant influence over management of the household and education of children. The Irish have a strong sense of family obligation, and this pattern continued when they immigrated to America after the famine years. As the Irish settled in urban areas, the roles of women increased. Irish women have more power in family life than women in most other ethnic groups (Dezell, 2001). The family lived with rigid rules maintained by social and moral pressures of the society. Traditionally, the husband did not want the wife exposed to outside values and gave commands, which the wife was expected to follow unquestioningly. Women were often expected to do their work without male assistance, in addition to working outside the home when economic circumstances dictated. The roles of Irish American families are changing with a move toward more egalitarian relationships in which men assist with household duties and child care.

PRESCRIPTIVE, RESTRICTIVE, AND TABOO BEHAVIORS FOR CHILDREN AND ADOLESCENTS

Kinship and sibling loyalty are important to the Irish. Families emphasize independence and self-reliance in children. Boys are allowed and expected to be more aggressive than girls, who are raised to be respectable, responsible, and resilient. Children are expected to have self-restraint, self-discipline, and respect, and obedience for their parents and elders.

In addition to having self-restraint and self-discipline, adolescents are expected to obey and show respect for their parents as well as church and community figures. Adolescent years are a time for experiencing emotional autonomy, independence, and attachment outside the family, while remaining loyal to the family and maintaining the traditional Irish belief in the importance of family. Peer group pressures at school may have a significant influence and are often incongruent with the belief systems of Irish Americans. While parents see this rebellion negatively, it can provide a functional benefit for teenagers by helping them to become autonomous, successful individuals of whom the family can be proud. Family relationships with teenagers contain mixed motivations of love and hatred. Because it is difficult for many Irish Americans to express their feelings, health-care providers can encourage openness between parents and teenagers.

FAMILY GOALS AND PRIORITIES

The traditional Irish family is nuclear, with parents and children living in the same household. Children are cherished, and primary socialization is aimed at making them productive members of society, providing necessary educational experiences, and conferring status on the family.

Whereas marriage in ancient Ireland was delayed until about age 30, in America, the Irish marry at an age comparable to that of the rest of the population. Early immigrants were under pressure to marry within the Irish community; the pressure was especially strong for Irish Catholics to marry other Irish Catholics. Today, marriage with other groups is more common; however, it is still more socially acceptable to marry within one's group, thereby continuing the transmission of culture within the Irish American community. While unmarried women are undervalued in many groups, single Irish women have status (Dezell, 2001).

Irish women may consider sexual relationships as a matter of "duty" to their husbands (Greeley, 1981). This belief may have its roots in tradition, where men and women had different roles, lived in separate worlds, and the sexes never learned to communicate with each other. This attitude is diminishing as gender roles become more egalitarian.

Irish respect the experience of elderly people and seek their counsel for decision making. Provisions are made in Irish homes for care of elderly family members, a task that becomes increasingly difficult when both parents work outside the home. The extended family is important to the Irish in America. Although sentimental emotions are not expressed freely and many Irish families have infrequent contact with extended family members, they are available to assist when needed. Early Irish immigrants provided assistance to elderly Irish through immigrant aid societies, which were fraternal or religious in nature. However, since the Great Depression and passage of the Social Security Act, financial assistance for care of the elderly is provided by social security, private pensions, and private insurance. Newer immigrants continue the patterns of earlier immigrants and work long hours to earn a living and send money to their homeland, so that other family members can join them in America.

The Irish value physical strength, endurance, work, the ability to perform work, children, and the ability to provide their children with the needed education to attain respectable socioeconomic status and professional accomplishments. Members of the clergy in all religions are respected. Additional status can be gained by remaining in traditional ethnic Irish neighborhoods. Middle-aged and older family members voice pride in their ethnic neighborhoods.

The Irish contributed to the growth of the Catholic Church in America by providing leadership, money, and membership numbers. They built and established Catholic schools and colleges, health-care institutions, and social service agencies. John Carroll, a descendant of an Irish immigrant, was the first Catholic bishop in the United States and the founder of Georgetown College, now Georgetown University.

ALTERNATIVE LIFESTYLES

No information on alternative lifestyles specific to Irish in America was found in the health-care literature. A net search revealed the Irish Lesbian and Gay Organization with links to other resources (*http://www.ilgo2000.com*). However, it has been reported that cases of acquired immunodeficiency syndrome (AIDS) related to homosexuality are low among the Irish. This may be related to the Catholic Church's teaching against homosexuality and the value placed on chastity among the Irish. Additionally, although no data could be found on divorce and single parenting among the Irish, one could expect that for some, a minor stigma continues for these groups.

Workforce Issues

CULTURE IN THE WORKPLACE

Most Irish immigrants came to America with a strong desire to work, survive, and send money to family back home. They experienced high mortality rates while working in industries and textile mills in New England and on the eastern seaboard. Irish immigrants were viewed as a cheap and willing source of hard labor.

Over time, the Irish have made a place for themselves in the workforce and are represented in all occupations and professional roles. The Irish have been described as good organizers who are skillful at establishing networks and making contacts. By the late 1960s, the Irish in America were over-represented in law, medicine, and the sciences and slightly underrepresented in the social sciences and business. Second- and third-generation Irish women are widely represented in occupational and professional fields and, compared with other groups, are over-represented in law, teaching, and clerical work. Often they moved from traditional service occupations to positions in education, health, and business.

Because cultural differences between Ireland and the United States are minimal, Irish assimilate into the American workforce easily. Many endure short-term deprivations such as living in a small rented apartment to save money for the down payment on a home and to achieve their long-term goal of improving family life. When change is necessary to improve the status quo, the Irish readily relinquish traditional beliefs and adjust to the workforce.

ISSUES RELATED TO AUTONOMY

Most past-oriented ethnic groups believe that the future is controlled by a higher power of fate and that humans must live in harmony with their surroundings. They promote respect for authority rather than questioning authority, and encourage group identity rather than individual identity. Even though the Irish are typical of past-oriented groups in other ways, they tend to question the status quo of the American workforce. When individual efforts were unsuccessful in improving work environments, the Irish joined forces and helped pave the way for change through early efforts of unionization. They are recognized as one of the groups responsible for the current union culture in the American workforce.

Many Irish Americans hold leadership positions and have made major contributions in their respective roles and professions. Within the labor movement, Terrance Vincent Powderly, the son of Irish immigrants, became the head of the Knights of Labor, the most powerful labor union of its day. Joe Curran founded the National Maritime Union and was its first president. Mike Quill organized the Transport Workers of America. Irish women were at the forefront of the American labor movement in the 19th century. Mary Harris Jones, also known as "Mother Jones," an immigrant from County Cork, was active in the labor movement into her 90s. Mary Kenney Sullivan was recruited by Samuel Gompers to be the first woman organizer of the American Federation of Labor (Dezell, 2001).

Most Irish people in America speak English, and because Ireland has a 99 percent literacy rate, newer Irish immigrants do not encounter language barriers in the workplace. The low contextual use of language, where most of the message is in the explicit mode rather than the implicit mode, enhances pragmatic communications in the workforce.

Biocultural Ecology

SKIN COLOR AND OTHER BIOLOGICAL VARIATIONS

Most Irish have either dark hair and fair skin or red hair, ruby cheeks, and fair skin; however, as with other ethnic groups, other variations exist in hair and skin color. The fair complexion of the Irish places them at risk for skin cancer. The Irish are taller and broader in stature than average European Americans, Asians, or Pacific Islanders.

DISEASES AND HEALTH CONDITIONS

Mining is an important economic activity in Ireland because many homes are heated with soft coal or peat. As a result, Irish miners are at increased risk for respiratory diseases. In addition, the cool maritime climate of Ireland increases susceptibility to respiratory diseases. Health-care providers should assess newer immigrants who worked in mining industries for respiratory health illnesses.

Heart disease and cancer are the leading causes of premature mortality in Ireland compared with the United States (Redmond, 2000). Mortality rates for cardiovascular disease and cancer are above the European Union (EU) average. Cardiovascular diseases, including coronary heart disease and stroke, account for two out of every five deaths in Ireland (Delvin, 1997). Irish Americans had the highest mortality rates for coronary heart disease of all foreign-born Americans in the 1950s and 1960s (Blessing, 1980). Health providers can make a significant impact on the health of Irish Americans by providing education and counseling regarding lifestyle and dietary changes to reduce risks associated with cardiovascular diseases.

Cancer is second to coronary heart disease as a major cause of mortality in Ireland and causes one in four deaths in a year (Delvin, 1997). Lung cancer mortality rates are above the EU average. Smoking has been identified as the major risk factor causing premature mortality from cancer in Ireland. Smoking cessation programs with group and one-to-one counseling are important activities that health providers can institute to assist Irish Americans to improve their health status.

Female life expectancy in Ireland is lower than the EU average. The Staffron Report on Women's Lifetime Health Needs addresses the health needs of older women (Irish Nursing Organization, 1999). Older women are described as "invisible" because later life for many women is a time of less influence, less enjoyment, and poorer health. The risk of coronary heart disease, a silent killer of women, increases after the age of 65. Osteoporosis is another significant health problem affecting older women. The report recommends mass screening programs for osteoporosis for women in their late 60s.

The major cause of infant mortality in Ireland is congenital abnormalities. Other conditions with a high incidence among Irish newborns are phenylketonuria (PKU), neural tube defects, and fetal alcohol syndrome (Geissler, 1995). Most states require screening of all newborns for PKU, but health-care providers may need to encourage women who give birth at home to seek PKU screening for their infants.

The Website for the Irish Nursing Organization contains useful information on health needs, and the journal, *The World of Irish Nursing*, is available online (*http://www.ino.ie*).

VARIATIONS IN DRUG METABOLISM

No reported studies on drug responses are specific to the Irish. Most studies of pharmacological responses that include people of Irish descent have used data aggregated under the category of whites. Because Irish diets are similar in carbohydrate, protein, and fat ratio to many other European American diets, until further research is reported, health-care providers might expect that the pharmacodynamics of drug metabolism among Irish are similar to those of other white ethnic groups.

High-Risk Behaviors

The use of alcohol, tobacco, and intravenous drugs are major health problems among the Irish and Irish Americans. Immigrants are identified as high-risk populations for many health conditions because they are confronted with many challenges in their adaptation to a new environment and lifestyle. Alcohol problems in Ireland are among the highest internationally. Irish Americans rank among the highest of all ethnic groups in alcohol use; 88 percent of the Irish Catholics in the United States drink compared with 67 percent of the overall population (Dezell, 2001). Alcoholism researchers generally agree that individuals' Irish ancestry puts them at risk for developing drinking problems (Dezell, 2001).

Greeley (1981) attributed problems with alcoholism to the **great potato famine** in Ireland, which was a bleak period in Irish history when marriage was postponed until a person's 30s because of insufficient income and when immigration to America was the only alternative for those who would not inherit the family farm. Drinking became both a recreation and an escape. The village pub became the center of the community, and heavy drinking and alcoholism spread throughout post-famine Ireland. This legacy of socializing in taverns continues in America. Irish pubs are popular establishments that have become synonymous with alcohol intake, lively music, and a vivacious time. This image of the Irish pub perpetuates the stereotype of Irish as heavy drinkers, but health-care providers should be careful not to ascribe this label to all Irish Americans.

Stivers (1976) claims that the Irish drank heavily in America because they were expected to be heavy drinkers. However, many factors, including family characteristics, social and economic conditions, and psychological orientation, influence alcoholism. Irish mothers, who rule the family by strong will and manipulation, may be a contributing factor to alcoholism in Irish men (Greeley, 1972). In addition, alcohol allows one to release aggressions and relinquish responsibility for one's actions, thus reducing stress. Because drinking may be a way of coping with problems, health professionals need to assist Irish clients in exploring more effective coping strategies and caution them against the dangers of mixing alcohol with medications.

Smoking, another high-risk behavior common among the Irish, is associated with the high incidence of lung cancer among men in Ireland, where lung cancer mortality rates are above the EU average. Although smoking is declining in the Irish American male population, smoking is increasing among females. The incidence of lung cancer in the United States is similar to that of Ireland with men having higher mortality rates associated with smoking than women. However, the rate of lung cancer among women is increasing as more women smoke. Health promotion efforts should be directed at decreasing the incidence of smoking among Irish Americans.

The incidence of AIDS among the Irish is primarily related to the use of intravenous drugs. As mentioned earlier, the incidence of AIDS associated with homosexual behavior is low (Robins, 1997). Health promotion should be directed at educating Irish in America about high-risk behaviors for the prevention of AIDS.

HEALTH-CARE PRACTICES

Many Irish ignore symptoms and delay seeking medical attention until symptoms interfere with the ability to carry out activities of daily living. Zola (1983), in a study of Irish and Italian Americans, reported that Irish limit and understate problems compared with Italians, who describe problems in detail. The Irish handle problems by using denial, which is culturally prescribed. The Irish view life as difficult and hard (Zola, 1983), which is understandable within the cultural context of a people who have experienced periods of deprivation.

The Irish believe that having a strong religious faith,

keeping one's feet warm and dry, dressing warmly, eating a balanced diet, getting enough sleep, and exercising are important for staying healthy. Health-care providers can optimize compliance for reducing health risks by emphasizing these important cultural values.

Nutrition

MEANING OF FOOD

Food is an important part of health maintenance and celebrations for Irish Americans. Within their religious framework, most Irish Catholics have a primary obligation to use food in moderation and in ways that are not injurious to their health. Traditional Catholic holidays celebrated with food include the Solemnity of Mary (Mother of God), January 1; Easter Sunday; Ascension Thursday, 40 days after Easter; the Feast of the Assumption, August 15; All Saints Day, November 1; the Feast of the Immaculate Conception, December 8; and Christmas, December 25. More devout Catholics fast and abstain from meat on Ash Wednesday, Good Friday, and all Fridays in Lent. Fasting is viewed as a discipline. Many holidays and special events are celebrated with specific foods appropriate to the occasion. Irish food is unpretentious and wholesome if eaten in recommended proportions.

COMMON FOODS AND FOOD RITUALS

Meat, potatoes, and vegetables are the staples of both the Irish and Irish American diets. Lamb, mutton, pork, and poultry are common meats. Seafood includes salmon, mussels, mackerel, oysters, and scallops. Popular Irish dishes include Irish stew made with lamb, potatoes, and onions. Potatoes are used in a variety of ways. *Colcannon* is made with hot potatoes, mashed with cabbage, butter, and milk, and seasoned with nutmeg. This dish may be served at Halloween. *Champ* is a popular dish made with mashed potatoes and scallions. The scallions are cut in small pieces, including the green tops, boiled in milk until tender, and then added to the mashed potatoes and served with butter. **Dulse** (also known as "Irish moss"), an iodine-rich seaweed found in northern latitudes, may be used in place of scallions. Potato cakes, made with mashed potatoes, flour, salt, and butter, are shaped into patties and fried in bacon grease. Potato cakes are served hot or cold with butter and sometimes molasses or maple syrup. Another popular dish is Dublin coddle, made with bacon, pork sausage, potatoes, and onions.

Oatmeal is popular in Ireland. During times of food shortages, oatmeal was a primary food, watered down to make it last longer. Soda bread, another popular food in Ireland and America, is made with flour, baking soda, salt, sugar, cream of tartar, and sour milk. In Ireland, it is usually made fresh daily. Broths and pudding are served frequently in Ireland. Ale, instead of beer, is a common beverage. Contrary to the popular belief in America, corn beef and cabbage is not a traditional food in Ireland.

Mealtime is an important occasion for the Irish family to socialize and discuss family concerns. Meals are eaten three times a day, with a large breakfast in rural areas, lunch around noon, and a late dinner. Some Irish Americas continue the afternoon tradition of "tea," a light sandwich or biscuit with hot tea. Because the Irish diet has the potential for being high in fats and cholesterol, health-care providers may need to assist clients with balanced food selections and preparation practices that reduce their risks of cardiovascular disease. Eating balanced meals is considered important even if it means the individual is late for an appointment. Vitamins are commonly used as a dietary supplement. Generally, fast foods are considered less healthy than home-prepared foods.

NUTRITIONAL DEFICIENCIES AND FOOD LIMITATIONS

No nutritional deficiencies or food intolerances were found in the literature that are specific to the Irish. However, low-weight Irish women are at increased risk for osteoporosis, and may need to increase the amount of calcium in their diet.

Most foods eaten in Ireland are available in America with the possible exception of **dulse**, which is used to clarify beer and some wines, and is also used as a suspension medium in pharmaceutical preparations. The Irish have a greater variety of foods available in America than in their home country.

Pregnancy and Childbearing Practices

FERTILITY PRACTICES AND VIEWS TOWARD PREGNANCY

Because fertility and sexuality practices for many Irish are influenced by Catholic religious beliefs, some Irish may have a tendency to view sexual relationships as a "duty." The only acceptable methods of birth control are abstinence and the rhythm method. Women practice other means of birth control, but no statistics are available on their exact numbers. Abortion is considered morally wrong and is against the law in Ireland. Women's groups have been vocal in Ireland and in America about concerns over women's rights, especially reproductive rights.

PRESCRIPTIVE, RESTRICTIVE, AND TABOO PRACTICES IN THE CHILDBEARING FAMILY

The birth of a baby is a joyous occasion for the Irish, with family and friends celebrating the birth with food and gifts. Consistent with many other cultural groups, a baby boy receives something blue; a baby girl receives something pink. If a gift is purchased before the birth and the sex of the baby was unknown, then the gift should be green or yellow.

Prescriptive beliefs for a healthy pregnancy include eating a well-balanced diet. The Irish believe that not eating a well-balanced diet or not eating the right kinds of food may cause the baby to be deformed. In addition, the Irish share the belief, common to many other ethnic groups, that the mother should not reach over her head during pregnancy because the baby's cord may wrap around its neck. A taboo behavior in the past, which some women still respect, is that if the pregnant woman sees or experiences a tragedy during pregnancy, a congenital anomaly may occur.

Eating a well-balanced diet after delivery continues to be a prescriptive practice for ensuring a healthy baby and maintaining the mother's health. Plenty of rest, fresh air, and sunshine are also important for maintaining the mother's health. The Irish believe that going to bed with wet hair or wet feet causes illness in the mother.

Death Rituals

DEATH RITUALS AND EXPECTATIONS

The typical Irish reaction to death is a combination of the pagan past and current Christian faith. The Celts denied death and ridiculed it with humor. The Irish are fatalists and acknowledge the inevitability of death. The American emphasis on technology and dying in the hospital may be incongruent with the Irish American belief that family members should stay with the dying person. After a death, family and friends make every effort to be present for the funeral.

RESPONSES TO DEATH AND GRIEF

A traditional practice in Ireland was for a deceased family member to be "laid out" in the home for a final farewell by the family. Ancient Gaelic women practiced "keening," or "loud wailing" at *wakes*, while men socialized while drinking and smoking. The wake continues as an important phenomenon in contemporary Irish families, and is a time of melancholy, rejoicing, pain, and hopefulness. The occasion is a celebration of the person's life. The wake represents the Irish people's stubborn refusal to believe death is the end (Greeley, 1977). Cremation is an individual choice, and there are no proscriptions against autopsy if required.

Spirituality

DOMINANT RELIGION AND USE OF PRAYER

The predominant religion of most Irish is Catholicism, and the church is a source of strength and solace for many Irish Americans. In times of illness, Irish Catholics receive the Sacrament of the Sick, which includes anointing, communion, and a blessing by the priest. The Eucharist, a small wafer made from flour and water, is given to the sick as the food of healing and health. Family members can participate if they wish. The obligation to fast and abstain from meat on specified days is relinquished during times of illness. Other religions common among Irish in America include various Protestant dominations, such as the Church of Ireland, Presbyterian, Quaker, and Episcopalian.

Prayer is an individual and private matter. In the health-care setting, clients should be given privacy for prayer whether or not a clergy member is present. In times of illness, the clergy may offer prayers with the sick, as well as with the family. Attending mass daily is a common practice among many traditional Irish Catholic families. For Irish Catholics who practice their religion regularly, holy day worship begins at 4 PM the evening preceding the holy day; all Sundays are considered holy days.

MEANING OF LIFE AND INDIVIDUAL SOURCES OF STRENGTH

Many Irish are fatalistic and view man as being subjected to the harshness of nature. To help overcome stresses associated with the harshness of nature, many Irish view life in a comic sense, using satire and self-burlesque (Dezell, 2001) as a means of keeping their problems in a proper perspective. In addition, they gain meaning in their life through home, religion, the church, and the pub, which are centers of life in Irish communities.

The Irish have a strong faith in life and a passion for freedom. Christianity existed in Ireland before the arrival of Ireland's patron saint, St. Patrick, in the 5th century. The theology and philosophy of Christianity was interwoven with the older Gaelic culture, creating a lasting identification between faith and the nation (Titley, 2000).

SPIRITUAL BELIEFS AND HEALTH-CARE PRACTICES

Religion is important for many Irish in their daily life and in times of sickness. Irish Catholics continue to receive sacraments when sick. Health-care providers should inquire whether sick individuals want to see a member of the clergy, even if they have not been active in church. Some Irish may wear religious medals to maintain health. These emblems provide them with solace and should not be removed by health-care providers.

Health-Care Practices

HEALTH-SEEKING BELIEFS AND BEHAVIORS

The Irish fatalistic outlook and external locus of control influences health-seeking behaviors. Many Irish people use denial as a way of coping with physical and psychological problems. Zola (1983), in a study of Irish and Italian Americans' perceptions of symptoms of illness, found that the Irish view of life is illustrated in the belief that "life was black and long suffering and the less said about it the better" (Zola, 1983: 104).

Many Irish limit and understate their symptoms when they are ill. For some Irish, illness behavior does little to relieve suffering and perpetuates a self-fulfilling prophecy of fatalism. Illness or injury may be linked to guilt and considered to be the result of having done something morally wrong. Restraint is a modus operandi in the Irish culture; temptation is ever-present and must be guarded against (Zola, 1983). Most Irish Americans believe one is obligated to use ordinary means to preserve life. Therefore, extraordinary means may be withheld to allow the person to die a natural death. The sick person and family define extraordinary means; finances, quality of life, and effects on the family usually influence the decision.

RESPONSIBILITY FOR HEALTH CARE

Although the Irish value good health, they often delay seeking treatment for health problems, hoping the problems will go away. Because Irish people may not be very descriptive about their symptoms, treatment may be more difficult. Early Irish American immigrants depended on fraternal organizations and religious institutions for assistance with health care in times of need. Today, most Irish Americans have some type of coverage for health care such as private insurance, Medicare, and Medicaid.

FOLK PRACTICES

Recent studies show that the use of traditional home remedies is increasing in the United States, and that most patients do not discuss these home remedies with their health-care providers (Eisenburg et al., 1993). Irish folk medicine practices include traditional remedies that have been passed down through generations and are considered effective in health promotion. These include eating a balanced diet, getting a good night's sleep, exercising, dressing warmly, and not going out in the cold air with wet hair. Other folk practices include wearing religious medals to prevent illness, using cough syrup made from honey and whiskey, taking honey and lemon for a sore throat, drinking hot tea with whiskey for a cold, drinking hot tea for nausea, drinking tea and eating toast for a cold, and putting a damp cloth to the forehead for a headache. Some folk practices may be harmful, such as the use of senna to cleanse the bowels every 8 days, eating a lot of oily foods, and avoiding seeing a physician.

No reports in the literature indicate that the Irish use over-the-counter medications more than any other group. Health-care providers should ask Irish Americans about their perceptions of their illness, its cause, treatments used (including prescription and over-the-counter medications and home remedies) and their effectiveness, and whether they know anyone else with a similar problem (Kleinman, 1980).

BARRIERS TO HEALTH CARE

Most Irish Americans have few barriers to health care. One self-imposed barrier is delaying treatment when symptoms occur. Irish Americans in lower socioeconomic classes experience health-care barriers such as lack of transportation, money, insurance, and knowledge about the availability of health-care resources.

CULTURAL RESPONSES TO HEALTH AND ILLNESS

The relationship of ethnicity and the experience of pain has been demonstrated in a number of studies (Neill, 1993; Zborowski, 1969; Zola, 1983). Zborowski (1969), in a classic study on pain and ethnicity, describes differences in the responses to pain of Irish, Italian, Jewish, and Yankee subjects. The behavioral response of the Irish to pain is stoic, usually ignoring or minimizing it. Irish deny pain and delay seeking medical treatment longer than Italians (Zola, 1983).

Irish immigrants have high rates of mental illness. Although children of Irish immigrants have fewer psychological problems than their parents, they lead all other second-generation Americans in frequency of mental health problems (Blessing, 1980). One explanation for high rates of mental illness may be associated with the Irish having difficulty describing emotions and expressing feelings. Health-care providers can encourage the expression of emotions and feelings before symptoms become a problem. In the past, the mentally and physically ill were taken care of in the home, not because of the stigma associated with mental illness and the family's desire to shield them, but rather because of the Irish family's preference for caring for each other whenever possible. Although some Irish attribute illness to sin and guilt, they readily excuse sick people from their obligations and become sources of support by assuming the normal roles of the sick until they are able to function again.

BLOOD TRANSFUSIONS AND ORGAN DONATION

Blood transfusions are acceptable to most Irish Americans. The literature does not reveal any information on organ donation and organ transplantation that is specific to the Irish. No religious or cultural proscriptions exist regarding this practice. Many Irish participate in organ donation, and indicate their willingness to do so on their driver's licenses. Health-care professionals should obtain this information on an individual basis, be sensitive to client and family concerns, explain procedures involved with organ donation and procurement, answer questions factually, and explain the risks involved.

Health-Care Practitioners

TRADITIONAL VERSUS BIOMEDICAL PRACTITIONERS

In most Irish families, nuclear family members are consulted first about health problems. Mothers and older women are usually sought for their knowledge of folk practices to alleviate common problems such as colds. The Irish are one of the few ethnic groups without a hierarchy of folk and traditional practitioners. When home remedies are not effective, the Irish seek care from biomedical practitioners.

Although the Irish are not noted for being overly modest, many may prefer to receive intimate care from someone of the same gender. In general, men and women may care for each other in health-care settings as long as privacy and sensitivity are maintained.

STATUS OF HEALTH-CARE PROVIDERS

Although the Irish do not readily seek health care for early symptoms, they do respect health-care professionals. Nursing, a predominately female profession in Ireland, is considered a worthwhile occupation. As in the United States, Irish nurses are not held in as high regard as physicians, which may be attributed to educational differences.

CASE STUDY   The O'Rourke family lives on a small farm in Iowa and comprises David, age 30; his wife Mary, age 29; and two children, Bridget, age 7, and Michael, age 6. Both David and Mary are second-generation Irish. Before purchasing their farm 5 years ago, David sold farm equipment in Ohio. The O'Rourkes are Catholic; Mary converted to Catholicism when they married.

David, who works long hours outdoors, is concerned about profitability from his corn crop because the size of the harvest, and thus his income, varies depending on the weather. Mary does not work outside the home because she wants to be with their children until they start school. However, because both children are now school age, Mary has discussed with David the possibility of working part time to supplement the family income. He would prefer that she stay at home, but Mary is anxious to return to the workforce and believes the timing is right.

Both David and Mary are happy with just two children and do not desire more. They use the rhythm method for family planning.

Eating a healthy breakfast is important to the O'Rourkes. Because eggs are readily available on the farm, they have fried eggs with potato bread and juice at least four times a week. Their main meal in the evening usually includes meat, potatoes, and a vegetable. David enjoys a glass of beer with dinner.

David has been a little edgy lately because of his concerns about the corn crop. He admits to having some minor chest pain, which he attributes to indigestion. His last visit to a physician was before their marriage. Mary knows David is concerned about finances and believes if she had a job it would help.

Bridget and Michael spend a lot of time outside playing and doing some minor chores for their parents. Both children enjoy school and are looking forward to returning in the fall. Bridget is starting to show concern over her appearance. She does not like her red hair and all the freckles on her face. Her teacher has noted that Bridget has trouble reading and may need glasses. Michael wants to be a farmer like his Dad, but worries about his Dad being tired at night.

The O'Rourkes have not taken a vacation since they were married. They go to the state fair in the summer, which is the extent of their trips away from home. They are active in the church and attend services every Sunday.

STUDY QUESTIONS

1 Describe the O'Rourke family structure in terms of individual roles.

2 Identify two potential family problems related to the O'Rourke's dietary practices.

3 Identify potential health risk factors for the O'Rourkes as a family unit and for each family member.

4 Explain the relationship between risk factors and ethnicity specific to the O'Rourke family and their Irish heritage.

5 Describe culturally competent health promotion strategies for the identified risk factors for the O'Rourke family.

6 Describe the O'Rourke family's fertility practices. Are they congruent with their Irish background and religious beliefs?

7 Describe the O'Rourke family's communication patterns.

8 What are predominant health conditions among Irish immigrants?

9 Explain the significance of the great potato famine for Irish Americans.

10 Name two genetic diseases common among Irish Americans.

11 Identify accepted fertility practices for Irish American Catholics.

12 Identify three sources of strength for the Irish American in times of illness.

13 Identify traditional home remedies commonly used by Irish Americans.

REFERENCES

Blessing, P. (1980). Irish. In S. Thernstrom (Ed.), *Harvard encyclopedia of American ethnic groups* (pp. 524–545). Cambridge, MA: Belknap Press.

Boatman, J. (1992). *A survey of the U.S. ethnic experience* (Vol. 1). Milwaukee, WI: University of Wisconsin-Milwaukee.

Byron, R. (1999). *Irish America.* Oxford: Oxford University.

Delvin, J. (1997). The state of health in Ireland. In J. Robins (Ed.), *Reflections on health: Commemorating fifty years of the Department of Health 1947–1997* (pp. 10–28). Dublin: Department of Health.

Dezell, M. (2001). *Irish America: Coming into the clover: The evolution of a people and a culture.* New York: Doubleday.

Eisenburg, D. M., Kessler, R. C., Foster, C., Norlock, F. E., Calkins, D. R., & Delbanco, T. L. (1993). Unconventional medicine in the United States. Prevalence, costs, and patterns of use. *New England Journal of Medicine, 328*(4), 246–252.

Geissler, E. (1995). *Pocket guide to cultural assessment.* St. Louis, MO: Mosby-Year Book.

Greeley, A. (1972). *That most distressful nation: The tanning of the American Irish.* Chicago: Quadrangle Books.

Greeley, A. (1977). *The American Catholic: A social portrait.* New York: Basic Books.

Greeley, A. (1981). *The Irish Americans.* New York: Harper & Row.

Griffin, W. (1981). *A portrait of the Irish in America.* New York: Charles Scribner's Sons.

Irish Nursing Organization. (1999). *Cover story.* World of Irish Nursing, April 1999. Retrieved April 30, 2002, from http://www.ino.ie.

Kleinman, A. M. (1980). *Patients and healers in the context of culture.* Berkeley: University of California Press.

McDonald, F. (1999). *Ireland: Eyewitness travel guides.* London: DK Publishing.

Neill, K. (1993). Ethnic pain styles in acute myocardial infarction. *Western Journal of Nursing Research, 15*(5), 531–547.

Redmond, A. (Ed.). (2000). *That was then, this is now: Changes in Ireland 1949–1999*. Dublin: Government of Ireland, Stationary Office.

Robins, J. (Ed.) (1997). *Reflections on health: Commemorating fifty years of the Department of Health 1947–1997*. Dublin, Ireland: Department of Health.

Stivers, R. (1976). *A hair of the dog: Irish drinking and American stereotype*. University Park, PA: Pennsylvania State University Press.

Titley, A. (2000). *A pocket history of Gaelic culture*. Dublin: The O'Brien Press.

U.S. Census Bureau. (2000). *We asked. You told us: Ancestry questionnaire content* (1990) CQC-14. Retrieved January 12, 2002, from http://www.census.gov/apsd/cqc/cqc14.pdf.

U.S. Department of Commerce. (1994). *Statistical Abstract of the United States 1994*. Washington, DC: U.S. Government Printing Office.

Zborowski, M. (1969). *People in pain*. San Francisco: Jossey-Bass.

Zola, I. K. (1983). *Socio-medical inquiries: Recollections, reflections, and reconsideration*. Philadelphia, PA: Temple University Press.

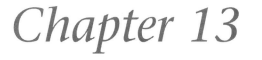

Chapter 13

People of Italian Heritage

SANDRA M. HILLMAN

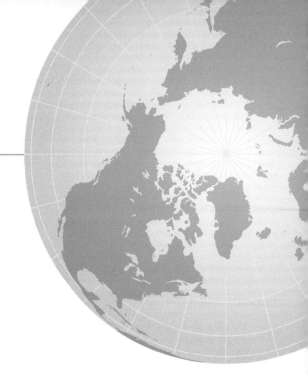

Overview, Inhabited Localities, and Topography

OVERVIEW

Italians in America, bound by the commonalities of language, home country, heredity, religion, and history, have found a permanent home in North America. Whereas much was written about Italians in America in the earlier part of this century, little has been written in the past 20 years. Italian American immigrant groups include (1) first-generation, mostly traditional, elderly Italians primarily living in enclaves; (2) second-generation, less traditional Italians living in suburban and urban neighborhoods with ethnic enclaves; (3) third-generation, usually more educated Italians primarily living in the suburbs; and (4) a relatively small group of newer immigrants with strong ties to their homeland. The first group reflects a somewhat despairing immigrant experience, whereas the remaining groups exemplify a happier, more resilient, and more contented experience. Because of the primary and secondary characteristics of culture (see Chapter 1) Italians are not a homogeneous group. This chapter describes the beliefs and practices of the Italians from the mainland of Italy, although Italians with a heritage from Sicily and Sardinia may share some of these characteristics

Italy, which includes Sicily and Sardinia, has a land-mass of 116,318 square miles, an area slightly smaller than New Mexico and slightly larger than Arkansas. With a population of 57.6 million, Italy is divided into 19 regions with 90 provinces. In the north, the Alps separate Italy from France, Switzerland, Austria, and Yugoslavia; on the west are the Ligurian and Tyrrhenian seas, on the east is the Adriatic Sea, and to the south are the Ionian and Mediterranean seas. The climate of Italy varies significantly according to its diverse topography. Northern Italy consists of the great plain and the valley of the river Po and surrounding Alps. Central Italy contains the Apennine Mountains, whereas **Mezzogiorno** (in the south) consists of lower mountains and stony hills with large areas bereft of trees, resulting in soil erosion and, in turn, deterioration of the soil into clay.

HERITAGE AND RESIDENCE

A country rich in history, Italy is famous for the marvels of ancient Rome, such as the Coliseum, Pantheon, libraries, museums, and St. Peter's Square; the Leaning Tower of Pisa; the canals and Piazza San Marco in Venice; the Ravenna opera; the ruins of Pompeii; the Portofino lace makers, wineries, and marble; and artists such as Michelangelo and Leonardo da Vinci. An Italian, Christopher Columbus, is credited with discovering North America, which is named after the Italian explorer, Amerigo Vespucci.

Early Italians, under the sponsorship of French, English, Portuguese, and Spanish governments, sought adventures as explorers, warriors, sailors, soldiers, and missionaries. The early Italians who came to America between the late 18th and 19th centuries were scattered throughout North America, with large concentrations in the Northeast and the lower Mississippi Valley. Early Italian immigrants came from an agricultural background and differed in several respects from later immigrants who began arriving at the close of the 19th century. Many of the later immigrants were political refugees who had a variety of skills and occupations, such as tradesmen, artists, musicians, and teachers. From the early to mid-1800s the majority came from northern Italy. After 1880, large numbers of Italian men came from the **Mezzogiorno**, and by 1901, southern Italians comprised 83 percent of the Italian immigrants in the United States. Of all Europeans who immigrated during those years, Italians had the smallest proportion of women and children.

Italian men were described as "birds of passage," whose goal was to stay for a few years, save their money, and return to their villages in Italy. Fleeing poverty in southern Italy in particular, many men left their families behind with the hope of returning to Italy once they had earned enough money (Chick-Gravel, 1999). Over 3.8 million Italians immigrated between 1899 and 1924, with the peak migration between 1901 and 1910. Many in this group were women and children. However, 2.1 million returned to their homeland during these same years, with only 1.7 million immigrants remaining. During the peak years of immigration, 97 percent of the Italians entered the United States through New York City, giving it the largest Italian population of any city in the country (Mangione & Morreale, 1993). Between 1965 and 1973, Italian immigration stabilized at around 25,000 people per year. Between 1974 and 1986, a steady decline occurred in Italian immigration, with less than 5000 new immigrants entering the United States (Mangione & Morreale, 1993). Most Italian Americans live in the states of New York, New Jersey, Massachusetts, Pennsylvania, and California. Major cities inhabited by Italian Americans include Chicago; New Orleans; New York; Philadelphia; Boston; Newark, New Jersey; and San Francisco (Mangione & Morreale, 1993). Italian enclaves, or "Little Italies" as they are called, can be found in New York City, Boston, Cleveland, and other major cities throughout the United States.

The great Italian migration to North America that began in the 19th century came to an end over the past 20 years. The current Italian population in America of 14.7 million ranks fifth in the United States. Canada hosts an additional 760,000 residents claiming Italian ancestry (Statistics Canada, 2001). Factors such as time in their new country, new experiences, and a new social environment are changing the offspring of these early immigrants. The Italian culture has had an impact on the cultural landscape of North America with its values and cuisine. Beyond pasta and pizza, Italian immigrants and their children have had and continue to make an impact on the arts, architecture, and commerce (Matusow, 1999).

REASONS FOR MIGRATION AND ASSOCIATED ECONOMIC FACTORS

In the early 1800s, Italy had an archaic, corrupt government, lacked an industrial base, and the mercantile system heavily taxed the population to raise capital for commerce. After unification, the national government imposed a legal system favoring the more industrialized north over the agricultural **Mezzogiorno** regions to the South. To meet impossible tax burdens, peasant farmers, **contadini**, mortgaged their lands. By 1900 a minority had most of the wealth, whereas the destitute majority paid almost all the taxes. Because of these economic hardships, many Italians mass-migrated to North America, where they often confronted equally severe economic hardships caused, in part, by language barriers. Many had to live in poverty until becoming established. Italians who immigrate today are less likely to live in poverty because most have relatives who assist them in getting established in their new environment. Italians continue to immigrate for job opportunities and to join family in North America.

EDUCATIONAL STATUS AND OCCUPATIONS

First-generation Italian immigrant parents insisted that their children conduct themselves according to the code of behavior and value system that kept Italian families intact for centuries. Under parental influence, most children did not stay in school long. Some completed high school and occasionally went to college, despite an Italian proverb that cautioned fathers against making their sons "better" than themselves. Although children usually paid their own way through college, their education often generated a sense of alienation between the educated offspring and the rest of the family. Although most early Italian immigrants were from the farmlands of Italy, lack of capital for land and equipment limited their ability to continue farming in the United States. The majority became contract laborers in urban areas such as New York, Boston, Baltimore, Chicago, Philadelphia, St. Louis, New Haven, San Francisco, Buffalo, and Rochester. A few were lured to the southern United States where they obtained employment in agriculture and, as soon as they could, bought land. These farmers created the small Italian farm communities that dot Louisiana, Texas, Mississippi, Alabama, Tennessee, Virginia, and Maryland today.

In work, as in all dimensions of life, the sense of pride among Italians is more visceral and passionate than subliminal and abstract. Italians in America seek to do something that can demonstrate their success to their families. Because of their general distaste for abstract values, ambivalent attitude toward formal schooling, and desire to remain close to family, a disproportionate number of second- and third-generation Italian Americans seek employment in blue-collar jobs. Even though Italian Americans have made great strides in many fields, only 20 percent have obtained professional status (Mangione & Morreale, 1993). For those who choose white-collar employment, men favor careers in law, engineering, music, pharmacology, and medicine; women favor teaching, nursing, clerical, and secretarial work. In recent years Italian Americans have not only caught up but also average slightly more schooling and higher incomes than non-Italians. Today Italian Americans are well represented in law, politics, research, technology, big business, and Wall Street. It was not until the late 1980s and early 1990s that Italian Americans gained prominence in the top ranks of the establishment (Matusow, 1999).

Communication

DOMINANT LANGUAGE AND DIALECTS

The official language of Italy is Italian, a Romance language derived from Latin. However, all socioeconomic groups in the 19 regions of Italy speak different dialects. The dialects of northern Italy contain numerous German words. Spanish, French, and German languages influence Neapolitan Italy. Piedmontese is strongly affected by the French and Spanish languages, whereas the dialects of Sicily have been strongly influenced by French, Spanish, Greek, Albanian, and Arabic languages. Sardinia has its own language, Sardinian. So numerous are the dialects that they are mutually incomprehensible to some extent. When an interpreter who speaks the client's specific dialect is unavailable, the interpreter should select words that have pure meanings from Tuscan Italian, which is used for formal writing.

First-generation Italians who immigrated to America brought the dialects of their region with them. Today, in some second- and third-generation Italian homes, these dialects are still spoken. However, many second-generation Italian Americans do not speak Italian well or at all. Either their parents encouraged them to learn English or, more often, the children refused to speak the mother tongue. Often, though, the next generation becomes curious about its background and tries to recover parts of its heritage. A number of third-generation Italian Americans are studying Italian in an effort to reconnect with their Italian heritage. Many would like to teach their children to speak Italian (Matusow, 1999).

Grammatically correct Italian is musical and romantic because vowels predominate over consonants, expressing the many subtleties of thoughts and feelings in a delicate manner. In many Italian households, discussions can become quite passionate, with voice volume raised and many people speaking at once. Health-care providers must understand this cultural characteristic when presenting health information for decision-making purposes.

CULTURAL COMMUNICATION PATTERNS

The willingness to share thoughts and feelings among family members is a major distinguishing characteristic of the Italian family. Positive and negative emotions and sentiments are permissible, encouraged, and color their daily lives. Many times a fluctuating emotional climate exists within the family, with expressions of affection erupting briefly into what appears to an outsider as anger or hostility. Conflict is usually confined to periodic outbursts and does not usually cause resentment or open and permanent ruptures. In fact, emotional neutrality to Italians denotes noninvolvement or the absence of affection. Non-Italian relatives by marriage are often singled out because they seem distant and unemotional. Italians are sentimental and not afraid to express their feelings.

Traditional Italians value close family ties, express warmth freely, and have deep feeling for each other. Frequent kissing reaffirms the emotional bond among Italians. The "typical" kiss is eastern European style, with a kiss on each cheek. They frequently touch and embrace family and friends. Touching between men and women, between men, and between women is frequently seen during verbal communication.

While nonverbal methods of communicating are common to all societies, Italians have elaborated, refined, and stylized gestures into an art form. It is said that the Italians from southern Italy are capable of carrying out a conversation without saying a single word. Gestures convey a range of feelings, from poetic eloquence to intense anger. These messages, however, are best conveyed in an economical, subtle, flowing, and almost imperceptible manner. For example, a slowly raised chin means "I don't know." Health-care providers need to observe Italian American clients for nonverbal cues to obtain the full meaning of verbal communication.

TEMPORAL RELATIONSHIPS

The literature provides different views of temporal relationships among Italian Americans; thus, one can posit that Italians are past, present, and future oriented. Past orientation is evidenced by the pride they take in their home country's rich Roman heritage. Within the context of fatalism and their present orientation, they do not allow their imagination to stray too far, occupy themselves with concrete problems and situations, and accept things the way they are. Finally, they are future oriented as evidenced by the importance given to planning ahead and saving financially for the future.

Time orientation varies by immigrant group. Whereas first-generation and newer immigrants view time as an approximation rather than categorically imperative, second- and third-generation Italian Americans adhere to clock time at least in the work situation and for appointments. For this group, deadlines and commitments are considered important and are adhered to firmly.

FORMAT FOR NAMES

Before the Napoleonic era, last names were not commonly used in southern Italy. After the Napoleonic era ended in 1814, the French often assigned to a family, or sometimes an entire village, the name of that village. The **contadini** peasant custom was to name first children for their grandparents and later children for their godparents. To avoid confusion, they instituted a practice of assigning nicknames according to some physical characteristic or their occupation. For example, Giovanni Pelo is translated as "Johnny one hair." This nickname was given because his body was covered with dark hair. This practice of assigning nicknames continues with many Italian American families. Otherwise, a person is called by the first or given name in social situations and by a title such as Miss, Ms., Mr., Mrs., or Dr. and his or her last or family surname in the health-care environment.

The order of first and last names is frequently reversed in Italy, without the use of a comma. Thus, Pietropaolo Vincenzo is often used when Vincenzo is the person's first name and Pietropaolo is the last name. More recent immigrants should be asked to clarify the order of the name to assure accurate health-care record keeping.

Middle names or initials are very seldom used, but compound first names (e.g., Pierfranco, Marialuisa, Giancarlo) are common, in which case the complete first name is used; it is considered impolite to abbreviate the first name (e.g., Pier, Maria, or Gian).

Family Roles and Organization

HEAD OF HOUSEHOLD AND GENDER ROLES

First-generation and newer immigrants, as well as traditional Italian families, recognize the father's authority as absolute; nothing is purchased and decisions are not made without his approval. The father's decision may be accepted as law even among his married children. To criticize one's father is considered a sacrilege. In many traditional Italian families today, the father continues to dominate family decisions as long as he remains in good health and is the chief breadwinner. He is known as the **padrone** or **capo di famiglia** (head of the family). In old age and illness, the eldest son supersedes him, but even then, the father retains much of his prestige. The "typical" traditional Italian father frequently demonstrates public and private affection for his children, but such demonstrations are less frequent in public for his wife.

Italian Americans discuss marriage largely in terms of power; thus, the divergence between the cultural ideal and the reality of marriage becomes obscure when one analyzes power issues between husbands and wives. Many husbands turn over their paychecks to their wives to run the home, and thus Italian women tend to have more power in economic decisions. Women also dominate decision making on childbearing issues and family social events. The Italian American husband believes that as the man he has the power as head of the family regardless of the wife's influence. As long as the wife verbally acknowledges that he is the head, he is satisfied. An early study of Italian American family roles reported that authority is concentrated either in the father or in both parents. Very few first-generation families expressed approval of the mother working outside the home. Even though traditional roles remain strong in second- and third-generation Italian American families, a trend toward more egalitarian relationships is evolving.

PRESCRIPTIVE, RESTRICTIVE, AND TABOO BEHAVIORS FOR CHILDREN AND ADOLESCENTS

Italian children who grow up in a home where the parents speak an Italian dialect are able to more readily absorb their culture. Although this creates closer family ties, it can produce a conflicting sense of identity when these children speak another language outside the home. Children are taught to have good manners and respect for their elders. Both boys and girls are encouraged to be independent and are expected to contribute to the family's support as soon as they are old enough to work. This work ethic continues in second- and third-generation families.

Adolescent girls are expected to remain virgins until they marry. Among first-generation Italians, an aunt or the teenage girl's mother acted as a chaperone when the girl went on a date. Today, second- and third-generation Italian American teenage girls have greater latitude and freedom in dating behavior, although the expectation of maintaining virginity remains important.

FAMILY GOALS AND PRIORITIES

L'ordine della famiglia (family order), a system of social attitudes, values, and customs, has remained a mainstay of Italian American culture. It is the main tie that holds the Italian American household together. The rules governing family membership are simple and explicit: fear God and respect the saints; the father is the father, and he is experienced; always honor and obey your parents; work hard, work honestly, work always, and you will never know hunger; trust family first, relatives second. The foundations of a good family life inherent in the traditional way are home ownership, good food, respect, and display of affection (Wells, New, & Richman, 1994).

Italian families maintain close relationships. Love and warmth, security, and the expression of emotions are the most common characteristics of an Italian family. Daughters have close ties with both parents, particularly as the parents grow older. Among first-generation Italians, the welfare of the family was considered the primary responsibility of each of its members. Although many second- and third-generation Italian Americans no longer live in an immediate Italian enclave, they return home frequently to maintain family, community, and ethnic ties.

While parents are alive, their home is most often the focus of family gatherings. Sons and daughters visit frequently during the week and after church on Sundays to share a large meal at the parents' house. Frequent contact with parents generally means contact with siblings and often aunts and uncles. Italian Americans are likely to see a parent daily or at least several times a week. If personal contact is not possible, frequent telephone contacts are made, sometimes several times a day. Love, respect, self-sacrifice, and mutual responsibility essentially summarize the diffuse sentiments most respondents express in regard to their parents.

The status of elderly Italians is one of continuity. Although they are more dependent in terms of their social and psychological needs, and more disengaged from work and roles connected with formal and informal associations, they are firmly entrenched in the extended family system. Even though they may have major worries about maintaining traditional family values, changes have not resulted in their exclusion from the lives of their children. Continuity in parental roles is an important factor in maintaining the high status of the elderly. For elderly women, motherhood and domestic roles change in intensity but do not lose their centrality. As grandmothers, their nurturing functions continue. For men, the loss of the work role does not noticeably affect their central role in the family. Instead, the absence of the work role permits greater family involvement.

To most elderly Italians, the ideal living situation is to maintain one's own home near one's children, because many believe they do not feel the same when they are not in their own homes. Parents receive respect, gratitude, and love in return for their many sacrifices. Having respect for the elderly is very important (Mason, 1997). With little variation, the prevailing view is that elders should reap rewards in old age for having had a single-minded dedication to parenthood during difficult times. Pesenti's study (1990) on family values and psychological adjustment among female Italian American and Jewish American immigrants in nursing homes suggested that elderly Italian women have greater filial expectations, are more traditional in family ideology, and have a poorer adjustment to nursing home life than Jewish women.

Most Italians have an actively functioning kinship and extended family system that is the primary focus of solidarity for the nuclear family. Relationships are not allowed to wither through lack of contact because through force of habit and the ritualization of occasions for high sociability, rarely a week passes that relatives do not play a central part in the average family's activities. Trying to distance oneself from such an all-embracing family system is easier said than done.

Primary relationships are usually lifelong. For example, many Italians of today's generation recall their childhoods in extended family systems where grandparents lived in the same house and aunts and uncles lived on the same block; this pattern still exists in some communities. As young children, cousins become well acquainted because their parents visit frequently. Because they live in close proximity, friendships form in their early years and continue throughout their lives. The elaboration of collateral relationships is one reason many Italian families are able to maintain a higher level of kinship solidarity than is evident for society at large. Because the extended family is close, and frequent visits are important, health-care providers may need to make special arrangements for visitation when Italian clients are in acute or long-term care facilities.

Social status for most Italian American families comes from family lineage. They cultivate power, wealth, and possessions when they can afford them. Titles are more important than names, which can be an asset in the health-care environment. If the health-care worker has a title of importance, using it may increase compliance with health treatments and regimens.

ALTERNATIVE LIFESTYLES

Despite values clearly defined around family obligations, Italians generally do not reject another family member because of an infraction or alternative lifestyle such as divorce, living together before marriage, or being involved in a lesbian or gay relationship. They may complain and argue with the deviant member, hoping for a change, but if their complaining and arguing fail to bring about the desired change, they still accept the individual and live with the consequences. When health-care providers need to make social support referrals for gays or lesbians, they can assist clients in contacting one of the gay and lesbian religious groups.

Workforce Issues

CULTURE IN THE WORKPLACE

For most Italian Americans, acquiring education, title, and money is of great importance. Italians believe strongly in the work ethic, are punctual, and rarely miss work commitments when suffering from a cold, headache, or minor illnesses. If completing their work requires staying later, they do so. Although the family is of utmost importance to Italians, work takes priority over family unless serious family situations arise. This cultural predisposition parallels the North American work ethic. The one thing Italians have in common is a sense of pride in their culture and in the achievements of their forbearers (Matusow, 1999).

ISSUES RELATED TO AUTONOMY

Italian immigrants and their descendants regard work as moral training for the young. Among Italians, work is viewed as a matter of pride, demonstrating that one has become a man or woman and is a full-functioning member of the family. This ethic is so strong that it governs behavior apart from monetary gain derived from employment. To the Italian, it is morally wrong not to be productively occupied. *Poveri si, ma perché lognisi?* (Poor yes, but why lazy?). Even though Italians have the utmost respect for their employer, they are emotional and passionate people, and when a confrontation arises, Italians are likely to get involved. For example, the first Italian immigrants working in New York City defended themselves against deplorable working conditions by forming one of the city's largest unions.

Because of language barriers, first-generation Italians and newer immigrants are more likely to accept assigned tasks without expecting any decision-making authority. Second- and third-generation immigrants, having a command of English, are more apt to seek positions of authority, take responsibility, and become managers or business proprietors. Italians who were born and educated in the United States usually have little difficulty communicating with others in the workforce. Newer immigrants and those with limited English language skills have the most difficulty assimilating into the workforce, a problem that is common to all non-English-speaking immigrants.

Biocultural Ecology

SKIN COLOR AND OTHER BIOLOGIC VARIATIONS

Because of Italy's proximity to Switzerland, Austria, and Germany in the North and to North Africa in the south, Italians as a group have varied physical characteristics. Those from a predominantly northern background have lighter skin, lighter hair, and blue eyes, whereas those from the south of Rome, particularly from Sicily, have dark, often curly hair, dark eyes, and olive-colored skin. Health-care practitioners should be aware of skin variations among Italian Americans, especially when assessing for anemia, cyanosis, lowered oxygenation levels, and jaundice in those who are darker skinned. In dark-skinned clients, the skin turns ashen instead of blue in the presence of cyanosis and decreased hemoglobin levels. To observe for the conditions, the practitioner must examine the sclera, conjunctiva, buccal mucosa, tongue, lips, nailbeds, palms of the hands and soles of the feet. To assess for jaundice, health-care providers need to look at the conjunctiva and in the buccal mucosa for patches of bilirubin pigment.

DISEASES AND HEALTH CONDITIONS

Early Italian immigrants to America lived and worked in poor, crowded conditions that made Italian families susceptible to anemia, bad teeth, pneumonia, meningitis, diphtheria, tuberculosis, and industrial accidents. Some first-generation Italians suffered from somatic complaints and physical ailments, which the immigrants sometimes attributed to **il mal occhio**, "evil eye" (see Folk Practices). Second-generation immigrants tend to develop neurological and psychotic symptoms attributable to guilt because they have broken away from the culture of their parents.

People of Italian ancestry have some notable genetic diseases, such as familial Mediterranean fever, Mediterranean-type glucose-6-phosphate dehydrogenase deficiency (G-6-PD), and β-thalassemia. Familial Mediterranean fever, recurrent polyserositis, was originally common in the Middle East only but is now seen in various parts of the world. This familial disease is characterized by short attacks of fever, peritonitis, pleuritis, and arthritis, with death caused by amyloidosis if the disease progresses. No specific diagnostic test is available; treatment is symptomatic. Mediterranean-type G-6-PD deficiency is an inherited, X-linked, recessive disorder most fully expressed in homozygous men with a carrier state found in heterozygous women. Red blood cell damage begins after intense or prolonged administration of sulfonamides, antimalarial agents, salicylates, or naphthaquinolones; after ingestion of fava beans; or in the presence of hypoxemia or acidosis. Supportive therapy includes withdrawing the causative agent and administering blood transfusions and oral iron therapy, which usually results in spontaneous recovery.

β-Thalassemia, of which there are two types, is prevalent in Greeks, Italians, Sephardic Jews, and Arabs. Both are caused by genetic defects in the synthesis of the hemoglobin A or B chain. Beta-chain production is depressed moderately in the heterozygous form, β-thalassemia minor, and severely depressed in the homozygous form, thalassemia major, which is also called Cooley's anemia, named after the American physician who described it. β-Thalassemia minor causes mild-to-moderate anemia, splenomegaly, bronze coloring of the skin, and hyperplasia of the bone marrow. Affected people are usually asymptomatic. Individuals with β-thalassemia major may experience severe anemia; death caused by high-output cardiac failure can occur in early childhood if this condition is left untreated. No cure exists, but palliative therapy includes repeated transfusions of packed red blood cells.

In addition to these genetic diseases, Italian Americans have a high incidence of hypertension and coronary artery disease related to smoking and their type A behavior. Bernstein, Flannery, and Reynolds (1993) reported that Italian Americans have significantly higher risks of nasopharyngeal, stomach, liver, and gallbladder tumors. Women exhibit a low risk for cancer of the oral cavity, esophagus, colon, rectum, and pancreas. Men exhibit a low risk for cancer of the larynx, lung, melanoma, breast, prostate, bladder, and non-Hodgkin's lymphoma. Kidd, Lancaster, and McCredie (1993) reported an increased incidence of ventricular septal defects in children of Italian heritage and that congenital heart disease in infants is associated with older maternal age at conception. Italian Americans are also at increased risk for multiple sclerosis (MS). This finding provides evidence that ancestry, genetics, and environment are a part of the complicated picture of MS.

VARIATIONS IN DRUG METABOLISM

The medical literature does not report any variations in drug metabolism or interactions specific to Italians or Italian Americans in general. However, health conditions such as Mediterranean-type G-6-PD deficiency and thalassemia have a profound effect on drug metabolism. Because conditions such as hypoxemia and acidosis, ingestion of fava beans, and the administration of sulfonamides, antimalarial agents, salicylates, and naphthaquinolones can exacerbate these conditions (Levy, 1993), health-care professionals must take extra precaution when prescribing these drug therapies for Italian Americans.

High-Risk Behaviors

Older Italian Americans may have significant health problems related to dental caries. Many first-generation Italians believe that it is useless to provide dental care to first teeth because they are temporary and are likely to impute caries in permanent teeth due to poor North American air. Although there is much education in the general population regarding the risks of smoking, many Italian American immigrants continue to smoke. Alcoholism also presents a risk in this group. Muhlin's (1985) comparison of alcohol-related and non-alcohol-related diagnoses among immigrants in New York state reports that 40 percent of Italian men, compared with 50 percent of Irish men, are hospitalized for alcohol-related diagnoses. Thus, health-care providers need to assess Italian Americans for dental problems caused by poor dental hygiene, cardiorespiratory diseases due to smoking, and possible alcohol abuse and alcohol-related diseases.

HEALTH-CARE PRACTICES

The beliefs of first-generation and newer Italian immigrants toward biomedical care are much the same as they are in Italy. Most of these immigrants believe they come to North America equipped with the best medical knowledge and ideas on the preservation of family health. Although many second- and third-generation Italian Americans are less traditional in health-care practices, many practice some of the traditional methods for staying well.

Several distinct patterns for making a decision to seek health care are reported among a sample of Catholic Italian Americans. These patterns include the occurrence of an interpersonal crisis, a perceived interference with social or personal relations, sanctioning, or a perceived interference with vocational or physical activity (Zola, 1973). Health-care providers must provide health counseling within these health-seeking and decision-making patterns. Providing culturally congruent care among Italian Americans is essential to compliance.

Nutrition

MEANING OF FOOD

To Italian Americans, food is symbolic of life and the principal medium of life, particularly family life. Respect for food is upheld even among the poor. The ceremony of eating is honored. Italians may convey to their children that the waste or abuse of food is a sin. In an emotional sense, food is a connection between an Italian child and the parents; food represents the product of the father's labor, prepared with care by the mother. In a symbolic sense, meals are a communion of the family, and food is sacred because it is the tangible medium of that communion.

Italian American mothers' "preoccupation with food" has a kernel of truth in it. There is something incredibly generous in the Italian nature, particularly when it comes to the preparation and sharing of food. An Italian mother may demonstrate her affection by feeding her family and anyone else she likes. To the average Italian mom, love is

a four letter word: *food*. The close association between food and mothering results in some predictable problems. Many Italians and traditional Italian Americans believe that bigger babies are healthier. The size of the baby is perceived as an index of the successful maintenance of maternal and wifely responsibilities. The expression *mangia, mangia,* or "eat, eat," on the lips of many immigrant mothers is still heard today.

COMMON FOODS AND FOOD RITUALS

The Italian diet, rich in vegetables, pasta, fruit, fish, and cheese, varies according to the region of Italy from which the individual originated. Northern Italian foods are rich in cream and cheese, resulting in a potential high intake of fat. Southern Italian foods are prepared in red sauces, spices, and added salt. Because of regional variations in food selections and preparation practices, it is important for health-care professionals to specifically inquire about the diet of their Italian American clients, preferably during intake assessments.

The staples of the Italian American diet are spaghetti, lasagna, ravioli, pasta with pesto, and manicotti. Vegetables, fresh fruit, and beans are common. Popular Italian foods include lentils, sausage, eggplant parmigiana, salami, olive oil, espresso and cappuccino coffee, wine, ice cream (gelato), pastries such as cannoli and biscotti, and cheeses such as provolone, ricotta, romano, and parmigiana. Other common dishes include escarole, Caesar salad, calzone, and pizza. Table 13–1 lists the Italian names of popular foods with their descriptions and ingredients.

One important concept to understand about many Italians and their relationship with food is that an outsider cannot enter an Italian home and discuss anything of consequence until at least some token meal is shared. Entering into the family communion is a prerequisite to partaking in any of its affairs. In the Italian tradition, each meal is significant. The noontime meal is traditionally taken whenever possible by the

Table 13–1 Italian Foods

Common Name	Description	Ingredients
Calamari	Squid, fried or on pasta	Floured squid fried in olive oil or in red sauce
Frittata	Italian omelet	Eggs, peppers, and onions cooked in olive oil
Minestrone	Soup with greens	Escarole and beans with garlic and other herbs
Parmigiana di melanzana	Eggplant parmesan	Eggplant, tomato sauce, bread crumbs, Parmesan cheese, and mozzarella cheese
Pasta con pesto	Sauce served over linguine	Sauce of basil, nuts, olive oil, and garlic
Pasta e fagioli	Macaroni and beans	Shell-shaped pasta, kidney beans, and tomato sauce
Pasta marinara	Pasta in tomato sauce	Tomato sauce
Pizza fritta	Fried dough with sugar and cinnamon	Bread dough fried in oil and sprinkled with sugar and cinnamon
Prosciutto	Thinly sliced ham	Delicate thin ham served with melon
Spaghetti aglio olio	Spaghetti with olive oil	Spaghetti, olive oil, garlic, and red pepper
Tortellini	Little rounds of pasta in white or red sauce	Pasta dough stuffed with meat and cheese
Veal scaloppine	Medallions of veal	Veal sautéed with wine, butter, and lemon

entire family. Dinner is a gathering of the family. Italian wine is taken at almost every meal, and a mixture of water and wine is given to children. The only outsiders to be invited are godparents and occasionally honored friends.

Breakfast has never been an important meal for Italians. Breakfast usually consists of a small cup of strong coffee and a sweet pastry, often taken at a local "bar." The major meal of the week was the one at which time and circumstances permitted the most leisurely and largest gathering of *la famiglia*. The Sunday dinner, which begins in midafternoon and lasts until early or even late evening, is a relaxed social gathering featuring tasty cheeses, fish, and salami. Although the routine of North American life has altered this schedule, especially of daytime weekday meals, many Italian Americans still adhere to the ceremonies of the evening and Sunday dinner.

Italians love ceremonies and feasts. The Italian historian Arrigo Petacco recalls that every day was a feast day to some patron saint, during which time the streets rang with shouts in every Italian dialect. Each feast day became an assertion of the southern Italian peasants' old world belief that magic rather than the religious sacraments was their way of dealing with the supernatural. Those afflicted in mind and body sought sorcerers rather than priests. Few Italians could resist the music, dancing, eating, drinking, and firework festivities associated with Italian feasts. In many parts of North American Italian communities, there is an annual religious festival honoring some favorite patron saint or the Madonna. The saint with the largest constituency is San Gennaro, the patron saint of Naples.

DIETARY PRACTICES FOR HEALTH PROMOTION

Italian immigrants brought many dietary practices to North America for keeping their families healthy. One of the most common practices for health promotion is eating a clove of garlic every night before going to bed to prevent upper respiratory infections. Garlic may also be worn around the neck when there is an epidemic of influenza or other upper respiratory ailments to prevent the wearer from getting the infection. Another health promotion practice, eating a fresh raw egg every morning, keeps the person strong. Fresh dandelions are used to make a salad or are boiled to make soup to give the person strength. Red wine mixed with water is given to children with meals to maintain healthy blood.

NUTRITIONAL DEFICIENCIES AND FOOD LIMITATIONS

Because the Italian diet is rich in fruits, vegetables, garlic, pasta, and olive oil, nutritional deficiencies are rare. First-generation Italians who lived in tenement housing initially suffered from nutritional deficiencies caused by a lack of money and dislike for American food. Native food practices have not changed much for Italian immigrants or for second- and third-generation Italian Americans. Italian foods are one of the most popular

choices for North Americans of all nationalities, making them easily accessible. In addition, because of the Italian propensity to cook with olive oil and garlic and serve pasta and a variety of vegetables, nutritionists have endorsed most Italian food as healthy.

Pregnancy and Childbearing Practices

FERTILITY PRACTICES AND VIEWS TOWARD PREGNANCY

Most first-generation Italian Americans did not practice birth control and rarely discussed matters related to sex. Premarital sex and adultery were absolutely forbidden. Second-generation Italian women often began using birth control years after their marriage. Sex was rarely discussed in the family, premarital sex was greatly restricted, and adultery was strictly taboo. However, many third-generation Italian Americans use birth control from the beginning of marriage, and sex is commonly discussed in the family. A weakened external restriction on premarital sex continues, but internal inhibitions remain strong. In the past, adultery was often seen as unacceptable but sometimes excusable.

The proportion of Italian American women, aged 35 to 44, with five or more children is second lowest in comparison to women of other ethnic groups in the same age range. A strong sense of modesty and embarrassment among Italian Americans may result in the avoidance of discussions related to sex and menstruation, hindering early diagnosis and primary prevention interventions.

Traditional ideas among Italian Americans regarding pregnancy have undergone slight but significant variations in the United States. The belief that a mother does not conceive while nursing continues to be held by many Italian women. Sprinkling salt under and around the bed of a newly married couple is believed to make them fertile.

PRESCRIPTIVE, RESTRICTIVE, AND TABOO PRACTICES IN THE CHILDBEARING FAMILY

Traditional beliefs related to pregnancy include the following: coffee spills may result in the baby being born with a birthmark where the coffee was spilled; women must abstain from sexual relationships while pregnant; and if the expectant mother's cravings for a particular food are not satisfied, a congenital anomaly may occur or the baby will be marked. In addition, if a pregnant woman is not given the food she smells, the fetus moves and a miscarriage results; if she turns or moves in a certain way, the fetus does not develop normally; and she should not reach over her head because harm may come to the baby. Many traditional Italians practice these beliefs.

Many traditional Italians fear hospital care in North America, except in the case of childbirth. Although many women still prefer having their children delivered at home by a family physician or a midwife, many Italian women deliver their babies in hospitals. A hospital delivery provides a means of avoiding the traditional sexual intercourse rites at the onset of labor—a tradition sometimes seen today. In the **via vecchia** (old way) if labor does not progress rapidly enough, a neighbor has to spit out the window. This ritualistic spitting has the power to break any magic spell that might have brought the ill fortune of a slow labor. People who believe in the **via nuova** (new way) do not practice this ritual spitting.

Among traditional Italian Americans, a postpartum woman is not allowed to wash her hair, take a shower, or resume her domestic chores for at least 2 or 3 weeks after birth so she can rest. The woman's mother and other female family members tend to the chores and assist with the care of the new baby. New mothers are expected to breast-feed to restore the health of the reproductive organs and keep the mother and baby free of infections.

Death Rituals

DEATH RITUALS AND EXPECTATIONS

In the Italian American family, death is a great social loss and brings an immediate response from the community. It means sending food and flowers (chrysanthemums), giving money, and congregating at the home of the deceased. As for other life events, among the first responses to death is food, which is brought by friends and distant relatives. Italians believe food is a source of comfort during troubled times.

Italian death rituals can be very demonstrative. The funeral procession to the cemetery is a symbol of family status. There is great pride in the size of the event, which is determined by the number of cars in the procession. Although there is a tendency today to decrease the elaborateness of the funeral, it remains very much a family and community event. Its ritual recognition de-emphasizes death. Grief over the deceased is eased if a biomedical explanation for the cause of death is given and if it is explained that the death was inevitable. Within the context of fatalism in Catholicism, many Italians view death as "God's will"; thus, a fatal diagnosis may not be discussed with the ill family member. More traditional families hold anniversary masses for the deceased and wear black for months or years. This is not as common among younger generations.

RESPONSES TO DEATH AND GRIEF

Emotional outpourings can be profuse and the activities around a funeral provide distinct examples of the Italian American way of ritualizing life events. Women may mourn dramatically, even histrionically, for the whole family. They do not merely weep; they may rage against death for the harm it has done to the family. Family members may moan and scream for the deceased throughout the church service. Screaming is an effort to ensure that Jesus, Mary, and the saints hear what the bereaved are thinking and feeling. Family members get up constantly to touch and talk to the deceased loved one. Children are taught to let the female kin express their feelings for them. The real time of sorrow comes at the end of the ceremony when the priest and nonfamily congregation say good-bye to the deceased. At this time, the family is on its own for a time with the loved one.

Older women may throw themselves onto the casket trying to prevent it from leaving the church. Then the priest intones the farewell: "May the angels take you into paradise, may the martyrs welcome you on your way." While men mourn, they do so in the fashion of **pazienza** (patience). Their constant, silent, and expressionless presence may be their only act of public mourning.

Today, second- and third-generation Italian American families still acknowledge the need for the mourning procession and the company of family and friends to grieve the loss of a loved one. Abundant tears and moaning are still recognized as the proper expression of grief. To many, giving up these customs means an improper expression of respect for the deceased. In fact, when the loss is great, such as in the death of a child or spouse, expressions of grief continue for years. Health-care providers working in hospices must be familiar with the Italian American's responses to death and grieving to effectively offer positive support.

Spirituality

DOMINANT RELIGION AND USE OF PRAYER

Rome is the world seat for the central administration of the Roman Catholic Church, the largest Christian denomination in the world. The predominant religion of Italians and Italian Americans is traditional Roman Catholicism, which includes folk religious practices that have changed little since the birth of Christ. Moreover, an amalgam of beliefs has evolved from diverse cultures that took up residence in Italy through the centuries. Thus, Italian Americans' spiritual and religious beliefs have their roots in pagan customs, magical beliefs, Muslim practices, Christian doctrines, and Italian pragmatism. The center of Roman Catholic worship is the celebration of Mass, the Eucharist, which is the commemoration of Christ's sacrificial death and of His Resurrection. Other sacraments are baptism, confirmation, confession, matrimony, ordination, and anointing of the sick. The workings of nature and the benefits and calamities caused by nature are attributed to (1) saints resembling pagan gods such as witches, ghosts, and demons; (2) the Christian God; (3) Satan; and (4) any and all possible combinations and alliances of these factors.

Most Italians pray to the Virgin Mary, the Madonna, and a number of saints. Many traditional first-generation and newer Italian American families display shrines to the Blessed Virgin in their backyards. Italian Americans view God as an all-understanding, compassionate, and forgiving being. Prayer and having faith in God and saints help Italian Americans through illnesses. Italian men bypass praying to the Madonna because women are perceived to have a closer relationship with her. Niceties of Catholic orthodoxy and enlightened learning are employed together with pagan practices. The lessons of common sense and science are freely mingled with those of magicoreligious beliefs. Health-care providers must respect and acknowledge such beliefs to gain the trust of their clients.

MEANING OF LIFE AND INDIVIDUAL SOURCES OF STRENGTH

Family and religious beliefs give strength to Italians, who see themselves first as family members and then as individuals. Family, whose primary focus is concern and a sense of pride in the **onore della famiglia** (family honor), helps individuals cope with the surrounding world and provides a sense of continuity.

Work and physical activity is considered essential for a full life. Italians love the arts and have made great contributions over the centuries in music, opera, and painting. They believe that life is to be experienced with **pazienza** (patience); they are happy and pride themselves on being clean, conscientious, and passionate people. Italian Americans prevail through their sheer determination, sustained by the solidarity of *la famiglia.*

SPIRITUAL BELIEFS AND HEALTH-CARE PRACTICES

Because Italian Americans have strong beliefs in Catholicism, when a loved one becomes ill they pray at home and in church for the person's health. In times of illness, health-care providers may need to help clients obtain the basic rites of the Sacrament of the Sick, which includes anointing, communion, and if possible, a blessing by the priest. A small wafer, the Eucharist, is considered a food for healing and of health. Even though Catholics are obligated to fast or abstain from meat and meat products on certain days of the year, the sick are not bound by this practice. Despite the church's exception for the sick, many first-generation immigrants choose to fast.

Health-Care Practices

HEALTH-SEEKING BELIEFS AND BEHAVIORS

The beliefs of first-generation and newer immigrants about health and health care are similar to beliefs in their homeland. In traditional terms, illnesses are attributable to (1) wind currents that carry disease, (2) contamination, (3) heredity, (4) supernatural (God's will) or human causes, and (5) psychosomatic interactions. In addition, superstition, a trait of Italian culture, plays a fundamental role in Italian Americans' choice of health-care practices. First-generation, and to a lesser degree, second- and third-generation Italian Americans may not accept institutional care either in sickness or in old age.

An example of a condition attributable to wind currents is as follows: leaving a body cavity such as the abdomen open too long during surgery exposes it to excess air and leads to a quicker death. Within the context of fatalism, diseases largely run their own course; thus, it is better to leave the investigation into health problems until a condition becomes so obvious that it cannot be neglected. The condition, evil eye, caused by supernatural human agents is discussed under Folk

Practices. Nervousness, hysteria, and many other mental illnesses are attributed to an evil spirit entering the body and remaining in the body until it is cast out by making its abiding place so unpleasant that it is forced to leave.

Gilford's study (1994) of Italian Australian working women found that these women discuss health and illness concerns as one way in which to express feelings of loss over the fertility of their youth and grief over the life they left behind in Italy. These losses are experienced physically and expressed metaphorically through conditions of "bad blood" and "nerves," and contribute to their increased vulnerability to a range of diseases, including cancer. For these women, the change of life is experienced as the end of life, and their fear of cancer is representative of their fear of social and physical death.

RESPONSIBILITY FOR HEALTH CARE

The concept of family, the most dominant influence on the individual, is viewed as the most credible source of health-care practices. Italians believe that the most significant moments of life should take place under their own roofs. The extended family may be the front-line resource for intensive advice on emotional problems. Mental health specialists are frequently perceived as inappropriate agents for meeting problems that are beyond the expertise of the family and local community. Most second- and third-generation Italians take responsibility for their own health care and engage in health promotion activities more than those of the first generation. Most also have health insurance coverage. From the family perspective, the mother assumes responsibility for the health of the children.

FOLK PRACTICES

Earlier immigrants from southern Italy had a mass of folk practices related to cures for organic and mental disorders. For difficult cases, they summoned a witch, barber, midwife, or herbalist. Because life was precarious and evils abounded, the **contadini** attempted to make sense of a dangerous world. Events were caused by forces and powers that were, in turn, controlled by agents. One had to find which agent was behind a certain force and then marshal a counterforce by soliciting a more powerful agent to oppose it. These agents are given one generic name, **il mal occhio** (the evil eye), which is also called *occhio cattivo* (bad eye); *occhio morto* (eye of death); and *occhio tristo* (wicked eye). Evil eye has its roots in ancient Greece and was introduced to Italy during colonization by the Greeks.

Individuals can protect themselves from the evil eye by using magical symbols and by learning the rituals of the **maghi** (witch). Amulets, miniature representations of natural or man-made weapons that fight off the evil eye, include teeth, claws, and replicas of animal horns that are worn on necklaces or bracelets, held in a pocket, or sewn into clothing. **Cornicelli** (little red horns) can still be purchased in Italian neighborhoods as good luck charms. First-generation and many second- and third-generation Italian Americans believe in obtaining as much protection from the evil eye as possible. An array of pictures and statues of the Madonna and saints are liberally distributed throughout their homes and supplement these red horns, which are often hung over a door. Many are still seen today. When Italian American clients bring these amulets with them into health-care settings, health-care providers should not remove them because they provide great solace to the clients.

All life-sustaining things of the earth are given special respect and, in particular, plants are thought to have special magical attributes. Common plant derivatives and items used in folk healing are olive oil, lemon juice, wine, vinegar, garlic, onion, lettuce, and tobacco. A crown of lemon leaves is believed to cure a headache, as are wild fennel, deadly nightshade, and sorrel. The leaves and flowers of the wild mallow herb, *malva*, are used to make tea, providing cool energy and positive effects on the lungs and stomach. When suffering from a fever, a person is given hot rather than cold drinks. For indigestion, a mixture of coffee grounds and sugar is taken. Grain sprouts, especially those grown in the dark, in consecrated ground, in the churchyard, or in a crypt are believed to protect against Satan and the forces of chaos.

The principal animals in folk prescriptions are the wolf, chicken, viper, lizard, frog, pig, dog, mouse, and sea horse. Body secretions such as saliva, urine, mother's milk, blood, and ear wax are commonly used as folk medicines. Some Italian mothers use early morning saliva to bathe the eyes of children with conjunctivitis. Baldness is treated with an application of warm cow's urine. Sulfur and lemon juice are mixed as an ointment for scabies, and potato or lemon slices are bound to the wrists to reduce fever.

BARRIERS TO HEALTH CARE

Most Italian Americans have few barriers to health services. However many, especially among the first generation, may underuse available resources because they have little faith in medical practitioners. In addition, the high cost of institutional care may be a deterrent for many. Newer immigrants, who have difficulty with the English language and are unfamiliar with the health-care system, can benefit from a cultural broker or case manager to help bridge these barriers.

CULTURAL RESPONSES TO HEALTH AND ILLNESS

Both age and gender mediate ethnic differences in the expression of pain for Italian Americans. Older Italian Americans, especially women, are more likely to report pain experiences, express symptoms to the fullest extent, and expect immediate treatment. Italians tend to be more verbally expressive with chronic pain than do other ethnic groups. Neill's study (1993) on pain in acute myocardial infarction indicates that clients of Jewish and Italian ancestry exhibit more expressive pain behaviors than clients of Irish or English ancestry.

Vincente's study (1993) examined Italian Americans' attitudes and beliefs about mental health services and mental health workers. The results suggested that Italian American professionals have the highest level of satisfac-

tion with their work, show the most tolerance for deviant behavior in the community, and hold a nontraditional view of psychiatry. Because Italian Americans tend to report more symptoms and report them more dramatically, health-care providers must be cautious not to overdiagnose emotional problems in Italian patients.

Most Italian Americans believe that people who have disabilities should be cared for at home by the family; thus, very few individuals are placed in long-term care facilities. Germans, followed by Italians, have the greatest acceptance for people with disabilities. Individuals with physiological or physical disabilities such as asthma, diabetes, heart disease, and arthritis are the most accepted, whereas people with disabilities such as AIDS, mental retardation, psychiatric illness, and cerebral palsy are the least accepted (Westbrook, Legge, & Pennay, 1993). A person with a physical or mental disability is not stigmatized in the Italian culture because the condition is believed to be God's will. Suppressing emotions and stress from fear, guilt, and anxiety can cause illness. For example, if a person does not vent these feelings, the person may burst.

For many Italians the sick role is not entered into without personal feelings of guilt; thus, individuals may keep sickness a secret from their family and friends, and are not inclined to describe the details because they blame themselves for the health problem. Families may be ashamed to let neighbors know of an incident that may impair the social status of a family member. This applies especially to afflicted daughters, and to a lesser degree to sons. A reputation of poor health unfavorably affects the value of a young woman's potential as a wife. When a family member is sick, other women in the family take over and assist until the sick person is well.

BLOOD TRANSFUSIONS AND ORGAN DONATION

Judicious use of medications and blood transfusions are permissible and morally acceptable as long as the benefits outweigh the risks to the individual; thus, Italian Americans have little objection to accepting a blood transfusion when needed. First-generation immigrants are, in general, not prone to donating their organs. Second- and third-generation Italian Americans may also reflect this perspective. Organ donation is morally permissible when the benefits to the recipient are proportionate to the loss of the organ to the donor, and when the organ does not deprive the donor of life or the functional integrity of the body. Otherwise, organ transplant is an individual decision.

Health-Care Practitioners

TRADITIONAL VERSUS BIOMEDICAL PRACTITIONERS

Mystical powers are not limited to saints. For traditional Italians, certain humans are believed to have immediate and potent access to magical powers. These are the *maghi*, "male witch" and the *maghe*, "female witch," who are granted various degrees of black magic power at birth. A man or woman with more limited powers is often called *un'uomo di fuori* (a different or "outside" man). A powerful sorcerer is called *lupo mannaro* (werewolf). These extraordinary people are thought to possess or influence the evil eye. They have the power to cast spells, cause or cure ailments, and change events by using their own force—even their gaze is thought to be potent. These traditional beliefs may be practiced by first-generation and newer Italian immigrants, but hold little value for second- and third-generation Italian Americans. Health-care providers should accept and incorporate these practices into their treatment plans, along with providing written instructions for biomedical treatments.

The barber's role in bloodletting was firmly established among first-generation Italian Americans. Native Italians who readily went to the barber for bloodletting may strenuously object to blood tests. The belief is that the barber draws off unhealthy blood, in contrast to blood taken for testing, where the needle is inserted into a healthy arm. Italians believe in the connection between soul and blood found in Leviticus: "for the life of all flesh is the blood thereof." The shaman (usually a male) is the family physician and a practical student of human relations.

STATUS OF HEALTH-CARE PROVIDERS

Early Italian immigrants looked questionably on book-trained physicians, having little trust in American health-care practitioners. With all the folk remedies for cure within easy reach, Italians did not eagerly accept physicians. They reasoned that when it was a question of seeking health advice, they would be foolish to pay money only to learn something unpleasant. Some health-care practitioners find themselves practicing in an invisible border, separating them from their Italian clients where differences of culture can lead to misunderstanding and impede gaining cooperation with prescribed therapy. Today, some physicians collaborate with shamans and herbalists to accommodate clients' cultural preferences. Respect for the customs and taboos of Italian immigrant clients can pay dividends in terms of increasing the health-care practitioner's effectiveness and efficiency.

Success in persuading children of Italian parents to take medicine depends on the trust the mother has in the health-care provider. If the health-care provider is Italian or makes an effort to understand the Italian culture, the mother is more compliant. Thus, assigning practitioners of the same culture, when possible, is advantageous.

CASE STUDY Rosa and Mario Gianquito live on the ground floor of a three-family house in Brooklyn, New York. Although they completed grammar school in Italy, they speak English and have little difficulty understanding most verbal communication. They have a daughter, Lucia, age 25, and a son, Anthony, age 28, who were born in this neighborhood but now live in Manhattan. Both children speak fluent Italian. Anthony is an attorney and does not visit with his sister very often. Lucia is a grammar school teacher,

married to an Italian man, Guido Venetto, who recently immigrated from southern Italy and is 10 years older than Lucia. Guido speaks mostly Italian at home but does speak broken English. In addition to smoking two packs of cigarettes a day Guido is emotionally abusive to Lucia. He is very jealous and does not want Lucia to go out after work with her friends or to spend much time visiting with her parents. Lucia has allergies, and the last time she visited the doctor he told her that her blood pressure was elevated. She has noticed lately that after standing all day at work she often has swollen ankles and leg pain.

Lucia's husband works 12 hours a day as a construction worker and expects her to cook old-country style Italian food, which requires that she use a great deal of salt. She is often depressed and feels isolated and powerless. She has been trying to have a baby for 3 years.

Rosa comes to visit her daughter when she can. She often brings homemade manicotti or tortellini when she comes. She is very concerned about Guido's behavior toward her daughter, but does not feel that she can challenge Guido because he is the *capo di famiglia*. Rosa is concerned about Lucia's swollen feet and suggests that she drink red wine and eat more garlic and dandelions. She tells Lucia to pray to the Virgin Mary to ask for help in conceiving a child and to make Guido treat her better.

Lucia and Guido attend the neighborhood Catholic Church on Sunday. Lucia always wears the **cornicelli** around her neck that her mother gave her to protect her from **il mal occhio**. Lucia says her faith and her family help her cope with life challenges with **pazienza**.

STUDY QUESTIONS

1 Identify three problems for a plan of care for Lucia.

2 Identify two health-teaching goals for this family that are congruent with family order and rituals.

3 Identify three socioeconomic factors that influence the health of the Venetto family.

4 How might the health-care provider involve Lucia in a mutual planning process for her holistic health-care needs including mind, body, and spirit?

5 Knowing that many first-generation Italians generally mistrust health-care providers, how would you encourage Lucia to engage in health promotion behaviors?

6 Discuss at least two preventive health maintenance teaching activities that respect the folk practices used to treat illness in this family.

7 Define the Italian's unique relationship with food and discuss implications this could have on the health of the Venetto family, particularly Lucia.

8 Discuss the status and role of elderly Italians in the extended family and explain the reluctance of Lucia's mother to come and visit with her.

9 Identify two practices common among Italian women that might affect conception and pregnancy.

10 Name two dietary health-care risks and two dietary health-care assets for Italians.

11 What are some of the primary religious practices and use of prayer for Italian people?

12 Define the terms *capo di famiglia, il mal occhio,* and *pazienza.*

REFERENCES

Bernstein, L., Flannery, J., & Reynolds, J. (1993). Cancer in Italian migrant populations in the United States. *IARC Science Publication, 123,* 95–102.

Chick-Gravel, S. (Reviewer) (1999). Italians in America, 1 & 2. Video cassettes. *School Library Journal, 5*(11), 62.

Gilford, S. (1994). *The Italian American catalogue.* New York: Doubleday & Co.

Kidd, S., Lancaster, P., & McCredie, R. (1993). The incidence of congenital heart defects (CHD) in the first year of life. *Journal of Pediatric Child Health, 29*(5), 344–349.

Levy, R. (1993). Ethnic and racial differences in response to medicines: Preserving individualized therapy in managed pharmaceutical programmes. *Pharmaceutical Medicine, 7,* 139–165.

Mangione, J., & Morreale, B. (1993). *La storia: Five centuries of the Italian American experience.* New York: Harper Collins.

Mason, A. S. (1997). Respect: an Italian-American story. *Commonweal, 124,* 11–16.

Matusow, B. (1999). Washington, Italian style. *Washingtonian, 34*(9), 44–49.

Muhlin, G. (1985). Ethnic differences in alcohol misuse: A striking reaffirmation. *Journal of Studies on Alcohol, 46*(2), 172–173.

Neill, K. (1993). Ethnic pain styles in acute myocardial infarction. *Western Journal of Nursing Research, 15*(5), 531–547.

Pesenti, P. (1990). *Family values and psychological adjustment among female Italian and Jewish immigrant nursing home residents.* Seton Hall University, School of Education 1990, p. 257, VMI order #PUZ9025093.

Statistics Canada. (2001). http://www.statcan.com.

Vincente, B. (1993). Attitudes of professional mental health workers to psychiatry. *International Journal of Social Psychiatry, 39*(2), 131–141.

Wells, N., New, R., & Richman, A. (1994). The "good mother": A comparative study of Swedish, Italian and American behavior and goals. *Scandinavian Journal of Caring Sciences, 8*(2), 81–86.

Westbrook, M., Legge, V., & Pennay, M. (1993). Attitudes towards disabilities in a multicultural society. *Social Science Medicine, 36*(5), 615–623.

Zola, I. (1973). Pathways to the doctor: From person to patient. *Social Science and Medicine, 7*(9), 677–689.

Chapter 14

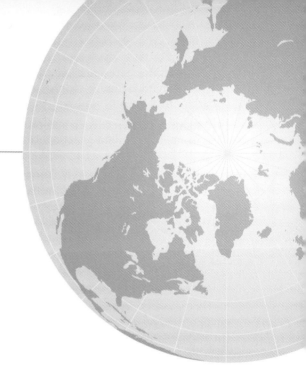

People of Japanese Heritage

NANCY C. SHARTS-HOPKO

Overview, Inhabited Localities, and Topography

OVERVIEW

Nihon, or **Nippon**, as Japan is called in the Japanese language, is a 1200-mile chain of islands in the northwestern Pacific Ocean. Japan borders Russia, Korea, and China, and its modern history has, until recently, been shaped by conflict with these countries. The population of more than 126 million resides mainly on the four largest islands (U.S. Department of State, 2000). The Japanese, who refer to themselves as **Nihonjin**, share a strong sense of nationalism and pride in ethnic purity. Japanese citizenship is not readily obtained, and foreign residents in Japan are required to register as aliens. The inclusion of even third-generation Korean residents in the category of foreigners has received considerable adverse international press in recent decades.

Japan's territory extends generally from northeast to southwest; the northern and westernmost areas have a climate similar to that found in the northern United States, while the Ryukyu Islands in the south are subtropical. The climate of the Tokyo region, where most of the population is clustered, is similar to that of Washington, D.C. Winters are moderate, with snows that seldom accumulate, while summers are hot and steamy.

This chapter reflects the author's experiences and observations while living and working in Japan for more than 2 years in the mid-1980s as a teaching missionary in a college of nursing, as well as on several visits since that time (Sharts Engel, 1989; Sharts-Hopko, 1995).

HERITAGE AND RESIDENCE

The original inhabitants of Japan most likely migrated from the Korean peninsula. The marked Chinese cultural influence began in the late 400s and included the system of writing, the calendar, Confucianism, Buddhism, and East Asian beliefs about health and illness. Following World War II, from 1945 to 1952, Japan was an occupied territory of the United States. As a bitter legacy of that war, the northernmost Kuril Islands are still claimed by Russia.

Japanese citizens residing in North America have tended to locate in large commercial and educational centers. With the establishment or purchase of factories in the midwestern and southern states by Japanese companies, communities of Japanese expatriates can now be found in smaller cities as well.

REASONS FOR MIGRATION AND ASSOCIATED ECONOMIC FACTORS

In the late 1800s, Japanese people began to migrate to the United States and Canada. From 1891 to 1924, more than 250,000 Japanese immigrated, settling primarily in the Territory of Hawaii and along the Pacific coast (Yanagisako, 1985). In 1998, the most recent year for which statistics are tabulated, 5647 Japanese nationals immigrated to the United States, adding to over one-half million Japanese immigrants since the late 1800s (Immigration & Naturalization Service, 2000). In addition, that year over 5.3 million Japanese visited the United States for short-term stays, including 4.7 million tourists and 83,000 students. Most of the rest were business travelers.

EDUCATIONAL STATUS AND OCCUPATIONS

Education is highly valued in Japan, where the illiteracy rate is nearly zero (U.S. Department of State, 2000). Completion of the 12th grade by more than 95 percent of young people ensures a highly competent workforce. For instance, calculus is part of the mandatory junior high school curriculum, and high school graduates complete 6 years of English. The school week includes a half day on Saturday. Many youngsters preparing for high school or college entrance examinations attend proprietary *juku*, or cram schools, in the evenings or on Sundays.

About 40 percent of all young people go on to higher education at over 1100 universities, junior colleges, and technical schools. Entrance examinations for high school and college are competitive. Because the alumni network primarily provides job placements, the school one attends determines to a great extent where one is employed after graduation.

While the concept of adults returning to college is new, self-improvement is a huge industry. Hobbies are taken very seriously, and often entail formal study. The traditional Japanese arts, such as the tea ceremony, *ikebana* (flower arranging), *bonsai*, *kimono* wearing, calligraphy, and even doll making are studied diligently by large numbers of women and by some retired men.

Sales of books, periodicals, and daily newspapers in Japan is the highest among industrialized nations (United Nations, 1993). The national broadcasting system, NHK, offers high-quality radio and television news and entertainment. *Issei* (first-generation Japanese immigrants) vary widely in their English language ability. *Nisei* (second-generation immigrants) and *sansei* (third-generation immigrants) are educated under the American educational system to the extent that they were permitted; for example, educational access was limited or segregated during the World War II internment of American citizens of Japanese ancestry. While the language barrier may be an obstacle to verbal instructions or explanations in English-speaking health-care settings, Japanese clients are likely to use written materials effectively.

Although Japanese culture reflects its recent agrarian past, at present only 2 percent of the population of Japan are engaged in agricultural occupations. In the United States, **issei** originally tended to work in agriculture or as small business owners. More recent immigrants work in business, the professions, service industries, and manufacturing. Second- and third-generation Japanese Americans tend to be highly educated professionals. Most Japanese nationals living in the United States are well-educated executives, visiting scholars, individuals with technical expertise, or students.

Communication

DOMINANT LANGUAGE AND DIALECTS

Japanese is the language of Japan with the exception of the indigenous **Ainu** people. The Japanese spoken in Tokyo is the national standard and that which is heard in media broadcasts. Because high school graduates in Japan complete 6 years of English, even newer Japanese immigrants and sojourners can speak, understand, read, and write the English language to some degree.

CULTURAL COMMUNICATION PATTERNS

One complexity of the Japanese language is the customizing of speech according to relative social status and gender. The Japanese sensitivity to relative status and the related need to constantly gauge one's behavior accordingly is one reason the circle of intimates with whom one can truly relax is quite limited. In addition, men tend to speak more coarsely and women with more gentility or refinement.

Light social banter and gentle joking are a mainstay of group relations, serving to foster group cohesiveness. Polite discussion unrelated to business, often over **o-cha**, green tea, precedes business negotiations. Relationship building and respect for personal privacy are important aspects of working relationships in all sectors.

In a densely populated society that values group harmony above all else, open communication is discouraged, making it difficult to learn what people think (Doi, 1971). In particular, among people of Japanese descent, saying "no" is considered extremely impolite; rather, one should let the matter drop.

A high value is placed on "face" and "saving face." Shame and its avoidance drive Japanese the way guilt and its avoidance is said to drive Westerners (Benedict, 1946). Asking someone to do something that he or she cannot do induces loss of face or shame. For people to be shown wrong is deeply humiliating. People feel shame for themselves and their group, but they are respected when they bear shame in stoic silence (French, 2001). Suicide over shame is a common theme in Japanese literature and lore. Because of ethnic homogeneity, an ingrained sensitivity to the feelings of others, and close contact with one's family, classmates, and work group, Japanese believe that vague, intuitive communication, called *hara wo yomu* (belly talk), is well understood by fellow group members.

In Japan, presenting a person with choices is regarded as a burden, and it is a kindness to spare people the burden of decision making. For example, a hostess may serve poured drinks to spare her guests the burden of deciding what they would like. A teacher may arrange employment for a former student; a physician will tell the client what to do about a health problem. These actions are motivated by concern for the well-being of the person in one's care. Japanese society is sometimes described as a web of **giri** (mutual obligations) that serves to ensure societal integrity and harmony.

Traditional Japanese people exhibit considerable control over body language. Anger or dismay may be quite difficult for Westerners to detect. Smiling and laughter are common shields for embarrassment or distress. However, one need only see tearful family partings at train stations to know that, contrary to Western assumptions, Japanese people do show their feelings.

Prolonged eye contact is not polite even within families. Social touching occurs among group members but not among people who are less closely acquainted. In general, body space is respected. Intimate behavior in the presence of others is taboo. In Japan, public kissing is occasionally decried in the newspapers.

When people greet one another, whether for the first time or for the first time on a given day, the traditional bow is performed. The depth of the bow, its duration, and the number of repetitions reflect the relative status of the parties involved and the formality of the occasion. An offer to shake hands by a Westerner is reciprocated graciously. With an introduction, *meishi* (business cards) are exchanged, enabling the parties to assess their relative status.

TEMPORAL RELATIONSHIPS

An awareness of Japanese history and legend, a high regard for the elderly, the value of family honor, and veneration of dead ancestors suggest a strong connection with the past. The overall orientation of the Japanese people, who are known for their postwar economic miracle, however, is toward the future. The population made huge sacrifices in the decades after the war for the good of the nation. Mothers encouraged their children to study hard so that their futures would be bright. Housewives are diligent savers for future family expenses. Companies plot their growth, and the government anticipates needs decades in advance. While Zen calls its practitioners to attend to the here and now, it actually has few adherents in Japan. Health-care providers may find that Japanese clients are astonishingly motivated in health-related decision making by considering their children's needs or the economic future for their family.

Punctuality is highly valued among the Japanese. Because people are so reliant on commuter trains, evening functions and city nightlife end rather early. In interesting contrast, the clinic system of health care pervades even the private sector in Japan. Clinic services are not expected to be efficient and hospital stays are lengthy.

FORMAT FOR NAMES

In Japan, family names are stated first, followed by given names. Seki Noriko would be the name of a woman, Noriko, of the Seki family. The family names of both men and women, married or single, are designated by the suffix, -*san*, but one does not use that designation when referring to oneself. Women generally assume their husband's family name upon marriage. School children may use given names when speaking to one another, also designated with the suffix -*san*. Work groups and business associates tend to use family names. Infants and young children are called by their first names followed by -*chan*. Schoolboys, and increasingly schoolgirls, may be referred to by their first or last names followed by -*kun*. Elders are referred to respectfully. The designation **sensei** (master) is a term of respect used with the names of physicians, teachers, bosses, or others in positions of authority.

Family Roles and Organization

HEAD OF HOUSEHOLD AND GENDER ROLES

The predominant family structure among the Japanese is nuclear. Only 11 percent of families include three generations (Ministry of Health and Welfare, 1999). In feudal Japan, a bride had very limited contact with her own family after marriage, and the mother-in-law dominated the household. Now, wives determine the household budget, their husbands' pocket money, investments, family insurance, real-estate decisions, and all matters related to child rearing.

Even today, with higher education widely available to women, the role of wife and mother is dominant. Young women in the workplace may have jobs with little substantive responsibility, even if they are college graduates (Orenstein, 2001). Over the last two decades Japanese women have started to rebel against social norms. Now 40 percent of women under 30 are single, and Japan demonstrates a precipitously low birth rate of 1.39, well below the replacement rate of 2.0, which has been the topic of numerous government white papers (Ministry of Health and Welfare, 1999; Behind the quest, 2001). The Ministry has identified one factor as the strong social pressure confronting women who try to continue working after motherhood, because of Japan's need for skilled workers.

Laws governing employment of women are restrictive, but their ongoing reform is controversial. Japan has a family leave policy but, in reality, it is difficult to return to work after childbearing. An equal rights amendment has been part of Japan's constitution since the U.S. occupation of Japan. While Japan has protected women's interests in matters such as property ownership and voting, women are treated far from equally in the workplace. On the other hand, within the past 4 years the Ministry of Health and Welfare has made the development of a system of child-care centers for working mothers a priority, though it is not yet adequate (Ministry of Health and Welfare, 1999). Other societal reforms, which may encourage women to bear more children, are under discussion. The Ministry has aptly identified traditional norms for women and their difficulty in pursuing careers after motherhood as major obstacles. For this generation, two incomes are increasingly needed to maintain a middle-class lifestyle.

Wives in Japan care for their husbands to a degree that Western women would not tolerate. Japanese men are presumed not to be capable of managing day-to-day matters. Japanese men may leave for work before 7 AM and return after 10 at night, Monday through Saturday. On Sundays, men may be so exhausted that they sleep a good part of the day, or they may be obligated to socialize with colleagues. Wives and children often stay behind when husbands are transferred by their companies within Japan or overseas. Not surprisingly, one focus of the Ministry of Health and Welfare for addressing the low birth rate is to convince men to assume more responsibility for childcare and housework. The paramount family concern is for the children's education.

Western observers would be wrong to presume that married Japanese couples do not love each other. But in Japan, love has not been valued highly as a prerequisite for a successful marriage, and men and women have tended to be more motivated by duty to fulfill societal expectations than by the desire for spousal companionship. On the other hand, in recent years domestic violence has begun to be openly acknowledged. One recent survey of nearly 200 randomly selected women found a 67 percent incidence of physical, psychological, and/or sexual abuse within the group (Weingourt et al., 2001). In a society marked by strict norms differentiating the public and public realms, couples have lacked resources to learn how to deal with tension and conflict.

Until recently, mothers in Japan had to be available on hours' notice to the school or PTA. This is changing, and in recent years the Ministry of Health and Welfare has begun to develop after school programs for children (Ministry of Health and Welfare, 1999). Still, it is the mother's responsibility to oversee the completion and quality of homework. When the children grow up and leave home, women tend to become involved in volunteer activities, community groups, travel, the arts, and self-improvement classes (Freed, 1993; Iwao, 1993). These are likely to be same-gender activities.

Health-care providers need to be aware of differences in spousal relationships when assessing the quality of family dynamics and communication, sexual health, and sensitivity to risk for sexually transmitted diseases. Health-care providers who work with college-age and young adults may find that Japanese youth are less autonomous than their American counterparts. Conflicts between traditional and American values may arise among these young people and within their families.

PRESCRIPTIVE, RESTRICTIVE, AND TABOO PRACTICES FOR CHILDREN AND ADOLESCENTS

The primary relationship within a Japanese family is the mother-child relationship, particularly that of mothers and sons. It is customary for a mother to sleep with the youngest child until that child is 10 years old or older, and when a new baby is born, the older sibling may sleep with the father or a grandparent. The primacy of the mother-son relationship and the absence of fathers contribute to the known problem of mother-son incest. Father-daughter incest occurs, but a stronger taboo prohibits public discussion of it (Kanazumi, 1997). Despite the occasional occurrence of family dysfunction in this area, health-care providers working with childbearing couples and children need to be aware of Japanese family sleeping practices and refrain from judgmental evaluation of them.

The maternal role is so important for women in Japan that it is not unusual for a young mother to spend hours watching her infant sleep. If she observes the reflexes of urination, she changes the diaper immediately. Babies are not allowed to cry; they are picked up instantly. Women constantly hold their babies in carriers on their chests and sleep with them (Sharts Engel, 1989). "Skinship," or direct contact, is a value. The psychology of infant development from the Japanese perspective is that babies are born into a state of aloneness, and they must be brought into symbiosis with their mothers (Doi, 1971).

This author has been told that it is a traditional religious belief that during the first few years of life, children belong to God. Young Japanese children, especially sons, are quite indulged by western standards, reflecting this belief (Higuchi, 1985). At the same time, children are socialized to study hard, make their best effort, and be good group members. They are taught to take care of each other, and girls are taught to take care of boys. Self-expression is not valued.

Corporal punishment is acceptable in Japan. Several cases of punishment by school officials, which resulted in the death of the children, have been reported in the international press. The Ministry of Health and Welfare (1999) has begun to address ways for families and schools to more effectively foster the development of Japanese children. In addition, in response to a 17-fold rise in child abuse reports from third parties over the last 10 years, a new law has greatly enhanced strategies for identifying and intervening in cases of child abuse (Child abuse, 2001). *Ijime* (bullying) is a behavior that generates much public discussion. Children who are bullied by schoolmates typically have different looks, interests, or family structures.

Adolescents in Japan have their rebellions. Rock music and pornography allow escape from social restrictions, and up to 20 percent of teens smoke (Smith & Umenai, 2000). During the affluent 1980s, use of illicit drugs increased, though not nearly to the degree seen in the United States (Greenfeld, 1994). Once young people graduate from high school, they may express themselves through their clothing, hair, and makeup. Vandalism is a minimal concern.

Teens and college students in Japan generally do not date. They typically join clubs, membership in which is taken seriously; most social activities, such as ski trips, are club activities. However, the extent of adolescent sexual activity has motivated the Japanese Medical Women's Association to train its members in the area of sex education (Female doctors, 2001). Forty percent of Japanese high school seniors have had sexual intercourse, and 1 percent of Japanese girls have had abortions by their late teens. Despite the level of sexual activity, Japan has the lowest incidence of teen birth in the world, with 4 per 1000 versus 64 per 1000 in the United States (UNICEF, 1996). American health-care providers cannot assume that dating holds the degree of concern for Japanese young people as it does for American teens; nor can they assume that Japanese youth are well-informed about sexuality and sexual health risks.

Other health concerns among young people include the pressure to conform within a peer group and to perform well in school, known factors in depression and suicide risk (Takakura & Sakihara, 2000). There is beginning awareness of eating disorders among Japanese youth (Nakamura et al., 2000).

After graduation from high school or college, young adults are traditionally expected to be employed through their network of school contacts or family friends. Young women typically live with their parents, while young men are likely to live in company housing until marriage, and even after.

FAMILY GOALS AND PRIORITIES

Promoting success in school is the mother's main focus in child rearing. Children compete for their junior and senior high school admission, and high schools vary in the caliber of universities to which their graduates are admitted. The schools from which individuals graduate determine such major issues as career prospects for men and the status of husbands whom young women are likely to marry.

Children are highly valued and motherhood traditionally has been revered in Japan. The recent extreme drop in the birth rate has taken the society by surprise, though in prior decades the expense of rearing and educating children triggered its beginning. Nothing is permitted to interfere with child-rearing responsibilities. Japanese women may be less likely than North American women to engage in activities that require them to leave their children with babysitters, including health-care appointments.

The ideal of romantic love plays less of a role in marriage in Japan than in the United States. About 30 percent of marriages are arranged, often by employers or family friends. The o-miai is the ritual of the first arranged meeting between prospective partners.

Japanese couples marry in their late 20s or early 30s, and less than 1.5 percent of the elderly have never married, compared to 6 percent in the United States (United Nations, 1999). The groom's goals for marrying tend to focus on advancement of his career and a desire to be cared for. For the bride, economic security and child rearing are traditional goals. A "honeymoon baby" is still common, and intended family size is often achieved early in the marriage. Few Japanese women bear children outside of marriage, and few married women choose to remain childless within marriage.

Japanese couples place less emphasis on companionship and sexual fulfillment than do North American couples. Despite what may be lower expectations for marriage than in the United States, the divorce rate has climbed steadily over the last two decades to a rate of 1.94 divorces per 1000 population, or exceeding 30 percent (Ministry of Health and Welfare, 1999). When Japanese husbands retire, often at age 55, with decades ahead of them, it can be quite disruptive for their wives. This age group has experienced a sharp increase in divorce.

Japan has traditionally cared for and respected its elders; customarily this was the role of the eldest son. While the sense of obligation of children toward their parents is still strong, urbanization makes its fulfillment more difficult (Ministry of Health and Welfare, 1999). Urban apartments housing families of four or five may total just 45 or 50 square meters of living space.

With the longevity of its people, Japan is aging more rapidly than any other nation. The government has begun to address how to care for the elderly, who are soon to exceed 20 percent of the total population.

Nursing homes are growing in number in Japan, though their public image is poor. North American health-care providers must be sensitive to Japanese clients' sense of obligation and commitment. Helping families network within the Japanese American community for both social support and for resources or good long-term care facilities are useful strategies.

Elements of social status include age, gender, educational background, and work group affiliation of oneself or one's husband. Though there is a peerage and some old families are known to be descendants of samurai, Japan is largely a meritocracy. Exceptions include Korean descendants or descendants of the **burakumin**, the "untouchable" caste who cared for the dead and tanned leather in feudal times. In this largely middle-class society, school children can reasonably expect to study hard and go on for higher education if that is the family goal.

Biases that may be evident among Japanese people who reside in North America are directed at minority groups such as African Americans, Jews, and individuals with limited education, as well as women in high-status positions. This prejudice is seldom overt, but it may threaten the comfort of Japanese people who are likely to encounter such diversity among health-care providers in North America.

ALTERNATIVE LIFESTYLES

In Japan, a small segment of women have long lived outside the usual constraints for their gender. Women of "the floating world," or the entertainment industry, enjoy a fair degree of autonomy. The most traditional of these, the geisha, live in all-female communal arrangements. Geisha are not prostitutes, and they are now recognized as a cultural treasure. The women in the entertainment industry fulfill men's need to relax in a society that is highly constrained by social norms. At hostess bars, women sit with male customers, pour their drinks, and listen to them. In earlier eras concubines were accepted within families, and today, infidelity is more tolerated in Japan than in North America.

A small proportion of the Japanese population remains single throughout life. Some men and women enter monastic life. The small proportion of heterosexual couples that live together outside of marriage find greater tolerance in urban settings in Japan. There is less tolerance for marriage of a Japanese person to a foreigner than in the United States. The existence of a gay and lesbian social network and of cross-dressing clubs is evident in English language publications in Tokyo. Another social trend starting to be addressed by feminist scholars is that of Japanese wives engaging in extramarital sex (Ueno, 1997).

The pornography industry thrives and prostitution is big business. Young women from Southeast Asian countries with no Japanese language ability, and whose passports have been taken away from them may be enslaved for prostitution (Matsui, 1997).

Rape and other sexual abuses are acknowledged in Japanese society, but they are just beginning to be openly discussed and studied (French, 2001; Kobayashi, 2001;

Weingourt et al., 2001). Education about avoiding rape and inappropriate touching, when approached in a matter-of-fact way, is appropriate for Japanese in North America.

Workforce Issues

CULTURE IN THE WORKPLACE

Japanese employees in North American institutions need to be carefully oriented to the legal and professional requirements of client autonomy, and accountability in reporting, solving, and documenting problems that occur. An overview of dominant American society values may prepare them for the directness of communication they will encounter.

The issue of malpractice liability, while growing in Japan, is far less prevalent than in the United States (Nakajima et al., 2001). A public advocacy group, the Group to Investigate Medical Accidents, is currently urging the government to legislate mandatory reporting of medical accidents by hospitals as well as to provide support for victims of malpractice (Medical group, 2001). American practices designed to avoid liability, such as informed consent, are not routinely implemented in Japanese health-care settings. Enhancement of client autonomy is not a priority in Japan, while meeting dependency and recuperation needs are.

Like most Japanese workers, nurses in Japan work long hours, often 10 hours per day 6 days per week. Their pay is low in relation to their cost of living, and nursing is not a highly respected profession. Staffing is complicated by federal restrictions on shift work among women, though change is underway because Japan, like North America, is experiencing a severe nursing shortage.

The mix of people providing nursing care in Japan represents many levels of education. Most nurses continue to graduate from diploma programs. In addition, 2-year programs prepare assistant nurses, comparable to licensed practical nurses, for registered nurse licensure. The Japan Nursing Association took the position that the baccalaureate degree is the appropriate professional entry level in 1982 (Anders, 1994). In the late 1980s the **Diet** (parliament) mandated that every prefecture must have a baccalaureate program, and the numbers have increased from 9 programs in 1986 to more than 95 now (M. Hishinuma, Dean, St. Luke's College of Nursing, Tokyo, Japan, personal communication, August 17, 2001). Now, in the face of the nursing shortage and the growing health-care needs of a rapidly aging population, aides are likely to be used more extensively.

With this explosion in collegiate programs and the fact that graduate nursing education was only begun in the early 1980s, the need for appropriately educated nursing faculty is great. After registered nurse preparation, an additional year's course prepares individuals for certification as midwives or as public health nurses. A recent nursing role is that of clinical specialist in a variety of settings. Over 30 masters and 8 doctoral programs in nursing now operate in Japan (Primomo, 2000).

Like nursing students, medical students enter medical school immediately after high school. A reform being implemented by the Ministry of Health and Welfare makes completion of a clinical residency after graduation from medical school mandatory; and a structure for the accreditation of residency programs is now being developed (Dr. Kenji Sakurai, President, St. Luke's International Hospital, Tokyo, personal communication, July 18, 2001).

ISSUES RELATED TO AUTONOMY

Japanese nurses are less likely to confront or question physicians or to suggest strategies than North American nurses. Workers tend to do what the head of the group tells them to do, and make every effort to doing it very well. Japanese health-care workers seeking to practice in the United States have studied English from grade 7 throughout professional school, and will have passed an examination certifying minimal competency, but their verbal skills may be weak. Specific approaches to documentation, such as problem-oriented record keeping, may be unfamiliar and need to be addressed specifically in employees' orientation.

Japanese workers are quite sensitive to the desires and expectations of colleagues and superiors. Because saying "no" or delivering bad news is extremely difficult, they may avoid issues or indicate that everything is fine rather than state the negative. Of course, sensitive Japanese workers, who are attuned to nonverbal cues, may understand the true situation. In addition, until recently Japanese workers tended not to leave work before their boss did. North American employers should explicitly discuss expectations about starting and quitting times with Japanese employees. Japanese workers do not assert individual rights. Japanese professionals working in the United States will accept the need to assert themselves if it is presented within the context of legal and professional requirements to protect their clients.

Biocultural Ecology

SKIN COLOR AND OTHER BIOLOGICAL VARIATIONS

Racial features of Japanese people include the epicanthal skin folds that create the distinctive appearance of Asian eyes, a broad and flat nose, and "yellow" skin that varies markedly in tone. Hair is straight and naturally black with differences in shade. Health-care providers who are not accustomed to assessing racially diverse client groups may need to rely on color changes in the mucous membranes and sclerae to assess oxygenation and liver function in Japanese clients. The average stature of Japanese adults is smaller than that of Americans, though the gap has steadily decreased as national wealth has increased and a greater percentage of the population are able to improve their dietary practices.

The **Ainu** people of northern Japan, of whom only about 15,000 are left, are a fair-skinned people. Their racial and linguistic origins remain uncertain (Reischauer

& Jansen, 1995). The Okinawan people of the Ryukyu Islands are darker-skinned than "mainlanders" and have a stockier build.

DISEASES AND HEALTH CONDITIONS

The leading causes of death in Japan include, in descending order: cancers, heart disease, stroke, pneumonia, accidents, motor vehicle accidents, suicide, renal disease, liver disease, diabetes, hypertension (related to the high sodium diet), and tuberculosis (Ministry of Health and Welfare, 1999). Asthma, related to dust mites in the **tatami** (straw mats that cover floors in Japanese homes) is one of the few endemic diseases along with illnesses related to air pollution in urban areas. Men have a life expectancy of 77.1 years, while women have a life expectancy of 83.99 years, making the Japanese the longest living people in the world.

VARIATIONS IN DRUG METABOLISM

In general, drug dosages may need to be adjusted for the physical stature of Japanese adults. In addition, racially linked genetic differences in drug metabolism can be important. More Asians than Caucasians are poor metabolizers of mephenytoin and related medications, potentially leading to increased intensity and duration of the drugs' effects (Levy, 1993). Asians tend to be more sensitive to the effects of some beta blockers, many psychotropic drugs, and alcohol. A greater proportion of Japanese people rapidly metabolize acetylate substances, which has an impact on metabolism of tranquilizers, tuberculosis drugs, caffeine, and some cardiovascular agents. Asians often require lower doses of some benzodiazepines and neuroleptics. Opiates may be less effective analgesics, but gastrointestinal side effects may be greater than among whites. Health-care providers need to take all clients' body mass into consideration in dosing; even with that precaution, clients' responses to drugs need to be monitored carefully.

High-Risk Behaviors

In Japan, 54 percent of Japanese men and 14.5 percent of Japanese women smoke cigarettes, though efforts by the government and professional associations are addressing smoking through education programs in schools and in the community (Izumi et al., 2001; Ohida et al., 2001). Smoke-free areas in offices and restaurants are rare.

The average intake per year of pure alcohol among Japanese is about one-third that of the French (Dahlby, 1994). Alcohol has ritual significance. For example, in the marriage ceremony the bride and groom drink **sake** (rice wine), which is also an appropriate offering at **Shinto** shrines, and at the *butsudan*, or household ancestral shrine. In addition, alcohol is part of many social rituals, such as picnics to celebrate cherry blossoms, autumn leaves, or moon viewing. Adults commonly drink beer and sake in the home, and children may be seen purchasing alcohol. College students engage in beer drinking when they socialize.

The most serious concerns about alcohol use reflect the informal work requirement for men in Japan to socialize after hours and on Sundays. Considerable alcohol may be consumed, and it is common to see intoxicated **salary men** (white collar workers) snoozing on the trains or stumbling home late in the evening. In part, this extensive use of alcohol reflects the stress of Japanese corporate life and the rigid protocols dictating social interactions. Once alcohol is consumed, workers can relax and speak freely; they are forgiven for what they say because of the alcohol. Though this practice has diminished in the economic downturn of the last decade, entertaining is expected in the Japanese business culture, and drinking is tolerated as an obligation to one's company.

Public acknowledgment of alcoholism is limited. The Ministry of Health's initiative, *Healthy Japan 21*, targets this and other lifestyle risk factors (Ministry of Health and Welfare, 1999). Over the last several decades, Maryknoll Missionaries have established alcohol treatment centers throughout the country, and were among the first to publicize the problem of alcoholism among housewives, opening the first treatment center for women in the mid-1980s. Health-care providers need to be aware of the prevalence of smoking and heavy alcohol consumption among Japanese people, particularly among men. An effective strategy for curtailing these abuses is to give individuals specific medical reasons why they must abstain, thus providing a socially acceptable excuse.

Students and workers in Japan make heavy use of over-the-counter stimulants. It is not unusual to see students and young **salary men** consuming high-dosage caffeine elixirs at the train station in the morning. The use of recreational drugs is not tolerated in Japan, though the problem did increase during the economic boom of the 1980s (Greenfeld, 1994). Punishment is harsh and swift, and there is no popular sentiment for liberalization. Likewise, guns are strictly controlled. The crime rate is quite low, and Tokyo streets are safe at all hours.

Groups of Japanese businessmen may be treated to a sex tour in Bangkok or other Southeast Asian cities. The implications for transmission of HIV to wives and children back home are clear, but societal acknowledgment of this risk has been slow to develop. In 1998, 422 new cases of HIV and 231 new cases of AIDS were reported in Japan; sex between men was identified as the main etiological factor (Ministry of Health and Welfare, 1999). Every health-care contact with Japanese businessmen or their wives is an opportunity to state the facts about infectious disease risk. The United States is perceived as a place that is high in HIV risk, and concerns among Japanese who come to the United States tend to focus on casual contact as a possible modality.

One growing concern related to health and behavior is the inactivity of children in Japan and the increase in obesity (Ministry of Health and Welfare, 1999). Success in the educational system demands long hours of study each day, thus precluding participation on sports teams or scouting. Mothers' time-honored strategy of rewarding academic diligence with candy and other treats contributes to the issue of the fitness of Japanese youth.

Another effect of this, combined with the unfluoridated water supply, is the prevalence of dental caries.

HEALTH-CARE PRACTICES

Japanese people are likely to attribute their generally high level of well being to the centuries-old tradition of the daily bath. The **o-furo** (Japanese bathtub) is deep enough for an adult to enjoy a leisurely soak in neck-deep water, and the temperature is typically set around 105°F. The purpose of the bath is relaxation. Scrubbing for cleanliness, and thorough rinsing are done before climbing into the tub. Families share the same water; in fact, they may soak together in the bath. Bath water is reheated for several days before the tub is drained, and the water may be recycled for washing clothes or watering plants. Herbs or bath salts with therapeutic properties are sometimes added.

Young people in Japan do not drive until age 18, and an expensive and lengthy course of instruction is mandatory. Driving under the influence of alcohol or reckless operation of a vehicle carry stiff penalties. Rigorous inspection standards mean that people drive recent models of vehicles that are fully equipped with standard safety features.

The Japanese exhibit a high degree of public safety consciousness. Traditional housing materials, and the close proximity of buildings, have made fire a common and large-scale hazard. Each neighborhood has modern fire stations. Japanese readily use public services. Explicit instructions for accessing the local police, fire station, paramedics, and emergency medical facility in a given North American community may be necessary, as well as the circumstances under which access is appropriate.

Nutrition

MEANING OF FOOD

Many social and business interactions begin or end (or both) with the serving of **o-cha** (coffee and snacks), or an **o-bento** (boxed lunch). Business entertaining can be lavish. Part of the atmosphere of congeniality depends on the artistic presentation of the food.

COMMON FOODS AND FOOD RITUALS

All food groups are well represented in Japan, even in small shops, and in Japan the national diet is steadily becoming more Western, particularly among young people. In a wealthy, cosmopolitan society in Japan one can find just about any food or drink in common use in North America and Europe.

Large-scale agricultural production within Japan provides rice, beef, poultry, pork, seafood, root vegetables, cabbage, persimmons, apples, and *mikan* (tangerines). Rice, or **gohan**, the mainstay of the traditional diet, is included in all three meals as well as snacks. The electric rice cooker is a household necessity.

A traditional breakfast includes fish, pickles, *nori* (various seaweeds used to flavor or garnish meals), a raw egg stirred into the hot rice, miso (soybean-based) soup, and tea. Some people prefer a western breakfast of toast or cold cereal and coffee.

School children lunch on their **o-bento**, packed with rice, pickles, and meat or fish. A popular lunch among working people is a steaming bowl of *ramen* (noodles) in broth, or cold noodles on a hot summer day. Instant broth, though high in sodium, is another popular quick lunch.

An example of a traditional dinner would be a pot of boiled potatoes, carrots and pork seasoned with *mirin* (sweet sake), garlic and soy sauce, or a stir-fried meat and vegetable dish. Japanese housewives and working people have easy access to an enormous range of take-out food or home-delivery service, including Japanese, Chinese and Western selections. American or Japanese fast-food hamburger chains can be found in all cities.

The daily intake of sweets can be high, and often includes European-style desserts, sweet breads and cookies, sweet bean cakes, soft drinks, and heavily sweetened coffee, which may contribute to the high incidence of tooth decay. In Japan, some offices still employ **office ladies**, one of whose chief responsibilities is to serve green tea or coffee to visitors and other workers, though this practice has diminished as a result of the recent recession.

For people in Japan, rice has a symbolic meaning related to the **Shinto** religion, analogous to the concept of the "bread of life" among Christians. One of the Emperor's duties is to ceremonially plant the first rice in the spring and harvest the first rice in the late summer. A staple of school children's **o-bento** is a white bed of rice garnished with a red plum pickle, reminiscent of the Japanese flag. Meals combine elements of land and sea.

Holidays and family celebrations are times for ritual use of food. *O-bon*, in the summer, is a holiday for remembering family members who have died (Shinto Online Network Association, 2001). Vegetables, especially *daikon* (large white radishes), are carved into animals, which are said to carry dead ancestors back to the afterlife after the holiday. Likewise, the new year's festival, **O-shogatsu**, is a 3-day celebration with food that has been prepared in advance. Japanese may ring in the new year by literally standing in line at a Shinto shrine to ring a gong, and then drinking a cup of warm sake. Another traditional new year's food is *mochi*, a ball of sticky rice dough that celebrants take turns pounding out with a heavy mallet. Red rice, or rice with red beans, is a celebratory food as are various sweet bean desserts. It is customary to begin a meal with the simple grace, *Itadakimasu*, and to end with the compliment, *Go-chiso-sama deshita*. Western food rituals, including birthday cakes, wedding cakes, Christmas cakes, and Valentine's chocolates have been incorporated into Japanese life.

DIETARY PRACTICES FOR HEALTH PROMOTION

Increasingly Westernized food tastes, resulting in higher fat and carbohydrate intake, have contributed to the rise in obesity in modern Japan and associated increases in diabetes, heart disease, and premature death (Ohta et al., 2001; Takakura et al., 2001). With this concern has emerged a diet industry including weight-loss clinics, programs, foods, and medications. In addition, there is growing public awareness that the sodium content of the traditional soups and sauces contributes to the high rate of cerebrovascular accidents (Sharts Engel et al., 1986). Public health campaigns have promoted the use of reduced-sodium *miso*, soy sauce, and table salt. General principles of nutrition are the same in America as in Japan, though the food preferences may differ.

Green tea, while high in caffeine, is a good source of vitamin C. Garlic and various herbs are widely used for their medicinal properties. In larger cities, health food stores offering organically grown produce are available, and 10 percent of the population now use dietary supplements (Ishihara et al., 2001).

NUTRITIONAL DEFICIENCIES AND FOOD LIMITATIONS

Asian people, including the Japanese, generally have difficulty digesting milk products due to lactose intolerance (Smolin & Grosvenor, 1994). Reduced-lactose milk is now available in supermarkets but, while ice cream is popular, dairy products are not prevalent in Japan. Calcium is supplied in other foods such as *tofu* (soybean curd) and small, unboned fish. Water supplies are not fluoridated, and dental caries continues to be widespread. Fluoridated dental products can be recommended to Japanese clients, with the rationale for their use provided. Iron deficiency anemia is a concern among young women, and can be alleviated with dietary counseling or dietary supplements. *Nori* is a traditional food source for iron.

Pregnancy and Childbearing Practices

FERTILITY PRACTICES AND VIEWS TOWARD PREGNANCY

After a national debate that lasted nearly 40 years, oral contraceptives became legal in Japan in 1999, after Viagra was quickly approved by the Japanese FDA (Takahashi & Negishi, 1999). Condoms remain the most common contraceptive method used in Japan. Most women have several abortions during their married fertile lives, but recent increases have occurred among women younger than 25 (Goto et al., 2000). Abortions are lucrative for physicians (Chamberlain, 1994). Buddhist temples also make money from aborted fetuses and miscarriages. Some temples have *Jizo* shrines, where women give offerings of gifts and money to attendants who watch over aborted or miscarried fetuses (Orenstein, 2002) (Fig. 14–1).

The decline in the Japanese birth rate, to 1.39 births per woman, is regarded as a national crisis (Ministry of Health and Welfare, 1999; Japan Nursing Association, 2001). At this rate, the population of Japan could be half its current size within this century, and the economic implications are devastating. An educated female population, in a society in which women are oppressed, has asserted itself in a way that has certainly caught the

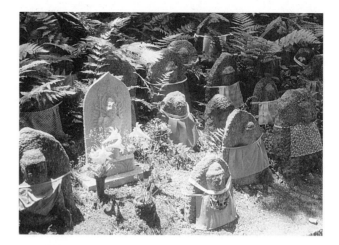

FIGURE 14–1   Misuko jizu are implored to protect the souls of aborted fetuses in the Japanese Buddhist tradition.

nation's attention. As a result, many social structures and policies regarding female labor laws, childcare and social support systems are under scrutiny. Japan's status as a "low birth rate country" has created great interest in assistive reproductive technology within the last few years, and the Ministry of Health and Welfare has targeted infertility treatment as a priority. In the past, male infertility was too shameful to address.

Pregnancy is highly valued within traditional Japanese culture as a woman's fulfillment of her destiny. Women may enjoy attention and pampering that they get at no other time. They may prepare themselves for the possibility of pregnancy when they become engaged and eliminate alcohol, caffeine, soft drinks, and tobacco (Sharts Engel, 1989).

The uniform of the pregnant woman is a loose jumper over a t-shirt, and knee socks. Keeping one's feet warm is said to promote uterine health. Underneath, an **obi** (sash) obtained from a Shinto shrine may be wrapped around the abdomen for warmth and protection. Because dogs give birth easily, the Chinese word for "dog" may be drawn on the **obi** by the obstetrician before he wraps it on the woman. A photograph of the Japanese Crown Princess (pregnant with the first successor after many years of failing to produce an heir), as she embarked for this ritual was published around the world as this chapter was being written.

In Japan, continuity of care has not been a value, because women often return to their mother's home for the last 2 months of their pregnancy and through the first 2 months postpartum. American health-care providers should explore a Japanese woman's expectations during pregnancy, and the possibility that she might return to Japan. Finding another Japanese woman who has experienced childbearing in the United States and who can share her experiences would be supportive of the pregnant client.

PRESCRIPTIVE, RESTRICTIVE, AND TABOO PRACTICES IN THE CHILDBEARING FAMILY

Health teaching for pregnant women in Japan emphasizes rest and restraint from stressful activities. Loud noises, such as a train or a sewing machine, are thought to be bad for the baby. Shinto shrines sell amulets for conception and easy delivery. Exercise classes for pregnant women became available in Tokyo in the mid-1980s.

In Japan it is still uncommon for husbands to attend the births of their children. Most births occur in hospitals with a physician delivering the baby. Certified nurse midwives serve as delivery room nursing staff. About one percent of births occur in free-standing midwifery clinics.

Medical procedures, such as enemas and episiotomies, are routinely used because they are thought to ease the baby's passage. In addition, Japanese midwives often use perineal massage. Japanese women are encouraged to eat full meals during labor so that they have energy for pushing. Traditional Japanese foods are preferred.

Currently, 15 percent of births in Japan are cesarean (Ministry of Health and Welfare, 1999). Physicians are skilled at mid- and high-forceps deliveries because cesarean delivery is viewed as hard on the mother. Vaginal deliveries are usually performed without medication. To give in to pain dishonors the husband's family, and mothers are said to appreciate their babies more if they suffer in childbirth. Japan enjoys the world's lowest infant mortality rate, at 3.2 per 1000 live births (United Nations, 2000). Maternal mortality, at 9.5 per 100,000 births, is most commonly caused by hemorrhage, and is associated with delivery in small single-physician birthing hospitals (Nagaya et al., 2000).

Japanese women residing in the United States are not likely to have a birth plan when admitted to a health-care facility. They are invested in avoiding a cesarean delivery, but they will use pain medications if they are encouraged to do so (Y. Nagato, Certified Nurse Midwife, Englewood, NJ, personal communication, June 14, 2001). Their husbands may choose not to attend the actual delivery, in which case they will need additional supportive nursing care.

The postpartum period, a time of recovery, is taken seriously. In Japan the woman may stay in the hospital for up to 1 week while learning to breast-feed and attending daily mother-care classes. Rooming-in is thought to disrupt the mother's rest, so at feeding times the baby is brought to her or she goes to the nursery. Traditional postpartal women do not bathe, shower, or wash their hair for at least the first week, probably reflecting prewar bathing conditions of unheated bath houses and contaminated water supplies. Since the new mother often stays with her mother, the new father may not see his baby until he comes to take the mother and baby back home from the grandmother's house after a few months. In Japan it is unusual to see infants in public before the age of 3 months.

Breast-feeding is taken so seriously that its duration is asked on the kindergarten admission forms. Maternal rest and relaxation are deemed essential for success. If the mother is asleep, the grandmother feeds the baby formula. Nipple confusion and inadequate milk supply are not problems that this author's midwife colleagues ever encountered. Lactation nurses are widely available, and breast massage is one of their strategies for promoting milk production and flow. This author's lactation nurse indicated that there is no point to encouraging women to nurse before the milk comes in. With greater employment among Japanese mothers, the subsequent decline in breast-feeding has been identified as a concern by the Ministry of Health and Welfare (1999).

Japanese women who give birth in the United States may resent the American expectation that they will resume self-care and child-care activities quickly. They believe it is harmful to them and their relationship with the baby. While American health-care providers cannot provide the length of hospital stay they would have enjoyed in Japan, they can explain the expectations for postpartal care, exercise sensitivity, and help plan for assistance upon discharge.

Death Rituals

DEATH RITUALS AND EXPECTATIONS

The taboo against open discussion of serious illness and death is still evident in Japanese society (Kawagoe & Kawagoe, 2000). In recent years the biomedical literature has begun to reflect open discourse on pain management in terminal illness, the need for greater national investment in intensive care services, the need to increase organ transplantation, and the need for end-of-life decision making. Hospice patients may not be told their diagnosis and prognosis in order to allow the patient to die in peace and to spare both the patient and the family the difficulty of having to discuss the situation. Ohnuki-Tierney (1984) posited that open discussion of a serious, but not fatal, illness could jeopardize the individual's career. In addition, the practice of ignoring that which is beyond one's control may reflect a traditional pragmatic fatalism.

RESPONSES TO DEATH AND GRIEF

When a Japanese person is dying, the family should be notified of impending death so they can be at the dying person's bedside. Traditionally, the eldest son has particular responsibility during this time. When death occurs, an altar is constructed in the home. Photographs of the deceased are displayed, and floral arrangements are placed within and outside of the home. A bag of money is hung around the neck of the deceased to pay the toll to cross the river to the hereafter (Shinto Online Network Association, 2001). An alternate version of this custom dictates that if the dead is satisfied with the amount of money, then the inheritance is freed for the survivors. Visitors bring gifts of money and food for the bereaved family.

Modern corporate life in Japan does not allow for taking more than a few days from work for official mourning. However, in terms of religious practice, the mourning period is 49 days, the end of which is marked by a family prayer service and the serving of special rice dishes. At this time the departed has joined those already in the hereafter. Perpetual prayers may be donated through a gift to the temple. In addition, special prayer services can be conducted for the 1st, 3rd, 7th, and 13th annual anniversaries of the death. The belief that the dead need to be remembered, and that failure to do so can lead the dead to rob the living of rest, is common. Proper funeral rites and reassurance that they are remembered during temple and family prayers alleviate the agitation of the dead.

Spirituality

DOMINANT RELIGION AND USE OF PRAYER

Japan does not have a clearly articulated theology or religious belief system. Tradition holds that the Japanese people are descendants of the Sun goddess, and that the emperor is a god (Keene, 1983), though the Occupation forces required Hirohito to publicly renounce this status after World War II ended. Some say that the demotion of the emperor from god to mortal has left the Japanese with a spiritual vacuum. Reischauer and Jansen (1995) believe this secularization of Japanese society began when Confucianism, imported during the 9th century, grew in influence during the 17th century. Confucian values, including faith in education, hard work, and the emphasis on interpersonal relationships and loyalty, continue to be important today.

Shinto, the indigenous religion, is the locus of joyful events such as marriage and birth. Many *matsuri* (festivals) are marked by offerings, parades through the streets, and a carnival on the grounds of the shrine. Buddhism, brought to Japan in the 6th century, has permeated Japanese artistic and intellectual life. Very few Japanese people regularly attend services, but most are registered temple members, if only to ensure a family burial plot. Most homes have a Buddhist altar, *butsudan*, where deceased family members are venerated (Shinto Online Network Association, 2001).

One percent of Japanese people are Catholic or Protestant in nearly equal numbers. Christianity has been known in Japan since the 16th century, and the Bible is claimed to be the most widely read book in Japan. Most Japanese do not identify themselves solely with one religion or another, and even a baptized Christian might have a **Shinto** wedding and a Buddhist funeral.

MEANING OF LIFE AND INDIVIDUAL SOURCES OF STRENGTH

The Buddhist belief in reincarnation is accepted by many Japanese, and the eternal life of the soul is also recognized in **Shinto** (Ohnuki-Tierney, 1984; Shinto Online Network Association 2001). Purification of the soul is one meaning ascribed to earthly life. Other valid interpretations include honoring one's family and country, working hard, being a good group member, or joining one's deceased ancestors (Woss, 1992) (Fig. 14–2).

SPIRITUAL BELIEFS AND HEALTH-CARE PRACTICES

Japanese religions play a significant role in health-care practices. People or objects such as cars are taken to shrines for purification from evil and to receive protective amulets. Some shrines and temples specialize in specific illnesses. **Kampo** (healers) often set up shop in

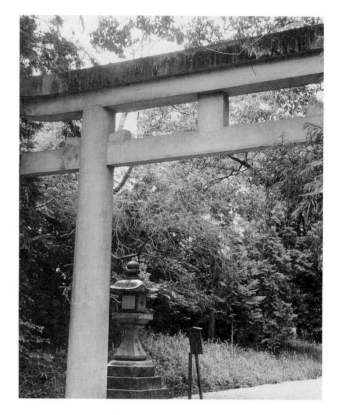

FIGURE 14–2 Torii are the gates that mark the entrance of all Shinto shrines.

the vicinity. At the temple or shrine a person might be seen scooping incense smoke onto an ailing body part. Prayer boards might bear requests for special healing. Gifts of devices used in childcare may be left with Buddha statues. Newborns are taken to a shrine for a blessing. Additional blessings take place on November 15, when a child is 3, 5, or 7 years old (the *shichi-go-san*) (Shinto Online Network Association, 2001). Visits to shrines and temples in Japan are social, recreational, and spiritual outings. Souvenirs and refreshments are usually available, and the hike into the prayer area provides exercise. People vary in the depth of their beliefs, but most agree that "it cannot hurt" (Ohnuki-Tierney, 1984).

Various types of diviners, soothsayers, and prophets, are available at shrines, temples, and even along the most fashionable streets in Tokyo. College-educated people make liberal use of them. Statues depicting folktale heroes, often animals, are thought to bring luck. Americans may have difficulty understanding and accepting the reliance of sophisticated and well-educated people on what may be viewed as superstitions. But these measures appear to be more sources of comfort than deciding factors in health-care decision making, and they should be accepted as such.

Health-Care Practices

HEALTH-SEEKING BELIEFS AND BEHAVIORS

The general health of the populations of Japan and the United States is similar with a shift in leading causes of morbidity and mortality from infections to chronic illnesses. However behaviors and underlying belief systems between Japan and the United States differ markedly. There is greater tolerance of self-indulgence even during minor illnesses in Japan. Because Japanese are less likely to express feelings verbally, this indulgence may be a way for people to affirm caring for one another nonverbally. Hypochondriasis among Japanese has been described in the medical literature. Bodily flaws, for example, birthmarks, are a source of concern, and ear piercing has never caught on among young women because it creates a physical imperfection.

The termination of pregnancy when the health of the fetus is in doubt is common, and medically compromised neonates are not treated aggressively when prognoses are not favorable (Sharts Engel, 1989; Sharts-Hopko, 1995). Values underlying these practices include concern for the common good of one's family and society and parental appreciation of extreme competitiveness of the educational system. Health-care providers working with Japanese obstetric clients may face values conflicts around these issues and need to balance legal obligations with cultural sensitivity.

In Japan, people seem less inclined to seek correction of minor orthopedic and dental variations than in middle-class American society, though immigrant families make full use of services offered in the United States. Health-care providers engaged in health promotion and screening need to be aware of this difference. Function, rather than appearance, may be a more appropriate emphasis.

The concept of **ki**, the life force or energy and how it flows through the body, is integral to traditional Chinese healing modalities, including acupuncture. Good health requires the unobstructed flow of **ki** throughout the body. Japanese people are sensitive to climate change, the emotional milieu, and their effects on physical health. The concepts of yin and yang are reflected in modern attitudes, as is the need to balance five energy sources: water, wood, fire, earth, and metal. These elements correspond to aspects of the universe such as the planets, the seasons, and specific body organs. Humankind is a part of nature, subject to its forces, and a person is an integrated whole. Strategies that help to restore balance include use of herbal medicines, bed rest, bathing, or having a massage. One traditional form of massage, **shiatsu**, or acupressure, involves redirection of energy along the Chinese meridians by application of light pressure to what we might recognize as acupuncture points.

While Chinese tradition calls for a restoration of balance when one is ill, **Shinto** calls for purging and purification. Both influences operate in modern Japan. In the past, **Shinto** was the source of principles of prevention, whereas Buddhist priests healed the sick. Centuries before the germ theory was known, **Shinto** effectively distinguished between spaces and body parts that were dirty versus those that were clean and pure. For example, taking off one's shoes at the doorway keeps one's home clean. Mothers carefully teach young children to fear dirt. It is customary in Japan to see people with colds wearing disposable surgical masks in public to shield others from their infection. Illness traditionally was

viewed as pollution, and any serious illness was taboo (Lock, 1980).

Preoccupation with germs and dirt is not likely to interfere with daily life. It may account for prejudices among some Japanese against certain categories of workers, including nurses. Americans who visit Japanese homes should note or even ask whether the family removes their shoes upon entering.

RESPONSIBILITY FOR HEALTH CARE

Newsstands and vending machines, particularly in commuter rail stations in Japan, provide large quantities of flavored caffeine elixirs, high-potency vitamin elixirs, and electrolyte replacement drinks. These products are promoted to give workers and students an edge in their daily work. Health-care providers need to ask specifically what remedies are being used, and why. Japanese clients in North America find general principles of nutrition to be the same as those taught in Japan, though their food preferences may differ.

The health of pregnant and nursing mothers and of children enjoyed the highest priority during the postwar modernization of services in Japan. Children are exposed to extensive screening and services through their schools and municipal health departments, and noncompliance by mothers is rare (Sharts Engel, 1989).

National insurance, recently revamped (Ministry of Health and Welfare, 1999), is available to any resident of Japan, including foreigners, for a sliding scale fee, and includes both medical and dental care. Treatment by osteopaths, chiropractors, and traditional practitioners is covered if clients have been referred by a physician; in fact, acupuncture, moxibustion (heat applied to acupuncture sites) and other traditional modalities of care are still part of the national university curriculum for physical therapists (Fig. 14–3). The elderly and people with certain chronic conditions receive free treatment, while low-income people may be eligible for subsidized services. The municipal government handles enrollments.

Japanese residents in America frequently carry Japanese health insurance. Japanese nationals working for American institutions or companies may be eligible

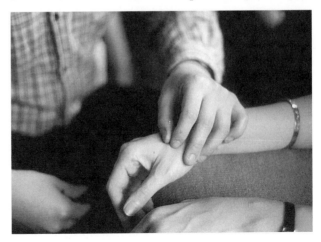

FIGURE 14–3 The author gets an acupuncture treatment from a blind physical therapist who is a graduate of Tsukuba National University.

for the same coverage as other employees, but they often need assistance in understanding how their benefits work. Students and others can continue their Japanese national health insurance, but they may need assistance in seeking care and negotiating the American billing and payment process.

Many American over-the-counter medications, or their Japanese equivalents, are widely available in Japanese pharmacies. In addition, many pharmacies stock traditional herbal **kampo** preparations. Enough stomach preparations are sold in Japan for every man, woman, and child to be treated more than monthly. The extent of gastric upset in Japan probably reflects a combination of stress, dietary practices, and drinking alcohol as well as constitutional behaviors (Ohnuki-Tierney, 1984).

Japanese people make liberal use of both modern medical and traditional providers of health care. Influenced by German and American medical science, the Japanese health-care system incorporates local primary care, neighborhood hospitals, specialty clinics, academic medical centers, and national research institutes. Most hospital beds are found in tiny, unregulated, physician-owned neighborhood clinics. A sophisticated public health system offers prenatal and well-child care, school health initiatives, visiting nursing services, home health services, senior centers, and health education at little or no cost to the public.

Japanese residents in the United States have Internet and mail order access to traditional medications, if they are not available locally. As with any client population, a complete health assessment includes inquiry about home therapies. The second generation of immigrants has tended to rely fully on the American health-care system.

FOLK PRACTICES

Morita therapy is an indigenous strategy for addressing *shinkei shitsu*, excess sensitivity to the social and natural environment. Introspection is seen as harmful, and **Morita therapy** focuses on constructive physical activity to help clients accept reality as it is (Ohnuki-Tierney, 1984). *Naikan* therapy is one of reflection on how much goodness and love is received from others. A third indigenous therapy, *Shinryo Naika*, focuses on bodily illnesses that are emotionally induced. Western-style psychiatry has been fully incorporated into Japanese health-care services only within the last several decades. In recent years, concerns about the increase of stress and violence in the society has focused attention on psychiatric problems (Ministry of Health and Welfare, 1999; Mino et al., 2001; Sumi, Tsuzuki, & Kanda, 2001; Tajima, 2001; Tseng et al., 2001).

Health-care providers need to be sensitive to workplace or family issues that may underlie illnesses among Japanese clients, as among all clients. If a provider believes that psychotherapy is indicated, the therapist must be someone familiar with the Japanese culture. Guidance in locating resources may be obtained through large academic medical centers or universities in coastal (particularly Pacific Coast) cities, as well as through professional associations, Japanese churches, or other religious organizations.

Health care is easily obtained in Japan. However, the system of referrals is unique. When a physician leaves medical school, he becomes part of that school's "family." He is unlikely to refer patients to specialists or hospitals outside the "family" of his fellow alumni or former professors. Personal acquaintance is essential for doing business in Japan, and it is reflected also in health-care practice.

Japanese people may be unlikely to assert themselves in American settings, and their efforts to do so may seem inappropriate to American health-care providers. Their high regard for the status of physicians decreases the likelihood of asking questions or making suggestions about their care. The idea that clients should be given care options may be alien. Health-care providers need to provide ample opportunity for dialogue and explain the choices that are offered. Japanese and Japanese American health-care providers may be an important resource in bridging gaps in understanding.

Japanese residents in the United States may need assistance in seeking care. Their verbal English skills may be an impediment to making their needs known and to understanding the care they are offered, though their ability to understand written information is very good. Japanese people tend to believe that they are physiologically different from non-Japanese people, and they may be skeptical of recommendations. Calling on the local Japanese community may be a useful strategy with these clients.

CULTURAL RESPONSES TO HEALTH AND ILLNESS

Pain, **itami**, may not be expressed, and bearing pain is considered a virtue and a matter of family honor. Medications that specifically relieve pain are used less frequently in Japan than in the United States, and narcotic use in particular is quite restricted. Addiction is a strong taboo in Japanese society. Biomedical researchers are beginning to study the comfort needs of dying patients (Morita et al., 2000). Hospice care emerged 20 years ago as a response to terminal illness, and providers struggle with traditional taboos regarding death and pain in meeting clients' needs (Kawagoe & Kawagoe, 2000).

American health-care providers may use a schedule of analgesic administration rather than an as-requested or patient-controlled approach, to ensure adequate pain management. Japanese clients may respond positively to the information that physiological status and healing are actually enhanced by pain control.

Mental illness is taboo, and psychiatry and psychiatric nursing were the last major specialties to be addressed in professional education (Ryder, 1984). Publicized crimes of violence, even among children, in recent years have raised public consciousness about mental health needs. Reform of the national health insurance program has expanded coverage for psychiatric illnesses (Ministry of Health and Welfare, 1999). Because emotional problems cannot be discussed freely, somatic manifestations are common and acceptable (Ohnuki-Tierney, 1984).

This author saw few handicapped children out in public during 2 years in Tokyo. However, exposure to a conversational English program for mildly mentally retarded adults through a YMCA revealed extremely humane treatment of those individuals. It is this author's impression that handicapped people have been a source of family shame or heartache, though they are treated kindly. Some communities have aggressive physical therapy programs such as a community health center that the author visited in the city of Kochi (Sharts Engel et al., 1986). Laws forbidding people with various disabilities from holding certain positions of employment are being reformed in the face of a shortage of skilled workers, including nurses (Japan Nursing Association, 2001). Japanese families residing in the United States would probably avail themselves of community resources if they were helped to access them, but not to the extent that many American families use them.

Assumption of the sick role is highly tolerated by families and colleagues, and a long recuperation period is encouraged by Japanese health-care providers. In Japan, a client with a myocardial infarction may be hospitalized for a month with outcomes comparable to those found in the United States. Rehabilitation to full activities of daily living after serious illness or injury is less aggressive than in the United States, though public pressure for reform in this area is growing (Liu et al., 2000).

BLOOD TRANSFUSIONS AND ORGAN DONATIONS

In Japan, the Red Cross is often seen collecting blood at public places such as commuter rail stations. People with negative blood types account for less than one percent of the population, and RhoGam is not usually stocked in Japanese hospitals, though it can be ordered within a few weeks.

Critical care technology has not received the emphasis in Japan that it has in the United States. Organ donation following brain death was legalized in 1997, and just a few hundred organ transplants have been done in Japan, probably reflecting traditional attitudes toward body integrity and purity (Kita et al., 2000). Critical care and organ transplantation and donation issues need to be approached sensitively with Japanese residents in the United States. Health-care providers must be cautious in initiating extraordinary measures with Japanese family members. Japanese people rely more heavily on the physician's opinion, and the family may have difficulty negotiating for cessation of treatment. The concept of advance directives has not been implemented in Japan, and families need to understand what this means upon admission to an American hospital.

Health-Care Practitioners

TRADITIONAL VERSUS BIOMEDICAL PRACTITIONERS

In modern health-care delivery, physicians are clearly in charge of the health-care team. Physicians may have a high degree of understanding of **kampo**, and may be quite accepting of clients' use of it (Anders, 1994; Tierney & Tierney, 1994). Likewise, traditional practitioners refer clients to the medical establishment. Japanese health practitioners who come to the United States face a different type of health-care system, with greater diversity and with domains of autonomy for many professionals. The authority of insurers to dictate care is novel for them, as is the extent of concern for malpractice liability.

STATUS OF HEALTH-CARE PROVIDERS

Physicians, referred to as **sensei**, are highly esteemed. Self-care as a philosophy is not evident in Japan. Being told what to do by the physician or **kampo** practitioner is expected, and his (or occasionally, her) authority is not questioned. Physicians control most health-care delivery in Japan. Hospital administration is not an established field. Rather, physicians run hospitals and own most of them.

Nurses in Japan in the mid-1980s repeatedly told this author that nursing is not as highly regarded in Japanese society as it is in the United States, reflecting traditional taboos against illness and impurity as well as the status of women. The proliferation of various types of health-care providers and technicians is less in Japan than in the United States (Anders, 1994; Tierney & Tierney, 1994). Japanese residents in the United States need considerable assistance in understanding how the health-care delivery system works and the functions of the different health-care providers whom they encounter. In particular, they need to understand the domains of autonomy of a diverse group of health professionals. Home care, and the orchestration of many community-based providers, may be overwhelming for Japanese residents who expect long recuperations in the hospital.

There are female physicians and male nurses in Japan. However, the professions and their interrelationships generally tend to reflect traditional gender roles and in their behavior toward one another (Tierney & Tierney, 1994). Nurses are even titled according to gender: **kango-san** if a male, and **kango-fu** if a female. The former means, roughly, "Mr. Nurse," while the latter means "nurse wife." Recently a male nurse has challenged the law prohibiting his becoming a midwife (Matsui, 2000). Japanese health professionals working in the United States need careful orientation to laws and institutional regulations about appropriate male-female interactions and professional requirements for accountability in communicating problems.

Japanese residents seeking health care in America may be surprised by the assertiveness and autonomy of nonphysician professionals. An overview of the details of their care and who will be doing various aspects of that care can be helpful.

CASE STUDY The following case study is a composite of actual situations. Marianne, who is American, and Ken Shimizu, who is Japanese, have worked in Tokyo for over 30 years as Methodist missionaries. They have annual furloughs and occasional sabbaticals during which they visit relatives and sponsoring organizations, and engage in continuing education in the United States. They met as college students in the United States, and their three grown children have established their own careers in the United States.

Ken's 98-year-old mother resides with Marianne and Ken. She is not Christian but has always been extremely supportive of Ken and Marianne's work. Ken teaches at a large Christian university while Marianne has served in various church-related positions over the years. As missionaries they live in subsidized post–World War II housing near Ken's university. Marianne has been a frugal housewife, preparing local foods in the Japanese style for her family.

Ken, who is nearly 60, recently learned that he has glaucoma. By the time it was discovered he had lost a significant amount of peripheral vision. While Marianne delivered all three children at a Christian hospital in Tokyo, she gets her annual physical examination when visiting relatives in the United States. She has never believed that the Japanese health system is as proactive as in the United States.

On her most recent visit to the United States, Marianne learned that she has hypertension. Her physician prescribed a medication that is readily available in Japan, but the physician was concerned about the level of stress in Marianne's life. Mother Shimizu is quite confused and requires considerable care, but it is unthinkable for Ken, the only child, to put his mother in a long-term care facility. Even if he would, the quality of facilities in Japan leaves much to be desired. Most of the responsibility for Mother Shimizu falls on Marianne, in addition to her work. Marianne's relatives are urging her to consider placing Mother Shimizu in a church-related life care community near Marianne's family in the United States, where Marianne and Ken would like to retire. Marianne's own parents lived in this facility at the end of their lives. She is considering these issues as she returns to Tokyo.

STUDY QUESTIONS

1 Identify some of the cultural issues that may lead to conflict in this international family.

2 What are the family resources for this international family?

3 What factors within the Japanese health system may account for the late diagnosis of Ken's glaucoma?

4 What practical issues might arise for the Shimizus if Mother Shimizu were placed in a long-term care facility in the United States?

5 What dietary factors may contribute to Marianne's hypertension?

6 In what ways might you consider Ken to be counter-cultural as a Japanese man?

7 What social pressures might Marianne have faced, given some of her choices, as a housewife in Japan?

8 What pressures will Ken likely experience as he considers how to meet the needs of both his mother and his wife?

9 Compare and contrast the fertility and mortality rates of Japan and the United States.

10 Do the traditional Japanese maintain sustained eye contact with strangers? Why or why not?

11 To which drugs might Japanese people have greater sensitivity than white ethnic populations?

12 How do most Japanese people meet their need for calcium?

REFERENCES

Anders, R. L. (1994). An American's view of nursing education in Japan. *Image: Journal of Nursing Scholarship, 26,* 227–230.

Behind the quest for more babies (2001, January 10). *The Japan Times Online.* Retrieved from http://www.japantimes.co.jp.

Benedict, R. (1946). *The chrysanthemum and the sword.* Tokyo: Charles E. Tuttle.

Chamberlain, G. L. (1994). Learning from the Japanese. *America, 171*(7), 14–16.

Child-abuse injuries up by 60 percent; reached record of 18,804 last year (2001, June 22). *The Japan Times Online.* Retrieved from http://www.japantimes.co.jp.

Dahlby, T. (1994). Kyushu: Japan's southern gateway. *National Geographic, 185*(1), 88–117.

Doi, T. (1971). (J. Bester, trans.) *The anatomy of dependence.* Tokyo: Kodansha International Ltd.

Female doctors to get training on sex education (2001, May 17). *The Japan Times Online.* Retrieved from http://www.japantimes.co.jp.

Freed, A. O. (1993). *The changing world of older women in Japan.* Manchester, CT: Knowledge, Ideas & Trends, Inc.

French, H. W. (2001, July 15). Fighting sex harassment, and stigma, in Japan. *New York Times,* pp. A1, A10.

Goto, A., Fujiyama-Koriyama, C., Fukao, A., & Reich, M. R. (2000). Abortion trends in Japan. *Studies in Family Planning, 31*(4), 301–308.

Greenfeld, K. T. (1994). *Speed tribes.* New York: Harper Collins.

Higuchi, K. (1985) (A. Tomii, trans.). *Bringing up girls.* Kyoto, Japan: Shoukadoh Booksellers Printing Co.

Immigration and Naturalization Service, U.S. Department of Justice. (2000). *1998 Statistical yearbook of the Immigration and Naturalization Service.* Retrieved from http://www.ins.usdoj.gov.

Ishihara, J., Sobue, T., Yamamoto, S., Sasaki, S., Akabane, M., & Tsugane, S. (2001). Validity and reproducibility of a self-administered questionnaire to determine dietary supplement users among Japanese. *European Journal of Clinical Nutrition, 55*(5), 360–365.

Iwao, S. (1993). *The Japanese woman.* New York: Free Press.

Izumi, Y., Tsuji, I., Ohkubo, T., Kuwahara, A., Nishino, Y., & Hisamichi, S. (2001). Impact of smoking habit on medical care use and its costs: a prospective observation of National Health Insurance beneficiaries in Japan. *International Journal of Epidemiology, 30*(3), 616–621.

Japan Nursing Association (2001, January). Japanese Nursing Association JNA News, No. 30. http://www.nurse.or.jp/jna/english.

Kanazumi, F. (1997). Interview. In S. Buckley (Ed.), *Broken silence: Voices of Japanese feminism* (pp. 70–81). Berkeley: University of California Press.

Kawagoe, H., & Kawagoe, K. (2000). Death education in home hospice care in Japan. *Journal of Palliative Care, 16*(3), 37–45.

Keene, D. (1983). Ise. In D. Richie (Ed.), *Discover Japan: Vol. 2. Words, customs and concepts* (pp. 196–197). Tokyo: Kodansha International, Ltd.

Kita, Y. et al. (2000). Japanese organ transplant law: a historical perspective. *Progress in Transplantation, 10*(2), 106–108.

Kobayashi, M. (2001). Infant abuse in Osaka: Health center activities from 1988 to 1999. *Pediatrics International, 43*(2), 197–201.

Levy, R. A. (1993). Ethnic and racial differences in response to medicines: Preserving individualized therapy in managed pharmaceutical programmes. *Pharmaceutical Medicine, 7,* 139–165.

Liu, M., Chino, N., & Takahashi, H. (2000). Current status of rehabilitation, especially in patients with stroke, in Japan. *Scandinavian Journal of Rehabilitation Medicine, 32*(4), 148–158.

Lock, M. M. (1980). *East Asian medicine in urban Japan.* Berkeley: University of California Press.

Matsui, Y. (1997). Interview. In S. Buckley (Ed.*), Broken silence: voices of Japanese feminism* (pp. 133-143). Berkeley: University of California Press.

Matsui, Y. (2000, August 8). One man's fight to be a midwife. *The Japan Times Online.* Retrieved from http://www.japantimes.co.jp.

Medical group laments lack of malpractice laws (2001, July 11). *The Japan Times Online.* Retrieved from http://www.japantimes.co.jp.

Ministry of Health and Welfare. (1999). Annual Reports on Health and Welfare 1998–1999, Social Security and National Life. Tokyo. Retrieved from http://www.mhlw.go.jp/english/wp.

Mino, Y. et al. (2001). Expressed emotion of families and the course of mood disorders: A cohort study in Japan. *Journal of Affective Disorders, 63*(1–3), 43–49.

Morita, T. et al. (2000). Pain and symptom management. Terminal sedation for existential distress. *American Journal of Hospice and Palliative Care, 17*(3), 189–195.

Nagaya, K. et al. (2000). Causes of maternal mortality in Japan. *Journal of the American Medical Association, 283*(20), 2661–2667.

Nakajima, K. et al. (2001). Medical malpractice and legal resolution systems in Japan. *Journal of the American Medical Association, 285*(12), 1632–1640.

Nakamura, Y. et al. (2000). Prevalence of anorexia nervosa and bulimia nervosa in a geographically defined area in Japan. *International Journal of Eating Disorders, 28*(2), 173–180.

Ohida, T. et al. (2001). Smoking prevalence and attitudes toward smoking among Japanese physicians. *Journal of the American Medical Association, 285*(20). Retrieved from http://jama.ama-assn.org/issues.

Ohnuki-Tierney, E. (1984). *Illness and culture in contemporary Japan.* Cambridge: Cambridge University Press.

Ohta, A. et al. (2001). Lifestyle and socio-demographic risk factors for death among middle-aged and elderly residents in Japan from a five-year follow-up cohort study. *Journal of Epidemiology, 11*(2), 51–60.

Orenstein, P. Mourning my miscarriage. (2002, April 21). *New York Times.* Retrieved from http://www.NYTimes.com.

Orenstein, P. (2001, July 1). Parasites in Prêt-à-Porter. *New York Times Magazine,* pp. 31–35.

Primomo, J. (2000). Nursing around the world: Japan—preparing for the century of the elderly. *Online Journal of Issues in Nursing, 5*(2). Retrieved from http://www.nursingworld.org/ojin.

Reischauer, E. O., & Jansen, M. B. (1995). *The Japanese today: Change and continuity.* Cambridge, MA: Harvard University Press.

Ryder, R. S. (1984). *Nursing reorganization in occupied Japan 1945–1952.* Unpublished doctoral dissertation, Columbia University Teachers College.

Sharts Engel, N. (1989). An American experience of pregnancy and childbirth in Japan. *Birth, 16*(2), 81–86.

Sharts Engel, N., Kojima, M., & Martinson, M. (1986). A community health center responds to the aging of Japan. *Journal of Geriatric Nursing, 12*(11), 12–16.

Sharts-Hopko, N. C. (1995). Birth in the Japanese context. *Journal of Obstetric, Gynecologic and Neonatal Nursing, 24,* 343–350.

Shinto Online Network Association. (2000). Shinto. http://www.jinja.or.jp/english.

Smith, M., & Umenai, T. (2000). Knowledge, attitude and practice of smoking among university students of allied health sciences in Japan. *Asia and Pacific Journal of Public Health, 12*(1), 17–21.

Smolin, L. A., & Grosvenor, M. B. (1994). *Nutrition: Science and applications.* Philadelphia: Saunders College Publications.

Sumi, K., Tsuzuki, S., & Kanda, K. (2001). Neurotic perfectionism, perceived stress, and self-esteem among Japanese men: A prospective study. *Psychological Reports, 88*(1), 19–22.

Tajima, O. (2001). Mental health care in Japan: Recognition and treatment of depression and anxiety disorders. *Journal of Clinical Psychiatry, 62*(Supp. 13), 39–44.

Takahashi, J., & Negishi, M. (1999, June 2). Cost, doubts mean rousing reception unlikely for pill. *The Japan Times Online.* Retrieved from http://www.japantimes.co.jp.

Takakura, M., & Sakihara, S. (2000). Gender differences in the association between psychosocial factors and depressive symptoms in Japanese junior high school students. *Journal of Epidemiology, 10*(6), 383–391.

Takakura, M. et al. (2001). Patterns of health-risk behavior among Japanese high school students. *Journal of School Health, 71*(1), 23–29.

Tierney, M. J., & Tierney, L. M. (1994). Nursing in Japan. *Nursing Outlook, 42*(5), 210–213.

Tseng, W. S. et al. (2001). Mental health in Asia: social improvements and challenges. *International Journal of Social Psychiatry, 47*(1), 8–23.

Ueno, C. (1997). Interview. In S. Buckley (Ed.), *Broken silence: Voices of Japanese feminism* (pp. 274–293). Berkeley: University of California Press.

UNICEF (1996). Progress of nations 1996. The industrial world. Japan has lowest teen birth rate. Retrieved from http://www.unicef.org/pon96/inbirth.htm.

United Nations, Department of Economic and Social Information and Policy Analysis/Statistical Division (1993). *Statistical yearbook 1990/1991* (38th ed.). New York: Author.

United Nations. (1999). *Economic and social commission for Asia and the Pacific. Statistics on women in Asia and the Pacific.* New York: Author.

United Nations (2000). *Economic and social commission for Asia and the Pacific. Statistics Division. Asia and the Pacific in Figures 2000.* Retrievef from http://unescap.org/stat/statdata/japan.htm.

U.S. Department of State. (2000). *Background Notes—Japan.* Updated July 2000. Retrieved from http://www.state.gov/r/pa/bgn.

Weingourt, R. et al. (2001). Domestic violence and women's mental health in Japan. *International Nursing Review, 48*(2), 102–108.

Woss, F. (1992). When blossoms fall: Japanese attitudes towards death and the other world: Opinion polls 1953–1987. In R. Goodman & K. Refsing (Eds.), *Ideology and practice in modern Japan* (pp. 72–100). New York: Routledge.

Yanagisako, S. J. (1985). Transforming the past: Tradition and kinship among Japanese Americans. Stanford: Stanford University Press.

Chapter 15

People of Jewish Heritage

JANICE SELEKMAN

Overview, Inhabited Localities, and Topography

OVERVIEW

The term *Jewish* refers to both a people and a religion; it is not a race. Throughout history, the terms *Hebrew, Israelite,* and *Jew* have been used interchangeably. In the Bible, Abraham's grandson, Jacob, was also called Israel. His 12 sons and their descendants became known as the children of Israel. The term Jew is derived from Judah, one of Jacob's sons. **Hebrew** is the official language of the state of Israel and is used for religious prayers by all Jews wherever they live. "Thus today, the people are called Jewish, their faith Judaism, their language Hebrew, and their land Israel" (Donin, 1972: 7).

Judaism is both a religion and a culture. The religion is practiced along a wide continuum that ranges from liberal **Reform** to strict **Orthodox**. Although **Reform** Jews might not engage in any special daily practices, they still observe holidays, religious rites, and selected dietary or cultural customs. The traditional **Orthodox** Jew attempts to adhere to most of the religious laws. There are also ultra-Orthodox groups. No caste system or social hierarchy exists within the Jewish community. However, instances occur within the ultra-Orthodox communities when individuals cannot make decisions without consulting their rabbis. Because the degree of religiosity may be the major force shaping Jewish culture and worldview, the reader may wish to read the section on Spirituality in this chapter first in order to obtain a better understanding of the wide spectrum of religious practice among Jews.

One of the issues that rages within **Orthodox** communities in Israel and frequently seeps into America is "Who is a Jew"? It is recognized that a child born to a Jewish mother is Jewish. As mixed marriages have increased in number, the debate has ensued over patrilineal descent. A child born from the union of a Jewish father and a non-Jewish mother is recognized as Jewish by those in the **Reform** movement but not by those in the **Orthodox** movement.

While the goal of this chapter is to provide an understanding of all Jewish Americans, the focus is on the needs of the more traditional religious individuals and their families. These descriptions may vary somewhat for Jewish people in other parts of the world.

HERITAGE AND RESIDENCE

There are 5.84 million Jews throughout the United States (The American Jewish Committee, 1994), which represents 2.3 percent of the total U.S. population. The states with the highest percentages of Jewish population are New York (9.1 percent), New Jersey (5.6 percent), Florida (4.6 percent), Massachusetts (4.5 percent), Maryland (4.3 percent), and Washington D.C. (3.9 percent) (The American Jewish Committee, 1994). Forty-nine percent of the Jewish American population lives in the Northeast. The updated census numbers will be available in early 2003.

Jews have had a presence in the New World since the earliest days of American history. A group of 23 **Sephardic** Jewish settlers came to New Amsterdam (New York) in America from Brazil around 1654 (Glazer, 1957). By 1776, approximately 2000 Jews lived in the 13 colonies (Fischel & Pinsker, 1992). Many fought in the colonial army during the Revolutionary War.

REASONS FOR MIGRATION AND ASSOCIATED ECONOMIC FACTORS

Migration of Jews from Europe began to increase in the mid-1800s, often because of the fear of religious persecution. However, the greatest influx of immigrants occurred between 1880 and 1920. Many of these immigrants came from Russia and eastern Europe after a wave of **pogroms** (anti-Jewish riots and murders) and anti-Jewish decrees (Glazer, 1957). Once in America, acculturation became their motivation to live in safety and practice their religion.

Most Jewish families in America today are descendants of these eastern European and Russian immigrants. They are referred to as **Ashkenazi** Jews. Ashkenazi Jews make up 82 percent of the world's Jewish population (Fischel & Pinsker, 1992). Many American Jews of **Ashkenazi** descent have stories of how some members of their families escaped to America, while others had relatives who were part of the six million Jews killed in the pogroms and the Holocaust. **Sephardic** Jews, on the other hand, are from Spain, Portugal, the Mediterranean area, North Africa, and South and Central America. They represent a more diverse group. A *Sabra* is a Jew who was born in Israel.

In the 1980s and 1990s, a significant increase occurred in the number of Jewish immigrants from Russia. Because the practice of religion was illegal there for over half a century, these Jews often have different practices and a different understanding of their religion than the previous generation. The same was true of the Falasha Jewish community in 1984. These black Jews from Ethiopia participated in a mass exodus from their country to Israel and then, for some, to America.

EDUCATIONAL STATUS AND OCCUPATIONS

Despite bias against Jews in every century, they have made major contributions to society, especially in the sciences and health care. Throughout their history, they have placed a major emphasis on education and social justice through social action.

Continued learning is one of the most respected values of the Jewish people, who are often called the "People of the Book" (Robinson, 2000). While this usually refers to the study of **Torah**, it includes both Jewish and secular learning. Formal education is promoted and advanced degrees are respected. In general, this population is well educated. For all Jewish adults over the age of 25, only 27.7 percent have a high school education or less, compared with 62.2 percent of the U.S. white population. Over 19 percent have some college education, 26.7 percent have completed college, and 26.4 percent have completed graduate studies. This last figure compares with only 8.7 percent of the total U.S. white population (Goldstein, 1992). Jews have won 39 percent of the Nobel prizes in the life sciences, 11 percent in chemistry, and 41 percent in physics (Fischel & Pinsker, 1992).

Because of the emphasis on education, a high percentage of Jewish Americans have succeeded in science, medicine, law, and dentistry. Thirty-nine percent of Jewish men, and over 36 percent of Jewish women, list their occupation as professional, compared with only 15 percent of the American white population. With respect to higher education, over 10 percent of professors in American colleges and universities are Jewish (Fischel & Pinsker, 1992).

Throughout their history, Jews were repeatedly forbidden to own land, and the Christian Church barred its members from money lending. As a result, Jews frequently became moneylenders, peddlers, and tailors because these were the only options available to them. The early Jews in America were businessmen and craftsmen (Fischel & Pinsker, 1992). They became well respected for their expertise in trade and commerce. Today, one-quarter of Jewish men are in retail sales.

Because of the emphasis on social action, volunteerism, and involvement in helping others are common vocations or avocations. The term *tzedakah* (righteousness and sharing) is commonly used to indicate charity, a central concept to Judaism. Jewish children are raised with the concept of giving *tzedakah* by sharing with others who have less than they have.

Communication

DOMINANT LANGUAGE AND DIALECTS

English is the primary language of Jewish Americans. Although Hebrew is the official language of Israel and is used for prayers, it is generally not used for conversation. Hebrew is read from right to left, and books are opened from the opposite side compared with English books.

Many elderly **Ashkenazi** Jews who immigrated early in the 20th century or who are first-generation Americans speak **Yiddish,** a Judeo-German dialect. Many Yiddish terms have worked their way into the English language, including the following: *kvetch* (someone who complains a lot); *chutzpah* (clever audacity); *bagel* (a circular roll with a hole in the middle); *challah* (braided white bread); *knish* (dumpling with filling); *nosh* (snack); *zaftig* (plump); *tush, tushie,* or *tuchus* (buttocks); *ghetto* (a restricted area where certain groups live); *klutz* (a clumsy person); *mentsch, mensh* (a respected person with dignity); *shlep* (drag or carry); *kosher* (legal or okay); and *oy, oy vey* (oh my), and *oy veys mier* (woe is me).

Common expressions include *l'chaim* (to life), which is said during a toast of wine; *shalom alechem* (peace be with you) a traditional salutation; *mazel tov* (congratulations), and *shabbat shalom* (a good and peaceful Sabbath) which is said from Friday evening at sunset until Saturday at sunset.

CULTURAL COMMUNICATION PATTERNS

No religious ban or ethnic characteristics prevent Jews from sharing their feelings. Communication practices are more related to their American upbringing than to their religious practices.

As a way to cope and a way to communicate with others, Jews frequently use humor. However, jokes are considered to be insensitive when they reinforce mainstream stereotypes about Jews, such as implying that Jews are cheap or pampered (e.g., Jewish American princess). Any jokes that refer to the Holocaust or concentration camps are also inappropriate. However, Jewish self-criticism through humor is acceptable.

The philosophy that actions speak louder than words is prominent throughout Jewish teachings. People are judged by their actions, not by what they say and feel, because only the actions last beyond the lives of individuals (Amsel, 1994).

Modesty is a primary value in Judaism, especially among the **Orthodox**. It is not only seen in the **Orthodox** style of dress, but also in one's actions. Modesty involves humility. Jews are encouraged not to "show off" or constantly try to impress others.

Hasidic Jewish men are not permitted to touch a woman other than their wives. They often keep their hands in their pockets to avoid touch. They do not shake hands with women, and their failure to do so when one's hand is extended should not be interpreted as a sign of rudeness. Because women are considered seductive, **Hasidic** men may not engage in idle talk with them nor look directly at their faces. Non-Hasidic Jews may be much more informal and may use touch and short spatial distance when communicating. Health-care providers should only touch **Hasidic** men when providing direct care. "Therapeutic touch" is not appropriate with these clients.

TEMPORAL RELATIONSHIPS

While Jews live for today and plan for and worry about tomorrow, they are raised with stories of their past, especially of the Holocaust. They are warned to "never forget," lest history be repeated. Therefore, their time orientation is simultaneously to the past, the present, and the future.

The Jewish calendar is based on both a lunar and solar year, with each month beginning with the birth of the new moon. The festivals and holidays are based on the phases of the moon, whereas the seasons are based on the solar year. The lunar year is 11 days shorter than the solar year. Therefore, an extra month is periodically added.

FORMAT FOR NAMES

The Jewish format for names follows the Western tradition. The given name comes first and is followed by the family surname. Only the given name is used with friends and in informal situations. In more formal situations, the surname is preceded by the appropriate title of Mr., Miss, Ms., Mrs., or Doctor.

Babies may be named after someone who has died or after a living person to keep the person's name alive. The format chosen depends on whether the family is of **Ashkenazi** or **Sephardic** heritage. In ultra-Orthodox circles, children are not referred to by their names until after the **bris** or **brit milah** (circumcision) (Robinson, 2000). Infants are also given a Hebrew first name that is used when they are older and are called to read from the Torah. An example would be Efraim ben Reuven (Frank son of Robert).

Family Roles And Organization

HEAD OF HOUSEHOLD AND GENDER ROLES

The family is the core of Jewish society, and the needs of all family members are respected. While the man is considered the breadwinner for the household, the woman is recognized for running the home and being responsible for the children. According to Jewish law, the father has the legal obligation to educate his children in Judaism, to teach them right from wrong, to teach them to swim, and to teach his sons a trade (Robinson, 2000). He must provide his daughters with the means to make them marriageable. The mother's role is to keep a Jewish home and to raise the children. With acculturation, little difference is seen today between Jewish and non-Jewish white families with regard to gender roles. In most Jewish families, both parents share the responsibilities of supporting the home and raising the children.

According to the Talmud, Jewish husbands are required to provide their wives with food, clothing, medical care, and conjugal relations, in addition to meeting other needs. They are prohibited from "beating their wives, forcing them to have sex, or restricting their free movement" (Robinson, 2000: 161).

Although traditional Jewish law is clearly male oriented, Jewish women have been at the forefront of activities to demand and protect all human rights, especially those of women. They were prominent in movements to gain women's suffrage, reproductive health-care rights, and equal rights for all segments of society. Women are now expected to achieve their maximal level of education and to seek gainful employment if they so desire. Both sexes are expected to give service to their community.

PRESCRIPTIVE, RESTRICTIVE, AND TABOO BEHAVIORS FOR CHILDREN AND ADOLESCENTS

Children are the most valued treasure of the Jewish people (Amsel, 1994). They are considered a blessing and are to be treated with respect and provided with love. Jewish children are to be afforded an education, not only in studies that help them progress in society, but also in studies that transmit their Jewish heritage and the laws. Jewish school-age children typically attend Hebrew school as least two afternoons a week after public school throughout the school year. Children play an active role in most holiday celebrations and services.

Respecting and honoring one's parents is one of the Ten Commandments. Children should be forever grateful to their parents for giving them the gift of life. Jewish parents are expected to be consistent and fair to all their children, avoiding favoritism. In addition, parents should not promise something to their children that they cannot deliver. They must be flexible and yet caring and attentive to discipline. The individuality of each child's special traits should be recognized (Amsel, 1994).

In Judaism, the age of majority is 13 years for a boy and 12 for a girl. At this age children are deemed capable of differentiating right from wrong and capable of committing themselves to performing the command-ments (Amsel, 1994). Recognition of adulthood occurs during a religious ceremony called a *bar* or *bat mitzvah* (son or daughter of the commandment). In America, this rite of passage is usually accompanied by a family cele-bration. However, because sons and daughters are still teenagers living at home, it is recognized that they are still the responsibility of their parents.

FAMILY GOALS AND PRIORITIES

The goal of the **Orthodox** family is to live their lives as prescribed by *halakhah*, which emphasizes main-taining health, promoting education, and helping others. In addition, "each person must find those qualities and characteristics that make him or her unique and then he or she must attempt to maximize potential by fully devel-oping those qualities" (Amsel, 1994: 234). The family is central to Jewish life and is essential to the continuation of Judaism from one generation to the next.

Marriage is considered the ideal human state for adults. The Bible states that man should not be alone. The two goals of this union are to propagate the race and companionship (Kolatch, 2000), allowing an individual to focus on another person. Marriages are monogamous and many restrictions limit whom one may marry. Sibling, parent-child, grandparent-grandchild, aunt-nephew, or uncle-niece combinations are prohibited (Robinson, 2000).

Sexuality is a right of both men and women. In addi-tion to procreation requirements, conjugal rights for women exist. Nonprocreative intercourse is required for married women who may be pregnant or are unable to conceive, and this is not considered as "wasting seed" (Kolatch, 2000). Sexual intercourse is viewed as a pure and holy act when performed mutually within the rela-tionship of marriage. With some exceptions, refusal of a husband to have sex with his wife is grounds for a divorce (Robinson, 2000). However, the act of sex, if performed in the wrong context, is considered disgusting and against Jewish values (Amsel, 1994). Premarital sex is not condoned.

Among the ultra observant, women must physically separate themselves from all men during their menstrual periods and for 7 days after (Robinson, 2000). No man may touch a woman nor sit where she sat until she has been to the *mikveh*, a ritual bath, after her period is over. Sexual contact for this group may therefore occur only during two weeks of each month.

Judaism supports the need for sex education. The Jewish community sees this as its responsibility. This belief has been re-emphasized during the acquired immunodeficiency syndrome (AIDS) epidemic, where the goal is to protect the next generation and provide them with accurate information so they can make informed choices.

The median age of Jewish Americans is 37.3 years, 4 years higher than for white non-Jewish Americans. And 17.2 percent of the Jewish population is age 65 and older. This reflects both a healthy aging population and a large number of aging immigrants. Just over 13 percent of the non-Jewish white population is over age 65. One-third of

Jewish elderly people are older than 74, and 10 percent are 85 years old and older (Fischel & Pinsker, 1992).

While it is recognized that the later years are a time of physical decline, the elderly receive respect, especially for the wisdom they have to share. The Talmud defines elders as those who have reached their 61st birthday (Robinson, 2000). Old age is a state of mind rather than a chronological age; one may continue to "give" to soci-ety in a variety of ways, other than employment. In addi-tion, one may never "retire" from practicing the commandments.

Honoring one's parents is a lifelong endeavor and includes maintaining their dignity by feeding, clothing, and sheltering them, even if they suffer from senility. Respect for elderly people is essential even when their actions are irrational. The care of an elderly family member is the responsibility of the family; when the family is unable to provide care due to physical, psycho-logical, or financial reasons, the responsibility falls to the community. This role has always been a hallmark of Jewish communal life (Robinson, 2000). A number of elderly Jewish people move to Florida or other warm states after retirement because the weather there is more conducive to maintaining their health and safety. One-third of all elderly people who are not institutionalized live alone.

Only 7 percent of Jewish American families have three generations living together (Fischel & Pinsker, 1992). It should be noted that a number of elderly immi-grants who experienced imprisonment in concentration camps during the Holocaust in the 1940s, or those more recently incarcerated in Russia, may refuse to enter a nursing home for fear of returning to an institutional environment that robs them of their freedom (Fischel & Pinsker, 1992).

ALTERNATIVE LIFESTYLES

The Jewish view on homosexuality varies with the branch of Judaism. The Bible, especially as interpreted by the **Orthodox**, prohibits homosexual intercourse (Kolatch, 2000); it says nothing specifically about sex between lesbians (Dorff, 1998). Within the ancient writ-ings, lesbians were not treated as harshly as male homo-sexuals. Some of the objections to gay and lesbian lifestyles include the inability of these unions to fulfill the commandment of procreation and the possibility that acting on the recognition of one's homosexuality could ruin a marriage. The liberal movement within Judaism, however, supports "full legal and social equality for homosexuals" (Washofsky, 2000: 320).

Workforce Issues

CULTURE IN THE WORKPLACE

Specific workforce issues may occur when staff are Jewish, especially when they are observant of the Sabbath. Jews who observe the Sabbath must have Friday evening and Saturday off. They may work on Sundays. Supervisors must be sensitive to the needs of Jewish staff and recognize the holiness of the Sabbath. It is also important for Jewish staff to be allowed to request the major Jewish holidays off. Remembering that all holidays begin the evening before, they must have off the evening shift and the following day. Staff should not be penalized by having to use this time off as unpaid holidays or vacation time, but should have the opportunity to exchange for the Christmas and Easter holidays, time usually afforded to Christian staff.

Jewish health-care providers are fully acculturated into the American workforce. Judaism's beliefs are congruent with the values that American society places on the individual and family, and because English is the primary language for Jewish Americans, there are no language barriers for communicating in the workplace.

ISSUES RELATED TO AUTONOMY

Jewish nurses have begun to speak out on their needs in the workplace. With the recent emphasis on cultural competence, including cultural sensitivity, many are now addressing this long-ignored area. In 1990, a National Nurses Council was established through Hadassah, the Zionist women's organization (Benson, 1994). This group promotes solidarity and empowerment to enhance sensitivity within the health-care community. Ways in which the professional nursing community demonstrates its insensitivity to Jewish nurses is by scheduling major nursing conferences during the High Holy Days in the fall or during Passover in the spring, or by serving pork products during catered affairs.

Biocultural Ecology

SKIN COLOR AND OTHER BIOLOGICAL VARIATIONS

Ashkenazi Jews have the same skin coloring as white Americans. They may range from fair skin and blonde hair to darker skin and brunette hair. **Sephardic** Jews have slightly darker skin tones and hair coloring, similar to those from the Mediterranean area. There are also Jewish groups throughout Africa who are black, most notably, the Jews originally from Ethiopia, known as *Falasha*.

DISEASES AND HEALTH CONDITIONS

Because Jews are integrated throughout the United States, no specific risk factors are based on topography. Genetic risk factors vary based on whether the family immigrated from **Ashkenazi** or **Sephardic** areas. There is a greater incidence of some genetic disorders among individuals of Jewish descent, especially those who are **Ashkenazi**. Most of these disorders are autosomal recessive, meaning that both parents carry the affected gene. Although the best known is Tay-Sachs disease, Gaucher's disease is more prevalent. Others include Canavan's disease, familial dysautonomia, torsion dystonia, Niemann-Pick disease, Bloom syndrome, Fanconi's anemia, and mucolipidosis IV (National Foundation for Jewish Genetic Diseases, 2001).

Gaucher's disease is the most common genetic disease affecting **Ashkenazi** Jews, with 1 in 10 carrying the gene (National Gaucher Foundation, 2001). Gaucher's disease is a lipid-storage disorder. This inborn error of metabolism results in a defective enzyme that normally breaks down glucocerebroside, a lipid byproduct of erythrocytes. The glucocerebroside accumulates in the body resulting in weakening and fracturing of the bones due to infarctions, anemia, and platelet deficiencies. While there are 34 different genetic mutations of the disease, 4 of them account for 95 percent of cases in **Ashkenazi** Jews. The disorder can be detected by a blood test for both those affected and for carriers. Gene therapy treatments are now being tested (National Gaucher Foundation, 2001).

The gene for Tay-Sachs disease (also called infantile cerebromacular degeneration) is carried by 1 in 27 **Ashkenazi** Jews and 1 in 250 Jews of **Sephardic** origin. This autosomal recessive condition is a lysosomal sphingolipid storage disorder caused by an absence of hexosaminidase A, resulting in an accumulation of a lipid called GM2 ganglioside in the neural cells. The onset of mental and developmental retardation begins in the middle of the first year of life, with progressive deterioration, increasing seizure activity, and death by approximately age 5 (National Tay-Sachs and Allied Diseases Association, 2001). Because of the ease of testing for carriers as well as testing the fetus during pregnancy, and because of a concerted effort among the Jewish American community to provide testing, the incidence of Tay-Sachs disease has decreased significantly over the past 25 years. Because the ultra-Orthodox are opposed to abortion, this group only recommends the testing before marriage (Washofsky, 2000). It should be noted that because there are 50 different mutations, testing can identify 95 percent of carriers with a Jewish background and 60 percent of non-Jewish individuals (National Tay-Sachs and Allied Diseases Association, 2001).

Canavan's disease is a rare fatal degenerative brain disease caused by a defective gene that impairs the formation of myelin. Approximately 1 in 40 **Ashkenazi** Jews carry the gene. The resulting symptoms begin in mid-infancy and include developmental delay, loss of vision, and a loss of reflexes resulting in death by the age of 10 years (Canavan Foundation, 2001).

Familial dysautonomia, or Riley-Day syndrome, is also an autosomal recessive genetic disease, with the gene located on chromosome 9q31. It causes dysfunction of the autonomic and peripheral sensory nervous systems. Affected children have decreased myelinated fibers on nerves that lead to afferent impulses but maintain a normal intelligence. Symptoms include a decrease in the number of taste buds; altered pain sensation; increased salivation and sweating; and abnormal sucking or swallowing difficulties, and vomiting resulting in failure to thrive; decreased tears, resulting in increased risk of corneal ulceration; and temperature and blood pressure fluctuations. Fifty percent live to the age of 30. One in 30 **Ashkenazi** Jews is a carrier (National Foundation for Jewish Genetic Diseases, 2001).

The following are also autosomal recessive conditions with a higher incidence among **Ashkenazi** Jews. The gene for torsion dystonia is carried by 1 in 70 **Ashkenazi** Jews in the United States. The disease leads to rapid progression in loss of motor control and twisting spasms of the limbs. Affected individuals lead a full life and have a normal intelligence. Niemann-Pick disease, Type A, is a severe neurodegenerative disorder that starts at 6 months of age. It involves an abnormal storage of sphingomyelin and cholesterol in organs caused by an enzyme deficiency and leads to central nervous system degeneration. While those with Type A usually die by age 3, those with Type B survive into their 50s and have a milder presentation, with the sphingomyelin building up in their liver, spleen, lymph nodes, and brain.

Bloom syndrome, a rare genetic condition, involves increased risk of respiratory and gastrointestinal infections, erythema, telangiectasia, photosensitivity, and dwarfism. While the intelligence of those who are affected is usually normal, they face an increased risk of infertility, malignancy, and diabetes. Fanconi's anemia results in pancytopenia and an increased risk of cancer. Many die before early adulthood. Type C is found more frequently among **Ashkenazi** Jews; 1 in 89 are carriers. Mucolipidosis IV is found in 1 of 100 **Ashkenazi** Jews. This lipid storage disease results in central nervous system deterioration during the first year with motor and mental retardation, as well as various eye disorders. The prognosis varies (National Foundation for Jewish Genetic Diseases, 2001).

Orthodox rabbis usually do not support genetic testing because it might cause couples to "refrain from marrying or having children, thus preventing them from fulfilling the *mitzvah* of procreation" (Washofsky, 2000: 266). The Reform movement supports a couple's right to make the decision as to whether or not to have the testing done. "If we have the means by which to discover this information, so vital to the emotional and psychological well-being of a couple, then we must use them; failure to do so cannot be morally justified" (Washofsky, 2000: 267).

Other conditions occur with increased incidence in the Jewish population. Inflammatory bowel disease (ulcerative colitis and Crohn's disease) is seen four to five times more often in white Jews than in other white groups (Cooke, 1991). Colorectal cancer appears to be seen with increased frequency in **Ashkenazi** Jews (6 percent) (American Cancer Society, 2001). While the incidence of breast cancer among Jews is similar to other Caucasians, "three distinct mutations in the BRCA1 and BRCA2 genes, found in one out of every 40 Jewish women of Ashkenazic background, increase a woman's odds of getting breast and ovarian cancers" (Wyce, 2001: 20).

VARIATIONS IN DRUG METABOLISM

One of the few drugs found to have a higher rate of side effects in people of Ashkenazic ancestry is clozapine, used to treat schizophrenia. Twenty percent of Jewish clients taking this drug developed agranulocytosis, compared with about one percent of non-Jewish clients. A specific genetic haplotype has been identified to account for this finding (Levy, 1993). Thus, health-care

providers must institute testing for agranulocytosis when Jewish clients are prescribed clozapine.

High-Risk Behaviors

According to Jewish law, individuals may not intentionally damage their bodies or place themselves in danger. The basic philosophy is that the body must be protected from harm. To the religious, the body is viewed as belonging to God; therefore, it must be returned to Him intact when death occurs. Consequently, any substance or act that harms the body is not allowed. This includes smoking, suicide, taking nonprescription or illegal medications, and permanent tattooing (Dorff, 1998; Washofsky, 2000).

Alcohol, especially wine, is an essential part of religious holidays and festive occasions and is a traditional symbol of joy. The Jewish attitude toward wine is ambivalent. The Bible speaks of the undesirable effects of wine on the person, as well as its positive use as a medicine. Consequently, wine is appropriate and acceptable as long as it is used in moderation. However, "Jewish alcoholics and drug abusers have a duty to seek help in recovering from their addiction" (Dorff, 1998: 251).

HEALTH-CARE PRACTICES

Because of the respect afforded physicians and the emphasis on keeping the body and mind healthy, Jewish Americans are health conscious. In general, they practice preventive health care, with routine physical, dental, and vision screening. This is also a well-immunized population. Health-care providers need to encourage these positive health promotion and disease prevention practices among Jewish clients.

Nutrition

MEANING OF FOOD

Eating is an important function among Jews. Besides satisfying hunger and sustaining life, it also teaches discipline and reverence for life (Klein, 1992). For those Jews who follow the dietary laws, a tremendous amount of attention is given to the slaughter, preparation, and consumption of food. In addition, the dinner table is often the site for numerous religious holiday celebrations and services, especially the Sabbath, Passover, Rosh Hashanah (Jewish New Year), and breaking the fast for Yom Kippur (Day of Atonement). The dietary practices of Jews serve as a spiritually refining act of self-discipline and a unifying factor as an instrument of ethnic identity.

COMMON FOODS AND FOOD RITUALS

Perhaps the food identified as "Jewish" that receives the most attention is chicken soup. This has frequently been referred to as "Jewish penicillin," and is often served with knaidle balls in it (dumplings made of matzoh meal). Though it has no intrinsic meaning or religious value, it is a staple in religious homes, especially on Friday evenings to usher in the Sabbath and during times of illness. It is frequently associated with a mother's warmth and love.

Other common foods include gefilte fish (ground freshwater fish molded into oblong balls and served cold with horseradish); challah (braided white bread); kugel (noodle pudding); blintzes (crepes filled with a sweet cottage cheese); chopped liver (served cold); hamentashen (a triangular pastry with different types of filling); and lox and bagel sandwiches. Lox is cold smoked salmon, served with cream cheese and salad vegetables, on a round roll (bagel) with a hole in it.

The laws regarding food are found in Leviticus and Deuteronomy. They are commonly referred to as the laws of **kashrut,** or the laws that dictate which foods are permissible under religious law. The term **kosher** means "fit to eat"; it is not a brand or form of cooking. Whereas some believe that the mandatory statutes were developed and implemented for health reasons, religious scholars dispute this view, claiming that the only reason for following the laws is that they are mandatory commandments of God. Therefore, the laws are followed as a personal attachment to the religion and as a belief that God has mandated them (Kolatch, 2000; Robinson, 2000). The laws' promotion of health is only a secondary gain.

Foods are divided into those that are considered **kosher** (permitted or clean) and those considered *treyf* (forbidden or unclean). A permitted animal may be rendered *treyf*, or forbidden, if it is not slaughtered, cooked, or served properly. Because life is sacred and animal cruelty is forbidden, **kosher** slaughter of animals must be done in a way that prevents undue cruelty to the animal and ensures the animal's health for the consumer. The jugular vein, carotid arteries, and vagus nerve must be severed in a single quick stroke with a sharp, smooth knife, causing the animal to die instantaneously. No sawing motion and no second stroke is permitted (Robinson, 2000). This also allows the maximal amount of blood to leave the body. Care must be taken that all blood is drained from the animal before eating it. Drinking of blood is prohibited. An animal that dies from old age or disease may not be eaten, nor may it be eaten if it meets a violent death or is killed by another animal (Birnbaum, 1998). In addition, flesh cut from a live creature may not be eaten.

Milk and meat may not be mixed together in cooking, serving, or eating. To avoid mixing foods, utensils used to prepare foods and the plates used to serve them are separated. Religious Jews who follow the dietary laws have two sets of dishes, pots, and utensils: one set for milk products (*milchig* in Yiddish) and the other for meat *(fleishig)*. Because glass is not absorbent, it can be used for either meat or milk products, although religious households still usually have two sets (Kolatch, 2000). Therefore, cheeseburgers, lasagna made with meat, and grated cheese on meatballs and spaghetti is unacceptable. Milk cannot be used in coffee if served with a meat meal. Nondairy creamers can be used instead, as long as they do not contain sodium caseinate, which is derived from milk.

A number of foods are considered *parve* (neutral), and may be used with either dairy or meat dishes. These include fish, eggs, anything grown in the soil (vegetables, fruits, coffee, sugar, and spices), and chemically produced goods (Robinson, 2000). A *U* with a circle around it is the seal of the Union of Orthodox Jewish Congregations of America and is used on food products to indicate that they are kosher. A circled *K* and other symbols may also be found on packaging to indicate that a product is **kosher**.

When working in a Jewish person's home, the health-care provider should not bring food into the house without knowing whether or not the client adheres to **kosher** standards. If the client keeps a **kosher** home, do not use any cooking items, dishes, or silverware without knowing which are used for meat and which are used for dairy products. Health-care providers must fully understand the dietary laws so they do not offend the client, can advocate for kosher meals if they are requested, and can plan medication times accordingly.

Mammals are considered clean if they meet the other requirements for their slaughter and consumption and have split (cloven) hooves and chew their cud. These animals include buffalo, cattle, goats, deer, and sheep. The pig is an example of an animal that does not meet these criteria. Although liberal Jews decide for themselves which dietary laws they will follow, many still avoid pork and pork products out of a sense of tradition and symbolism. Serving pork products to a Jewish client, unless specifically requested, is insensitive.

Birds of prey are considered "unclean" and unacceptable because they grab their food with their claws. Poultry that is acceptable includes chicken, one of the most frequently consumed forms of protein, turkey, goose, and duck. Fish can be eaten if it has both fins and scales. Nothing that crawls on its belly is allowed, including clams, lobsters and other shellfish, tortoises, and frogs (Robinson, 2000).

In religious homes, meat is prepared for cooking by soaking and salting it to drain all the blood from the flesh. Broiling is acceptable, especially for liver, because it drains the blood (Robinson, 2000). Care must be taken in serving cheese to ensure that no animal substances are served at the same time. Breads and cakes made with lard are *treyf,* and breads made with milk or milk by-products (for example, casein) cannot be served with meat meals. Eggs from nonkosher birds, milk from nonkosher animals, and oil from nonkosher fish are not permitted. Butter substitutes are used with meat meals. Honey is allowed because it is produced from the nectar of flowers.

Kosher meals are available in most hospitals. They arrive on paper plates and with sealed plastic utensils. Health-care providers should not unwrap the utensils or change the foodstuffs to another serving dish. Frozen **kosher** meals are available on a commercial basis. If health-care providers have difficulty locating a supplier, they should contact a local rabbi. Determining a client's dietary preferences and practices regarding dietary laws should be done during the admission assessment.

DIETARY PRACTICES FOR HEALTH PROMOTION

As mentioned previously, although many Jewish dietary practices afford the secondary gain of preventing disease, their intention is not for health promotion, but rather for observance of a commandment. This is also true of the practice of washing one's hands before eating. Religious Jews wash their hands while reciting a prayer.

NUTRITIONAL DEFICIENCIES AND FOOD LIMITATIONS

No nutritional deficiencies are common to individuals of Jewish descent. As with any ethnic group, nutritional deficiencies may occur with individuals in lower socioeconomic groups because of the expense of certain foods.

In addition to the dietary laws discussed previously, additional dietary laws are followed at specified times. For example, during the week of Passover, no bread or product with yeast may be eaten. Matzoh (unleavened bread) is eaten instead. Any product that is fermented or can cause fermentation (souring) may not be eaten (Kolatch, 2000). Rather than attend synagogue, the family conducts the service (seder) around the dinner table during the first two nights and incorporates dinner into a service that includes all participants and retells the story of Moses and the Exodus from Egypt.

The Jewish calendar has a number of fast days. The most observed is the holiest day of the year, Yom Kippur. On this Day of Atonement, Jews abstain from food and drink as they pray to God for forgiveness for the sins they have committed during the past year. They eat an early dinner on the evening the holiday begins and then fast until after sunset the following day. It should be noted that ill people, the elderly, the young, and the physically incapacitated are absolved from fasting and may need to be reminded of this exception to Jewish law; this is also true for pregnant and nursing women (Lutske, 1995). Maintaining an ill person's health supersedes the act of fasting. If concerns arise, a consultation with the client's rabbi may be necessary.

Pregnancy and Childbearing Practices

FERTILITY PRACTICES AND VIEWS TOWARD PREGNANCY

God's first commandment to man is, "Be fruitful and multiply." Children are considered a gift and a duty, with men considered more important by the ultra-Orthodox because they can say *kaddish* (the prayer for the dead) for their parents. In other branches of Judaism, both sexes may recite the *kaddish*. Families are encouraged to have at least two children (Kolatch, 2000).

Couples who are unable to conceive should try all possible means to have children. This includes infertility counseling and interventions, including egg and sperm donation. "Orthodox opinion is virtually unanimous in prohibiting...artificial insemination when the semen donor is a man other than the woman's husband" (Washofsky, 2001: 234); some **Orthodox** Jews view this as adultery while others argue that it cannot be considered adultery if no sexual intercourse has occurred. When all natural attempts have been made, adoption may be pursued. Having children allows religious parents to fulfill many of the commandments (Dorff, 1998).

The lower number of pregnancies occurring among Jewish Americans and the high intermarriage rate has resulted in a decreased Jewish population. By age 45, Jewish women averaged 1.6 children compared to 2.1 children born to non-Jewish white women in the same age range. Data from 1970 indicated that Jewish women had an average of 2.4 children. Because one-third of all Jews were killed during the Holocaust, some believe that today's Jews "have a special moral obligation to bring one more child into the world than they would have normally" (Amsel, 1994: 314).

Prevention of pregnancy in the more **Orthodox** view implies deferring the commandment to be fruitful and multiply. Unless pregnancy jeopardizes the life or health of the mother, contraception is not looked on favorably among the ultra-Orthodox (Dorff, 1998). Liberal Judaism recognizes that children have the right to be wanted and that they should be born into homes where their needs can be met. Therefore, the use of temporary birth control may be acceptable. Condom use is supported, especially if unprotected sexual intercourse would pose a medical risk to either spouse (Dorff, 1998). Reform Judaism supports the access of minors to reproductive health services that are unrestricted by parental notification or permission, including dispensing contraceptives (Vorspan, 1992).

To the **Orthodox**, it is important to know the mechanism of action of the birth control. Coitus interruptus and masturbation are not acceptable because they result in the needless expenditure of semen, although most Jews consider the former practice a normal, healthy activity (Kolatch, 2000). Barrier techniques are not acceptable because they interfere with the full mobility of the sperm in its natural course. The birth control pill does not result in any permanent sterilization, nor does it prevent semen from traveling its normal route. Therefore, use of this method is the least objectionable to most branches of Judaism. "Today, almost all rabbinic authorities permit the use of contraceptive devices...in cases where pregnancy may imperil the life of the mother or where it is certain that the newborn might be afflicted with a serious congenital disease or abnormality" (Kolatch, 2000: 153). Sterilization implies permanence, and **Orthodox** Jews probably oppose this practice, unless the life of the mother is in danger. There is less objection to women being sterilized than men (Dorff, 1998). Reform Judaism leaves the choice of what to use and if to use contraceptives up to the parents.

Recognizing that Judaism's primary focus is the sanctity of life, it is important to identify when life begins. The fetus is not considered a living soul or person until it has been born. Birth is determined when the head or "greater part" is born (Robinson, 2000). Until that time, it is merely part of the mother's body and has no independent identity.

The mother and her health are paramount. If her physical or mental health is endangered by the fetus, all branches of Judaism see the fetus as an aggressor and require an abortion (Dorff, 1998; Kolatch, 2000). While saving the mother's life is certainly grounds for abortion, random abortion is not permitted by the **Orthodox** branch because the fetus is part of the mother's body and one must not do harm to one's body. However, Jewish law does allow for a reduction of fetuses in the case of multiple gestation when the potential viability of one or more are threatened by the others (Dorff, 1998).

Reform Judaism believes that a woman maintains control over her own body and it is up to her whether to abort a fetus. Although no connotation of sin is attached to abortion, the decision is not to be made without serious deliberation. Most Jews favor a woman's right to choose regarding abortion.

PRESCRIPTIVE, RESTRICTIVE, AND TABOO PRACTICES IN THE CHILDBEARING FAMILY

A Hasidic husband may not touch his wife during labor and may choose not to attend the delivery, because he is not permitted by Jewish law to view his wife's genitals. These behaviors should never be interpreted as insensitivity on the part of the husband. During the delivery of a child to an ultra-Orthodox family, the following interventions should be initiated: the mother should be given hospital gowns that cover her in the front and back to the greatest extent possible. She may prefer to wear a surgical cap so that her head remains covered (because the hair is considered a private part of her body). The father should be given the opportunity to leave during procedures and during the birth or, if he chooses to stay, the mother can be draped so that the husband may sit by his wife without viewing her perineum, including by way of mirrors, in order to protect her dignity. Because he is not permitted to touch his wife, he may offer only verbal support. The female nurse may need to provide all of the physical care. Pain medication during delivery is acceptable.

For male infants, circumcision, which is both a medical procedure and a religious rite, is performed. The history of this ritual dates back to Abraham and Isaac in the Book of Genesis. A **brit milah** (sometimes referred to as a **bris**) means a covenant between the Jewish people and God and is symbolized through the circumcision (Lau, 1997). The procedure and the ceremony are performed on the eighth day of life by a person called a **mohel**, an individual trained in the circumcision procedure, asepsis, and the religious ceremony. Although a rabbi is not necessary, it is also possible to have the procedure done by a physician with a rabbi present to say the blessings.

Attending a **brit milah** is the only mitzvah for which religious Jews must violate the Sabbath, so that the **brit** can be completed at the proper time (Robinson, 2000). The **brit milah** is a family festivity, and many relatives are invited. In most cases today, the ceremony is performed in the home; however, if the child is still in the hospital, it is important for the hospital to provide a room for a small private party to celebrate. While the

medical community sometimes debates the practice of circumcision, to even suggest to Jewish parents that the practice is "barbaric" is insensitive.

A circumcision may be delayed for medical reasons. These may include unstable condition due to prematurity, life-threatening concerns during the early weeks after birth, bleeding problems, or a defect of the penis, which may require later surgery. At birth, a child is free of all sin; failure to circumcise carries no eternal consequences should the child die.

Death Rituals

DEATH RITUALS AND EXPECTATIONS

Death is an expected part of the life cycle. Yet each day is to be appreciated and lived as if it was one's last day. Religious Jews start each day with a prayer of appreciation for having lived another day. The goal is to appreciate things and people while one still has them. Death is defined as the cessation of breathing and a heartbeat (Dorff, 1998). Many also accept a flat electroencephalogram (EEG) as determining death. Traditional Judaism believes in an afterlife where the soul continues to flourish, although many dispute this interpretation, and it is not mentioned in the Torah (Dorff, 1998). Most Jews do not give much thought to life after death and are unconcerned about it; their focus is on how one conducts one's present life.

Active euthanasia, where something is given or done to result in death, is forbidden for religious Jews. One of the Ten Commandments is "Thou shalt not kill," and euthanasia is considered murder. A dying person is considered a living person in all respects. Sufficient pain control should be provided, even if it decreases the person's level of consciousness (Dorff, 1998). Withholding food from a deformed child to speed its death is considered active euthanasia and is forbidden.

Passive euthanasia, or "refusal to intervene in the process of a person's natural demise" (Dorff, 1998: 177) may be allowed depending on its interpretation. Nothing may be used or initiated that prevents a person from dying naturally or that prolongs the dying process. Therefore, anything that artificially prevents death (cardiopulmonary resuscitation, ventilators, and so forth) may possibly be withheld, depending on the wishes of the patient and his or her religious views. Regardless of the decisions made, pain control must be maintained.

Taking one's own life is prohibited and is viewed as a criminal act and morally wrong because it is forbidden to harm any human being, including oneself. To the ultra-religious, suicide removes all possibility of repentance. Adult Jews who commit suicide, who are not insane or depressed, and who belong to ultra-religious factions of Judaism are not afforded full burial honors (Dorff, 1998; Lamm, 2000). They are buried on the periphery of the Jewish cemetery and mourning rites are not observed, unless the individual was not mentally competent. However, the more liberal view is to emphasize the needs of the survivors, and all burial and mourning activities proceed according to the usual traditional rites and wishes of the family. Children are never considered to have intentionally killed themselves and are afforded all burial rights.

The dying person should not be left alone. It is considered respectful to stay with a dying person, unless the visitor is physically ill or their emotions are out of control (Lamm, 2000). Judaism does not have any ceremony similar to Catholic sacrament of the sick. Any Jew may ask God's forgiveness for his or her sins; no confessor is needed. Some Jews feel solace in saying the *Shema* in Hebrew or English. This prayer confirms one's belief in one God. At the time of death, the nearest relative can gently close the eyes and mouth and the face is covered with a sheet. The body is treated with respect and revered for the function it once filled. Health-care providers may need to ask the closest relative of the deceased specifically about the practices to follow after death.

Ultra-Orthodox Jews follow a ritual that is not conducive to hospital protocols and is more commonly observed for those who die at home. After the body is wrapped, it is briefly placed on the floor with the feet pointing toward the door. A candle may be placed near the head. However, this does not occur on the Sabbath or holy days. The dead body is not left alone until the funeral, so as not to leave the body defenseless.

Autopsy is usually not permitted among religious Jews because it results in desecration of the body, and it is important that the body be interred whole. Allowing an autopsy might also delay the burial, something that is not recommended. On the other hand, however, autopsy is allowed if its results would save the life of another patient who is immediately at hand. Many branches of Judaism currently allow an autopsy if (1) it is required by law; (2) the deceased person has willed it; or (3) it saves the life of another, especially an offspring (Dorff, 1998). The body must be treated with respect during the autopsy.

Any attempt to hasten or retard decomposition of the body is discouraged. Cremation is prohibited because it unnaturally speeds the disposal of the dead body. Embalming is prohibited because it preserves the dead (Lamm, 2000). However, in circumstances where the funeral must be delayed, some embalming may be approved. Cosmetic restoration for the funeral is discouraged.

Jewish funerals and burials follow certain practices; they usually occur within 24 to 48 hours after the death. The funeral service is directed at honoring the departed by only speaking well of him or her. It is not customary to have flowers either at the funeral or at the cemetery; this was a Christian custom used to offset the odor of decaying bodies. The casket should be made of wood with no ornamentation. The body may only be wrapped in a shroud to ensure that the body and casket decay at the same rate. A wake or viewing is not part of a Jewish funeral. The prayer said for the dead, **kaddish**, is usually not said alone. Actually, the prayer says nothing about death, but rather it praises God and reaffirms one's own faith.

After the funeral, mourners are welcomed to the home of the closest relative. Outside the front door is water to wash one's hands before entering, which is symbolic of cleansing the impurities associated with contact with the dead. The water is not passed from person to person, just as it is hoped that the tragedy is not passed. At the home, a meal is served to all the guests. This "meal of condolence" or "meal of consolation" is traditionally provided by the neighbors and friends.

Shiva (Hebrew for "seven") is the 7-day period that begins with the burial. *Shiva* helps the surviving individuals face the actuality of the death of the loved one. During this period when the mourners are "sitting *shiva*," they do not work. When health-care providers are the ones experiencing the loss, it is important for supervisors to understand the mourning customs. In some homes mirrors are covered to decrease the focus on one's appearance; no activity is permitted to divert attention from thinking about the deceased; and evening and morning services may be conducted in the closest relative's home. Condolence calls and the giving of consolation are appropriate during this time.

After *shiva*, the mourning period varies based on who has died. Mourning for a relative lasts 30 days, and for a parent, 1 year. Judaism does not support prolonged mourning (Amsel, 1994). A tombstone is erected within 1 year of the death, at which time a graveside service is held. This is called an "unveiling." The anniversary of the death according to the Jewish calendar is called *yahrzeit*, and at this time, candles are lit and the **kaddish** is said.

Understanding some specific practices related to death and dying may have an impact on other aspects of health care. These include death of premature infants and the care of amputated limbs. Mourning is not required for a fetus that is miscarried or stillborn. This is also true of any premature infant who dies within 30 days of birth. However, parents are required to mourn for full-term infants who die at birth or shortly thereafter (Washofsky, 2000). While the baby should be named, not all of the traditional burial customs are followed (Lamm, 2000).

Within Orthodoxy, when a limb is amputated before death the amputated limb and blood-soaked clothing are buried in the person's future gravesite (Lamm, 2000). Because the blood and limb were part of the person, they are buried with the person. No mourning rites are required. In the case of an amputation, the health-care provider may need to assist with arrangement for burial of the body part.

RESPONSES TO DEATH AND GRIEF

The period following a death has discrete segments to assist mourners in their adjustment to the loss. The period of time between the death and the burial is short, and is the time for the emotional reaction to the death. The burial may only be delayed if required by law, if relatives must travel great distances, or if it is the Sabbath or a holy day. Mourners are absolved from praying during this time. Crying, anger, and talking about the deceased person's life are acceptable. A common sign of grief is the tearing of the garment that one is wearing before the funeral service. In liberal congregations, a black ribbon with a tear in it is a symbolic representation of mourning. During *shiva*, the mourner sets the tone and initiates the conversation. Because there are such discrete periods of mourning, Judaism tells the mourner that it is wrong to mourn more than 30 days for a relative and a year for parents.

Spirituality

DOMINANT RELIGION AND USE OF PRAYER

Judaism is over 3000 years old. Its early history and laws are chronicled in the Old Testament. Jews consider only the Old Testament as their Bible. They have a history of being singled out as a people and have often been persecuted; expelled from countries; "black-balled" from jobs, housing, and admission to college; rounded up and killed; and mass-exterminated.

Judaism is a monotheistic faith that believes in one God as the creator of the universe. The watchword of the faith is found in Deuteronomy (6:4), "Hear O Israel, the Lord is our God, the Lord is One." No physical qualities are attributed to God, and making and praying to statues or graven images are forbidden in the second commandment. "The Jewish conception of God is of a moral God who demands moral, ethical living and justice for all mankind. He is a universal God, whose sovereignty is over all the world" (Donin, 1972: 22).

Many Jews in America have immediate family members who were killed in the pogroms in Russia in the early 1900s and in the Holocaust in eastern Europe. Yet throughout this persecution, Judaism has lived and flourished. The spiritual leader is the **rabbi** (teacher). He (or she, in liberal branches) is the interpreter of Jewish law. Rabbis are not considered to be any closer to God than common people. All Jews pray directly to God. They do not need the rabbi to intercede, to hear confession, or to grant atonement. Some of the major principles that guide Judaic bioethics are as follows:

- Man's purpose on earth is to live according to certain God-given guidelines
- Life possesses enormous intrinsic value, and its preservation is of great moral significance
- All human lives are equal
- Our lives are not our own exclusive private possessions (Glick, 1994: 19)

The first five books of the Bible, also known as the five books of Moses, are handwritten in Hebrew on parchment scrolls called **Torah.** These scrolls are kept in the "Holy Ark" within each synagogue under an "eternal light." The **Torah** directs Jews on how they should live their lives; it provides guidance on every aspect of human life. The rest of the Bible includes sacred writings and teachings of the prophets.

The 613 commandments within the **Torah** (also called Mitzvot) and the oral law derived from the biblical statutes determine Jewish law, or **halakhah.** These commandments ask for a commitment in behavior and also address ethical concerns. Thus, the commandments reflect the will of God, and religious Jews feel it is their duty to carry them out to fulfill their covenant with God. This makes Judaism not only a religion but also a way of life (Amsel, 1994).

Current practice of Judaism in America spans a wide spectrum. While there is only one religion, there are three main branches or denominations of Judaism. The **Orthodox** are the most traditional. They adhere most strictly to the **halakhah** (Code of Jewish Law) of traditional Judaism and try to follow as many of the laws as possible while fitting into American society. They observe the Sabbath by attending the synagogue on Friday evening and Saturday morning and by abstaining from work, spending money, and driving on the Sabbath. Orthodox Jews observe the Jewish dietary laws; men wear a **yarmulke** or **kippah** (head covering) at all times in reverence to God, whereas women usually wear long sleeves and modest dress. In many **Orthodox** synagogues, the services are primarily in Hebrew and men and women sit separately. In America, 6.1 percent of the Jewish population consider themselves **Orthodox** (Singer, 1992).

Orthodox Jews and some **Conservative** men and women use the *tefillin* or "phylacteries" during morning prayer services. These are two small black boxes with parchment containing biblical passages that are connected to long leather straps. These are wrapped around the arms and forehead as reminders of the laws of the Torah. The *tallis* (or *tallit*) is a rectangular prayer shawl with fringes. This is also only used during prayer but is frequently used by both **Conservative** and **Orthodox** Jews. Ultra-Orthodox men wear a special garment under their shirts year-round; the *tzitzit* has long fringes as a reminder of the laws of the Torah.

A **mezuzah** is a small container with scripture inside. Its origin was as a sign ensuring God's protection; it serves as a reminder of the presence of God, His commandments, and a Jew's duties to Him. Jewish homes have a **mezuzah** on the doorpost of the house. A number of individuals also wear a **mezuzah** as a necklace. Other religious symbols include the Star of David, a six-pointed star that has been a symbol of the Jewish community since the 1350s (Fig. 15–1), and the menorah (candelabrum).

The **Conservative** branch (35.1 percent of American Jews) is not quite as strict in its tradition (Singer, 1992). While **Conservative** Jews observe most of the **halakhah**, they do make concessions to modern society. Many drive to the synagogue on the Sabbath, and men

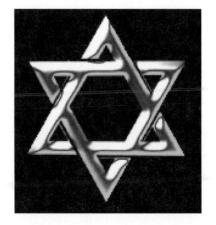

FIGURE 15–1   The Star of David is the symbol most commonly associated with Judaism today. The Star is thought to bring good luck.

and women sit together. Many keep a kosher home, but they may or may not follow all of the dietary laws outside the home. Women are ordained as rabbis and are counted in a *minyan*, the minimum number of 10 that is required for prayer. These practices are unacceptable to the Orthodox. While a yarmulke is required in the synagogue, it is optional outside of that environment.

The liberal or progressive movement is called **Reform** (38 percent of the Jews in America). **Reform** Jews claim that post biblical law was only for the people of that time, and only the moral laws of the Torah are binding (Fischel & Pinsker, 1992). They practice fewer rituals, although they frequently have a *mezuzah* (parchment with a religious passage within a small receptacle) posted on the doorpost of their homes, celebrate the holidays, and have a strong ethnic identity. They consider education and ethics of paramount importance in one's personal life and try to link Jewish religious values with American political liberalism. They may or may not follow the Jewish dietary laws, but they may have specific unacceptable foods (for example, pork), which they abstain from eating. Men and women share full equality, and they engage in many social action activities. **Reform** Jews do not celebrate the extra day added to many Jewish holidays.

Of the many small groups of ultra-Orthodox fundamentalists; the **Hasidic** (or **Chasidic**) Jews are perhaps the most recognizable. They usually live, work, and study within a segregated area. They are usually easy to identify by their full beards, uncut hair around the ears *(pais)*, black hats or fur *streimels*, dark clothing, and no exposed extremities. Women, especially those who are married, also keep their extremities covered and may have shaved heads covered by a wig and often a hat as well.

A relatively new denomination, **Reconstructionism** (1.3 percent of American Jews), is a mosaic of the three main branches. It views Judaism as an evolving religion of the Jewish people and seeks to adapt Jewish beliefs and practices to the needs of the contemporary world. In addition to these groups, many Jews do not indicate any affiliation.

The Jewish house of prayer is called a **synagogue**, temple, or *shul*. It is never referred to as a church. However, Jews may pray alone or may pray as a group anywhere that 10 Jews, over the age of 13 who have had their *bar mitzvah*, are gathered together for prayer. This group is called a **minyan. Orthodox** Jews pray three times a day: morning, late afternoon, and evening. They wash their hands and say a prayer on awakening in the morning and before meals.

Religious clients in hospitals may want their prayer items (**yarmulke** or *kippah, tallit, tzitzit, tefillin*) and may request a **minyan.** Hospital policies regarding the number of visitors in the sick person's room may have to be ignored in such instances.

One of the most common religious practices related to patients involves "visiting the sick" *(bikkur cholim)*. This commandment is one of the social obligations of Judaism and ensures that Jews look after the physical, emotional, psychological, and social well-being of others. It provides hope as well as companionship. However, it is important for visitors to consider the patient's welfare. This means not staying too long, tiring the patient, or coming only to satisfy one's own needs.

MEANING OF LIFE AND INDIVIDUAL SOURCES OF STRENGTH

The preservation of life is one of Judaism's greatest priorities. Even the laws that govern the Sabbath may be broken if one can help save a life. Each individual is considered special, and the individuality of the human experience is one of the precepts of the faith. Good health is considered an asset. In this regard, individuals who are ill must *not* fast during Yom Kippur (Robinson, 2000).

SPIRITUAL BELIEFS AND HEALTH-CARE PRACTICES

One of the Ten Commandments is to remember the Sabbath day and keep it holy. The Sabbath begins 18 minutes before sunset on Friday. Lighting candles, saying prayers over challah and wine, and participating in a festive Sabbath meal, usher in this weekly holy day. It ends 42 minutes after sunset (or when three stars can be seen) on Saturday, with a service called *Havdalah*. The Sabbath serves as a release from weekday concerns and pressures. During this time, religious Jews do no manner of work, including answering the telephone, operating any electrical appliance, driving, or operating a call bell from a hospital bed.

If an **Orthodox** client's condition is not life threatening, medical and surgical procedures should not be performed on the Sabbath or holy days. However, "illness, extremely foul weather, or great distance from the synagogue are legitimate reasons for not attending the services" (Donin, 1972: 75). Although the Sabbath is holy, matters involving human life take precedence over it (Robinson, 2000). Therefore, a gravely ill person and the work of those who need to save him are exempted from following the commandments regarding the Sabbath.

In addition to the Sabbath, a number of Jewish holidays are celebrated with special traditions. Rosh Hashanah (Jewish New Year) and Yom Kippur (Day of Atonement) are called the high holy days, and are usually in September or early October. They mark a 10-day period of self-examination and repentance. Rosh Hashanah is started by eating apples and honey to wish for a sweet year, and on Yom Kippur, one fasts for a day to cleanse and purify oneself. Fasting for Yom Kippur may be broken for reasons of critical illness, labor and delivery, or for children under the age of 12. The holiday includes the blowing of the *shofar* (a ram's horn) and the greeting, "May you be inscribed in the book of life for a good year."

Other major holidays include Passover, the Feast of the Unleavened Bread, which lasts 8 days and celebrates the Jews' Exodus from Egypt and freedom from slavery; Sukkot, a festival of the harvest where individuals may live in temporary huts built outside their homes or **synagogues** for a week; and Shavuot, which celebrates the giving of the Ten Commandments. Minor holidays

Table 15–1 Jewish Holidays: 2002–2006

Holiday	2002–2003	2003–2004	2004–2005	2005–2006
Rosh Hashanah	9/7–8	9/27–28	9/16–17	10/4–5
Yom Kippur	9/16	10/6	9/25	10/13
Sukkot	9/21–22	10/11–12	9/30–10/1	10/18–19
Chanukah	11/30–12/7	12/20–27	12/9–15	12/26–1/2
Purim	2/26	3/18	3/25	3/14
Passover	4/17–24	4/6–13	4/24–5/1	4/13–20
Shavuot	6/6–7	5/25–26	6/13–14	6/2–3

Jewish holidays always begin at sundown the evening before the date recorded on this type of calendar; holidays end at sundown on the date shown.

include Chanukah, an 8-day holiday, and Purim, both of which celebrate religious freedom. Table 15–1 provides a list of Jewish holidays for the years from 2002 through 2005.

Health-Care Practices

HEALTH-SEEKING BELIEFS AND BEHAVIORS

According to those who interpret Jewish law, all people have a duty to keep themselves in good health. This encompasses physical and mental well-being, and includes not only early treatment for illness but also prevention of illness. Judaism teaches its members to "choose life." "To refuse lifesaving medical treatment is to commit suicide, to choose death over life" (Washofsky, 2000: 223). All denominations recognize that religious requirements may be laid aside if a life is at stake or if an individual has a life-threatening illness. However, once it is clear that an individual is dying and that medical treatment is no longer working, individuals may choose not to interfere with death. Hospice care is fully consonant with Jewish beliefs (Dorff, 1998).

In ultra-Orthodox denominations of Judaism, taking medication on the Sabbath that is not necessary to preserve life may be viewed as "work" (i.e., an action performed with the intention of bringing about a change in existing conditions), and is unacceptable. This belief may result in some people with conditions such as asthma not recognizing the severity of their condition; they may also be unaware of the laws that allow them to take their necessary medications. These patients need to be taught about the potential life-threatening sequelae of their condition as well as the exceptions to Jewish law that permit them to take their medications.

In the Jewish faith, all individuals have value regardless of their condition. This includes individuals with developmental disabilities and AIDS. Judaism opposes discrimination against people with physical, mental, and developmental conditions (Dorff, 1998).

RESPONSIBILITY FOR HEALTH CARE

While it is the responsibility of health-care providers to heal, individuals must seek the services of the physi-cian to ensure a healthy body. Once individuals have the knowledge to heal, it is their obligation to do so. To abstain from healing would be equivalent to murder. Jews believe that God provides human beings with wisdom, and it is up to them to use that wisdom to create a better world. This includes the discovery of new medications and treatments to eliminate or modify disease and suffering. Jews also believe that God gives humans freedom of choice.

Because the preservation of life is paramount, all ritual commandments are waived when danger to life exists. Physical and mental illnesses are legitimate reasons for not fulfilling some of the commandments. Because adult Jews are often well read, they may try many of the treatment modalities about which they have read. This could have both positive and negative consequences. The literature reveals no studies regarding Jews' self-medicating practices.

FOLK PRACTICES

Jewish folklore practices are historically and biblically based. Specific practices are explained in the sections of this chapter on Nutrition and Spiritual Beliefs and Health-Care Practices.

BARRIERS TO HEALTH CARE

Except for the unavailability of health insurance for some people, there are no major barriers to health care for Jews in contemporary America. In early colonial America, Jews were only allowed to stay in the colonies on the condition that they support their own poor and care for their own sick (Fischel & Pinsker, 1992). The Jewish community helped those in need, including new immigrants, and assisted fellow Jews in becoming self-sufficient. This practice continued so that "the 230,000 Jews in the United States in 1880 absorbed 3 million immigrants in the next 50 years" (Fischel & Pinsker, 1992: 106).

CULTURAL RESPONSES TO HEALTH AND ILLNESS

The verbalization of pain is acceptable and common. Individuals want to know the reason for the pain, which they consider just as important as obtaining relief from pain. The sick role for Jews is highly individualized and may vary among individuals according to the severity of symptoms. As prescribed in the **halakhah**, the family is central to Jewish life; therefore, family members share the emphasis on maintaining health and assisting with individual responsibilities during times of illness.

Many Jews have become physicians, psychoanalysts, psychiatrists, and psychologists. In addition, many of their clients are Jewish. The maintenance of one's mental health is considered just as important as the maintenance of one's physical health. Mental incapacity has always been recognized as grounds for exemption from all obligations under Jewish law (Dorff, 1998). This designation includes psychiatric conditions. However, requirements for those who are rational but have cognitive deficiencies are decided on an individual basis.

According to Jewish law, individuals must be taught the **Torah** regardless of their age or level of disability. This speaks to the unique value of each individual.

BLOOD TRANSFUSIONS AND ORGAN DONATION

Jewish law views organ transplants from four perspectives: the recipient, the living donor, the cadaver donor, and the dying donor. Because life is sacred, if the recipient's life can be prolonged without considerable risk, then transplant is ordained. For a living donor to be approved, the risk to the life of the donor must be considered. One is not obligated to donate a bodily part unless the risk is small. Examples include kidney and bone marrow donations (Lamm, 2000). The action of donating an organ to save another is considered a great mitzvah.

Organ donation at the time of death is acceptable if it saves a person's life; in this respect, it is actually an honor to the dead person (Dorff, 1998). The concern has always been that the patient will be killed for the purpose of getting the organs sooner. **Conservative** and **Reform** Judaism approve using the flat EEG as the determination of death so that organs, such as the heart, can be viable for transplant. Burial may be delayed if organ harvesting is the cause of the delay. Health-care providers may need to assist Jewish clients to obtain a **rabbi** when making a decision regarding organ donation or transplant.

The use of a cadaver for transplant is usually approved if it is to save a life. No one may derive economic benefit from the corpse. Although desecration of the dead body is considered purposeless mutilation, this does not apply to the removal of organs for transplant. Use of skin for burns is also acceptable, although no agreement has been reached on the use of cadaver corneas (Abraham, 1994).

Health-Care Practitioners

The ancient Hebrews are credited with promoting hygiene and sanitation practices and basic principles for public health care. From the practice of visiting the sick and the desire to initiate measures to prevent the spread of disease, Lillian Wald, a Jewish nurse, developed the Henry Street Settlement as a prototype of public health nursing for those in need (Benson, 1993).

STATUS OF HEALTH-CARE PROVIDERS

Physicians are held in high regard. While physicians must do everything in their power to prolong life, they are prohibited from initiating measures that prolong the act of dying (Rosner, 1993). Once standard therapy has failed, or if additional treatments are unavailable, "the physician's role changes from that of curer to that of carer. Only supportive care is required at that state and includes care such as food and water, good nursing care, and maximal psychosocial support" (Rosner, 1993: 10).

CASE STUDY Selecting a "typical" Jewish client is difficult. An ultra-Orthodox Jew has a particular set of special needs. Yet, it is more common to see a Jew who is a middle-of-the-road Conservative.

Sarah is an 80-year-old woman who is a first-generation American. She was raised in a traditional Conservative home. Her husband died after 50 years of a strong marriage. She has three children. While her home is not kosher, she practices a variation of kosher-style eating, avoiding pork and not making dishes that combine meat and milk.

Two months ago, she was diagnosed with pancreatic cancer. Surgery was attempted, but the cancer was already in an advanced stage. Chemotherapy was started, but the cancer has progressed and is not responding to the medications. She is having difficulty eating because of the pressure of the tumor on the gastrointestinal track. Discussions are being held to determine whether or not treatments should be stopped and whether hospice care should be initiated.

Her hospital room is always filled with visitors.

STUDY QUESTIONS

1 What must you anticipate in discussing with Sarah her wishes regarding the continuation of medical care?

2 How would you respond to her initial decision to have surgery and initiate chemotherapy?

3 What questions do you need to ask in the initial patient interview to assess her degree of religious practice, and how will you determine her spirituality needs?

4 What is your understanding of the reason she has so many visitors in her room?

5 Is hospice care appropriate for this patient?

6 Sarah dies with her family at her bedside. What interventions can you take at the time of death to demonstrate religious sensitivity to the family? What questions do you need to ask the family?

7 Describe three genetic or hereditary diseases common with Ashkenazi Jews.

8 Describe the Jewish ritual of circumcision.

9 Discuss the laws of Kashrut in regard to food practices for observant Jewish clients.

10 What should the health-care provider keep in mind when entering a Jewish home to provide care?

11 Distinguish between the terms Sephardic and Ashkenazi.

12 How might a non-Jewish and Jewish coworker share holidays in the workforce.

13 What is the official language the Jewish people use for prayer?

REFERENCES

Abraham, A. (1994). Organ transplantation and Jewish law. In H. Branover & I. Attia (Eds.), *Science in the light of Torah.* Northvale, NJ: Jason Aronson.

American Cancer Society. http://www.Cancer.org/eprise/main/docroot/cri/cri_2_3x.

The American Jewish Committee (1994). *American Jewish year book.* New York: Author.

Amsel, N. (1994). *The Jewish encyclopedia of moral and ethical issues.* Northvale, NJ: Jason Aronson.

Benson, E. (1994). Jewish nurses: A multicultural perspective. *Journal of the New York State Nurses Association, 25*(2), 8–10.

Benson, E. (1993). Public health nursing and the Jewish contribution. *Public Health Nursing, 10*(1), 55–57.

Birnbaum, P. (1998). *Encyclopedia of Jewish Concepts.* New York: Hebrew Publishing Co.

Canavan Foundation. Retrieved November 2, 2001, from http://www.canavanfoundation.org.

Cooke, D. (1991). Inflammatory bowel disease: Primary health care management of ulcerative colitis and Crohn's disease. *Nurse Practitioner, 16*(8), 27–39.

Donin, H. (1972). *To be a Jew: A guide to Jewish observance in contemporary life.* New York: Basic Books.

Dorff, E. (1998). *Matters of life and death: A Jewish Approach to modern medical ethics.* Philadelphia: The Jewish Publication Society.

Fischel, J., & Pinsker, S. (1992). *Jewish-American history and culture: An encyclopedia.* New York: Garland Publishing.

Glazer, N. (1957). *American Judaism.* Chicago: University of Chicago Press.

Glick, S. (1994). *Trends in medical ethics in a pluralistic society: A Jewish perspective.* University of Cincinnati, Judaic Studies Program, Cincinnati, Ohio.

Goldstein, H. (1992). Commentary: Better ways to compare schools? *Journal of Educational Statistics, 16,* 89–92.

Klein, I. (1992). *A guide to Jewish religious practice.* New York: Jewish Theological Seminary of America.

Kolatch, A. (2000). *The second Jewish book of why.* Middle Village, NY: Jonathan David.

Lamm, M. (2000). *The Jewish way in death and in mourning.* Middle Village, NY: Jonathan David.

Lau, I. (1997). *Practical Judaism.* Jerusalem: Feldheim.

Lutske, H. (1995). *The book of Jewish customs.* Northvale, NJ: Jason Aronson.

Levy, R. (1993). Ethnic and racial differences in response to medicines: Preserving individualized therapy in managed pharmaceutical programmes. *Pharmaceutical Medicine, 7,* 139–165.

National Foundation for Jewish Genetic Diseases. http://www.nfjgd.org/Factsheets/Fsindex.htm.

National Gaucher Foundation. http://www.gaucherdisease.org.

National Tay-Sachs and Allied Diseases Association, Inc. http://www.ntsad.org.

Robinson, G. (2000). Essential Judaism: A complete guide to beliefs, customs, and rituals. New York: Pocket Books.

Rosner, F. (1993, July/August). Hospice, medical ethics and Jewish customs. *American Journal of Hospice and Palliative Care,* 6–10.

Singer, D. (1992). *American Jewish year book 1992.* Philadelphia: The Jewish Publication Society.

Vorspan, A. (1992). *Tough choices: Jewish perspectives on social justice.* New York: UAHC (Union of American Hebrew Congregations) Press.

Washofsky, M. (2000). *Jewish Living: A guide to contemporary reform practice.* New York: UAHC (Union of American Hebrew Congregations) Press.

Wyce, M. (2001, Summer). Genetic profiling: Who will be seen as damaged goods? *Inside,* 18–22.

Chapter 16

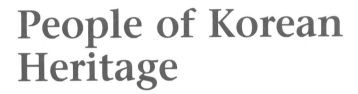

People of Korean Heritage

LARRY D. PURNELL and SUSIE KIM

Overview, Inhabited Localities, and Topography

OVERVIEW

Information in this chapter focuses on the commonalties among people of Korean ancestry with historical reference to the mother country, South Korea. Therefore, the use of the term *Korea* refers to the Republic of Korea. Because some information may not be pertinent to every Korean immigrant, it should be used as a guide for health-care providers rather than as a mandate of facts. Differences in beliefs and practices among Koreans in Korea, the United States, and other countries vary according to the primary and secondary characteristics of culture (see Chapter 1). An understanding of Korean culture and history gives health professionals the insight needed to perform culturally appropriate assessments, plan effective care and follow-up, and to work effectively with Koreans in the workforce.

Korea is a peninsula separated by North Korea to the north at the 38th parallel, and is surrounded by the former Soviet Union to the northeast, the Yellow Sea on the west, and the Sea of Japan to the east. South Korea has a landmass of 98,480 km² (38,031 mi²), which is about the size of the state of Indiana, and a population of 48 million. Korea has one percent of the landmass of the United States, but has one-sixth as many people, making it 16 times more densely populated than the United States (Kohls, 2001). The mega-modern metropolitan area of Seoul, the capital, has a population of 19 million people. A new international state-of-the art airport is

located in Incheon, 60 km from the center of Seoul. Other large cities are Busan (Pusan) and Daegu (Taegu). Planes, trains, and buses link all South Korean major cities, making travel easy and efficient. With the recent increase in the number of automobiles and the construction of highways, motorways are becoming more congested. Major industries are electronics, machinery, agricultural products, textiles, and shipbuilding.

The continental and monsoon climate of Korea is fairly consistent throughout the peninsula, except during the winter months. North Korea has cold, snowy winters, with an average temperature in January of 17°F. South Korea is milder, with an average January temperature of 23°F. During the summer months, the monsoon winds create an average temperature of 80°F, with high humidity throughout the peninsula. Precipitation occurs mostly during the summer months and is heavier in the south. The peninsula is mountainous with only 20 percent of the terrain located in lowlands. Such topography encourages the development of concentrated living areas. Most cities and residential areas are located along the coastal plains and the inland valleys opening to the west coast. The filming in Korea of the movie and highly popular television series, *M.A.S.H.*, has popularized this small nation, making it more familiar to people around the world.

HERITAGE AND RESIDENCE

Korea is one of the two oldest continuous civilizations in the world, second only to China. Koreans trace their heritage to 2333 BC. In the first century AD, tribes from central and northern Asia banded together to form this "Hermit Kingdom," littering the countryside with palaces, pagodas, and gardens. Over the ensuing centuries, the Mongols, Japanese, and Chinese invaded the Korean peninsula. Japan forcibly annexed Korea in the early 20th century, ruling it harshly and leaving ill will that persists to this day. As a result of the Potsdam Conference after WWII, the United States took over the occupation of South Korea, with the USSR occupying North Korea. By 1948, Korea's new government was recognized by the UN, only to be followed by the North Korean Communist forces invading South Korea in 1950. The result was the Korean War, which lasted until 1953 and caused mass devastation, from which the country has made a remarkable recovery. Open aggression between North and South Korea again occurred in 1998 and 1999. In 2000, the two Koreas signed a vague, yet hopeful, agreement that the two countries would be reunited. Some believe that it will take 20 years for unification to occur. The United States continues to maintain a strong military presence throughout South Korea.

In 1988, the year Seoul hosted the Olympic games, elections were held, and relations were re-established with China and the Soviet Union. Intermittent corruption among political officials has continued to surface, threatening internal relationships and the economy. In 1997, South Korea's economy tumbled dramatically, resulting in economic and democratic reforms. With unwavering persistence, Koreans have rebuilt their major world economy, reflecting a 9 percent annual growth rate and 4.4 percent rate of inflation (Lonely Planet) (Fig. 16–1).

REASONS FOR MIGRATION AND ASSOCIATED ECONOMIC FACTORS

The first major immigration from Korea occurred between 1903 and 1905, when more than 7000 men arrived in Hawaii. The U.S. Immigration Act of 1924 practically closed the door to Japanese and Koreans. During the civil rights movements of the 1950s and 1960s, new immigration laws repealed the earlier limitations on Asian immigration. Koreans continue to immigrate to America to pursue the American dream, to increase socioeconomic opportunities, and to attend colleges and universities. Additionally, many Koreans and Americans marry, making both Korea and America their homes. Korea ranks fourth in the number of Asian immigrants to the United States, with 1.3 million, closely following the Philippines, China, and Vietnam (Shin & Shin, 1999). Of the more than 44,000 Koreans in Canada, over half live in Ontario (Statcan.com, 2001).

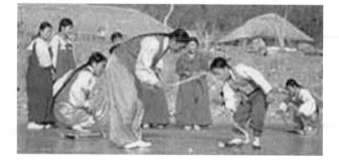

FIGURE 16–1 Traditional Korean dancers.

EDUCATIONAL STATUS AND OCCUPATIONS

Koreans place a high value on education, a statement emphasized many times in this chapter. Most of the population pursues higher education, and South Korea has more citizens with PhDs per capita than any other country in the world. There are several reasons why Koreans place such high value on educational attainment. Confucianism provides Korea with a strong family structure, norms of frugality and hard work, and places a high value on education, which is the means of raising one's status. National Korean studies report college-educated individuals earn twice the income of high school graduates and three times the income of primary or middle school graduates (Sorensen, 1994). Korean students receive family pressure to perform well in the intense competition for passing entrance examinations required by high schools and universities.

Before the late 19th century, education was primarily for those who could afford it. State schools educated the youth from the *yangban* (upper class), focusing on Chinese classics in the belief that these contained the tools of Confucian morality and philosophy that also apply in politics. In the late 1800s, the state schools were opened to all citizens. Early Christian missionary work introduced the Western style of modern education to Korea. Initially, many Koreans were skeptical of the radical curriculum and instruction for females, but the popularity of this style grew rapidly.

After the takeover of Korea by the Japanese in 1910, two types of schools emerged, one for Japanese and another for Koreans. The Korean schools focused on vocational training, which prepared Koreans only for lower-level positions. Japanese colonial education was designed to keep Koreans subordinate in all ways to ethnic Japanese (Sorensen, 1994). In 1949, a South Korean law implemented the same educational system as that of the United States. This 6-3-3-4 ladder (6 years in elementary school, 3 years in junior high, 3 years in high school, and 4 years in college) continues today in contemporary South Korea. Anticommunism and morality are taught throughout elementary and secondary schools.

In the United States, many Koreans own their own businesses, which vary from mom-and-pop stores and gas stations, to grocery stores and real estate agencies, to retail shops. Their reputation for hard work, independence, and self-motivation has given them the reputation of the "model minority." However, this has caused a backlash in some communities, such as Washington, D.C., where they have been compared with other minority groups. The message has become: "If the Koreans can do it, why not other groups?" The turmoil and riots that took place in Los Angeles in April 1992 between the African American community and Korean American merchants is another example of conflicts that arise from such labeling.

Many Korean businesses are located in African American neighborhoods because of low capital investment requirements and limited resources of the owners. Korean merchants begin dealing in inexpensive consumer goods as a practical way to start a business in a capitalistic society. Koreans often assist each other in establishing businesses, pooling their money, and taking turns with rotating credit associations providing each family with the opportunity for financial success.

Communication

DOMINANT LANGUAGE AND DIALECTS

The dominant language in Korea is Korean, or *han'gul*, which originated in the 15th century with King Se Jong, and is believed to be the first phonetic alphabet in East Asia. The Korean language belongs to the Ural-Altaic language family, which includes Turkic, Mongolian, and Tungusic as major branches (Comrie, Matthews, & Polinsky, 1996). Chinese and Japanese have influenced the Korean language, which has 14 consonants and 10 vowels. During their annexation in the early 20th century, the Japanese forbade public use of the Korean language, requiring the use of the Japanese written and spoken language. Dialects do not exist in Korean, but slang terminology is characteristic of specific age groups and regions.

Most Koreans in the United States can speak, read, write, and understand English to some degree. However, some Americans may have difficulty understanding the English spoken by Koreans, especially those who learned English from Koreans who spoke with their native intonations and pronunciations.

In Korea, four levels of speech characterize the degree of intimacy between conversants. These varying levels are called *honorifics*, reflecting differences in social status based on gender, age, and social positions. Verb endings aid in delineating social rank and age; for example, there is no word in Korean for brother or sister, only younger or older brother or sister.

CULTURAL COMMUNICATION PATTERNS

The sharing of thoughts, feelings, and ideas is very much based on age, gender, and status in Korean society. Traditionally, the Korean community values the group over the individual, men over women, and age over youth. Those holding the dominant position are the decision-makers that share thoughts and ideas on issues.

The concept of **kibun** helps provide a better understanding of Korean interpersonal relationships. No equivalent English word explains the true meaning of the term **kibun**. The closest words are related to mood, feelings, and state of mind. A high value is placed on harmony and the maintenance of a peaceful environment. Understanding **kibun** in relation to another person's feelings, and keeping your **kibun** in balance, are essential in interpersonal relations. For example, if one needs something done and notices that the other person's **kibun** is not in harmony, it would be foolish to think this person could be helpful in meeting those needs. Having the ability to assess one's **kibun** is called *nunchi*, which literally means "eye measure." **Kibun** can be disrupted when a younger person disrespects an elder or

when one of lower status insults one of perceived higher status. Koreans have developed this nonverbal form of communication to an art form.

Koreans are comfortable with silence. Confucianism teaches that "silence is golden." Therefore, small talk may appear senseless and insincere to Korean Americans. Chores and daily activities are carried out efficiently and in a matter-of-fact fashion without unnecessary exchange of words. However, the American author of this chapter (L. Purnell) did not experience this on his travels in Korea. Faculty, students, and housekeeping staff alike engaged him in "small talk" on a daily basis. Thus, the social fabric and cultural norms of Koreans are changing as they interact with Western societies and culture.

Visitors from America may be uncomfortable with Koreans' spatial distancing while communicating. Whereas European Americans value personal space, Koreans are comfortable touching strangers in public places. Koreans stand close to one another and do not excuse themselves if they bump into someone on the street because they do not know the person and, therefore, would not speak to the stranger. In a store or bank, the salesperson may comfortably look over peoples' shoulders and breathe directly down their necks. Americans may find this rude, but it is quite common and socially accepted in Korea. Touching among friends and social equals is also common and does not carry a sexual connotation as it might in Western societies.

More social etiquette rules apply when it comes to touching family members or those of higher social status. Hugging and kissing are uncommon among parents and children as well as among children and older aunts or uncles. If the elderly person initiates the touching, this gives the younger person permission to reciprocate. Touch in the realm of health care is readily accepted because it is for the betterment of one's health. However, more acculturated Koreans are quite comfortable with, and often initiate, embraces and kisses with their Western cohorts.

Age, gender, and social status are determinants in the use of eye contact in Korean society. Koreans show respect for those in senior positions by not looking them directly in the eye. A woman performing a bank transaction does not look a male teller in the eyes, yet she can look a female teller in the eyes. Similarly, elders and professionals such as professors, physicians, and ministers are not looked directly in the eye.

Feelings are infrequently communicated in facial expressions. Smiling a lot shows a lack of intellect and disrespect. One would not smile to a stranger on the street nor try to joke during a serious conversation. Joking and amusement have their designated times. In Korea, men frequent bars after work and may express their sense of humor in this setting. Men and women alike appreciate and encourage jokes and laughter in appropriate settings. Given these cultural communication patterns, health-care providers should not interpret these nonverbal behaviors as meaning that Korean clients are not interested in, or do not care about information presented during health teaching and health promotion interventions.

TEMPORAL RELATIONSHIPS

Traditional Koreans are past oriented. Much attention is paid to the ancestry of a family. Yearly, during the Harvest Moon in Korea, *chusok* (respect) is paid to ancestors by bringing fresh fruits from the autumn harvest, dry fish, and rice wine to gravesites. However, the younger and more educated generation is more futuristic and achievement oriented.

In Korea, palm readers are visited to determine the best home to purchase, the date for having a wedding, and when new businesses should open. The busiest time of the year for the palm reader is just before the Chinese New Year. Koreans are eager to know their fortune for the coming year. Many believe that misfortunes occur because ancestors are unhappy. During these times, families show respect to ancestors by more frequent visits to their gravesites in the hope of appeasing the spirits. Shamans are also used in Korea to rid homes and new places of business from spirits, and may be used by Koreans of all socioeconomic levels.

The Korean conception of time depends on the circumstances. Koreans embrace the Western respect for time for important appointments, making transportation connections, and working hours, all of which are recognized as situations where punctuality is necessary. Yet, socially, Korean Americans arrive at parties and visit family and friends within 1 to 2 hours of the agreed-upon time. This is socially acceptable when the person or family is waiting at home. If the social meeting is being held in a public setting, a half-hour time span for arrival at the meeting place can be expected.

FORMAT FOR NAMES

The number of surnames in Korea is limited, with the most common ones being Kim, Lee, Park, Rhee or Yi, Choi or Choe, and Chung or Jung. Korean names contain two Chinese characters, one of which describes the generation and the other the person's given name. The surname comes first; however, because this may be confusing to many Americans, some Koreans in the United States follow the Western tradition of using the given name first, followed by the surname. Adults are not addressed by their given names unless they are on friendly terms; individuals should be addressed by their surname with the title Mr., Mrs., Ms., Dr., or Minister.

Given the diversity and acculturation of Korean Americans, health-care providers need to determine Korean clients' language ability, comfort level with silence, and spatial distancing characteristics. Additionally, Koreans should be addressed formally until they indicate otherwise.

Family Roles and Organization

HEAD OF HOUSEHOLD AND GENDER ROLES

Fundamental ideas about morality and the proper ordering of human relationships among Koreans are closely associated with kinship values derived mainly from Confucian concepts of filial piety, ancestor worship, funerary rites, position of women, the institution of marriage, kinship groups, social status and rank, and respect for scholars and political officials. Although constitutional law in South Korea declares equality for all citizens, not all aspects of society have accepted this. The Confucian worldview deems society as an "ordered inequality." Korean women have long been degraded in Korean society. Women were seen as appendages of the male family members rather than as competent human beings. A woman's identity was determined by her role as someone's daughter, wife, or mother, as well as her responsibility for protecting the family with whom she was identified. While many may still practice these gender relationships, more educated women and men no longer adhere to these Confucian values.

Soh (1993) presented a Korean study of sexual equality and the role of Korean women in politics. She examined the social actions of male-female political interactions in the National Assembly of South Korea. Soh found that social actions were compartmentalized into public versus private and formal versus informal situations. Women were active in legislative life working for the improvement of women's rights and status. Women in appointed positions kept lower profiles and voted in support of the elected political party.

Discussing domestic violence violates Korean cultural norms. Despite this taboo, Song (1990) interviewed 150 Korean women. His findings supported a strong relationship between traditionalism and rigid gender roles, with 60 percent of the women having been abused. Seventy percent of the abused women experienced bruises; 38 percent received black eyes; 19 percent had broken bones or teeth; 17 percent had concussions; and 14 percent received minor cuts or burns. Interestingly, verbal and psychological abuses were not included in the definition of battered. Similar to abused women in the United States, social and economic factors were relevant in deciding whether or not to leave the violent situation, but these women also had to deal with the language barrier and lack of knowledge of community resources and support services. For this particular study group, violence was most likely to occur between the third and fifth year of residency in the United States. When a group of elderly Korean women were asked to give their perceptions about elder abuse based on case scenarios, they were substantially less likely to perceive a given situation as abusive than were elderly African American and Caucasian American women (Moon & Williams, 1993).

A clear role division (*turyotan yokhal punop*) traditionally exists between men and women in Korea. Men are the primary financial providers, unless the family is from a lower socioeconomic class and the woman has to work. Otherwise, women are expected to stay home and care for the children and domestic affairs. Some Korean women are said to have a power over their children called *ch'imapparam* (skirt wind). This means that when the skirt wind blows, it is impossible for a child to ignore the wishes of the mother. The overall style of parenting in Korea is authoritative in nature, although class differences among Korean parents may play a more influential role in determining parenting styles and family roles.

PRESCRIPTIVE, RESTRICTIVE, AND TABOO BEHAVIORS FOR CHILDREN AND ADOLESCENTS

In contrast to the Western culture, wherein mothering is individually fashioned and relies on the expertise of health-care providers, in the highly ritualistic Korean culture mothering is molded by societal rules and information is less frequently sought from health-care providers. In this context, mothers tend to view infants as passive and dependent, and seek guidance from folklore and the extended family (Choi, 1995). In Korea, children over the age of 5 are expected to be well behaved because the whole family is disgraced if a child behaves in an embarrassing manner. Most children are not encouraged to state their opinions. Parents usually make the decisions.

"Teaching to the test" is common in Korea, but the role of teachers is also to encourage self-study. The future of Korean students is determined by their teachers' recommendations, and this pressure can be extremely intense for students who are not doing well. The teaching style is one in which students listen and learn what is being taught. Regardless of private doubts, a student rarely questions a teacher's authority. Korean children in American must be taught the teaching style in American schools, where questioning is positive and is valued as class participation. Even if Korean American students understand the style of teaching, it can be difficult to know the appropriate timing for asking questions. Because of language difficulties, some Korean students must formulate their questions in their heads first, and by the time they get the courage to ask their question, the subject has changed or their question may no longer seem relevant. Those in health education should be sensitive to these issues.

The pressure of doing well in school and attending a university of high quality leaves Korean adolescents little room for social interactions. Activities that interfere with one's education are considered taboo for adolescents. In Korea, students frequently attend study groups after school or special tutoring sessions paid for by their families in preparation for examinations to enter a university. Short coffee breaks or snacks at local coffee shops or noodle houses are permissible, but then it is "back to the books."

Dating is uncommon among high school students in Korea. Once young adults have entered a university, they receive their freedom and are then permitted to make their own decisions about personal and study time. Group outings are common for meeting the opposite sex. Dating may occur from these group meetings and consists of movies, dinner, and walks in the park. Neither the school system nor the family assumes responsibility for sex education. Girls in elementary school are given a class regarding their menstrual cycle, but no information is given regarding sexual relations. Information is exchanged by word of mouth from friend to friend as the students piece details together.

Issues arise between Korean American parents and children in relation to conflicting values and communication. With rapid acculturation, Korean American children often take on the values of the dominant society or culture. Thus, parents are challenged when their children do not accept traditional values and ideals that they may still hold dear.

FAMILY GOALS AND PRIORITIES

In Korea, the family is described as "corporate," where family members have specific rights and duties within their family. A Korean cannot belong to more than one corporate family, and a family member replaces the roles of another family member who dies. This traditional corporate family is dissolving among both Koreans and Korean Americans. Usually both parents work to provide every opportunity possible for their families. As each family member learns to adjust to the changing roles, conflict can result. Children adapt most easily to the new culture and may even take on the dominant culture's values.

Lee and Lee (1990) studied the adjustment of Korean immigrant families in the United States in relation to roles, values, and living conditions between husbands and wives and parents and children. The findings showed a transition from an independent family structure, in which the woman had little knowledge of the man's activities outside the home, to a joint family structure. Many activities were carried out together with an interchange of roles at home. Conflict centered on undefined role expectations. In Korea, the roles of men and women were very clear. However, upon immigrating to the United States, men and women were faced with conflicting roles in the new culture and had to struggle to redefine them. Other conflict areas were the couple's ability to speak English, the woman's inability to drive, the degree of acculturation, limited social contact, and the stressors of living in a new culture.

In Korea, education is a family priority. The outcome of a highly educated child was a secure old age for the parents. Because of the dependent relationship between parents and their children, parents were more willing to make drastic sacrifices for the advancement of their children's education. Today, status is achieved rather than inherited in Korea. Education in Korea is a determinant of status, independent of its contribution to economic success.

Harmony is another priority of Korean families. This goal is achieved by creating accord among immediate and extended family members and between the body and mind.

Traditionally in Korea, parents expected their children to care for them in old age. *Hyo* (filial piety), which is the obligation to respect and obey parents, care for them in old age, give them a good funeral, and worship them after death, was a core value of Korean ethics. The obligation to care for one's elderly parents is written into civil code in Korea. The burden was on the eldest son, who was obliged to reside with his parents and carry on the family line. Such an arrangement made the generations dependent on each other. The son felt obligated to care for his parents because of the sacrifices they made for him. Similarly, he made the same sacrifices for his children and expected them to provide for him and his wife in their old age. Many of these traditions in Korea have changed. Some of the eldest children immigrated, leaving the responsibility for their parents to the siblings who remained in Korea.

Some elderly Koreans were brought to the United States without their friends and with minimal or no English skills. They often felt obligated to assist the family in any way possible by preparing meals or taking care of the children when the parents were not home. Decision making for elders was hampered in their new culture. Korean elders were frequently consulted on important family matters as a sign of respect for their life experiences. The elders' role as decision makers in the United States has shifted with the younger generation of Korean Americans wanting the final decision-making authority in their young families.

Traditionally, Koreans give great respect to their elderly. Old age begins when one reaches the age of 60, with an impressive celebration prepared for the occasion. The historical significance of this celebration is related to the Chinese lunar calendar. The lunar calendar has 60 cycles, each with a different name. At the age of 60, the person is starting the calendar cycle over again. This is called **hwangap**. This celebration was more significant in the past when life expectancy in Korea was much lower than it is today. Despite a change in the direct role of elderly people in their families, elderly Koreans are socially well respected in Korea. In public, an elderly woman is called *Halmoni*, "grandmother," and those who are not blood relatives call an elderly man *Harabuji*, "grandfather." The elderly are offered seats on buses out of respect and honor.

Traditionally, the extended Korean family played an important role in supporting its members throughout the life span. With the breakup of the extended family, Korean Americans support each other through secondary organizations such as the church. The church assists new immigrants with the transition to life in the United States. The church is a resource for information about childcare, language classes, and social activities. Korean Americans without family support may seek other Korean Americans who live in the area. With Korean Americans dispersed throughout the United States, however, this task can be difficult.

While some Koreans inherit social status, many have the ability to change their status through their education and professions. Traditional Korean culture espouses respect not only for elders but also for those of valued professions. In modern Korea, professors, bureaucrats, business executives, physicians, and attorneys receive a high level of respect. A well-published professor may have higher status than a physician or an attorney. Historically, those with the highest education were handsomely paid. Even though the salary differences between university professors and other professions have narrowed significantly in recent years in Korea, the status of the intellectual remains high. Similarly, the bureau-

cratic officer has a high social status, wielding much respect and influence.

ALTERNATIVE LIFESTYLES

Alternative lifestyles are frowned upon in Korean culture. Women who divorce may suffer social stigma, the degree of which depends on the situation. A woman who made her own decision to marry, versus one in an arranged marriage, suffers less alienation because the arranged marriage involves not only the marital partners but also both their families. Because great detail and time go into arranging marriages, families suffer great dishonor when a divorce occurs. Mixed marriages, between a Korean and a non-Korean, are highly disregarded by some, and the Korean government makes it very difficult for these marriages to occur. Korean women who have married American servicemen are often the objects of Korean jokes and are ridiculed by some.

Living together before marriage is not customary in Korea. If pregnancy occurs outside marriage, it may be taken care of quietly and without family and friends being aware of the situation. In the United States, pregnancy outside of marriage may not carry such a great stigma among the more acculturated.

Homosexuality is not accepted in Korean culture. Those who have relations with a person of the same sex must remain "in the closet." Personal disclosure to friends and family jeopardizes the family name and may lead to ostracism. The community may stigmatize both the family and the individual, making it difficult to conduct their personal lives.

Workforce Issues

CULTURE IN THE WORKPLACE

Korean Americans come from a culture that places a high value on education. Many arrive in America with a minimum of a high school education. The skills and work experiences they had in Korea are often not accepted by American businesses, forcing them to take jobs in which they may be over skilled while they save money to start their own businesses. Korean American women frequently need to find jobs to assist the family financially, which may cause role conflicts between more traditional husbands and wives.

Korean Americans have a strong work ethic. They work long hours each week for the advancement of family opportunities. Family is the priority for Korean Americans but, on the surface, this may not always be apparent when long hours are devoted to work. The goal is to save money for education and other opportunities, so the family can provide for their children in the future.

The number of Korean medical personnel working in the American health-care system is unknown. Significant numbers of Korean nurses and physicians are practicing in the United States and Canada; many have received part or all of their education in the United States. Yi and Jezewski's study (2000) of 12 Korean nurses' adjustment to hospitals in the United States identified five phases of adjustment. The first three phases, relieving psychological stress, overcoming language barriers, and accepting American nursing practice take 2 to 3 years. The remaining two phases, adopting the styles of American problem-solving strategies and adopting the styles of American interpersonal relationships, take an additional 5 to 10 years. Accordingly, orientation programs need to address language skills, practice differences, and communication and interpersonal relationships to help Koreans adjust to the American workforce. These same phases may occur with other Korean health professionals.

ISSUES RELATED TO AUTONOMY

Those in supervisory positions need to recognize the roles and relationships that exist between Koreans and their employers. A supervisor is treated with much respect in work and in social settings. Informalities and small talk may be difficult for Korean immigrants. It is often unacceptable for an employee to refuse a request of an employer even if the employee does not want or feel qualified to complete the request. Supervisors should make an effort to promote open conversation and the expression of ideas among Korean Americans. Those who have adjusted to the American business style may be more assertive in their positions, but an understanding of this work role gives supervisors the tools to more readily use Korean Americans' skills and knowledge.

As with any new language, it is often difficult to understand American slang and colloquial language. Employers and other employees should be clear in their communication style and be understanding of miscommunications. Ethnic biases are often directed at Korean Americans who speak English with an accent. Employers' and coworkers' preconceived notions of immigrants can also be a deterrent to Korean Americans in the workforce.

Biocultural Ecology

SKIN COLOR AND OTHER BIOLOGICAL VARIATIONS

Koreans are an ethnically homogeneous Mongoloid people who have shared a common history, language, and culture since the 7th century AD when the peninsula was first united. Common physical characteristics include dark hair and dark eyes, with variations in skin color and degree of hair darkness. Skin color ranges from fair to light brown with those residing in the southern part of South Korea being darker. Epicanthal skin folds create the distinctive appearance of Asian eyes.

DISEASES AND HEALTH CONDITIONS

Schistosomiasis and other parasitic diseases are endemic to certain regions of Korea. Therefore, health-care providers should consider parasite screening, when appropriate, with Korean immigrants. South Korea continues to manufacture and use asbestos-containing products and has not taken the precautions necessary to adequately protect employees and meet international standards; thus, Korean immigrants to the United States need to be assessed for asbestos-related health problems (Johanning, Goldberg, & Kim, 1994).

The high prevalence of stomach and liver cancer, tuberculosis, hepatitis, and hypertension in South Korea predispose recent immigrants to these conditions. High rates of hypertension lead to an increase in cardiovascular accidents and renal failure. The high incidence of stomach cancer is associated with environmental and genetic factors (Sawyer & Eaton, 1992). As with other Asians, there is a high occurrence of lactose intolerance among people of Korean ancestry. Dental hygiene and preventive dentistry have recently been emphasized in health promotion in South Korea. Because of the high incidence of gum disease and oral problems, however, these problems deserve attention.

VARIATIONS IN DRUG METABOLISM

Growing research in the field of pharmacogenetics has found variations in drug metabolism among ethnic groups. Studies suggest that Asian populations require lower dosages of psychotropic drugs (Levy, 1993). Other studies have shown variations in drug metabolism and interaction with propranolol, isoniazid, and diazepam among Asians in comparison to European Americans and other ethnic groups (Meyer, 1992). Although these studies primarily focus on people of Chinese and Japanese heritage, health-care professionals should be aware and attentive to the possibility of drug metabolism variations among Korean Americans.

High-Risk Behaviors

Because Koreans place great emphasis on education, many subject their children to intense pressure to do well in school. A survey conducted among middle and high school students in Korea demonstrated such pressures. Three-quarters of the students reported having considered running away or committing suicide because of their lack of success in school (Sorensen, 1994). Another study conducted at Seoul National University, the apex of universities in South Korea, reported that 14 percent of the students admitted to the class of 1980 experienced nervous disorders, character blocks, or nervous breakdowns (Sorensen, 1994). Similar pressures have been seen in the United States, where suicide has occurred with Korean high school and college students because of intense pressure to do well in school.

Korea has a high incidence of alcohol consumption, up from 7.0 L in 1980 to 8.1 L per adult per capita, which is similar to that of the United States and Ireland at 7.8 L per adult per capita. However, among adult men in Korea, consumption is 18.4 L per capita, one of the highest rates of alcohol consumption in the world (Park, Oh, & Lee, 1998). Korean business transactions commonly transpire after the decision makers have had several drinks. Koreans believe that people let their masks down when they drink and that they truly get to know someone after they have had a few drinks. Socioeconomic changes in Korea have resulted in differences in alcohol-related social and health problems, with a change from drinking mild fermented beverages with meals to drinking distilled liquors without meals. In the United States, 62 percent of Korean American men and 39 percent of Korean American women drink alcoholic beverages, with beer being the most common alcoholic beverage consumed (Yu, 1990a).

In Korea, women drink far less than men. Sons' drinking patterns are similar to their fathers' patterns. There is a substantial generational difference among females, with daughters abstaining from alcohol less frequently than their mothers and drinking more and more often than their mothers (Weatherspoon, Park, & Johnson, 2001). In the United States and in Korea, drinking and vehicular accidents among Koreans and Korean Americans are a cause for concern.

One-third of Korean Americans living in the Los Angeles area smoke, and Korean American men (37 percent) smoke more than Korean American women (20 percent) (Yu, 1990a). In their study Lee, Sobal, and Frongillo (2000) found that bicultural Korean men were least likely to smoke, while acculturated and bicultural women were more likely to smoke than traditional women. In Korea, a few women do smoke, and for those who do smoke, smoking in public, such as on the street, is considered taboo.

Cho and Faulkner (1993) studied the cultural conceptions of alcoholism among Korean and American university students. Students had to decide whether the person described in a vignette was an alcoholic or not and why. The results showed that American-born students tended to define alcoholism in terms of social and interpersonal problems related to drinking, whereas Korean-born students defined alcoholism in terms of physical degeneration and physiological addiction. The authors cautioned against the misuse of American concepts and diagnostic scales in the cross-cultural arena. Cultural factors should be examined closely in relation to the study, diagnosis, and treatment of alcohol problems.

HEALTH-CARE PRACTICES

Seat belts are infrequently worn in South Korea, although there has been recent pressure to use them. Korean Americans understand the legal mandates in the United States and comply with seat belt and child restraint laws.

Hobbies such as hiking and golf are enjoyed in South Korea. Korean Americans do not identify hiking as a frequent pastime, either because of environmental constraints or because of living situations. Golf remains a significant activity among Korean Americans who are financially able to play the sport.

Nutrition

MEANING OF FOOD

Food takes on a significant meaning when one has been without food. Many Koreans over the age of 50 who fought in the Korean War experienced a time when their next meal was not guaranteed. Because of a devastated economy and agricultural base, barley and *kimchee*,

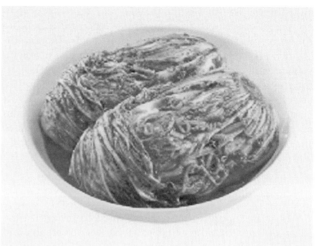

FIGURE 16–2   Kimchee—A spicy pickled cabbage that is a staple of the Korean diet.

a spicy pickled cabbage, were dietary staples during the war.

COMMON FOODS AND FOOD RITUALS

Korean food is flavorful and spicy. Rice is served with 5 to 20 small side dishes of mostly vegetables and some fish and meats. The variety of seasonings in Korean cooking includes red and black pepper, garlic, green onion, ginger, soy sauce, and sesame seed oil. The traditional Korean diet includes steamed rice; hot soup; *kimchee*; and side dishes of fish, meat, or vegetables served in some variation for breakfast, lunch, and dinner. Breakfast is traditionally considered the most important meal.

Kimchee, a spicy fermented cabbage, is made from a variety of vegetables but is primarily made from a Chinese, or Napa, cabbage (Fig. 16–2). Spices and herbs are added to the previously salted cabbage, which is allowed to ferment over time, and is served with every meal in a variety of forms. A list of some common Korean American dishes follows:

Beebimbap is a combination of rice, finely chopped mixed vegetables, and a fried egg served in a hot pottery bowl. Hot pepper paste is usually added.

Bulgolgi is thinly sliced pieces of beef marinated in soy sauce, sesame oil, green onions, garlic, and sugar, and served after being barbecued.

Chopchae are clear noodles mixed with lightly stir-fried vegetables and meats.

Rice is usually served in individual serving bowls, which are set to the left of the diner. Soup is served in another bowl, placed to the right of the rice. Chopsticks and large soup spoons are used at all meals. Korean Americans may use forks and knives, depending on their degree of assimilation into American culture. Meals are frequently eaten in silence, using this opportunity to enjoy the food. When Koreans migrate to the United States, they increase their consumption of beef, dairy products, coffee, soda, and bread as well as decrease their intake of fish, rice, and other grains. However, the incorporation of a larger quantity of Western food items does not make a less healthy diet. They continue to consume diets that are consistent with their traditional Korean food patterns, with 60 percent of calories coming from carbohydrates, and 16 percent of calories from fat (Kim et al., 2000). To increase compliance with dietary prescriptions, health teaching should be geared to the unique Korean American food choices and practices.

It is important to understand the ritual offering of food and drink to guests. Koreans offer a guest a drink on first arriving at their home. The guest declines courteously. The host offers the drink again and the guest again declines. This ritual can occur three to five times before the guest accepts the offer. This interaction is done out of respect for the hosts and their generosity to share with their guest and to express an unwillingness to impose on the hosts. It would be considered rude and selfish to accept an offer when first asked.

DIETARY PRACTICES FOR HEALTH PROMOTION

Most dietary practices for health promotion apply to pregnancy, which is discussed later in this chapter. Someone suffering from the common cold will be served soup made from bean sprouts. Dried anchovies, garlic, and other hot spices are added to the hot soup, which assists in clearing a congested nose.

NUTRITIONAL DEFICIENCIES AND FOOD LIMITATIONS

Kim et al. (1993) examined the nutritional status of elderly Chinese, Korean, and Japanese Americans. Along with a dietary interview and anthropometric measurements, a 24-hour recall technique was used to obtain dietary data. The results of the study showed that elderly Korean Americans had the poorest diets, particularly with inadequate amounts of vitamins A and C. Korean American women had a low intake of protein. The results also suggested that elderly Asian Americans are at high risk for calcium deficiencies. The authors concluded that a large-scale national nutritional survey is needed for Asian Americans to plan health programs based on the specific needs of selected populations.

Korean Americans, as with most other Asians, are at a high risk for lactose intolerance. Thus, milk and other dairy products are not part of the traditional Korean diet, emphasizing the need to assess for calcium deficiencies.

Korean Americans living in or near large metropolitan cities have access to Korean markets and restaurants. When no Korean stores are available, Chinese or Japanese markets may contain some of the foods Koreans enjoy. When no Asian markets are available, the American grocery store suffices.

Pregnancy and Childbearing Practices

FERTILITY PRACTICES AND VIEWS TOWARD PREGNANCY

To curtail population growth in Korea, the government promotes the concept of two children per household. The government supported the use of contraception when a 10-year family planning program was adopted in the early 1960s, resulting in a mass public education program on contraception. When contraceptive devices became easily available in Korea, fertility control spread widely among married women. Contraceptive devices are covered by the present national health insurance of Korea. Before the 1950s abortion was illegal, although induced abortions were performed widely. Today abortion is legal and is widely used in Korea. Abortion is not highly publicized in Korea, yet there is an unspoken acceptance of the practice. The government keeps a hands-off policy, which has not met with major opposition. Women are not expected to get their husband's consent nor are underage youth required to have their parents' acknowledgment. The government does not pay for abortions; rather, patients pay a set price from personal funds.

Pritham and Sammons (1993) investigated Korean women's attitudes toward pregnancy and prenatal care with regard to their beliefs and interactions with health-care professionals from the United States. A survey of 40 unemployed Korean women between the ages of 18 and 35 was conducted at an American military medical care facility in a major metropolitan area of Korea. Attitudes toward childbearing practices and relationships with health-care providers were elicited. The results indicated that these women were happy about their pregnancies. Only one-third of the respondents agreed with the traditional preference for a male child. About 40 percent of the women reinforced strong food taboos and restrictions, and acknowledged the need to avoid certain foods during pregnancy. Twenty percent disagreed with the use of prenatal vitamins, and 25 percent indicated only needing a 10- to 15-lb weight gain in pregnancy. The women generally had sound health habits in relation to physical activity and recognized the harm of smoking while pregnant. The study sample was homogeneous and small, limiting the ability to generalize about the findings.

Pregnancy in the Korean culture is traditionally a highly protected time for women. Both the pregnancy and the postpartum period have been ritualized by the culture. A pregnancy begins with the **tae-mong**, which is a dream of the conception of pregnancy. Once a woman is pregnant, she starts practicing **tae-kyo,** which literally means "fetus education." The objective of **tae-kyo** is to promote the health and well-being of the fetus and mother by having the mother focus on art and beautiful objects. If the pregnant woman handles unclean objects or kills a living creature, it can lead to a difficult birth (Howard & Barbiglia, 1997). Some women wear tight abdominal binders beginning at 20 weeks gestation or work physically hard toward the end of the pregnancy to increase the chances of having a small baby (Howard & Barbiglia, 1997). Additionally, expectant mothers should avoid duck, chicken, fish with scales, squid, or crab because eating these foods may affect the child's appearance. For example, eating duck may cause the baby to be born with webbed feet (Howard & Barbiglia, 1997).

A study in Honolulu supports the belief that Korean women attribute a variety of complaints to naeng (chill), a cold imbalance of the womb that brings on a heavy vaginal discharge and can make women who experience it sterile. The researcher emphasized that an intimate condition such as naeng may be lost in translation in non-Korean contexts (Kendall, 1987).

PRESCRIPTIVE, RESTRICTIVE, AND TABOO PRACTICES IN THE CHILDBEARING FAMILY

Ludman, Kang, and Lynn (1992) conducted a study that explored the food beliefs and diets of 200 pregnant Korean American women. The food items most frequently consumed were *kimchee* (82.5 percent), rice or noodles (81.5 percent), and fresh fruit (79 percent). Foods avoided during pregnancy included coffee (19.8 percent), spicy foods (9.9 percent), chicken (6.9 percent), and crab (6.9 percent). A list of 20 food items was then given to the women, who were asked to respond whether they consumed the food or not and, if not, to indicate their reasons. A number of respondents indicated that they did not eat rabbit (91.5 percent), sparrow (91.5 percent), duck (89.5 percent), goat (84 percent), or blemished fruit (63 percent) because of dislike or lack of availability. The reason most frequently given for not eating blemished fruit was that it might produce a skin disease on the infant or cause an unpleasant face. The study showed that although many Korean American women are aware of traditionally taboo foods, they did not avoid consuming them. An awareness of these beliefs can give health professionals a basis for nutritional education for Korean American women.

Birthing practices both among Koreans and Korean Americans are highly influenced by Western methods. Women commonly labor and deliver in the supine position. After the delivery, women are traditionally served seaweed soup, a rich source of iron, which is believed to facilitate lactation and to promote healing of the mother. Bed rest is encouraged after pregnancy for 7 to 90 days. Women are also encouraged to keep warm by avoiding showers, baths, and cold fluids or foods.

The postpartum period is seen as the time when women undergo profound physiological, psychological, and sociological changes; this period is known as the *Sanhujori* belief system. In this dynamic process, the postpartum women should care for their bodies by augmenting heat and avoiding cold, resting without working, eating well, protecting the body from harmful strains, and keeping clean. (Howard & Barbiglia, 1997). In Western society, where there may be a lack of extended family members from whom to seek assistance, Korean women may be faced with a cultural dilemma.

Park and Peterson (1991) studied Korean American women's health beliefs, practices, and experiences in relation to childbirth. Using structured questions, a nonrandom sample of 20 female volunteers was interviewed in Korean. Those interviewed subscribed to a holistic view, which emphasized both emotional and physical health. Only one-half of the women interviewed rated themselves healthy. The authors related this to the stresses of immigration and pregnancy. Preventive practices were not found among members of this group. Only one woman regularly received Pap smears and did breast self-examinations. A common finding was that most women participated in a significant rest period during puerperium. Those who did not rest lacked help for the home. All the women ate brown seaweed soup and steamed rice for about 20 days after childbirth to cleanse the blood and to assist in milk production. Because pregnancy is a hot condition and heat is lost during labor and delivery, some women avoided cold foods and water after childbirth to prevent chronic illnesses such as arthritis. The baby should be wrapped in warn blankets to prevent harm from cold winds. Herbal medicines are also used during puerperium to promote healing and health (Howard & Barbiglia, 1997).

Health-care professionals can improve the health of Korean American women by providing factual information about Pap smears and teaching breast self-examination. Pregnant Korean American women should be asked about their use of herbal medicine during pregnancy so that harmless practices can be incorporated into biomedical care. Recommendations for improving postpartum care among Korean American women include (1) developing an assessment tool which health-care providers can use to identify traditional beliefs early in a pregnancy, (2) developing a bilingual dictionary of common foods, (3) developing pamphlets with medical terms used in the U.S. health-care system, and (4) providing time for practicing English skills (Park & Peterson, 1991).

Death Rituals

DEATH RITUALS AND EXPECTATIONS

Traditionally in Korea, it was important for Koreans to die at home. It was considered bad luck to bring a dead body home if the person died in the hospital. Consequently, viewing of the deceased occurred at home if the individual died at home or at the hospital if the individual died at the hospital. Several days or more were set aside for the viewing, depending on the status of the deceased. The eldest son was expected to sit by the body of the parent during the viewing. Friends and relatives paid their respects by bowing to a photograph of the deceased in the same room in which the body rested. The guests were then offered the favorite foods of the deceased. Today, most Korean Americans are not accustomed to viewing the body of the deceased. More commonly, relatives and friends come to pay respect by viewing photographs of the deceased.

Although Korean Americans view life support more positively than European Americans, the majority in one study did not want such technology. Additionally, they were less likely to have made a prior decision about life support. Older and more educated Koreans were less likely to favor truth telling, believing that patients should not be told that they have a terminal illness (Blackhall et al., 1999).

An ancestral burial ceremony follows with the body being placed in the ground facing south or north. Both the place and position of the deceased is important for the future fortune of the living relatives. Koreans believe that if the spirit is content, good fortune will be awarded to the family. Unlike Western graves, a mound of dirt covers the gravesite of the deceased in Korea.

Cremation is an individual and family choice and is practiced more commonly in Korea for those who have no family. For example, when unmarried people die without any children to perform ancestral ceremonies, they are often cremated and their ashes scattered over a body of water.

Rice wine is traditionally sprinkled around the grave. Korean families bow two to four times in respect at the gravesite, and then the men, in descending order from the eldest to the youngest drink rice wine. Some Korean Americans dedicate a corner of their home to honor their ancestors because they cannot go to the gravesite.

Circumstances where "do not resuscitate" orders are an issue need to be addressed cautiously. Families trust physicians and may not question other options. Because death and dying are fairly well accepted in the Korean culture, prolonging life may not be highly regarded in the face of modern technology. Korean hospitals focus on acute care. Families are expected to stay with family members to assist in feeding and personal care around the clock. Thus, many Korean Americans may expect to care for their hospitalized family members in health-care facilities.

RESPONSES TO DEATH AND GRIEF

Mourning rituals, with crying and open displays of grief, are commonly practiced and socially accepted at funerals, and signify the utmost respect for the dead. The eldest son or male family member who sits by the deceased sometimes holds a cane and makes a moaning noise to display his grief. The cane is a symbol of needing support. Health-care personnel may need to provide a private setting for Korean Americans to be able to grieve in culturally congruent ways.

Spirituality

DOMINANT RELIGION AND USE OF PRAYER

Confucianism was the official religion of Korea from the 14th to the 20th century. Buddhism, Confucianism, Christianity, shamanism, and **Chondo-Kyo** are practiced in Korea today. **Chondo-Kyo** (religion of the Heavenly Way) is a nationalistic religion founded in the 19th century that combines Confucianism, Buddhism, and Daoism. Among Korean Americans, the most recent estimates of organized religions include Christianity (48.2 percent), Buddhism (48.8 percent), and **Chondo-Kyo** (0.2 percent) (LonelyPlanet.com). In the United States, the church acts as a powerful social support group for Korean immigrants. Yu (1990b) speculated that with the growth of other organizations that facilitate the transition for Korean immigrants, they might have less need for churches as the major source of emotional support and practical information on life in the United States.

Kim (1990) studied Korean Christian churches in the Pacific Northwest in an attempt to prove the importance of the structure and function of the church as a secondary association for Korean immigrants in the United States. Many of the churches were young in terms of both years of operation and the age of the membership. Most had been in operation between 5 and 10 years. Most of the churches were hierarchically organized, and only a couple of the churches reported having female pastors. A

variety of services other than prayer meetings were offered, such as English and Korean language programs; income tax seminars; health education, including AIDS prevention; information on U.S. citizenship and laws, driver's licenses, and job searches; and assistance with elderly family members. Kim reinforced the role of churches in preserving Korean culture and, consequently, ethnic identity. Kim also stressed the importance of retaining one's ethnic identity in the Korean culture. Korean immigrants experience a dramatic transition and are frequently faced with the forces of racism and individualism.

Koreans in America might not pray in the same fashion as Westerners, but the spirits demand homage for many people. Korean churches often have prayer meetings several times a week, some with early morning prayers. Buddhist temples have spirit rooms attached to them. Although Buddhists believe the spirit enters a new life, the beliefs of the shamans are so strong that the Buddhist church incorporated an area of their church for those who believe that ancestral spirits need honoring and homage. With such a variety of spiritual beliefs, caregivers must assess each Korean client individually for religious beliefs and prayer practices.

MEANING OF LIFE AND INDIVIDUAL SOURCES OF STRENGTH

Family and education are central themes that give meaning to life for Korean Americans. These themes were previously covered under the sections Family Roles and Organization and Educational Status and Occupations. The nuclear and extended families are primary sources of strength for Korean Americans in their daily lives. These concepts were previously covered under Family Roles and Organization.

SPIRITUAL BELIEFS AND HEALTH-CARE PRACTICES

Shamanism is a powerful belief in natural spirits. All parts of nature contain spirits: rivers, animals, and even inanimate objects. The many religions of Koreans create numerous ideologies about what happens with the spirits of the deceased. Christians believe the spirit goes to heaven; Buddhists believe the spirit starts a new life as a person or an animal; and Shamanists believe the spirit stays with the family to watch over them and guide their actions and fortunes. Such a variety of faith systems provide a great diversity in beliefs of the Korean people. Given this diversity of spiritual beliefs among Koreans, each client needs an individual assessment in regard to spiritual and health-care practices.

Health-Care Practices

HEALTH-SEEKING BELIEFS AND BEHAVIORS

Beliefs that influence health-care practices include religious beliefs (see Dominant Religion and Use of Prayer) and dietary practices (see Nutrition). Health-care providers need to be aware that the theme dominating these beliefs is a holistic approach, which emphasizes both emotional and physical health.

Health-care practices among Koreans in America are primarily focused on curative rather than preventive measures. Health promotion in Korea is a relatively new public health focus. In Korea, education on dental hygiene, sanitation, environmental issues, and other preventive health measures is being encouraged. Visits to the physician for an annual physical examination, Pap smears, and breast self-examination are uncommon. Among Koreans, traditional patterns of health promotion include harmony with nature and the universe, activity and rest, diet, sexual life, covetousness, temperament, and apprehension (Lee, 1993).

RESPONSIBILITY FOR HEALTH CARE

One American study reported that only 13.5 percent of Korean American men and 11.3 percent of Korean American women had a digital rectal exam (DRE) for occult blood. Regression analysis indicated that gender, education, knowledge of the warning signs of cancer, and length of residence in the United States were significantly related to having undergone DRE. The researchers determined that this group of Korean Americans did not see health-care providers or health brochures as valuable sources of information and to target this group, efforts should be coordinated with church and community leaders and by developing brochures in the Korean language (Kim et al., 1998).

Because of modesty during physical examinations and women's preferences that women perform intimate examinations, many Korean women defer having Pap tests (Wismer et al., 1998), especially if male physicians are non-Korean (Nursing faculty of Keimyung University, Deegu, Korea, personal communications, October 2001). This reluctance for undergoing Pap tests directly relates to cervical cancer's rating as the number one female cancer diagnosed among women in Korea (Lee, 2000). Modesty has also been associated with low rates of mammography among Korean Americans (Maxwell, Bastani, & Warda, 1998) as well as limited knowledge about breast self-examination and causes of breast cancer (Han, Williams, & Harrison, 2000).

Recent Korean immigrants come from a country where universal health insurance was implemented in the late 1980s. A government mandate established employer-based health insurance for medium and large firms. Regional health insurance systems, subsidized by the government, were later established for small firms, farmers, and the self-employed. Yu (1990b) found that 55 percent of the Koreans surveyed in Los Angeles and Orange counties have medical insurance; however, the rates vary according to income, with higher rates among the high-income group and lower rates among the low-income group.

The use and availability of over-the-counter medications varies tremendously between the United States and Korea. Many prescription drugs in the United States, such as antibiotics, anti-inflammatory and cardiac medications, and certain pain control medications can be purchased over-the-counter in Korea at any *yak bang* (pharmacy). For example, when feeling "tired" or "fatigued" the elderly in Korea may perform home infusions of dextrose and water or albumin.

Self-medication with herbal remedies is also practiced. Ginseng is a root used for anything from a remedy for the common cold to an aphrodisiac. Seaweed soup is used as a medicine. Chinese herbs are used to control the degree of "wind" that may be in the body. Other herbal medications are taken for preventive or restorative purposes such as *haigefen* (clamshell powder) which has high levels of lead (Markowitz et al., 1994), causing abdominal colic, muscle pain, and fatigue. Accordingly, health-care professionals should query their patients about their use of traditional Korean medicine, and must be aware that herbal medicine may be used in conjunction with Western biomedicine.

FOLK PRACTICES

Hanyak, traditional herbal medicine used for creating harmony between oneself and the larger cosmology, is a healing method for the body and soul. *Hanbang,* the traditional Korean medical care system, works on the principle of a disturbed state of **ki**, cosmological vital energy. Symptoms are often interpreted in terms of a psychological base. Treatments include acupuncture, acumassage, acupressure, herbal medicines, and moxibustion therapy. The therapeutic relationship between *hanui* (oriental medicine doctors) and their clients is genuine, spontaneous, and harmonious. Clients who use both Western and traditional Korean practitioners may experience conflicts because of the lack of cooperation between *hanui* and biomedical practitioners (Pang, 1989). In 1993 in Korea, a pharmaceutical act supported pharmacists in prescribing and dispensing herbal drugs, creating a lucrative business and increasing conflicts among *hanui* physicians and pharmacists (Cho, 2000).

Shamans are used in healing rituals to ward off restless spirits. Shamans originated with the religious belief of shamanism, the belief that all things possess spirits. A shaman, **mundang**, is usually a woman who has special abilities for communicating with spirits. The shaman is used to treat illnesses after other means of treatment are exhausted. The shaman performs a *kut*, a shamanistic ceremony to eliminate the evil spirits causing the illness. Such a ceremony may take place when a young person dies to prevent his or her spirit from staying tied to the earth. Others believe a shaman can eliminate evil spirits, which may be causing difficulty with financial transactions. Although shamans have been around for many years, Koreans consider them part of the lowest class. Health-care providers need to determine whether or not Koreans in America are using folk therapies and should include nonharmful practices with biomedical therapies and prescriptions.

BARRIERS TO HEALTH CARE

Because many Korean Americans use various options for healing, Western medical practices may be used in conjunction with acupressure, acupuncture, and herbal medicine. Barriers for Koreans in America may result from the expense of non-Western therapies because insurance companies often do not cover alternative therapies.

As for many other American residents, the lack of insurance creates barriers to health care. Paying for health care out-of-pocket is expensive and not feasible for many Korean American families. Language, modesty, cultural attitudes toward certain illnesses, and communication problems also serve as impediments for access to health care.

CULTURAL RESPONSES TO HEALTH AND ILLNESS

Perceptions of pain vary widely among Koreans. Some Koreans are stoic and are slow to express emotional distress from pain. Others are expressive and discuss their smallest discomforts. Family and friends are useful resources for learning some of the historical coping mechanisms of sick individuals. Nonverbal cues and facial expressions must be monitored for those who are stoic rather than expressive. Pain assessments should be conducted regularly and patient education may be necessary for stoic individuals.

Mental illness in the Korean culture is stigmatized. Kim and Grant (1997) conducted a study of Korean American women and their reluctance to use mental health professionals in the United States. Their study supported that these women experienced gender role disruption, evidence of depressive symptoms, and subsequent risk of substance abuse, suicide, battering, loss of employment, deficits in parenting, and low use of mental health professionals. A study in Korea of 3711 respondents showed that 23.1 percent of men and 27.4 percent of women were at risk for depression, which is a higher rate than in the United States and Western countries. In this study, female gender, fewer than 13 years of education, and disrupted marriage were significant predictors of severe, definitive symptoms of depression (Cho, Nam, & Suh, 1998). Pang (1990) explored the cultural construction of *hwa-byung* among a group of Korean immigrant women in the United States using a convenience sample. *Hwa-byung*, a traditional Korean illness, occurs from the suppression of anger or other emotions (Donnelly, 2001). *Hwa* means "fire and anger," whereas *byung* means "illness." All the women in the study knew the meaning of *hwa-byung*, and 80 percent reported having experienced the illness. The emotions they reported suppressing were sadness, depression, worry, anger, fright, and fear. Most of the emotions described were related to conflicts with close relatives or family, such as sons and daughter or significant others. These were expressed as physical complaints, ranging from headaches and poor appetites to insomnia and lack of energy. The complaints were chronic in nature, and a variety of remedies were used to alleviate the symptoms. Most of the women suggested that *hwa-byung* was difficult to cure and accepted the symptoms as inevitable. For these elderly Korean women *hwa-byung* was a mode for constructing illness as a personal, social, and cultural adaptive response (Pang, 1990). These women expressed life's

hardships by channeling their emotional illnesses into physical symptoms.

A community study of Korean Americans addressed the prevalence, clinical significance, and meaning of *hwa-byung* (Lin et al., 1992). The results indicated a high percentage of Korean Americans (11.9 percent) who identify themselves as suffering from *hwa-byung.* A strong association was shown between *hwa-byung* and major depressive disorders. Although *hwa-byung* is found predominately among elderly Korean women with little education, this study's findings did not support this notion. The ability to generalize these findings, however, is limited because assignment to the study groups was not completely random and because the sample size was small.

The area of special education historically has not been well studied or researched in Korea. Families who have children with mental or physical disabilities often question what they have done wrong to make their ancestors angry. Families feel stigmatized for such a misfortune, and cannot accept their children's disfigurement or low intellect. Korea lacks social support to assist families in caring for children with mental or physical disabilities. Some families abandon these children in their desperate need for support with long-term care and expenses. Other children are kept from the public eye in the hope of saving the family from stigmatization.

Seo et al. (1992) explored the historical and future needs of special education in South Korea. Korea is faced with high teacher-pupil ratios, a reliance on self-contained programs, negative attitudes toward the disabled, and lack of advocacy for them. Of the 600,000 children aged 6 to 17 years who were disabled, only 15 percent received service in special private or public schools or classes. Negative attitudes toward the disabled influence the idea of mainstreaming mildly disabled students in South Korea. Korean Americans may hold these same views regarding the mentally and physically disabled and need special support in obtaining assistance.

In Korea, once hospitalized people are physically stable, they are discharged to their homes to be with the family. Bowel training and physical therapy activities are not the responsibility of the hospital. The families must care for family members at home with the support of other family members. Long-term care for chronic problems or for rehabilitation is rare in Korea. Thus, Korean Americans are familiar with the concept of family home care. Depending on their adaptation to the American health-care system, and families' contact with American health-care professionals, some Korean Americans adjust their ideologies on the sick role.

BLOOD TRANSFUSIONS AND ORGAN DONATION

No beliefs held by Korean Americans prevent the acceptance of blood transfusions. Organ donation and organ transplantation are rare, reflecting traditional attitudes toward integrity and purity. These issues need to be approached sensitively with Korean Americans and may be influenced by the individual's religious beliefs.

Health-Care Practitioners

TRADITIONAL VERSUS BIOMEDICAL PRACTITIONERS

In general, no taboos exist that prevent health-care practitioners from delivering care to the opposite gender. Female physicians are definitely preferred for maternity care and female problems because women feel more comfortable discussing gynecologic and obstetric issues with female physicians. However, more traditional Koreans frequently prefer health-care providers who speak Korean, are older, and are of the same gender, although many will seek health care from others who do not meet these requirements if their preferred care provider is not available. Miller (1990) studied the use of traditional health practitioners, acupuncturists, and herbalists among a group of 102 Korean immigrants. The findings indicated that Korean immigrants with higher incomes were more likely to use traditional Korean practitioners.

The area of social work is new in Korea. The hospitals have no positions for such a role. A few educational programs exist in Korea for social workers, but much development is needed in the area of social support. Because these roles may be new to many Koreans, health-care providers may need to encourage Korean Americans to use these services.

STATUS OF HEALTH-CARE PROVIDERS

Because traditional Korean culture accords high respect for men, elderly people, and physicians, the ideal physician is an older man with gray hair. This shows that he has experience and wisdom and is able to make the best decisions. With such a high status in Korea, physicians expect respect from all other health professionals. Usually, nurses are expected to carry out physicians' orders explicitly. This is not to say that the nurse cannot question orders, but great time and effort go into consulting other nurses before questioning physicians in the most respectful way. However, as nurses are becoming more educated in Korea they are becoming more assertive and more closely mirror Western practice patterns.

With an emphasis on increasing the educational level of nurses, they too are gaining stature and respect in Korean culture. Baccalaureate, masters, and doctoral programs are available for nurses in Korea. Although exact numbers are not available, there are approximately 600 doctorally prepared nurses in Korea as of 2001.

CASE STUDY Joon Kim, age 31, and Yung-Hee Kim, age 30, immigrated from Korea 5 years ago. They came to the United States as newlyweds and moved in with family members in Los Angeles. When they had saved enough money, they were able to find a small one-bedroom apartment where they have lived for 4 years. Yung-Hee finished secondary school in Korea, and Joon graduated from a university with a degree in business. They have two children, Soony, their 4-year-old daughter, and Suk-Choo, their 2-year-old son.

Both children were born in the United States and are cared for by an elderly family member while the other family members work.

When they arrived in the United States, Joon was unable to find a job using his business skills because of his poor proficiency in English. Although Joon is able to speak minimal English, he is not confident in his abilities in this new culture. Joon eventually obtained a job working at a dry cleaner for family friends. Yung-Hee found a job working for a Korean grocer. She assists in restocking shelves and managing inventory.

Yung-Hee became pregnant shortly after arriving in the United States. This had not been planned and finances were of great concern. Half way through her first pregnancy, Joon hit Yung-Hee after an argument about finances. Yung-Hee had a black eye, which was concealed with makeup and not discussed with anyone. Battering occurred sporadically throughout the next several years and seemed to heighten with financial woes and pregnancy. Yung-Hee gave Joon several warnings about leaving with the children, but she felt she had nowhere to turn for support.

Soony will begin kindergarten in the fall, yet her English language skills are lacking. Korean is spoken at home, and the children have been brought up in a Korean community in which minimal English is spoken. Soony has never been to a dentist, and two of her teeth are decaying. Suk-Choo was born with a mild form of mental retardation. Public health nurses repeatedly suggested early intervention programs, but the family was embarrassed about their child's "problem." They blamed themselves, and Joon felt especially guilt ridden for having hit his wife during her pregnancies. He enjoys drinking beer while watching television and frequently gets intoxicated on the weekends.

The Kims are a religious family and attend their community's Protestant church regularly. They are involved in many church activities.

STUDY QUESTIONS

1 Discuss some approaches a public health case manager might take in relation to the health of the Kim family.

2 Identify three areas of health teaching for this Korean American family.

3 Discuss two implications for Soony's poor understanding of the English language.

4 Identify how traditional role relations in Korean American families might affect Yung-Hee's alternatives in an abusive situation.

5 Name three health problems a health-care professional should be aware of when assessing the Kim family.

6 Discuss how the role of the church can be used in terms of health education.

7 Discuss the role of alcohol in Korean American society.

8 How might a health-care professional approach the topic of alcoholism with the Kim family?

9 Where do Koreans primarily live in the United States?

10 Discuss social support issues for Korean families not living in highly populated Korean areas of the United States.

11 How might the model minority theory affect the Kim family in terms of health resources? Identify health problems common among Korean immigrants.

12 As a home health caregiver, how might you handle the Korean American offer of food on your arrival?

13 Discuss contraceptive practices in the Korean American childbearing family.

REFERENCES

Blackhall, L. et al. (1999). Ethnicity and attitudes toward life sustaining technology. *Social Science Medicine, 48*(12), 1779–1789.

Cho, B. (2000). The politics of herbal drugs in Korea. *Social Science Medicine, 51*(4), 505–509.

Cho, Y. I., & Faulkner, W. R. (1993). Conception of alcoholism among Koreans and Americans. *International Journal of the Addictions, 28*(8), 681–694.

Cho, M., Nam, J., & Suh, G. (1998). Prevalence of symptoms of depression in a nationwide sample of Korean adults. *Psychiatric Residence, 81*(3), 341–352.

Choi, E. (1995). A contrast of mothering behaviors in women from Korea and the United States. *Journal of Obstetrics, Gynecological and Neonatal Nursing, 24*(4), 363–369.

Comrie, B., Matthews, S., & Polinsky, M. (1996). *The atlas of languages.* London: Quarto Publishing, Inc.

Donnelly, P. L. (2001). Korean American family experiences of caregiving for their mentally ill adult children: An interpretative study. *Journal of Transcultural Nursing, 12*(4), 292–301.

Han, Y., Williams, R., & Harrison, R. (2000). Breast cancer screening knowledge, attitudes, and practices among Korean-American women. *Oncology Nursing Forum, 27*(10), 1589–1591.

Howard, J., & Berbiglia, V. (1997). Caring for childbearing Korean women. *Journal of Obstetrical, Gynecological, and Neonatal Nursing, 26*(6), 665–671.

Johanning, E., Goldberg, M., & Kim, R. (1994). Asbestos hazard evaluation in South Korean textile production. *International Journal of Health Services, 24*(1), 131–144.

Kendall, L. (1987). Cold wombs in balmy Honolulu: Ethnography among Korean immigrants. *Social Science Medicine, 25*(4), 367–376.

Kim, H. (1990). Korean Christian churches in the Pacific Northwest: Resources for Korean ethnic identity? In H. C. Kim & E. H. Lee (Eds.), *Koreans in America: Dreams and realities* (pp. 177–192). Seoul: Institute of Korean Studies.

Kim, Y., & Grant, D. (1997). Immigration patterns, social support, and adaptation among Korean immigrant women and Korean American women. *Cultural Diversity in Mental Health, 3*(4), 235–245.

Kim, K. et al. (1998). Colorectal cancer screening: Knowledge and practices among Korean Americans. *Cancer Practices, 6*(3), 167–175.

Kim, K. et al. (2000). Nutritional status of Korean Americans: Implications for cancer risk. *Oncology Nursing Forum, 27*(10), 1573–1583.

Kim, K. K. et al. (1993). Nutritional status of Chinese-, Korean-, and Japanese-American elderly. *Journal of the American Dietetic Association, 93*(12), 1416–1422.

Kohls, R. L. (2001). *Learning to think Korean.* Yarmouth, ME: Intercultural Press.

Lee, D. C., & Lee, E. H. (1990). Korean immigrant families in America: Role and value conflicts. In H. C. Kim & E. H. Lee (Eds.), *Koreans in America: Dreams and realities* (pp. 165–177). Seoul: Institute of Korean Studies.

Lee, M. (2000). Knowledge, barriers, and motivators related to cervical cancer screening among Korean-American women. A focus group approach. *Cancer Nursing, 23*(3), 168–175.

Lee, Y. (1993). Health promotion: Patterns of traditional health promotion in Korea. *Kanhohak Tamgu, 2*(2), 21–36.

Lee, S., Sobal, J., & Frongillo, E. (2000). Acculturation and health in Korean Americans. *Social Science Medicine, 51*(2), 159–173.

Levy, R. (1993). Ethnic and racial differences in response to medicines: Preserving individualized therapy in managed pharmaceutical programmes. *Pharmaceutical Medicine, 7*, 139–165.

Lin, K. et al. (1992). Hwa-Byung: A community study of Korean Americans. *Journal of Nervous and Mental Disease, 180*(6), 386–391.

Lonely Planet. http://www.LonelyPlanet.com.

Ludman, E. K., Kang, K. J., & Lynn, L. L. (1992). Food beliefs and diets of pregnant Korean American women. *Journal of the American Dietetic Association, 92*(12), 1519–1520.

Markowitz, S. et al. (1994). Lead poisoning due to haigefen. The porphyrin content of individual erythrocytes. *Journal of the American Medical Association, 271*(12), 932–934.

Maxwell, A., Bastani, R., & Warda, U. (1998). Misconceptions and mammography use among Filipino- and Korean American women. *Ethnic Diversity, 8*(3), 377–384.

Meyer, U. (1992). Drugs in special patient groups: Clinical importance of genetics in drug effects. In M. Melmon & T. Morrelli (Eds.), *Clinical pharmacology: Basic principles in therapeutics* (8th ed., pp. 62–83). New York: Pergamon Press.

Miller, J. (1990). Use of traditional Korean health care by Korean immigrants to the United States. *Sociology and Social Research, 75*(1), 38–48.

Moon, A., & Williams, O. (1993). Perceptions of elder abuse and help-seeking patterns among African-American, Caucasian-American, and Korean-American elderly women. *Gerontologist, 33*(3), 386–395.

Pang, K. Y. (1989). The practice of traditional Korean medicine in Washington, DC. *Social Science Medicine, 28*(8), 857–884.

Pang, K. Y. (1990). Hwa-Byung: The construction of a Korean popular illness among Korean elderly immigrant women in the United States. *Culture, Medicine, and Psychiatry, 14*, 495–512.

Park, S., Oh, S., & Lee, M. (1998). Korean Status of alcoholics and alcohol-related health problems. *Alcohol and Clinical Expression Research, 22*(3, Suppl), 170S–172S.

Park, K. Y., & Peterson, L. M. (1991). Beliefs, practices, and experiences of Korean women in relation to childbirth. *Health Care for Women International, 12*(2), 261–269.

Pritham, U. A., & Sammons, L. N. (1993). Korean women's attitudes toward pregnancy and prenatal care. *Health Care for Women International, 14*, 145–153.

Sawyer, E., and Eaton, L. (1992). Gastric cancer in the Korean American: Cultural implications. *Oncology Nursing Forum, 19*(4), 619–623.

Seo, G. et al. (1992). Special education in South Korea. *Exceptional Children, 2*, 213–218.

Shin, K., & Shin, C. (1999). The lived experience of Korean immigrant women acculturating into the United States. *Health Care for Women International, 20*(6), 603–617.

Soh, C. S. (1993). Sexual equality, male superiority, and Korean women in politics: Changing gender relations in a "patriarchal democracy." *Sex Roles, 28*(1), 73–90.

Song, Y. I. (1990). The silent suffering of abused Korean immigrant women. In H. C. Kim & E. H. Lee (Eds.), *Koreans in America: Dreams and realities* (pp. 87–104). Seoul: Institute of Korean Studies.

Sorensen, C. W. (1994). Success and education in South Korea. *Comparative Education Review, 38*(1), 10–35.

Statcan.com. (2001). Canada: Ethnic Origins (1993). Ottawa, Canada: Minister of Industry, Science, and Technology.

Weatherspoon, A., Park, J., & Johnson, R. (2001). A family study of homeland Korean alcohol use. *Addictive Behavior, 26*(1), 101–113.

Wismer, B. et al. (1998). Rates and independent correlates of Pap smear testing among Korean American women. *American Journal of Public Health, 88*(4), 656–660.

Yi, M., & Jezewski, M. (2000). Korean nurses' adjustment to hospitals in the United States of America. *Journal of Advanced Nursing, 32*(3), 721–729.

Yu, E. Y. (1990a). Korean community profile: Life and consumer patterns. *Korea Times*, p. 3.

Yu, E. Y. (1990b). Korean American community in 1989: Issues and prospects. In H. C. Kim & E. H. Lee (Eds.), *Koreans in America: Dreams and realities* (pp. 112–126). Seoul: Institute of Korean Studies.

Chapter 17

People of Mexican Heritage

RICHARD ZOUCHA and LARRY D. PURNELL

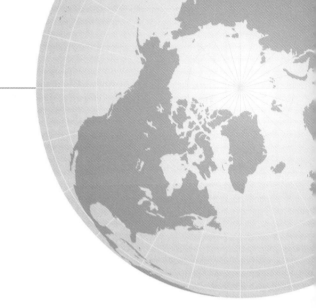

Overview, Inhabited Localities, and Topography

OVERVIEW

People of Mexican heritage are a very diverse group and are not easy to describe. Although no specific set of characteristics can fully describe people of Mexican heritage, some commonalities distinguish them as an ethnic group, with many regional variations that reflect subcultures in Mexico and in the United States. A common term used to describe Spanish-speaking populations, including people of Mexican heritage, is **Hispanic.** However, many Hispanic people prefer to be identified by descriptors more specific to their cultural heritage, such as Mexican, Mexican American, Latin American, Spanish American, **Chicano, Latino,** or **Ladino.** The Latino National Political Survey conducted in 1989 to 1990 (McDonald, 1993) reported that the most popular self-referent of 62 percent of people of Mexican heritage born in the United States and 86 percent of the immigrant population was *Mexican.* As a broad ethnic group, people of Mexican heritage often refer to themselves as **la gente de la raza,** which means "the people of the race." The Spanish word for race has a different meaning from the American interpretation of race. *La raza* is another designation for people of Mexican origin in the United States (Gonzales, 1999).

HERITAGE AND RESIDENCE

Mexico, with a population of 100,350,000, is considered a blend of Spanish white and Indian, Native American, or African (Williams, 1984). Mexican Americans are descendants of Spanish and other European whites; Aztec, Mayan, and other Central American Indians; and Inca and other South American Indians. Some individuals can trace their heritage to North American Indian tribes in the southwestern part of the United States.

Mexico City, one of the largest cities in the world, has a population of over 20 million. Mexico is undergoing rapid changes in business and health-care practices. Undoubtedly, these changes have and will continue to accelerate with the passage of the North American Free Trade Agreement and people are more able to move across the border to seek employment and educational opportunities.

Historically, people of Mexican heritage lived on the land that is now known as the southwestern United States for generations, long before the first white settlers came to the territory. By about 1853 approximately 80,000 Spanish-speaking settlers lived in the area lost by Mexico during the Texas Rebellion, Mexican War, and the Gadsden Purchase. After the annexation of the northern part of Mexico to the United States, the settlers were not officially considered immigrants but were often viewed as foreigners by the incoming white Americans (Rosales, 1996). By 1900, Mexican Americans numbered approximately 200,000. However, during the "Great Migration" between 1900 and 1930 an additional 1 million Mexicans entered the United States. This may have been the greatest immigration of people in the history of humanity (Gonzales, 1999).

Hispanics, the fastest growing ethnic population in the United States, include over 35 million people, or 12.5 percent of the population. Fifty-eight percent are of Mexican heritage with an increase in 1990 from 13.5 million to 20.6 million in 2000 (U.S. Census Bureau, 2001). Mexican Americans reside predominantly in

California, Texas, Illinois, Arizona, Florida, New Mexico, and Colorado. However, the major concentration of Mexican Americans totaling over 18 million are found in the south and west portions of the United States (U.S. Census Bureau, 2001). Ninety percent of Mexican Americans live in urban areas such as San Diego, Los Angeles, New York City, Chicago, and Houston, whereas less than 10 percent reside in rural areas.

REASONS FOR MIGRATION AND ASSOCIATED ECONOMIC FACTORS

Historically, many Mexicans left Mexico during the Mexican revolution to seek political, religious, and economic freedoms (Gonzales, 1999). Following the Mexican revolution, strict limits were placed on the Catholic Church and until recently clerics were not allowed to wear their church garb in public. For many, this restricted the expression of faith and was a minor factor in their immigration north to the United States (Meyer & Beezley, 2000). Since and during the "Great Migration," limited employment opportunities in Mexico, especially in rural areas, has encouraged Mexicans to migrate to the United States as sojourners, immigrants, or with undocumented status who are often derogatorily referred to as **wetbacks** *(majodos)* by the white and Mexican American populations.

Of the more than 5 million undocumented people in the United States, over 54 percent come from Mexico. Before the Immigration Reform and Control Act of 1986, hundreds of thousands of Mexicans crossed the border, found jobs, and settled in the United States. Although the numbers have decreased since 1986, border towns in Texas and California still experience large influxes of Mexicans seeking improved employment and educational opportunities. According to Gonzales (1999) the tide of illegal immigration to the United States has increased as evidenced by the apprehension of at least 1.5 million Mexicans annually and 100,000 to 200,000 people entering illegally.

Even though the economy of Mexico has grown, the buying power of the peso has decreased and inflation rates have increased faster than that of wages (Rangel, 1999); thus, a large percentage of the population continues to live in poverty (CIA, 1998). Recent Mexican immigrants are more likely to live in poverty, are more pessimistic about their future, and are less educated than previous immigrants (Gonzales, 1999). Many Mexicans are among the very poor with little hope of improving their economic status. Between the years 1999 and 2000 in the United States, the poverty rates for Hispanics fell from 22.8 percent to 21.2 percent (U.S. Census Bureau, 2001).

EDUCATIONAL STATUS AND OCCUPATIONS

Many second- and third-generation Mexican Americas have significant job skills and education. By contrast, many, especially newer immigrants from rural areas, have poor educational backgrounds and may place little value on education because it is not needed to obtain jobs in Mexico. Once in the United States, they initially find

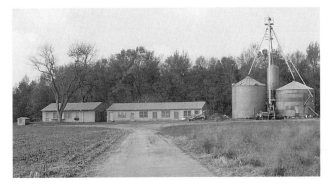

FIGURE 17–1 A migrant worker camp on Maryland's eastern shore. The Sanchez family (discussed in the Case Study at the end of the chapter) lives in such a camp, as do many Mexican American farm workers in the United States.

work similar to that which they did in their native land, including farming, ranching, mining, oil production, construction, landscaping, and domestic jobs in homes, restaurants, and hotels and motels. Economic and educational opportunities in the United States are attainable, which allows immigrants to pursue the great American dream of a perceived better life (Kemp, 2001). Many Mexicans and Mexican Americans work as seasonal migrant workers, who may relocate several times each year as they "follow the sun." Sometimes their unwillingness or inability to learn English is related to their intent to return to Mexico; however, this may hinder their ability to obtain better-paying jobs (Fig. 17–1).

The mean educational level in Mexico is 5 years. Until 1992, Mexican children were required to attend school through the sixth grade, but since the Mexican School Reform Act of 1992, a ninth-grade education is required. A common practice among parents in poor rural villages is to educate their children in what they need to know. This group often finds immigration to the United States to be their most attractive option. For many Mexicans, high school and a university education is unavailable and in many cases unattainable.

Hispanics are the most undereducated ethnic group in the United States, with only 57 percent aged 25 years or older having a high school education compared with 88.4 percent for non-Hispanic whites. However, that number has increased from 43 percent to 57 percent completing high school from 1993 to 2000 (U.S. Census Bureau, 2001). Some migrant worker camps have free or low-cost bilingual educational programs to assist Mexican Americans in learning to read and write in both languages. Only 10.6 percent of Mexican Americans aged 25 years or older have a college degree. However, the number of Hispanics who completed 4 years of college doubled between 1990 and 2000 (U.S. Census Bureau, 2001).

Communication

DOMINANT LANGUAGE AND DIALECTS

Second to Spain, Mexico is the largest Spanish-speaking country in the world (U.S. Department of Commerce,

2000). The dominant language of Mexicans and Mexican Americans is Spanish. However, Mexico has 54 indigenous languages and more than 500 different dialects. Knowing the region from which a Mexican American originates may help to identify the language or dialect the individual speaks. For example, major indigenous languages besides Spanish include Nahuatl and Otami, spoken in central Mexico; Mayan, spoken in the Yucatan peninsula; Maya-Quiche, spoken in the state of Chiapas; Zapotec and Mixtec, spoken in the valley of Oaxaca; Tarascan, spoken in the state of Michoacan; and Totonaco, spoken in the state of Veracruz. Many of the Spanish dialects spoken by Mexican Americans have similar word meanings. However, the dialects of Spanish spoken by other groups may not have the same word meanings. Because of the rural isolationist nature of many ethnic groups and the influence of native Indian languages, the dialects may be so diverse in selected regions that it may be difficult to understand the language, regardless of the degree of fluency in Spanish.

Radio and television programs broadcasting in Spanish in both the United States and Mexico have helped to standardize Spanish. For the most part, public broadcast communication is primarily derived from Castilian Spanish. This standardization reduces the difficulties experienced by subcultures with multiple dialects. When speaking in a nonnative language, health-care providers must select words that have relatively pure meanings in the language and avoid the use of regional slang.

Contextual speech patterns among Mexican Americans may include a high-pitched, loud voice and a rate that seems extremely fast to the untrained ear. The language uses apocopation, which accounts for this rapid speech pattern. An apocopation occurs when one word ends with a vowel and the next word begins with a vowel. This creates a tendency to drop the vowel ending of the first word and results in an abbreviated rapid-sounding form. For example, in the Spanish phrase for How are you?, *¿Cómo está usted?* may become *¿Comestusted?*. The last word, *usted,* is frequently dropped. Some may find this fast speech difficult to understand. However, if one asks the individual to enunciate slowly, the effect of the apocopation or truncation is less pronounced.

To help bridge potential communication gaps, health-care providers need to watch the client for cues, paraphrase words with multiple meanings, use simple sentences, repeat phrases for clarity, avoid the use of regional idiomatic phrases and expressions, and ask the client to repeat instructions to ensure accuracy. Approaching the Mexican American client with respect and *personalismo* (being friend-like) and directing questions to the dominant member of a group (usually the man) may help to facilitate more open communication. Zoucha (1998) found that becoming personal with the client or family is essential in building confidence and promoting health. The concept of *personalismo* may be difficult for some health-care professionals because they are socialized to form rigid boundaries between the caregiver and the client and family (Zoucha & Zamarripa, 1997).

CULTURAL COMMUNICATION PATTERNS

While some topics such as income, salary, or investments are taboo, Mexican Americans generally like to express their inner beliefs, feelings, and emotions once they get to know and trust a person. Meaningful conversations are important, often become loud, and seem disorganized. To the outsider, the situation may seem stressful or hostile, but this intense emotion means the conversants are having a good time and enjoying each other's company. Within the context of *personalismo* and **respeto**, respect, health-care providers can encourage open communication and sharing and develop the client's sense of trust by inquiring about family members before proceeding with the usual business. It is important for health-care providers to engage in "small talk" before addressing the actual health-care concern with the client and family (Zoucha & Zamarripa, 1997).

Mexican Americans place great value on closeness and togetherness, including when they are in an in-patient facility. They frequently touch and embrace and like to see relatives and significant others. Touch between men and women, between men, and between women are acceptable. To demonstrate respect, compassion, and understanding, health-care providers should greet the Mexican American client with a handshake. On establishing rapport, providers may further demonstrate approval and respect through backslapping, smiling, and affirmative nods of the head. Given the diversity of dialects and the nuances of language, culturally congruent use of humor is difficult to accomplish and therefore should be avoided unless health-care providers are absolutely sure that there is no chance of misinterpretation. Otherwise, inappropriate humor may jeopardize the therapeutic relationship and opportunities for health teaching and health promotion.

Mexican Americans consider sustained eye contact when speaking directly to an older person as rude. Direct eye contact with teachers or superiors may be interpreted as insolence. Avoiding direct eye contact with superiors is a sign of respect. This practice may or may not be seen with second- or third-generation Mexican Americans. It is imperative that health-care providers take cues from the client and family.

TEMPORAL RELATIONSHIPS

Many Mexican Americans, especially those from lower socioeconomic groups, are necessarily present oriented. Many individuals do not consider it important or have the income to plan ahead financially. The trend is to live in the "more important" here and now, because *mañana* (tomorrow) cannot be predicted. With this emphasis on living in the present, preventive health care and immunizations may not be a priority. *Mañana* may or may not really mean tomorrow; it often means "not today" or "later."

Some Mexicans and Mexican Americans perceive time as relative rather than categorically imperative. Deadlines and commitments are flexible, not firm. Punctuality is generally relaxed, especially in social situations. This concept of time is innate in the Spanish language. For example, one cannot be late for an appointment; one can only arrive late! In addition, a few immigrants from rural environments where adhering to a strict time clock is unimportant may not own a clock or even be able to tell time.

Because of their more relaxed concept of time, Mexican Americans may arrive late for appointments, although the current trend is toward greater punctuality. Health-care facilities that use an appointment system for clients may need to make special provisions to see clients whenever they arrive. Health-care providers must carefully listen for cues when discussing appointments. Disagreeing with health-care providers who set the appointment may be viewed as rude or impolite. Therefore, some Mexican Americans will not tell you directly that they cannot make the appointment. In the context of the discussion, they may say something like "my husband goes to work at 8:00 A.M. and the children are off to school, then I have to do the dishes...." The health-care professional should ask: "Is 8:30 A.M. on Thursday okay for you?" The person might say "yes" but the health-care professional must still intently listen to the conversation and then possibly negotiate a new time for the appointment.

FORMAT FOR NAMES

Names in most Spanish-speaking populations seem complex to those unfamiliar with the culture. A typical name is La Señorita Olga Gaborra de Rodriguez. Gaborra is the name of her father, and Rodriguez is her mother's surname. When she marries a man with the surname name of Guiterrez, she becomes La Señora (denotes a married woman) Olga Guiterrez de Gaborra y Rodriguez. The word *de* is used to express possession, and the father's name, which is considered more important than the mother's name, comes first. However, this full name is rarely used except on formal documents and for recording the name in the family Bible. Out of respect, most Mexican Americans are more formal when addressing nonfamily members. Thus, the best way to address Olga is not by her first name but rather as Señora Guiterrez. Titles such as *Don* and *Doña* for older respected members of the community and family are also common.

Health-care providers must understand the role of the elderly when providing care to people of Mexican heritage. To develop confidence and *personalismo,* an element of formality must exist between health-care providers and the elderly. Becoming overly familiar by using physical touch or using first names may not be appreciated early in a relationship (Kemp, 2001). As the health-care professional develops confidence in the relationship, becoming familiar may be less of a concern. However, using the first name of an elder client may never be appropriate (Zoucha, 1998).

Family Roles and Organization

HEAD OF HOUSEHOLD AND GENDER ROLES

The typical family dominance pattern in traditional Mexican American families is patriarchal, with evidence of slow change toward a more egalitarian pattern in recent years (Grothaus, 1996). Change to a more egalitarian decision-making pattern is primarily identified with more educated and higher socioeconomic families. **Machismo** in the Mexican culture sees men as having strength, valor, and self-confidence, which is a valued trait among many. Men are seen as wiser, braver, stronger, and more knowledgeable regarding sexual matters. The female takes responsibility for decisions within the home and for maintaining the family's health. Women are expected to be devoted mothers and receive great respect from their husbands and children (Grothaus, 1996).

PRESCRIPTIVE, RESTRICTIVE, AND TABOO PRACTICES FOR CHILDREN AND ADOLESCENTS

Children are highly valued because they ensure the continuation of the family and cultural values (Locke, 1999). They are closely protected and not encouraged to leave home. Even **compadres** (godparents) are included in the care of the young. Each child must have godparents in case something interferes with the parents' ability to fulfill their child-rearing responsibilities. Children are taught at an early age to respect parents and older family members, especially grandparents. Physical punishment is often used as a way of maintaining discipline and is sometimes considered child abuse in the United States.

FAMILY GOALS AND PRIORITIES

The concept of *familism* is an all-encompassing value among Mexicans, where the traditional family is still the foundation of society. Family takes precedence over work and all other aspects of life. In many Mexican families it is often said "God first, then family." The dominant Western health-care culture stresses including the client and family in the plan of care. Mexicans are strong proponents of this family-care concept, which includes the extended family. By including all family members, health-care providers can build greater trust and confidence and, in turn, increase compliance with health-care regimens and prescriptions (Zoucha & Husted, 2000).

Blended communal families are almost the norm in lower socioeconomic groups and in migrant worker camps. Single, divorced, and never-married male and female children usually live with their parents or extended families, regardless of economics. Extended kinship is common through *padrinos,* godparents who may be close friends, are usually considered family members (Zoucha & Zamarripa, 1997). Thus, the words brother, sister, aunt, and uncle do not necessarily mean that they are related by blood For many men, having children is evidence of their virility and is a sign of machismo.

When grandparents and elderly parents are unable to live on their own they generally move in with their children. The extended family structure and the Mexicans' obligation to visit sick friends and relatives encourage large numbers to visit hospitalized family members and friends. This practice may necessitate that health-care providers relax strict visiting policies in health-care facilities.

Social status is highly valued among Mexican Americans, and a person who holds an academic degree or position with an impressive title commands great respect and admiration from family, friends, and the community. Good manners, a family, and family lineage, as indicated by extensive family names also confer high status for Mexicans.

ALTERNATIVE LIFESTYLES

Thirty-four percent of Latino families in the United States live in poverty and are headed by a single female parent. This percentage is lower than that for other minority groups in the United States (U.S. Census Bureau, 2001). Because the Hispanic cultural norm is for a pregnant woman to marry, Mexicans are more likely to marry at a young age. Yet, common law marriages *(unidos)* are frequently practiced and readily accepted, with many couples living together their entire lives.

Although homosexual behavior occurs in every society, no information was found in the medical literature regarding same-sex Mexican American couples living together as a family unit. Newspapers from Houston, Texas; Washington, D.C.; and Chicago, Illinois report on the efforts of Hispanic lesbian and gay organizations in the areas of human immunodeficiency virus (HIV) and acquired immunodeficiency syndrome (AIDS, *La SIDA* in Spanish) and life partner benefits. In Mexico, antihate groups raised serious concerns about killings of homosexual men, causing many to remain closeted (Redding, 1999). In Mexico, machismo plays a large part in the phobic attitudes toward gay behavior. Harassment and police brutality against gay men and transvestite prostitutes are common in larger cities like Mexico City and Guadalajara (Schaefer, 1998). Larger cities in the United States may have *Ellas,* a support group for Latina Lesbians; El Hotline of Hola Gay, which provides referrals and information in Spanish; or Dignity, for gay Catholics. Health-care providers who wish to refer gay and lesbian clients to a support group may use such agencies.

Workforce Issues

CULTURE IN THE WORKPLACE

In the United States, Hispanics are the most underrepresented minority group in the health-care workforce. Although 12.5 percent of the American population is of Hispanic origin, only 4.2 percent of physicians and 1.6 percent of registered nurses are from Hispanic heritage (National Sample Survey of Registered Nurses, 1996). Cultural differences that influence workforce issues include values regarding family, pedagogical approach to education, emotional sensitivity, views toward status, aesthetics, ethics, balance of work and leisure, attitudes toward direction and delegation, sense of control, views about competition, and time.

People educated in Mexico are likely to have been exposed to pedagogical approaches that include rote memorization and emphasis on theory with little practical application taught within a rigid, broad curriculum. American educational systems usually emphasize an analytical approach, practical applications, and a narrow, in-depth specialization. Thus, additional training may be needed for some Mexicans when they come to the United States.

Because family is a first priority for most Mexicans, activities that involve family members usually take priority over work issues. Putting up a tough business front may be seen as a weakness in the Mexican culture. Because of this separation of work from emotions in American culture, most Mexican Americans tend to shun confrontation for fear of losing face. Many are very sensitive to differences of opinion, which are perceived as disrupting harmony in the workplace. People of Mexican heritage find it important to keep peace in relationships in the workplace.

For many Mexicans, truth is tempered by diplomacy and tact. When a service is promised for tomorrow, even when they know the service will not be completed tomorrow, it is promised to please, not to deceive. Thus, for many Mexicans, truth is seen as a relative concept, whereas for most European Americans, truth is an absolute value and people are expected to give direct yes and no answers. These conflicting perspectives about truth can complicate treatment regimens and commitment to the completion of work assignments. Intentions must be clarified and at times altered to meet the needs of the changing and multicultural workforce.

For most Mexicans work is viewed as a necessity for survival and may not be highly valued in itself, while money is for enjoying life (Kras, 1989). Most Mexican Americans place a higher value on other life activities. Material objects are usually necessities and not ends in themselves. The concept of responsibility is based on values related to attending to the immediate needs of family and friends (Kras, 1989) rather than on the work ethic. For most Mexicans, titles and positions may be more important than money.

Many Mexicans believe that time is relative and elastic, with flexible deadlines, rather than stressing punctuality and timeliness. In Mexico, shop hours may be posted but not rigidly respected. A business that is supposed to open at 8:00 A.M. opens when the owner arrives; a posted time of 8:00 A.M. may mean the business will open at 8:30 A.M., later, or not at all. The same attitude toward time is evidenced in reporting to work and in keeping social engagements and medical appointments. If people believe that an exact time is truly important, such as the time an airplane leaves, then they may keep to a schedule. The real challenge for employers is to stress the importance and necessity of work schedules and punctuality in the American workforce.

ISSUES RELATED TO AUTONOMY

Many Mexican Americans respond to direction and delegation differently from European Americans. Many newer immigrants are used to having traditional auto-cratic managers who assign tasks but not authority, although this practice is beginning to change with more American-managed companies relocating in Mexico. A Mexican worker who is not accustomed to responsibility may have difficulty assuming accountability for deci-sions. The individual may be sensitive to the American practice of checking on employees' work.

Mexicans who were born and educated in the United States usually have no difficulty communicating with others in the workplace. When better-educated Mexican immigrants arrive in the United States, they usually speak some English. Newer immigrants from lower socioeconomic groups have the most difficulty accultur-ating in the workplace and may have greater difficulty with the English language.

Biocultural Ecology

SKIN COLOR AND OTHER BIOLOGICAL VARIATIONS

Because Mexican Americans draw their heritage from Spanish peoples and various North American and Central American Indian tribes and Africans, few physical char-acteristics give this group a distinct identity. Some indi-viduals with a predominant Spanish background might have light-colored skin, blond hair, and blue eyes, whereas people from indigenous Indian backgrounds may have black hair, dark eyes, and cinnamon-colored skin. Intermarriages among these groups have created a diverse gene pool and have not produced a typical-appearing Mexican.

Cyanosis and decreased hemoglobin levels are more difficult to detect in dark-skinned people, whose skin appears ashen instead of the bluish color seen in light-skinned people. To observe for these conditions in dark-skinned Mexicans, the practitioner must examine the sclera, conjunctiva, buccal mucosa, tongue, lips, nailbeds, palms of the hands, and soles of the feet. Jaundice, likewise, is more difficult to detect in darker-skinned people. Thus, the practitioner needs to observe the conjunctiva and the buccal mucosa for patches of bilirubin pigment in dark-skinned Mexicans.

DISEASES AND HEALTH CONDITIONS

Common health problems in Mexico are malnutri-tion, malaria (in some places), cancer, alcoholism, drug abuse, obesity, hypertension, diabetes, heart disease, adolescent pregnancy, dental disease, and HIV and AIDS (Geissler, 1998). In Mexican American migrant worker populations, infectious, communicable, and parasitic diseases continue to be major health risks. Substandard housing conditions and employment in low-paying jobs have perpetuated higher rates of tuberculosis in Mexican Americans. Intestinal parasitosis, amoebic dysentery, and bacterial diarrhea (*Shigella*) are common diseases among Mexican immigrants (Ackerman, 1997).

Research has revealed an increase in the incidence of malaria in the border towns of the southwestern part of the United States. Newer Mexican immigrants from coastal lowland swamp areas where mosquitoes are more prevalent may also have a higher incidence of malaria. People from high mountain terrains may have increased red blood cell counts on immigration to the United States (Gavagan & Brodyaga, 1998). Health-care providers must take these topographic factors into consideration when performing health screening for such symptoms as anemia, lassitude, failure to thrive, and weight loss among Mexican immigrants (Uphold & Graham, 1998).

Cardiovascular disease is the leading cause of death and disability in Mexican American communities (Sundquist & Winkleby, 1999). However, current research shows that despite the adverse cardiovascular risk profile, including the incidence of obesity, diabetes, and untreated hypertension, Mexican Americans have a lower rate of coronary heart disease mortality than nonwhite Hispanics (Pandey et al., 2001). Cardiovascular risk factors are influenced by behavioral, cultural, and social factors (Sundquist & Winkleby, 1999). In addition, poor health, low social support, lack of educational and occupational opportunities, low access to health care, and discrimination add to the risk factors associated with cardiovascular disease.

Mexican Americans have five times the rate of diabetes mellitus, with an increased incidence of related complications when compared with European American cohort groups. Additionally, health-care professionals working with Mexican immigrants and Mexican Ameri-cans should offer screening and teach clients preventive measures regarding pesticides and communicable and infectious diseases because many work with chemicals and live in crowded housing conditions.

VARIATIONS IN DRUG METABOLISM

Because of the mixed heritage of many Mexican Americans, it may be more difficult to determine a ther-apeutic dose of selected drugs. Several studies report differences in absorption, distribution, metabolism, and excretion of drugs, including alcohol in some Hispanic populations. The mixed heritage of Mexican Americans makes it more difficult to generalize drug metabolism. Few studies include only one subgroup of Hispanics; and therefore, health-care providers need to consider some notable differences when prescribing medications. Hispanics require lower doses of antidepressants and experience greater side effects than non-Hispanic whites.

High-Risk Behaviors

Alcohol plays an important part in the Mexican culture. Many of this group's colorful lifestyle celebra-tions include alcohol consumption. Men drink in greater proportion than women, but both sexes begin drinking at early ages and consume large quantities of alcoholic beverages (Chavez et al., 1993).

Because of these drinking patterns, alcoholism represents a crucial health problem for many Mexicans. The number one admitting diagnosis for Mexican Americans in the psychiatric setting is alcoholism (Monrroy, 1983). Low acculturation and distorted application of the chivalric norm of machismo may influence the high alcoholism rates in this group. Less acculturated Hispanics are more likely to consume alcoholic beverages than more acculturated Hispanics. Even the more acculturated Hispanics consume more alcoholic beverages than non-Hispanic whites, expecting alcohol to make them more emotional and socially extroverted (Marin, Posner, & Kenyon, 1993). Low acculturation and distorted self-image problems have special implications for counseling (Zimmerman & Sodowsky, 1993). Many deny the physiological problems of alcoholism. Hispanics suffer higher rates of automobile accidents and other types of injuries associated with alcohol consumption (Marin, Posner, & Kenyon, 1993). In another study contrasting the drinking patterns of Latinos and non-Latino whites in San Francisco, Perez-Stable, Marin, and Marin (1994) reported that Latinos of both sexes consume less alcohol than non-Latino whites, but Latino men are more likely to drink to excess and engage in binge drinking.

Marijuana is the number two drug used by Mexican Americans because it is readily available in their native land and easily accessible from people who work in farming and ranching occupations. Some adults who can afford them use cocaine and heroin, and the younger population uses inhalants (Eden & Aguilar, 1989).

The trend toward decreasing cigarette smoking in the United States may not extend to the Mexican American culture, where cigarette-smoking rates remain steady (Escobebe & Remington, 1989). However, Perez-Stable, Marin, and Marin (1994), in their San Francisco study, reported that Latino smokers of both sexes smoke fewer than half as many cigarettes per day as non-Latino whites. The differing results from these two studies attest to the fact that health-care providers should not draw general conclusions regarding high-risk behaviors.

HEALTH-CARE PRACTICES

Responsibility for health promotion and safety may be a major threat for those of Mexican heritage accustomed to depending on the family unit and traditional means of providing health care. Continuing disparities in health and health-seeking behaviors have been reported in several studies. Lower socioeconomic conditions are responsible for Latina women being overweight, exhibiting hypertension, experiencing high cholesterol levels, and having increased smoking behaviors (Blantan et al., 1993). In addition, Latina women are less likely to have pap smears, medical examinations, or clinical breast examinations compared with non-Latino whites (Perez-Stable, Marin, & Marin, 1994). Latino men are less likely to have cancer screening or physical examinations than their non-Latino white counterparts. High-risk health behaviors such as drinking and driving, cigarette smoking, sedentary lifestyle, and nonuse of seat belts increase with fewer years of educational attainment. Through educational programs and enforcement of state laws,

more Mexicans are beginning to use seat belts; however, it is still common to see children traveling unrestrained in automobiles.

Nutrition

MEANING OF FOOD

As in many other ethnic groups, Mexicans and Mexican Americans celebrate with food. Mexican foods are rich in color, flavor, texture, and spiciness. Any occasion—births, birthdays, religious holidays, official and unofficial holidays, and anniversaries of deaths—is seen as a time to celebrate with food and enjoy the companionship of family and friends. Because food is a primary form of socialization in the Mexican culture, Mexican Americans may have difficulty adhering to a prescribed diet for illnesses such as diabetes mellitus and cardiovascular disease. It is important for health-care professionals to seek creative alternatives and to negotiate types of food consumption with individuals and families in relation to these concerns.

COMMON FOODS AND FOOD RITUALS

The Mexican American's diet is extremely varied and may depend on the individual's region of origin in Mexico. Thus, one needs to ask the individual specifically about his or her dietary habits. The staples of the Mexican American diet are rice (*arroz*), beans, and tortillas, which are made from corn (*maíz*) treated with calcium carbonate. However, in many parts of the United States, only flour tortillas are available. Even though the diet is low in calcium derived from milk and milk products, tortillas treated with calcium carbonate provide essential dietary calcium. Popular Mexican American foods are eggs (*huevos*); pork (*puerco*), chicken (*pollo*), sausage (*salchicha*); lard (*lardo*); mint (*menta*); chili peppers (*chile*), onions (*cebollas*), tomatoes (*tomates*), squash (*calabaza*); canned fruit (*fruta de lata*); mint tea (*hierbabuena*), chamomile tea (*té de camomile* or *manzanilla*); carbonated beverages (*bebidas de gaseosa*), beer (*cerveza*), cola-flavored soft drinks, sweetened packaged drink mixes (*agua fresa*) that are high in sugar (*azucar*); sweetened breakfast cereals (*cereales de desayuno*); potatoes (*papas*), bread (*pan*), corn (*maíz*); gelatin (*gelatina*), custard (*flan*), and other sweets (*dulces*). Other common dishes include chile, chile con carne, enchiladas, tamales, tostadas, chicken mole, arroz con pollo, refried beans, tacos and soups (*caldos*). Soups (*caldos*) are varied in nature and may include chicken, beef, and pork with vegetables.

Mealtimes vary among different subgroups of Mexican Americans. Whereas many individuals adopt North American schedules and eating habits, many continue their native practices, especially those in rural settings and migrant worker camps. For these groups, breakfast is usually fruit, perhaps cheese, or bread alone or in some combination. A snack may be taken in midmorning before the main meal of the day, which is eaten from 2 to 3 P.M., and in rural areas especially, may last for 2 hours or more. Mealtime is an occasion for socialization and keeping family members informed about each other. The evening meal is usually late and is taken between 9 and 9:30 P.M. Health-care providers must consider Mexican Americans' mealtimes when teaching clients about medication and dietary regimens related to diabetes mellitus and other illnesses.

DIETARY PRACTICES FOR HEALTH PROMOTION

A dominant health-care practice for Mexicans and many Mexican Americans is the hot and cold theory of food selection. This theory is a major aspect of health promotion and illness and disease prevention and treatment. According to this theory, illness or trauma may require adjustments in the hot and cold balance of foods to restore body equilibrium. The hot and cold theory of foods is described under the section Health-care Practices later in this chapter.

NUTRITIONAL DEFICIENCIES AND FOOD LIMITATIONS

In lower socioeconomic groups, wide-scale vitamin A deficiency and iron deficiency anemia exist (Mendoza et al., 1992). Some Mexican and Mexican Americans have lactose intolerance, which may cause problems for schools and health-care organizations that provide milk in the diet for its high calcium content.

Because major Mexican foods and their ingredients are available throughout the United States, native food practices may not change much when Mexicans emigrate. Of course, Mexican foods are extremely popular throughout the United States and are eaten by many Americans because of the strong flavors, spiciness, and color. Table 17–1 lists the Mexican names of popular foods, their description, and ingredients. Individual adaptations to these preparations commonly occur.

Pregnancy and Childbearing Practices

FERTILITY PRACTICES AND VIEWS TOWARD PREGNANCY

Mexican American birth rates are 3.45 per household in comparison with 2.6 per household among other minority groups (Chapa & Valencia, 1993). Multiple births are common, especially in the economically disadvantaged groups. Men see a large number of children as proof of their virility. Optimal childbearing age for Mexican women is between 19 and 24 years. Fertility practices of Mexican Americans are connected with their predominant Catholic religious beliefs and their tendency to be modest. The only acceptable methods of birth control are abstinence and the rhythm method. Some women practice the belief that prolonged infant breast-feeding is a method of birth control. Theoretically, most other types of birth control, on the surface, are unacceptable. Abortion is considered morally wrong and is practiced (theoretically) only in extreme circumstances to keep the mother's life intact. However, legal and illegal abortions are common in some parts of Mexico and the United States. Despite the strong influence of the Catholic Church over fertility practices, Catholicism does not prevent some Mexican American women from using contraceptives, sterilization, or abortion for unwanted pregnancies.

Diaphragms, foams, and creams are not commonly used for birth control practice, mostly because they are not approved by Catholic doctrine and partly because of the belief that women are not supposed to touch their genitals. Birth control pills are unacceptable because they are an artificial means of birth control. Physicians' offices and clinics that see large numbers of migrant workers on the Delmarva Peninsula on the east coast report that many younger female clients are using Norplant for birth

Table 17–1 *Mexican Foods*

Common Name	Description	Ingredients
Arroz con pollo	Chicken with rice	Chicken baked, boiled, or fried and served over boiled or fried rice
Chili	Chili	Same as the United States but tends to be more spicy
Chili con carne	Chili with meat	Chili with beef or pork
Chili con salsa	Chili with sauce	Chili with a sauce that contains no meat
Dulces	Sweets	Candy and desserts usually high in sugar, lard, and eggs
Enchiladas	Enchiladas	Tortilla rolled and stuffed with meat or cheese and a spicy sauce
Papas fritas	Fried potatoes	Potatoes usually fried in lard
Flan	Flan	Popular dessert made of egg custard and may be filled with fruit or cheese
Gelatina	Gelatin	Popular dessert made with sugar, eggs, and jelly
Pollo con molé	Chicken molé	Chicken with a sauce made of hot spices, chocolate, and chili
Salchica or chorizo	Sausage	Sausage almost always made with pork and spices
Tacos	Tacos	Tortilla folded around meat or cheese
Tamales	Tamales	Fried or boiled chopped meat, peppers, cormeal, and hot spices
Tortilla	Tortilla	A thin unleavened bread made with cornmeal and treated with lime (calcium carbonate)
Tostadas	Tostadas	Toast that may have a spicy sauce

control. Men are reluctant to use condoms because they are associated with prostitutes and because of the belief that they should be used only for disease control. A woman may reject the use of a condom and find it offensive because it means that she is "dirty." Family planning is one area in which health-care providers can help the family to identify more realistic outcomes consistent with current economic resources and family goals.

Foreign-born Mexicans are less likely to give birth to low birth weight babies than U.S.-born Mexican women, even though U.S.-born mothers are usually of higher socioeconomic status and receive more prenatal care. Research suggests that better nutritional intake and lower prevalence of smoking and alcohol use are some reasons for these protective outcomes (American Public Health Association, 2002).

Because pregnancy among Mexican Americans is viewed as natural and desirable, many women do not seek prenatal evaluations. In addition, because prenatal care is not available to every woman in Mexico, some women do not know about the need for prenatal care. With the extended family network and the woman's role of maintaining the health status of family members, many pregnant women seek family advice before seeking medical care. Thus, *familism* may deter and hinder early prenatal checkups. To encourage prenatal checkups, health-care providers can encourage female relatives and husbands to accompany the pregnant woman for health screening and incorporate advice from family members into health teaching and preventive care services. Using videos with Spanish-speaking Hispanics is one culturally effective way for incorporating health education, especially for those who have a limited understanding of English. In addition, incorporating cultural brokers known to the Mexican American family may help to empower clients and reduce conflict for Mexicans.

PRESCRIPTIVE, RESTRICTIVE, AND TABOO PRACTICES IN THE CHILDBEARING FAMILY

Beliefs related to the hot and cold theory of disease prevention and health maintenance influence conception, pregnancy, and postpartum rituals. For instance, during pregnancy, a woman is more likely to favor hot foods, which are believed to provide warmth for the fetus and enable the baby to be born into a warm and loving environment. Cold foods and environments are preferred during the menstrual cycle and in the immediate postdelivery period. Many pregnant woman sleep on their backs to protect the infant from harm, keep the vaginal canal well lubricated by having frequent intercourse to facilitate an easier birth, and keep active to ensure a smaller baby and to prevent a decrease in the amount of amniotic fluid (Burk, Wieser, & Keegan, 1995). An important activity restriction is that pregnant women should not walk in the moonlight because it might cause a birth deformity. To prevent birth deformities, pregnant women may wear a safety pin, metal key, or some other metal object on their abdomen (Villarruel & Ortiz de Montellano, 1992). Other beliefs include avoiding cold

air, not reaching over the head to prevent the baby's cord from wrapping around its neck, and avoiding lunar eclipses because they may result in deformities.

In more traditional Mexican families the father is not included in the delivery experience and should not see the mother or baby until after both have been cleaned and dressed. This practice is based on the fear that harm may come to the mother, baby, or both. Integrating men into the birthing of a child is a process that requires changing social habits in relation to cultural aspects of life and gender roles. For many, the presence of men during delivery is considered an uninvited intrusion into the Mexican culture. Among less traditional and more acculturated Mexican Americans, men participate in prenatal classes and assist in the delivery room. However, in one of the author's (L. Purnell) personal experiences, men who provide support during delivery may receive friendly gibing from their male counterparts for taking the role of the wife's mother. In any event, health-care providers must respect Mexicans decision to not have men in the delivery room.

During labor, traditional Mexican women may be quite vocal and are taught to avoid breathing air in through the mouth because it can cause the uterus to rise up. Immediately after birth, they may place their legs together to prevent air from entering the womb (Olds, London, & Ladewig, 2000). Health-care providers can help the Mexican pregnant woman have a better delivery by encouraging attendance at prenatal classes.

The postpartum preference for a warm environment may restrict postpartum women from bathing or hair washing for up to 40 days (Reinert, 1986). Although postpartum women may not take showers or sit in a bathtub, this does not mean that they do not bathe. They take sitz baths, wash their hair with a washcloth, and take sponge baths. Other postpartum practices include wearing a heavy cotton abdominal binder, cord, or girdle to prevent air from entering the uterus; covering one's ears, head, shoulders, and feet to prevent blindness, mastitis, frigidity, or sterility; and avoiding acidic foods to protect the baby from harm (Olds, London, & Ladewig, 2000).

When the baby is born, special attention is given to the umbilicus; the mother may place a belt around the umbilicus (*ombliguero*) to prevent the naval from popping out when the child cries. Cutting the baby's nails in the first 3 months is thought to cause blindness and deafness (R. M. Solorzano, M.D., personal communication, September 1995).

Health-care providers need to make special provisions to provide culturally congruent health teaching for lactating women who work with or are exposed to pesticides, such as dichlorodiphenyldichlorothene (DDE), the most stable derivative from the pesticide DDT. High DDE levels among lactating women have a direct correlation with a decrease in lactation and increase in breast cancer, especially in women who have had more than one pregnancy and previous lactation (Gladen & Rogan, 1995). Education level and degree of acculturation are key issues when developing health education and interventions for risk reduction.

Death Rituals

DEATH RITUALS AND EXPECTATIONS

Mexicans often have a stoic acceptance of the way things are and view death as a natural part of life and the will of God (Luckmann, 1999). Death practices are primarily an adaptation of their religion. Family members may arrive in large numbers at the hospital or home in times of illness or an approaching death. In more traditional families, family members may take turns sitting vigil over the sick or dying person. Autopsy is acceptable as long as the body is treated with respect. Burial is the common practice; cremation is an individual choice.

RESPONSES TO DEATH AND GRIEF

When a person dies, the word travels rapidly, and family and friends travel from long distances to get to the funeral. They may gather for a **velorio**, a festive watch over the body of the deceased person before burial. Some Mexican Americans bury the body within 24 hours, which is required by law in Mexico.

More traditional grieving families may engage in protection of the dying and bereaved such as small children who have difficulty dealing with the death (Andrews & Boyle, 1999). Mexican Americans encourage expressions of feeling during the grieving process. In these cases, health-care providers can assist the person by providing support and privacy during the bereavement.

Spirituality

DOMINANT RELIGION AND USE OF PRAYER

The predominant religion of most Mexicans and Mexican Americans is Catholicism. The major religions in Mexico are Roman Catholic, 89 percent; Protestant, 6 percent; and other, 5 percent of the population. Over the last several years, other religious groups such as Mormons, Jehovah's Witnesses, Seventh Day Adventists, Presbyterians, and Baptists have been gaining in popularity in Mexico. Although many Mexicans and Mexican Americans may not appear to be practicing their faith on a daily basis, they may still consider themselves devout Catholics, and their religion has a major influence on health-care practices and beliefs. For many, Catholic religious practices are influenced by indigenous Indian practices.

Newer immigrant Mexican Americans may continue their traditional practice of having two marriage ceremonies, especially in lower socioeconomic groups. A civil ceremony is performed whenever two people decide to make a union. When the family gets enough money for a religious ceremony, they schedule an elaborate celebration within the church. Common practice, especially in rural Mexican villages and some rural villages in the southwestern United States, is to post a handwritten sign on the local church announcing the marriage, with an invitation for all to attend.

Frequency of prayer is highly individualized for most Mexican Americans. Even though some do not attend church on a regular basis, they may have an altar in their homes and say prayers several times each day, a practice which is more common among rural isolationists.

MEANING OF LIFE AND INDIVIDUAL SOURCES OF STRENGTH

The family is foremost to most Mexicans, and individuals get strength from family ties and relationships. Individuals may speak in terms of a person's soul or spirit (*alma or espiritu*) when they refer to one's inner qualities. These inner qualities represent the person's dignity and must be protected at all costs in times of both wellness and illness. In addition, Mexicans derive great pride and strength from their nationality, which embraces a long and rich history of traditions.

Leisure is considered essential for a full life, and work is a necessity to make money for enjoying life. Mexican Americans pride themselves on good manners, etiquette, and grooming as signs of respect. Because the overall outlook for many Mexicans is one of fatalism, pride may be taken in stoic acceptance of life's adversities.

SPIRITUAL BELIEFS AND HEALTH-CARE PRACTICES

Most Mexicans enjoy talking about their soul or spirit, especially in times of illness, while many health-care providers may feel uncomfortable talking about spirituality. This tendency may communicate to Mexicans that the health-care provider has suspect intentions, is insensitive, and is not really interested in them as individuals. It may be common for a person needing care in the home or hospital to have a statue of a patron saint or a candle with a picture of the saint. Rosaries may be present and at times the family may pray as a group. Depending on the confidence maintained with the family and client, a health-care professional may be asked to join in the prayer. If time permits, it is very appropriate to pray with the family even if only for a few minutes. This action promotes confidence in the relationship and can have a positive impact on the health and well being of the client and family (Zoucha & Zamarripa, 1997).

Health-Care Practices

HEALTH-SEEKING BELIEFS AND BEHAVIORS

The family is the most credible source of health information and the most significant impediment to positive health-seeking behavior. Mexican Americans' fatalistic worldview and external locus of control are closely tied to health-seeking behaviors. Because expressions of negative feelings are considered impolite, Mexicans may be reluctant to complain about health problems or to place blame on the individual for poor health. If a person becomes seriously ill, that is just the way things are; all events are acts of God (Luckmann, 1999). This belief system may impair the dominant view of communications and hinder health teaching, health promotion, and disease prevention practices. Therefore, it is imperative for health-care professionals to plan health-promoting activities and teaching that is consistent with this belief but encourages health. For instance, if a person believes that the illness is due to a punishment from God, it may be possible to ask to be forgiven by God, thereby restoring health. This may be an opportune time to call a priest or minister for official recognition of forgiveness.

RESPONSIBILITY FOR HEALTH CARE

To many Mexicans good health may mean the ability to keep working and have a general feeing of well-being (Zoucha, 1998). Illness may occur when the person can no longer work or take care of the family. Therefore, many Mexicans may not seek health care until they are incapacitated and unable to go about the activities of daily living. Unfortunately, many people of Mexican heritage may not know and understand the occupational dangers inherent in their daily work. Migrant workers are often unaware of the dangers of pesticides and the potentially dangerous agricultural machinery. Health-care professionals must serve as advocates for these people regarding occupational safety. Often the companies do not tell the workers of the dangers of the work or the workers may not understand due to the inability of the company officials to speak the language of the workers.

The use of over-the-counter medicine may pose a significant health problem related to self-care for many Mexican Americans. In part this is a carryover from Mexico's practice of allowing over-the-counter purchases of antibiotics, intramuscular injections, intravenous fluids, birth control pills, and other medications that require a prescription in the United States. Often Mexican immigrants bring these medications across the border and share them with friends; in addition, friends and relatives in Mexico send drugs through the mail. To protect clients from contradictory or potentiating effects of prescribed treatments, health-care providers need to ask clients about prescription and nonprescription medications they may be taking.

FOLK PRACTICES

Mexican Americans engage in folk medicine practices and use a variety of prayers, herbal teas, and poultices to treat illnesses. Many of these practices are regionally specific and vary between and among families. The Mexican *Ministerio de Salud Publica y Asistencia Social* (Ministry of Public Health and Social Assistance) publishes an extensive manual on herbal medicines that are readily available in Mexico. Lower socioeconomic groups and well-educated upper- and middle-class Mexicans to some degree practice traditional and folk medicine. Many of these practices are harmless, but some may contradict or potentiate therapeutic interventions. Thus, as with the use of other prescription and nonprescription drugs discussed earlier, it is essential for health-care providers to be aware of these practices and to take

them into consideration when providing treatments (Rivera-Andino & Lopez, 2000). The provider must ask the Mexican American client specifically whether they are using folk medicine.

To provide culturally competent care, health-care practitioners must be aware of the hot and cold theory of disease when prescribing treatment modalities and when providing health teaching. According to this theory, many diseases are caused by a disruption in the hot and cold balance of the body. Thus, eating foods of the opposite variety may either cure or prevent specific hot and cold illnesses and conditions. Physical or mental illness may be attributed to an imbalance between the person and environment. Influences include emotional, spiritual, and social state, as well as physical factors such as humoral imbalance expressed as either too much hot or cold. As health-care providers, it is important to understand that if people of Mexican heritage believe in the "hot and cold" theory it does mean that they do not believe or use professional Western practices (Zapata & Shippee-Rice, 1999). Unless a level of trust and confidence is maintained, Mexicans who follow these beliefs may not express them to health professionals (Zoucha & Husted, 2000).

"Hot" and "cold" are viewed as specific properties of various substances and conditions, and sometimes opinions differ about what is "hot" and what is "cold" in the Mexican community. In general, it can be viewed that cold diseases or conditions are characterized by vasoconstriction and a lower metabolic rate. "Cold" diseases or conditions include menstrual cramps, *frio de la matriz*, coryza (rhinitis), pneumonia, *empacho*, cancer, malaria, earaches, arthritis, pneumonia and other pulmonary conditions, headaches, and musculoskeletal conditions and colic. Common hot foods used to treat cold diseases and conditions include cheeses, liquor, beef, pork, spicy foods, eggs, grains other than barley, vitamins, tobacco, and onions (Neff, 1998).

"Hot" diseases and conditions may be characterized by vasodilation and a higher metabolic rate. Pregnancy, hypertension, diabetes, acid indigestion, *susto*, *mal de ojo*, *bilis* (imbalance of bile which runs into the blood stream), infection, diarrhea, sore throats, stomach ulcers, liver conditions, kidney problems, and fever may be examples of hot conditions. Common cold foods used to treat hot diseases and conditions include fresh fruits and vegetables, dairy products (even though fresh fruits and dairy products may cause diarrhea), barley water, fish, chicken, goat meat, and dried fruits (Neff, 1998).

Folk practitioners are consulted for several notable conditions. *Mal de ojo* (bad eye or evil eye) is a folk illness that occurs when one person (usually older) looks at another (usually a child) in an admiring fashion. Another example of *mal de ojo* is if a person admires something about a baby or child, such as beautiful eyes or hair. Such eye contact can be either voluntary or involuntary. Symptoms are numerous, ranging from fever, anorexia, and vomiting to irritability. The spell can be broken if the person doing the admiring touches the person while they are admiring them. Children are more susceptible to this condition than women, and women are more susceptible than men. To prevent *mal de ojo*, the child wears a bracelet with a seed (*ojo de venado*) or a bag of seeds pinned to the clothes (Zapata & Shippee-Rice, 1999).

Another childhood condition often treated by folk practitioners is *caida de la mollera* (fallen fontanel). The condition has numerous causes, which may include removing the nursing infant too harshly from the nipple or handling an infant too roughly. Symptoms range from irritability to failure to thrive. To cure the condition, the child is held upside down by the legs.

Susto (magical fright or soul loss) is associated with epilepsy, tuberculosis, and other infectious diseases and is caused by the loss of spirit from the body. The illness is also thought to be caused by a fright or by the soul being frightened out of the person. This culture-bound disorder may be psychological, physical, or physiological in nature. Symptoms may include anxiety, depression, loss of appetite, excessive sleep, bad dreams, feelings of sadness, and lack of motivation. Treatment sometimes includes elaborate ceremonies at a crossroads with herbs and holy water to return the spirit to the body (C. Zamarripa, Fort Worth, TX, personal communication, March 2002).

Empacho, blocked intestines, may result from an incorrect balance of hot and cold foods, causing a lump of food to stick in the gastrointestinal track. To make the diagnosis, the healer may place a fresh egg on the abdomen. If the egg appears to stick to a particular area, this confirms the diagnosis. Older women usually treat the condition in children by massaging their stomach and back to dislodge the food bolus and to promote its continued passage through the body.

The use of herbs, roots, and teas vary among Mexicans and Mexican Americans and depends on the area from which they originate. One online source for a variety of herbs and teas is *http://www.riceinfo.edu/projects/ Hispanichealth/Courses/mod7/mid7.html*.

Health-care practitioners are cautioned against diagnosing psychiatric illnesses too readily in the Mexican population. The syndromes *mal ojo* and *susto* are culture bound and are potential sources of diagnostic bias.

BARRIERS TO HEALTH CARE

Thirty-two percent of Mexican Americans, compared with 14 percent of the U.S. population in general, do not have health insurance (U.S. Census Bureau, 2001). A number of factors may account for this high percentage of uninsured individuals. First, many Mexican Americans constitute the working poor and are unable to purchase insurance. Second, many are migratory and do not qualify for Medicaid. Third, many have an undocumented status and are afraid to apply for health insurance. Fourth, even though insurance is available in their native homeland, it is very expensive and not part of the culture.

Whereas wealthier Mexican Americans have little difficulty accessing health care in the United States, lower socioeconomic groups may experience significant barriers, including inadequate financial resources, lack of

insurance and transportation, limited knowledge regarding available services, language difficulties, and the culture of health-care organizations. Like many other immigrant groups who lack a primary provider, they may use emergency rooms for minor illnesses. Health-care providers have the opportunity to improve the care of Mexican Americans by explaining the health-care system, incorporating a primary care provider whenever possible, using an interpreter of the same gender, securing a cultural broker, and assisting clients in locating culturally specific mental health programs (Zoucha & Husted, 2000).

CULTURAL RESPONSES TO HEALTH AND ILLNESS

Good health to many Mexican Americans is to be free of pain, able to work, and spend time with the family. In addition, good health is a gift from God and from living a good life (Zoucha, 1998).

Mexicans and Mexican Americans tend to perceive pain as a necessary part of life, and enduring the pain is often viewed as a sign of strength. Men commonly tolerate pain until it becomes extreme (Luckmann, 1999). Often pain is viewed as the will of God and is tolerated as long as the person can work and care for the family. These attitudes toward pain delay seeking treatment; many hope that the pain will simply go away. Research has shown that many Mexican Americans experience more pain than other ethnic groups, but that they report the occurrence of pain less frequently and endure pain longer (Villarruel & Ortiz de Montellano, 1992). The following six themes have emerged that describe culturally specific attributes of Mexican Americans experiencing pain:

> Mexicans accept and anticipate pain as a necessary part of life.
> They are obligated to endure pain in the performance of duties.
> The ability to endure pain and to suffer stoically is valued.
> The type and amount of pain a person experiences is divinely predetermined.
> Pain and suffering are a consequence of immoral behavior.
> Methods to alleviate pain are directed toward maintaining balance within the person and the surrounding environment (Villarruel & Ortiz de Montellano, 1992).

By using these themes, health-care providers can evaluate Mexicans experiencing pain within their cultural framework and provide culturally specific interventions.

Because long-term care facilities in Mexico are rare and tend to be crowded, understaffed, and expensive, many Mexican Americans may not consider long-term care as a viable option for a family member. In addition, because of the importance of extended family, Mexican Americans may prefer to care for their family members with mental illness, physical handicaps, and extended physical illnesses at home. In Mexican American culture, someone with a mental illness is not looked on with scorn or blamed for their condition because mental illness, like physical illness, is viewed as God's will. It is common to accept those with mental illness and care for them in the context of the family until the illness is so bad that they cannot be managed in the home (Zoucha & Husted, 2000).

Mexicans can readily enter the sick role without personal feelings of inadequacy or blame. A person can enter the sick role with any acceptable excuse and be relieved of life's responsibilities. Other family members willingly take over the sick person's obligations during his or her time of illness.

BLOOD TRANSFUSIONS AND ORGAN DONATION

Extraordinary means to preserve life are frowned on in the Mexican and Mexican American cultures, and ordinary means are commonly used to preserve life. Extraordinary means are defined and determined by the individual, taking into account such factors as finances, education, and availability of services.

Blood transfusions are acceptable if the individual and the family agree that the transfusion is necessary. Organ donation, although not deemed morally wrong, is not a common practice and is usually restricted to cadaver donations, because donating an organ while the person is still alive means that the body is not whole. Acceptance of organ transplant as a treatment option is seen primarily among more educated people. One reason that organ transplant is unacceptable with some groups is the belief that *mal aire* (bad air) enters the body if it is left open too long during surgery and increases the potential for the development of cancer.

Health-Care Practitioners

TRADITIONAL VERSUS BIOMEDICAL PRACTITIONERS

Educated physicians and nurses are often seen as outsiders, especially among newer immigrants. However, health-care professionals are viewed as knowledgeable and respected because of their education (Zoucha, 2002). To overcome this initial awkwardness, health-care providers should attempt to get to know the client on a more personal level and gain confidence before initiating treatment regimens. Engaging in small talk unrelated to the health-care encounter before obtaining a health history or providing health education is advised. Health-care providers must respect this cultural practice to achieve an optimal outcome from the encounter.

Folklore practitioners, who are usually well known by the family, are usually consulted before and during biomedical treatment. Numerous illnesses and conditions are caused by witchcraft. Specific rituals are carried out to eliminate the evils from the body. Lower socioeconomic and newer immigrants are more likely to use folk practitioners, but well-educated upper- and middle-class people also visit folk practitioners and *brujas* (witches),

on a regular basis (Torres, 2001). Although often no contradictions or contraindications to folk remedies exist, health-care providers must always consider clients' use of these practitioners to prevent conflicting treatment regimens.

Even though the Catholic Church preaches against some types of folk practitioners, they are common and meet yearly for several days in Catemaco, Veracruz. Folk practitioners include the **curandero**, who may receive their talents from God or serve an apprenticeship with an established practitioner. The **curandero** has great respect from the community, accepts no monetary payment (but may accept gifts), is usually a member of the extended family, and treats many traditional illnesses. A **curandero** does not usually treat illnesses caused by witchcraft.

The **yerbero** (also spelled **jerbero**) is a folk healer with specialized training in growing herbs, teas, and roots and who prescribes these remedies for prevention and cure of illnesses. A **yerbero** may suggest that the person go to a botanica (herb shop) for specific herbs. In addition, these folk practitioners frequently prescribe the use of laxatives.

A **sobador** subscribes to treatment methods similar to those of a Western chiropractor. The **sobador** treats illnesses, primarily affecting the joints and musculoskeletal system, with massage and manipulation.

Even though Mexicans like closeness and touch within the context of family, most tend to be modest in other settings. Women are not supposed to expose their bodies to men or even to other women. Female clients may experience embarrassment when it is necessary to touch their genitals or may refuse to have pelvic examinations as a routine part of a health assessment. Men may have strong feelings about modesty as well, especially in front of women, and may be reluctant to disrobe completely for an examination. Mexican Americans often desire that members of the same gender provide intimate care (C. Zamarripa, Fort Worth, TX, personal communication, March 2002). Health-care providers must keep in mind clients' need for modesty when disrobing or being examined. Thus, only the body part being examined should be exposed, and direct care should be provided in private. Whenever possible, a same gender caregiver should be assigned to care for Mexican Americans.

STATUS OF HEALTH-CARE PROVIDERS

Mexican American clients have great respect for health-care providers because of their training and experience. They expect health-care providers to project a professional image and be well groomed and dressed in attire that reflects their professional status (Zoucha, 2002). While having great respect for health-care providers, some Mexican Americans may distrust them out of fear that they will disclose their undocumented status. Health-care practitioners who incorporate folk practitioners, the concept of *personalismo*, and respect into their approaches to care of Mexican American clients will gain their clients' confidence and be able to obtain more thorough assessments.

Health-care providers can demonstrate respect for Mexican American clients by greeting the client with a handshake, touching the client, or holding the client's hand, all of which help to build trust in the therapeutic relationship. Providing information and involving the family in decisions regarding health; listening to the individual's concerns; and treating the individual with *personalismo*, which stresses warmth and personal relationships, also fosters trust.

CASE STUDY Mr. Sanchez is a 61-year-old Mexican American who was recently diagnosed with osteomyelitis requiring 6 to 8 weeks of intravenous antibiotic treatment in the home. Mr. Sanchez is married and has three adult children: two daughters ages 35 and 27, a son age 33, and four grandchildren ages 14, 12, 9, and 5. The youngest daughter lives with Mr. and Mrs. Sanchez. The two older children are married and live within 1 mile of the Sanchez family. Mr. Sanchez's 85 year-old mother, Doña Reyna Sanchez (called Mama Reyna), lives with them. All members of the family were born in the United States with the exception of Mama Reyna, who was born in San Juan Obispo, Mexico. Mr. Sanchez has worked in a steel mill for the last 40 years. All members of the family speak Spanish and English with the exception of Doña Sanchez who speaks mainly Spanish.

The Sanchez family are practicing Catholics as is evidenced by the religious items hanging on the walls. A small shrine is dedicated to our Lady of Guadalupe with a candle nearby. Mrs. Sanchez and Mama Reyna recently returned from a *manda* to pray for the safe recovery of Mr. Sanchez and for the health of the family. The family attends Mass every Sunday and then they have breakfast as a family. Mr. Sanchez believes that his health is in the hands of God.

The Sanchez family lives in a modest three-bedroom home, which they bought about 35 years ago. The home is located in a predominately Mexican American community. Mr. and Mrs. Sanchez are active in the church community and have other family members and friends who live in the neighborhood. The Sanchez home is usually occupied by many people and has always been known as the gathering place in the community.

Mr. Sanchez is the sole provider of the family except for a small social security check from Doña Reyna. Mrs. Sanchez worked for short periods as a secretary for the church, but she is not working at the present time. Doña Sanchez has been the caretaker of the family and has always known the ways of folk practices and home remedies. Members of the family and community seek Doña Reyna's skills of healing. Even though she has the gift of healing and knowledge of herbs, the family practices both folk and Western health care. Mrs. Sanchez, the wife, has always taken care of the family looking out for the emotional, spiritual, and physical well being. In caring for family and friends, she shows concern, love, and attention to the needs of the ill person. Mrs. Sanchez will be caring for Mr. Sanchez during his treatment for osteomyelitis.

STUDY QUESTIONS

1 | What type of health-care provider is Doña Reyna?

2 | When the home health nurse comes to administer the intravenous medication to Mr. Sanchez and teach about the care of the line, who should be included in the teaching?

3 | Explain the significance of family and kinship for the Sanchez family.

4 | Identify two stereotypes about Mexican Americans that were dispelled in this case with the Sanchez family.

5 | Describe the importance of religion for the Sanchez family.

6 | Name three things that need to be assessed that would allow the nurse to promote culturally congruent care.

7 | Identify strategies for assessment and treatment for the Sanchez family.

8 | If the family believes in the "hot and cold" theory of illness, is Mr. Sanchez's illness hot or cold? How would it be treated?

9 | Identify four major health problems of Mexican Americans in the United States.

10 | Explain the importance of *familism* in the Mexican American culture.

11 | What folk treatments might be prescribed for osteomyelitis using the hot and cold theory of treatment?

REFERENCES

Ackerman, L. K. (1997). Health problems of refugees. *Journal of the American Board of Family Practice, 10*(5), 337–348.

American Public Health Association. (2002). *Maternal health risks of immigrant women from Latin America.* Retrieved March 18, 2002, http://www.apha.org.

Andrews, M., & Boyle, J. (1999). *Transcultural concepts in nursing care* (3rd ed.) Philadelphia: JB Lippincott.

Blantan, M. L. et al. (1993). Latin and African women: Continuing disparities in health. *International Journal of Health Services, 23*(2), 555–584.

Burk, M., Wieser, P., & Keegan, L. (1995). Cultural beliefs and health behaviors of pregnant Mexican-American women: Implications for primary care. *Advances in Nursing Science, 17*(4), 37–52.

Central Intelligence Agency (CIA). *World factbook 2001.* Retrieved March 18, 2002, http://www.odci.gov/cia/publications/factbook.

Chapa, J., & Valencia, R. R. (1993). Latino population growth, demographics, characteristics, and educational stagnation: An examination of recent trends. *Hispanic Journal of Behavioral Science, 15*(2), 165–187.

Chavez, L. S. et al. (1993). Alcohol-related mortality. In T. M. Becker et al. (Eds.), *Racial and ethnic patterns of mortality in New Mexico* (pp. 108–117). Albuquerque: University of New Mexico Press.

Eden, S., & Aguilar, R. (1989). The Hispanic chemically dependent client: Considerations for diagnosis and treatment. In G. Lawson & A. Lawson

(Eds.), *Alcoholism and substance abuse in special populations* (pp. 291–295). Rockville, MD: Aspen.

Escobebe, L. G., & Remington, P. L. (1989). Birth cohort analysis of prevalence of cigarette smoking among Hispanics in the United States. *Journal of the American Medical Association, 261*(1), 66–69.

Gavagan, T., & Brodyaga, L. (1998). Medical care for immigrants and refugees. *American Family Physician, 57*(5), 1061–1068.

Geissler, E. (1998). *Pocket guide to cultural assessment* (2nd ed.). St. Louis, MO: Mosby.

Gladen, B., & Rogan, W. (1995). DDE and shortened duration of lactation in a northern Mexican town. *American Journal of Public Health, 85*(4), 504–508.

Gonzales, M. (1999). *Mexicanos*. Bloomington: Indiana University Press.

Grothaus, K. L. (1996). Family dynamics and family therapy with Mexican Americans. *Journal Psychosocial Nursing and Mental Health Services, 34*(2), 31–37.

Kemp, C. (2001). *Hispanic health beliefs and practices: Mexican and Mexican-Americans (clinical notes)*. Retrieved May 23, 2002, http://www3.baylor.edu/~Charles_Kemp/hispanic_health.htm.

Kras, E. (1989). *Management in two cultures: Bridging the gap between U.S. and Mexican managers*. Yarmouth, ME: Intercultural Press.

Locke, D. (1999). *Increasing multicultural understanding: A comprehensive model*. Newbury Park, CA: Sage.

Luckmann, J. (1999). *Transcultural communication in nursing*. Albany, NY: Delmar.

Marin, G., Posner, S. F., & Kenyon, J. B. (1993). Role of drinking status and acculturation. *Hispanic Journal of Behavioral Science, 15*(3), 343–354.

McDonald, M. (1993, January 13). Term limits: Hispanic? Latino? A national debate proves no one name pleases everyone. *Dallas Morning News*, D13, D15.

Mendoza, F. S. et al. (1992). In A. Furino (Ed.), *Health policy and the Hispanic* (pp. 97–115). Boulder, CO: Westview Press.

Meyer, M., & Beezley, W. (2000). *The Oxford history of Mexico*. Oxford: Oxford University Press.

Monrroy, L. S. (1983). Nursing care of Raza/Latino patients. In M.S. Block & L. S. Monrroy (Eds.), *Ethnic nursing care: A multicultural approach* (pp. 115–145). St. Louis, MO: Mosby.

National Sample of Registered Nurses. (1996). http://bhpr.hrsa.gov/nursing/sampsurvpre.htm.

Neff, N. (1998). Folk medicine in Hispanics in the Southwestern United States. Retrieved March 9, 2002, from http://www.riceinfo.edu/projects/Hispanichealth/Courses/mod7/mid7.html.

Olds, S., London, M., & Ladewig, P. (2000). *Maternal newborn nursing: A family-centered approach* (5th ed.) Redwood City, CA: Addison Wesley.

Pandey, D. K. et al. (2001). Community-wide coronary heart disease mortality in Mexican Americans equals or exceeds that in non-Hispanic whites: The Corpus Christi Heart Project. *American Journal of Medicine, 110*(2), 81–87.

Perez-Stable, E. J., Marin, G., & Marin, B. V. (1994). Behavioral risk factors: A comparison of Latinos and non-Latino Whites in San Francisco. *American Journal of Public Health, 84*(6), 971–976.

Rangel, E. (1999, November 5). Working toward the middle. *The Dallas Morning News*, pp. D1, D10.

Redding, A. (1999). Mexico: Update on treatment of homosexuals. Resource center of the Immigration and Naturalization Service, U.S. Department of Justice. Retrieved March 9, 2002, from http://worldpolicy.org/Americas/sexorient/mexgay-99.html.

Rivera-Andino, J., & Lopez, L. (2000). When culture complicates care. *RN, 63*(7), 47–49.

Reinert, B. (1986). The health care beliefs and practices of Mexican-Americans. *Home Health-Care Nurse, 4*(5), 23–31.

Rosales, F. (1996). *Chicano!* Houston, TX: Arte Publico Press.

Schaefer, C. (1998). *Danger zones: Homosexuality, national identity and Mexican culture*. Tucson: University of Arizona Press.

Sundquist, J., & Winkleby, M. A. (1999). Cardiovascular risk factors in Mexican American adults: A transcultural analysis of NHANES III 1988–1994. *American Journal of Public Health, 89*(5), 723–730.

Torres, E. (2001). *The folk healer: The Mexican American tradition of curanderismo*. Albuquerque, NM: Nieves Press.

Uphold, C., & Graham, M. (1998). *Clinical guidelines in family practice* (3rd ed.) Gainesville, FL: Barmarrae Books.

U.S. Census Bureau. (2001). *Population division*. http://www.census.gov.

U.S. Department of Commerce. (2000). *Statistical abstract of the U.S. 2000*. Washington, DC: U.S. Government Printing Office.

Villarruel, A. M., & Ortiz de Montellano, B. (1992). Culture and pain: a Mesoamerican perspective. *ANS Advances in Nursing Science, 15*(1), 21–32.

Williams, E. (1984). *From Columbus to Castro: The history of the Caribbean*. New York: Vintage Press.

Zapata, J., & Shippee-Rice, R. (1999). The use of folk healing and healers by six Latinos living in New England: A preliminary study. *Journal of Transcultural Nursing, 10*(2), 136–142.

Zimmerman, J. E., & Sodowsky, G. R. (1993). Influences of acculturation on Mexican-American drinking practices: Implications for counseling. *Journal of Multicultural Counseling and Development, 21*(1), 22–35.

Zoucha, R. D. (1998). The experience of Mexican Americans receiving professional nursing care: An ethnonursing study. *Journal of Transcultural Nursing, 9*(2), 34–44.

Zoucha, R. (2002). Confidence in the nursing relationship with Mexican Americans: An ethnonursing study.

Zoucha, R., & Husted, G. L. (2000). The ethical dimensions of delivering culturally congruent nursing and health care. *Issues in Mental Health Nursing, 21*(3), 325–340.

Zoucha, R., & Zamarripa, C. (1997). The significance of culture in the care of the client with an ostomy. *Journal of Wound Ostomy Continence Nursing, 24*(5), 270–276.

Chapter 18

Navajo Indians

OLIVIA STILL and DAVID HODGINS

Overview, Inhabited Localities, and Topography

OVERVIEW

American Indians are the original inhabitants of North America. Although these groups are referred to as Native Americans and Alaskan Natives, many prefer to be called American Indians or names more specific to their cultural heritage. The amount of Indian blood necessary to be considered a tribal member or American Indian varies with each tribe. Navajo Indians claim the distinction of being the largest tribe: at least one-fourth Navajo blood is required to be considered a member of the tribe. Even among Native Americans, there is controversy concerning what constitutes an American Indian. This chapter primarily describes the cultural attributes, values, beliefs, and health-care practices of the Navajo.

The **Bureau of Indian Affairs (BIA)** recognizes over 500 different American Indian tribes that extend throughout Alaska and Canada, from Maine to Florida, and from the east coast to the west coast. Subdivisions of American Indians include the Plains Indians, the Pueblos, and the Five Civilized Tribes. These Five Civilized Tribes are further subdivided into Eastern and Western bands. The Pueblo, Navajo, and Apache are located in New Mexico and Arizona, whereas the Pima and Papago tribes are located in southern Arizona. Each of these American Indian cultures is unique; however, some share similar views regarding cosmology, medicine, and family organization. (See Table 18–1 for a comparison of Indian and non-Indian cultural value systems.)

The Navajo reservation is located on a high desert plateau with sparse grazing due to very poor soil. Water, often scarce, is a valuable commodity. Sometimes, individuals have to haul water obtained from natural springs or windmills for long distances.

HERITAGE AND RESIDENCE

The Navajo, the largest American Indian **tribe**, consists of approximately 200,000 people and has one of the largest reservations in the United States, covering portions of Arizona, Utah, and New Mexico. In New Mexico, the Navajo are scattered in settlements intermingled with the Pueblo Indians and Mormon settlers. The Navajo Indians are nomadic and wander great distances searching for adequate grazing grounds for their sheep. Their **cosmology** states that they came from the first world, the black world full of demons, and came through different worlds until they finally entered the fourth world, the present turquoise world. Thus, the value of the turquoise stone is established as an important reminder of their beliefs. In addition, animals play a vital role in Navajo mythology. For example, the coyote is considered a trickster who plays pranks on other animals and humans.

REASONS FOR MIGRATION AND ASSOCIATED ECONOMIC FACTORS

In the early 1800s, many American Indian tribes were forced to migrate or were contained in forts by the military. Some Navajo were forced to walk from Eastern reservations to Fort Sill, Oklahoma. Because of the proximity of the Eastern reservation to major cities, these Navajos had earlier contact with Western civilizations. The earliest governmental agencies, trading centers, schools, and roads were on the Eastern reservation. The Western reservation remained isolated until the last 20 to 25 years. When the Navajos were released from Fort Sill, they returned to the reservation.

Because of severe economic conditions and high unemployment rates, significant migration occurs into and out of the reservations. Commercial activities on reservations are limited to businesses owned by Navajo Indians or partnerships in which a Navajo must own the

Table 18–1 *Comparison of Cultural Value Systems*

In comparing patterns of behavior between Indian culture and non-Indian culture, one should recognize that the differences are relative and not absolute. Some of these differences are as follows:

Tribal Traditional Cultural Values	Middle-Class, Urban Values
Group, clan, or tribal emphasis	Individual emphasis
Present oriented	Future oriented
Time, always with us	Time, use every minute
Age	Youth
Cooperation	Competition
Harmony with nature	Conquest of nature
Giving, sharing	Saving
Pragmatic	Theoretical
Mythology	Scientific
Patience	Impatience
Mystical	Skeptical
Shame	Guilt
Permissiveness	Social coercion
Extended family and clan	Immediate family
Nonaggressive	Aggressive
Modest	Overconfident
Silence	Noise
Respect others' religion	Convert others to religion
Religion, way of life	Religion, a segment of life
Land, water, forest belong to all	Land, etc., private domains
Beneficial, reasonable use of resource	Avarice, greedy use of resource

Source: Sando, Joe S. (1976). *Pueblo Indians.* San Francisco: Indian Historian Press, with permission.

controlling interest. On some reservations, the business owner must be from the same tribe, whereas on other reservations, other groups may not own any interest in a business. Such restrictions severely limit employment. Occasionally big businesses contract with the reservation for mining, timbering, and electrical power services. These companies usually employ Navajo residents to the maximum extent possible.

Most Indians from the western and northern tribes tend to remain on the reservation. Many of those who leave the reservation experience culture shock resulting from a rapid and drastic change in their environment. They usually return because of lack of social support systems and loss of identity and self-esteem. Many Indians return to their reservation on a regular basis to refresh and renew themselves through Blessingway ceremonies.

In contrast to the poor economic environment of some tribes, an unusual example is the Osage tribe in Oklahoma, which has oil leases. Each tribal member has head rights and receives an income from these leases. In addition, the Navajo band of *Dzilth na ol dith le* also has

oil leases, which makes their group more likely to have money. More recently, to increase revenues on reservations, many tribes have instituted gaming in the form of bingo, poker, black jack, video poker, and slot machines. The Navajo tribe has resisted this practice until recently, when the Navajo tribal council approved gaming and other activities. Even though the tribal council approved this, they did not bring it to the vote of the people and are instituting it without the approval of the tribal members.

EDUCATIONAL STATUS AND OCCUPATIONS

Educational levels for American Indians are lower than those of similar populations, creating another barrier to employment. American Indians have consistently been identified as the most underrepresented of all minority groups in colleges and universities. Before the 1970s, an increase occurred in educational achievement among American Indians; however, since then there has been a downward curve (Preito, 1989). Overall, 55.3 percent of American Indians have completed high school (Discharry, 1986.)

Traditional educational values for most American Indians are reflected in learning the tribal culture and clarifying their roles in the **clan** and the community. Competitiveness is generally discouraged among American Indian populations. In contrast to some other cultures, the American Indian culture views group activities as more important than individual accomplishments. With few support systems from American society, many American Indians quit school and return to the reservation, even in the face of severe economic difficulties. An additional practice that influenced poor educational achievement was the past practice of the BIA that took children from their parents and placed them in boarding schools where many were forbidden to speak their native language.

Occupations selected by American Indians vary, and the health-care field severely lacks Navajo professionals. Nursing is perceived as an undesirable profession because Navajo beliefs consider it inadvisable to be around sick people. Additionally, since the culture of nursing is based on middle-class values related to competition, it is difficult for American Indian students to adjust in the nursing environment. As a result, the need for American Indian workers to staff hospitals and other health-care facilities remains high. Navajos choosing to work in a hospital must sometimes have a special cleansing ceremony to protect themselves. Many American Indian students choose careers such as social workers, laborers, artists, and weavers.

Art is an important occupation and takes such forms as rug weaving, basket weaving, pottery making, and beadwork. Rug weaving and jewelry making are the most common forms of art among the Navajo. They are also noted for **sand paintings**, which traditionally were used in healing ceremonies by medicine people and not originally intended for sale. Original sand paintings, created on the hogan floor, were gathered and returned to the earth (Medicine Man, Coho, personal communication, August 1994).

Communication

DOMINANT LANGUAGE AND DIALECTS

The dominant language varies with each American Indian tribe. The Navajo language was not reduced to writing until the 1970s; consequently, most elderly Navajo speak only their native language and few are literate in the English language. The few elderly Navajo who are bilingual speak limited Spanish or English. The younger populations are usually bilingual, with their native tongue being spoken primarily in the home. Both the Navajo and Zuni tribes had assistance from non-American Indians in developing the written form of their language.

Dialects also differ among tribes. The Navajo and the Apache have similar dialects, Athbascan, and are able to understand one another to a limited extent. These dialects are similar to variations in English found among the northern and southern regions in the United States. Even though a common language is spoken, the tribes have difficulty understanding one another related to regional accents and the use of slang expressions. Health-care providers must be extremely careful when attempting to use Navajo, because minor variations in pronunciation may change the entire meaning of a word or phrase. Differences in pronunciation, particularly while speaking with an elderly Navajo, may cause a misunderstanding. Such misunderstandings make subsequent caring for the individual difficult. Thus, it is often safer to use an interpreter.

Talking loudly among Navajo Indians is considered rude. When American Indians talk outside their group, voice tones are quiet, but not monotone. Their language is full of inflections with different meanings, making the language melodious with a quiet volume.

CULTURAL COMMUNICATION PATTERNS

Nonverbal communication styles have different connotations within each tribe. For example, the willingness of Indians to share their thoughts and feelings varies from group to group and from individual to individual. In addition, there is no set pattern regarding their willingness to share tribal ceremonies. However, suspicion always exists because earlier government and church groups banned tribal ceremonies and events. Navajos generally do not share inner thoughts and feelings with anyone outside their clan. It sometimes takes nontribal health-care providers a long time to build trust with American Indians.

Navajo Indians are comfortable with long periods of silence. Interest in what an individual says is shown through attentive listening skills. Chisholm (1983) reported that to establish a positive social relationship, the rule of silence is considered a serious matter that calls for caution, careful judgment, and plenty of time. It is important to allow time for elderly Navajo to respond to questions. Failing to allow adequate time for information processing may result in an inaccurate response or no response. One may be considered immature if answers are given quickly or one interrupts another who is forming a response.

The elderly Navajo are more somber and less likely to laugh aloud except in family settings. For example, a nurse complained, "I don't know why the family comes in here for they only sit there. They don't even say a word to the person and then they get up and walk out." What this nurse failed to realize was that they were supporting the individual, not through talking, but just by being present. The nurse's view reflects her cultural bias that saying something is essential for demonstrating support, but in reality, for American Indians, silence is being supportive. An awareness of nonverbal communication is extremely helpful for health-care providers who wish to establish mutually satisfying relationships.

Touch among the Navajo is unacceptable unless one knows the person very well. In some tribes, touch is very important because many forms of traditional medicine involve massaging and rubbing by the traditional healer, a family member, or both. However, if a Western health-care provider were to do this even within the context of treatment, it would not be permissible. If contact is made, it is in the form of a handshake. Close observation of body language is very important for determining cues related to the permissibility of touch.

In the Navajo tribe, shaking hands is the traditional greeting. However, their handshake is different from that of other populations where a firm handshake is expected. In the Navajo world, the handshake is light, more of a passing of the hands. This type of handshake in the European American society is known as a "dead fish handshake." Traditionally, Navajo's greet by saying *Yay ta hey*, literally translated as "all is well" or "it is well," and by shaking hands.

Among the Navajo, it is considered rude for people to point with their fingers. Rather than pointing a finger to indicate a direction, individuals shift their lips toward the desired direction. Seeing this nonverbal behavior for the first time can be puzzling for non-American Indian health-care providers.

Physical distance between conversants differs among friends and strangers. One quickly learns that the acceptable personal space for American Indians is greater than that of most European American cultures.

Direct eye contact is considered rude and possibly confrontational for the Navajo. Even close friends do not maintain eye contact, and this rule does not change with socioeconomic status. This is in direct opposition to some other populations where maintaining direct eye contact is essential to trust.

The American Indian is often referred to as having a deadpan expression. This is only true with strangers but not among their own group, where smiling and laughing are quite common. However, in unfamiliar settings, behaviors may be different.

TEMPORAL RELATIONSHIPS

The time sequences of importance for American Indians are present, past, and future in comparison with the time sequences important to most European Americans, which are present, future, and past (Burke,

Kisilevsky, & Maloney, 1989). Most American Indian tribes are not future oriented. Very little planning is done for the future because their view is that many things are outside of one's control and may affect or change the future. In fact, the Navajo language does not include a future tense verb. Time is not viewed as a constant or something that one can control, but rather as something that is always with the individual. Thus, to plan for the future is sometimes viewed as foolish. Past events are an important part of the American Indian's heritage as evidenced in verbal histories passed down from generation to generation. The present is addressed as a here-and-now issue.

The term *Indian time* has little meaning in a European American worldview, but it assumes particular importance for those who supervise an American Indian workforce, where time has no meaning or importance. Events do not always start on time, but rather time starts when the group gathers. To help prevent frustration in scheduling events, time factors need to be taken into consideration and the speaker made aware of these unique time perceptions. Appointments may not always be kept, especially if someone else in the clan needs help.

FORMAT FOR NAMES

Elderly people are addressed as grandmother or grandfather, or mother or father by members in their clan. Otherwise, they are called by a nickname. A health-care provider can call an older Navajo client "grandmother" or "grandfather" as a sign of respect.

Family Roles and Organization

HEAD OF HOUSEHOLD AND GENDER ROLES

The Navajo society and most other American Indian tribes are matrilineal. The land is not owned, but grazing rights are passed from mothers to daughters. While men are seen as important, the grandmothers and mothers are at the center of Navajo society. In Navajo tradition, the relationship between brother and sister is often more important than the relationship between husband and wife. These defined roles have been maintained over centuries. Some tribes are bilineal and share equally in the decision making. When providing family care, it is important to note that no decision is made until the appropriate elderly woman is present. If the health-care provider does not find the appropriate gatekeeper, time is lost and the problem must be addressed again at a later time.

Traditionally, Navajo men are expected to care for the livestock, the corral, and the fields. Men move with their sheep grazing over large areas. Women care for and stay close to the hogan, are independent, and often weave (Fig. 18–1). In recent times, changes from traditional roles have created stress and cultural disintegration as some family members have migrated off the reservation.

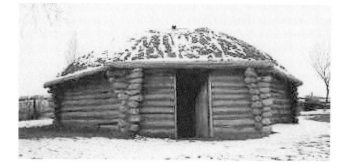

FIGURE 18–1   A typical hogan on a Native American reservation.

PRESCRIPTIVE, RESTRICTIVE, AND TABOO BEHAVIORS FOR CHILDREN AND ADOLESCENTS

Children are looked on with joy and proudly welcomed into the family. Ritual ceremonies and practices occur at various stages for both children and adolescents. Even though children may be named at birth, their names are not revealed until their first laugh, when they are considered to officially have a soul and self-identity. This protects the children and keeps them in tune with the Holy People. The "first laugh ceremony" is celebrated with food, which encourages the child to be a generous individual. Anthropologists believe that the tradition of not naming the infant until this time came about because of high infant mortality in the past.

During the cradleboard phase of child rearing, infants are kept in the cradleboard until they begin walking. The cradleboard protects them when they start to crawl and is introduced to siblings and inattentive adults. However, hip dysplasia may be exacerbated by the cradleboards. In recent years, the use of diapers has decreased the incidence of hip dysplasia because diapers bind the hips in a slightly abducted position.

The postcradleboard period consists of weaning, toilet training, and disciplining, which are frequently left to the grandmother. Thus, the language and culture are well entrenched as traditions are passed to grandchildren. If the grandmother is unavailable, an aunt or a sister assumes this role. Weaning is started during this phase if the mother is pregnant. However, if the mother is not pregnant, weaning is more gradual.

Navajo women in the past almost exclusively practiced breast-feeding, but within the last 15 to 20 years, the use of formula has become popular. As a result, an increased incidence of bottle caries has been observed among Navajo children, because many babies go to bed with a bottle of juice or soda pop. This practice causes children to lose their teeth by the age of 4 years. One health promotion priority is to educate parents about this early to prevent dental caries and to encourage a return to breast-feeding.

A primary social premise is that no person has the right to speak for another. Thus, Navajo children are frequently allowed to make decisions that other cultures might consider irresponsible. For example, children may be allowed to decide if they want to take their medicine. This practice may present an ethical concern for some health-care providers. Such practices support perceptions among health-care providers that children are undisciplined. Children who do not listen to their parents or elders accept the consequences regardless of their age. As clients, Navajo children are usually shy and wary of strangers.

An important ceremonial ritual in Navajo society for teenage girls is the onset of menarche, which is celebrated with special foods that symbolize passage into adulthood. Men are usually excluded from this celebration, with only aunts and grandmothers participating. Some tribes have a specific rite of passage for young men, but the Navajo do not. Older children may be more comfortable with physical closeness rather than actual contact. In addition, older children are taught to be stoic and uncomplaining.

FAMILY GOALS AND PRIORITIES

Family goals are a priority in the American Indian culture. Family bonds remain strong, even marriage joins the couple with another family. When a couple marries in the Zuni tribe, it is the man who goes to live in the woman's house. In Navajo tradition, families have separate dwellings but are grouped together by familial relationships. The Navajo family unit consists of the nuclear family and relatives such as sisters, aunts, and their female descendants. Family goals do not center on wealth or the attainment of possessions. In fact, if one person has more wealth than other relatives, the member who has more has a responsibility to assist relatives who have less.

The elderly Navajo are looked on with clear deference. A man with many dependents, though poor, is listened to with respect. The elderly Navajo play an important role in keeping rituals and in instructing children and grandchildren. Even though the elderly are respected, elder neglect is on the rise, possibly as a result of the increased survival of individuals with chronic disease and improved longevity. Younger adults are faced with the responsibility of caring for relatives over a longer period of time. In addition, there are few nursing homes, and hospitals are forced to keep patients until a nursing home placement is found. When nursing home placement is found, it may be at a great distance from the family, making it difficult for family visits. Hence, elders are often taken from the nursing home, even though the family is not in a position to care for their needs. Patients end up being readmitted to the hospital and a revolving door syndrome develops.

Extended family members are important in Navajo society, particularly the mother's family. A sister's children are considered the same as her own children. If a mother dies or for some other reason cannot care for her children, it is assumed that the grandmother or sister will raise the children as her own.

Social status is determined by age and life experiences. Generally, individuals are discouraged from having more than their peers, and those who display more material wealth are ignored. Status derives from not standing out in the clan or tribe.

ALTERNATIVE LIFESTYLES

Alternative lifestyles are not discussed among the Navajo. However, special individuals exist who are not looked on with disfavor, but rather are accepted as being different. In Zuni society and some northern tribes, some men take on women's roles. There are no pressures for them to change. Single-parent households are becoming more prevalent and are an accepted practice, with family members providing assistance with child rearing. It is common for a mother to have children from different fathers.

Workforce Issues

CULTURE IN THE WORKPLACE

Many American Indians remain traditional in their practice of religious activities. Navajo are compelled to attend these ceremonies and often must take time from work to do so. For example, the burial ceremony of the Zuni requires individuals to take off 3 days from work. The needs of the individual must be weighed against organizational requirements in the development of a reasonable solution. Many people in the community function informally as cultural brokers and assist by helping non-American Indian staff to understand important cultural issues. Sensitivity on the part of the employer is of utmost importance. The **Indian Health Service (IHS)** has developed a method for addressing these needs. Besides allowing employees to use annual leave, employees may earn religious compensatory time. Respected non-Indian staff are sensitive to American Indian cultural issues. The American Indian staff reciprocates this respect during traditional European American holidays.

European Americans who are upset or in conflict often want to talk through the issue that has caused the conflict. This may not be the case with American Indians. Many American Indians avoid people with whom they are in conflict. Persistence in dealing immediately with the conflict causes additional ill feelings. This may continue to the point that the American Indian loses his or her temper and expresses anger toward the other person. The European American, in the eyes of the American Indian, exhibits rude behavior by continuing to press for resolution. The American Indian method of resolving anger and conflict among themselves is much different. If one tribal member has a disagreement with another, that member does not address the second party face to face. Rather the member tells a third person, who then relays the information to the second party. The conflict is resolved through a third-party compromise.

ISSUES RELATED TO AUTONOMY

Group activities are an important norm in the Navajo culture. One individual should not be singled out for answering a question because one's mistakes are generally not forgotten by the group. For example, if an individual is quick to answer and is wrong, the entire group laughs. Later, the group talks about the mistake and again laughs about it. Conversely, when remarks are made concerning an individual without group participation, revenge may be sought in a passive-aggressive manner. The transgression is not forgotten. Conversely, in American society, mistakes may be forgiven as an acceptable method of learning as long as the mistakes are not repeated. Administrators who respect these differences are more effective.

This concept is also true in the classroom. The instructor who allows adequate time for observation has a greater chance of success with American Indian students. Improved success is achieved if the American Indian is allowed to observe the task several times before being asked to demonstrate it. Their first effort at completing the task in front of a group should occur without error. This is especially true when delivering care to their own people. Mistakes that have been made are discussed in the community. Because educational levels may be low, work assignments should be made in clear concrete terms.

Issues of superior-subordinate roles exist, and are related to age. Younger supervisors may not be respected because they are not perceived as possessing the life experiences necessary to lead. In like situations, major decisions are made by the group with the assistance of the group leader, who is generally the senior woman. Thus, a young male manager on the reservation may face resistance when attempting to direct a work group.

Because English may not be their primary language, one must often allow extra time for a verbal response from most Navajo. This extra time is required to think about a response and translate it into English. When translating from the native Indian language into English, adjectives and adverbs sometimes follow the noun or verb, making it appear that the person is speaking backwards.

Most American Indian students are not good test takers, which poses a special problem. Although the individual may have the knowledge necessary to complete an examination, the translation of the knowledge into written form is especially difficult. When tested verbally on the same material, students pass the examination. To the extent possible, examinations that consist of return demonstration and that do not use abstract terminology are preferred. Thus, in the ethnocultural context of teaching Navajo students and staff, actions should be directed toward assisting, supporting, or enabling the individual or group to improve a human condition or way of life.

Biocultural Ecology

SKIN COLOR AND OTHER BIOLOGICAL VARIATIONS

Skin color among American Indians varies from light brown to very dark brown depending on the tribe. To assess for oxygenation in darker-skinned people, health-care professionals must examine the client's mucous membranes and nailbeds for capillary refill. Anemia is detected by examining the mucous membranes for pallor and the skin for a grayish hue. To assess for jaundice, it is necessary to examine the sclera rather than to rely on skin hue. Newborns and infants commonly have Mongolian spots on the sacral area. Health-care professionals unfamiliar with this trait may mistake these spots for bruises and suspect child abuse.

Each of the American Indian tribes has varying degrees of Asian traits. In facial appearance, the Athabascan tribes, such as the Navajo, appear Asian, with epithelial folds over the eyes. The Navajo are generally taller and thinner than other American Indian tribes. The Navajo have traditionally been good runners and excel in relay races and long-distance running. Health-care providers must remember that these characteristics are not seen with everyone; variations in this population do exist.

DISEASES AND HEALTH CONDITIONS

The water on the Navajo reservation is often impure and unchlorinated, making those who drink it susceptible to waterborne bacteria such as *Shigella*. Some notable risk factors are related to the topography of the Navajo reservation: *Salmonella* is common because of the lack of refrigeration, and hypothermia because of frequent snow storms and conditions that limit their ability to gather wood. For example, most of the dirt roads quickly become impassable with rain or snow.

Common diseases related to living in close contact with others include upper respiratory illnesses and acute otitis media (Indian Health Service, 2000). In the 1950s, many families suffered from tuberculosis, but more recent cases are related to isolated family groups. Comparing the 1994 to 1996 Indian age-adjusted death rates with all races of the United States population in 1995 reveals the following higher death rates in the American Indian population:

- Alcoholism 627 percent higher
- Tuberculosis 533 percent
- Diabetes mellitus 249 percent
- Unintentional injuries 204 percent
- Suicide 72 percent
- Pneumonia and influenza 71 percent
- Homicide 63 percent
- Gastrointestinal disease 42 percent
- Infant mortality 22 percent
- Heart disease 13 percent

Even more alarming, the most recent data presently being gathered by the National Center for Health Statistics documents that the mortality disparities are worsening. Other health problems include the plague, tick fever, and recently the Muerto Canyon Hanta virus. Many of these illnesses are due to the area's rodent population, consisting of prairie dogs and deer mice.

Type I diabetes mellitus is almost nonexistent in American Indians; however, type II diabetes mellitus is the third most prevalent disease affecting all American Indian tribes. In the year 2000, the **IHS** and tribal clinics recorded almost 500,000 outpatient visits for diabetes (U.S. Department of Health and Human Services, 1998).

The incidence of diabetes varies among tribes. Navajo's rate of diabetes has steadily increased and is approaching 30 percent. Poor control and dietary compliance is associated with major long-term complications such as blindness and kidney failure. These complications in American Indians occur at a greater rate than in European American populations. Dialysis clinics have been opened in all of the major Navajo communities such as Chinle, Tuba City, Kayenta, and Shiprock.

Because of the prevalence of diabetes among Indians, Congress has delegated funds exclusively for diabetes research and education in this population. The National Institutes for Health and the diabetes team on several reservations are presently engaged in research with high school students to determine the age of onset of type II diabetes. Thus far, the youngest student is age 8; however, controversy exists over whether this case is type I or type II diabetes.

Historically, most diseases affecting American Indians were infectious. In the past, contact with settlers who had communicable diseases eliminated entire tribes because they had no acquired immunity for some infectious diseases that were common among other American populations.

Cardiovascular diseases are on the increase among the Navajo. The incidence of myocardial infarction, nearly nonexistent until recent times, is increasing, as is the incidence of renal disease and gallbladder disease. Transports to tertiary care hospitals are occurring at a rate of ten per month from one hospital. In 1998 the numbers were one or two a month.

Studies with the Navajo have identified a high incidence of **severe combined immunodeficiency syndrome (SCIDS)**, an immunodeficiency syndrome unrelated to AIDS, that results in a failure of the antibody response and cell-mediated immunity (World Health Organization Scientific Group, 1986). An epidemiological study is underway to determine the prevalence of SCIDS in the Navajo population. Factors being examined include space, time, pedigree, and immunologic status. Affected infants who survive initially are sent to tertiary care facilities. Survivors must receive gamma globulin on a regular basis until a bone marrow transplant can be performed. Thus far, studies indicate that SCIDS is unique to this Navajo population.

Navajo neuropathy, researched since 1974, is also unique to this population. Characteristics of this disease include poor weight gain, short stature, sexual infantilism, serious systemic infections, and liver derangement. Manifestations include weakness, hypotonia, areflexia, loss of sensation in the extremities, corneal ulcerations, acral mutilation, and painless fractures. Sural nerve biopsies show a nearly complete absence of myelinated fibers, which is different from other neuropathies that present a gradual demyelination process. Individuals who survive have many complications and are generally ventilator dependent. None have been known to survive past the age of 24.

In 1985, a study reported a new type of hereditary sensorimotor neuropathy in six Navajo children from three families (Carter, Pugh, & Monterrosa, 1996). Of these children, four had Charot joints of the knees and ankles, two had less severe, painless and deforming foot fractures, and five had deficiencies in seating and some degree of heat intolerance. All had hyperkeratosis of the palms of the hands and diminished response to pressure.

The annual incidence of Navajo neuropathy on the Navajo Reservation between 1972 and 1986 was 20 cases per 100,000 births. In 1993 Johnson reported eight more children with the disease, all from the western half of the reservation. An autosomal recessive gene originating from a single common ancestry may explain this. A founder effect has been proposed as the genetic basis of Navajo neuropathy (Kerth, personal communication, 1997). A potential candidate gene for Navajo neuropathy is currently under investigation.

Albinism occurs in the Navajo and Pueblo tribes. An additional disease that affects Navajos who live in the Rainbow Grand Canyon area is genetically prone blindness that develops in individuals during their late teens and early 20s. Many of these hereditary and genetic diseases are believed to result from a limited gene pool. As a result of the increased availability of Western medicines, improved sanitary conditions, increased community surveillance, early case finding, and improved education, survival has increased and chronic diseases related to lifestyle are surfacing.

VARIATIONS IN DRUG METABOLISM

Research has documented adverse reactions to medication in Navajo populations (Hodgins & Still, 1989). Lidocaine reactions occur in 29 percent of the Navajo population as compared with 11 to 15 percent of European Americans. Little research has been completed that distinguishes absorption differences of specific medications in American Indian populations.

High-Risk Behaviors

Most American Indian tribes exhibit high-risk behaviors related to alcohol abuse, along with its subsequent morbidity and mortality. Alcohol use is more prevalent than any other form of chemical abuse. Health problems related to alcoholism include motor vehicle accidents, homicides, suicides, and cirrhosis (Indian Health Service, 2000). Many accidents are attributed to driving while under the influence of alcohol. Although alcohol is illegal on most reservations, alcohol is purchased off the reservation by many, and bootleggers make money selling alcohol on reservations at grossly inflated prices. The northern tribes living on the Rosebud Sioux reservation have a higher alcoholism rate than most other American Indian tribes. This is often attributed to an unemployment rate of 50 percent among these tribes.

Spousal abuse is common and is frequently related to alcohol use. The wife is the usual recipient of the abuse, but occasionally the husband is abused. Emergency rooms have documented cases of husbands being beaten by their wives with baseball bats in response to their drinking. The effects of alcohol abuse are also evidenced in newborns as fetal alcohol syndrome, in teenagers as pregnancies and sexually transmitted diseases, and in adults as liver failure. One research study on school achievement among Native Americans linked weekly and daily alcohol abuse with low high school graduating rates of only 33 to 40 percent. Incarcerated Native American youths in major urban centers begin drinking at an earlier age than other youths, had more binge drinking episodes, and used more illegal drugs (Social Issues Research Center, 2002).

Although smoking is not as prevalent as in some other cultures, the use of smokeless tobacco has steadily increased among teenagers and those in their early 20s. Cocaine is rarely used by Navajo Indians because of its high cost and limited accessibility.

Suicide is becoming more prevalent among the adolescent population. Attempted drug overdoses occur in an effort to get even with someone. In Tuba City, two sisters decided to commit suicide together because they felt there was no alternative to their present life.

Acquired immunodeficiency syndrome (AIDS), thus far, has not presented a major problem on the Navajo reservation. However, health officials believe that when it does occur, it will spread rapidly because high rates of other sexually transmitted diseases occur in Navajo communities. To help combat these diseases, an increased emphasis on community-based programs has been initiated to provide improved education for adults and teenagers.

HEALTH-CARE PRACTICES

A number of programs among the Navajo promote public awareness and encouragement for positive health-seeking behaviors. These include programs encouraging seat belt and helmet use for those who bicycle or ride motorcycles. Unfortunately, the success of these programs has been limited. Seat belts are required by state law as well as by tribal law enforcement agencies. Although many adults comply with these laws, noncompliance is high among younger Indians. Unfortunately, children are often permitted to ride in the back of open trucks, resulting in serious and sometimes fatal injuries when they fall off or are thrown from vehicles.

Health promotion programs have been initiated in an attempt to reestablish healthy behaviors. These programs also promote runs, relay races, and aerobic classes. The Navajo have visited this program in an attempt to develop a similar program. The younger generation has responded well to wellness programs. However, promoting these programs among the elderly tribal members has met with limited success.

Nutrition

MEANING OF FOOD

Food has major significance beyond nourishment in American Indian populations; it is offered to family and friends or may be burned to feed higher powers and those who have died. Life events are celebrated with food. Food is the center of all dances and many healing and religious ceremonies.

The importance of food is evident when a family sponsors a dance. Sponsors of this event are expected to feed the participants and their entire families. Food preparation takes several days. Women cook large amounts of food, which may include green chili stew, mutton, and fry bread, cooked over an outdoor fireplace.

COMMON FOODS AND FOOD RITUALS

Sheep are a major source of meat, and sheep brains are considered a delicacy by the Navajo. Traditionally, in sheep camps where the herds are tended, food is limited to what can be cooked outside. Fry bread and mutton are cooked in lard. Access to fresh fruits or vegetables is minimal except during the fall. Squash is common at harvest time.

In years past, it was taboo for the Navajo to eat chicken. This is no longer the case, and now chicken is an integral part of their diet. In fact, chicken is so popular that commercial fast-food chicken establishments have emerged on the Navajo reservation. A concurrent increased incidence of gallbladder disease is attributed to this dietary practice. Clients as young as 11 years old are having cholecystectomies.

Corn is an important staple in the diet of Navajo and other American Indian tribes. Rituals such as the green corn dance of the Cherokees and harvest time rituals for the Zuni surround the use of corn. Corn pollen is used in the Blessingway and many other ceremonies by the Navajo.

DIETARY PRACTICES FOR HEALTH PROMOTION

Food is not generally associated with promoting health or illness among the Navajo. The establishment of diabetic projects in all American Indian service units has prompted teaching that integrates the optimal selection, preparation, and quantities of native foods to encourage good health habits. This is especially important for elderly tribe members, who are less likely to change their diets but may be willing to change methods of preparation or amounts eaten. Herbs are used in the treatment of many illnesses to cleanse the body of ill spirits or poisons.

NUTRITIONAL DEFICIENCIES AND FOOD LIMITATIONS

American Indian diets may be deficient in vitamin D because many individuals suffer from lactose intolerance or do not drink milk. Many individuals in the Navajo tribe and some other isolated tribes lack electricity for refrigeration. Therefore, they have difficulty storing fresh vegetables or milk. Malnutrition, such as kwashiorkor and marasmus, occurred in the Navajo as late as the 1960s and 1970s. After some ceremonies, individuals may not eat salt or particular foods. For example, during initiation into some American Indian societies, young boys have a restricted diet. It is important for the health-care provider to assess whether a ceremony has been recently performed and ask if there are specific food restrictions.

Pregnancy And Childbearing Practices

FERTILITY PRACTICES AND VIEWS TOWARD PREGNANCY

Traditional American Indians do not practice birth control and, thus, do not limit the size of their families. The birth rate among American Indians is 96 percent higher than the birth rate in the overall U.S. population. Large families are looked on favorably because, in times past, many children died at an early age. Survival rates of American Indian children have greatly improved within the last few years.

In the past, many traditional Navajo women did not seek prenatal care because pregnancy was not considered an illness. Today, more pregnant women seek prenatal care at **IHS** facilities. Health-care providers can improve the health of Navajo women and children by encouraging prenatal care. (See Table 20–2 for a cultural nursing intervention assessment tool for expectant Navajo women.)

Twins are not looked on favorably and are frequently believed to be the work of a witch, in which case one of the babies must die. Recent observations reveal that this no longer happens, but sometimes the mother may have difficulty caring for two infants. For example, twins may be readmitted to the hospital for neglect and failure to thrive. In such instances, culturally sensitive counseling assists adoption. Despite a social worker's assistance, some mothers may not be able to cope with twins, and eventually tribal members adopt the children.

PRESCRIPTIVE, RESTRICTIVE, AND TABOO PRACTICES IN THE CHILDBEARING FAMILY

Arthur (1976) described Navajo pregnancy ceremonies, taboos, and herbal medicine practices in the prebirth phase of pregnancy recognition. In this phase, the extended family and community assists the mother in recognizing the pregnancy as a reality. During the

Table 18–2 Nursing Care and Beliefs of Expectant Navajo Women: Cultural Nursing Intervention Assessment Tool

1 Do you want blood, urine, or other specimens returned?

_____ Yes _____ No Comments:

2 Do you wish to use herbs during labor and after delivery?

_____ Yes _____ No Comments:

3 According to your beliefs, what foods are you not allowed to eat?

4 During labor, would you like a medicine woman present to perform a ceremony if necessary?

_____ Yes _____ No Comments:

5 During labor, do you want your long hair braided?

_____ Yes _____ No Comments:

6 During labor, what position do you want to deliver in?

_____ Squatting position _____ Lying-down position

_____ Side-lying position _____ Use stirrups

_____ Any position that is comfortable for me

Comments:

7 During labor, do you want to use the sash belt to hold onto for delivery?

_____ Yes _____ No Comments:

8 Who will be with you during labor and delivery?

9 After delivery, do you or someone in your family want to massage the baby?

_____ Yes _____ No Comments:

10 Do you want to save the afterbirth (placenta)?

_____ Yes _____ No Comments:

11 Do you want to save the baby's umbilical cord?

_____ Yes _____ No Comments:

12 After delivery, do you want to save the baby's first stool?

_____ Yes _____ No Comments:

13 Do you want to _____ breast-feed or _____ formula feed your baby? If you want to do both ways of feeding, please tell us the reason?

14 What kinds of things do you expect nurses to do for you during labor and delivery?

Source: Ursula Wilson, July 1987. IHS inservice seminar, Tuba City Indian Health Center, Tuba City, AZ, with permission.

precradleboard phase, a **hogan** is designated for the birth, and a religious practitioner ties to the **hogan** a red sash for a girl and a buckskin rope for a boy. These are used to give the mother support during delivery. At this time, the pregnant woman becomes one with Mother Earth, Father Sky, and the Universe with the Holy People; therefore, she is actually reliving the creation plan of humankind (Arthur, 1976). It is especially important to adhere to the many prescriptive and restrictive taboo practices related to pregnancy, which involve both husband and wife. See Table 18–3, Navajo Taboos Regarding Expectant Women, and Table 18–4, Taking Care of Yourself during Pregnancy: Navajo Rules for Expectant Couples, which were developed by Urusla Wilson in 1987.

Many Navajo women are reluctant to deliver their babies in hospital settings. They know that people have died in hospitals and thus perceive that pregnant women should not be around the dead or in a place where people have died. To provide culturally competent care, many facilities, with the assistance of individuals like Ursula Wilson, are reinstituting more traditional American Indian methods of birthing into the hospital setting. These adaptations include birthing rooms that are more acceptable to Navajo women. The blending of Western traditional methods with American Indian practices has greatly improved the health care of American Indian women.

During the labor process, the mother wears birthing necklaces made of juniper seeds and beads to assist with a safe birth. Woven belts or sashes are used to help push the baby out (see Table 18–4). This practice is also used by Navajo midwives in caring for their clients.

A taboo practice among the Navajo is purchasing clothes for an infant before birth. Outsiders may inter-pret this practice as the mother not wanting the baby. In reality, preparing for the baby before birth is forbidden by Indian tradition.

Many different rituals related to postpartum care exist for each tribe. Table 18–4 lists some Navajo taboos during the postpartum period. The cultural assessment tool (see Table 18–2) developed by Ursula Wilson can be adapted to the practices of other tribes to acknowledge general American Indian beliefs and values regarding labor and delivery.

Immediately after birth, the placenta is buried as a symbol of the child being tied to the land. Sometimes it is burned in a fire. This is considered a safe place because fire is sacred and protects the baby against evil spirits. After birth, the baby is given a mixture with juniper bark to cleanse its insides and rid it of mucus. In addition, a ceremonial food of corn pollen and boiled water is given. Corn symbolizes healthy nutrients and an enduring nature.

Death Rituals

DEATH RITUALS AND EXPECTATIONS

Death rituals vary among tribes. The body must go into the afterlife as whole as possible. In some tribes, amputated limbs are given to the family for a separate burial. These limbs are later exhumed and buried with the body. The Navajo do not bury the body for approxi-mately 4 days after death. A cleansing ceremony must be performed after an individual dies or the spirit of the dead person may try to assume control of someone else's spirit. Frequently, family members are reluctant to deal with the body because those who work with the dead

Table 18–3 *Navajo Taboos Regarding Expectant Women*

1 Don't wear two hats at once; you'll have twins (or two wives).
2 Don't hit babies in the mouth; they'll be stubborn and slow to talk.
3 Don't have a weaving comb (rug) with more than five points; your baby will have extra fingers.
4 Don't have a baby cross its fingers; its mother will have another one right away.
5 Don't swallow gum while you are pregnant; the baby will have a birthmark.
6 Don't kill animals while your wife is pregnant; the baby will look like a bird.
7 Don't stand in the doorway when a pregnant woman is present.
8 Don't make a slingshot while you are pregnant; the baby will be crippled.
9 Don't go to ceremonies while pregnant; it will have a bad effect on the baby.
10 Don't eat a lot of sweet stuff while you are pregnant; the baby won't be strong.
11 Don't sleep too much when you are about to have a baby; the baby will mark your face with dark spots.
12 Don't look at a dead person or animal while you are pregnant; the baby will be sickly because of bad luck.
13 Don't jump around if you are pregnant or ride a horse; it will induce labor.
14 Don't cut gloves off at the knuckles, the baby will have short round fingers.
15 Don't cut a baby's hair when it is small; it won't think right when it gets older.
16 Don't put on a Yei mask while your wife is pregnant; the baby will have a big head and look strange.
17 Don't let a baby's head stay to one side in the cradle board; it will have a wide head.
18 Don't watch or look at an accident while your wife is present; it will affect the baby.
19 Don't sew on a saddle while your wife is pregnant; it will ruin the baby's mouth.

Source: Ursula Wilson, July 1987. IHS inservice seminar, Tuba City Indian Health Center, Tuba City, AZ, with permission.

Table 18–4 *Taking Care of Yourself during Pregnancy: Navajo Rules for Expectant Couples*

DURING PRENATAL PERIOD

Mind/Soul

Do's
- Keep the peace
- Keep thoughts good
- Talk with "corn pollen sprinkled" words
- Say morning (dawn prayers)
- Have shielding prayers done if you have nightmares

Don'ts
- Argue with partner or others
- Scold children
- Allow bad thoughts to occupy mind for long period of time
- Talk negatively or with criticism

Body

Do's
- Eat foods good for baby
- Get up early and walk around
- Have a Blessingway ceremony for a safe delivery

Don'ts
- Drink milk or eat salt or foods taken away by Navajo ceremonies
- Lay around too much
- Tie knots
- Attend funerals or look at body of deceased person
- Be with sick people for long or go to crowded place
- Attend healing ceremonies for sick people like "Yei Bei Chai Dance"
- Look at dead animals or taxidermic trophies
- Look at eclipse of moon or sun
- Make plans for baby or prepare layette sets until after birth
- Don't lift heavy things
- Don't kill living things or cut a sheep's throat
- Don't weave rugs or make pottery

DURING LABOR

Mind/Soul

Do's
- Think about a good delivery
- Have medicine people do "Singing Out Baby" chants
- Have medicine person perform "Unraveling" songs if necessary

Don'ts
- Let too many people observe labor; only people who are helping you in some way

Body

Do's
- Loosen your hair
- Drink corn meal mush
- Wear juniper seed beads
- Burn cedar
- Hold onto sash belt when ready to push
- Have someone apply gentle fundal pressure during pushing effort
- Get in squatting position for pushing
- Drink herbal tea to relax if necessary
- Drink herbal tea to strengthen contractions if necessary

Don'ts
- Braid or tie hair in a knot
- Tie knots

AFTER BIRTH OF BABY (POSTPARTUM PERIOD)

Do's
- Bury the placenta
- Drink juniper/ash tea to cleanse your insides
- Drink blue cornmeal mush
- Smear baby's first stool on your face
- Breast-feed your baby
- Wrap sash belt around waist for 4 days after delivery

Don'ts
- Drink cold liquids or be in cold draft
- Smell afterbirth blood for too long
- Show signs of displeasure if baby soils on you or during diaper change
- Burn placenta or afterbirth blood fluids
- Have sexual intercourse for 3 months after delivery

Source: Ursula Wilson, July 1987. IHS inservice seminar, Tuba City Indian Health Center, Tuba City, AZ, with permission.

must have a ceremony to protect themselves from the deceased's spirit. If the person dies at home, the **hogan** must be abandoned or a ceremony must be held to cleanse it. Individuals who choose embalming as a profession are rare, and people tend to avoid the area where the dead lived. Before a tribal member is buried they place a ring on the index finger of each hand and place their shoes on the wrong feet. This allows them to recognize the individual if they come back and present themselves at ceremonial dances. Health-care providers should not wear rings on their index fingers, as elderly people will not want to be around them.

One death taboo involves talking with clients concerning a fatal disease or illness. Effective discussions require that the issue be presented in the third person, as if the illness or disorder occurred with someone else. The health-care provider must never suggest that the client is dying. To do so would imply that the provider wishes the client dead. If the client does die, it would imply that the provider might have evil powers.

RESPONSES TO DEATH AND GRIEF

Because their fear of the power of the dead is very real, excessive displays of emotion are not looked on favorably among some tribes. The Navajo are not generally open in their expression of grief and touching the body. Grief among the Pueblo is expressed openly and involves much crying among extended family members. Even if the deceased is a distant relative and has not been seen in years, much grief is expressed. Health-care providers must support survivors and permit family bereavement and grieving in a culturally congruent and sensitive manner that respects the beliefs of each tribe.

Spirituality

DOMINANT RELIGION AND USE OF PRAYER

American-Indian religion predominates in many tribes. Missionaries continue their efforts to convert American Indians to Christian religions, such as the Church of Jesus Christ of Latter Day Saints, Jehovah's Witnesses and, to a lesser extent, Evangelical groups. When illnesses are severe, consultations with appropriate religious organizations are sought. Sometimes hospital admissions are accompanied by traditional ceremonies and consultation with a pastor. Even if people are strong in their adopted beliefs, they honor their parents and families by having a traditional healing ceremony. The current director of the **IHS** has issued a memorandum that reaffirms the rights of American Indians to conduct ceremonies in health-care facilities. This memorandum also directs **IHS** health-care providers to be attuned to the total needs of clients in order to provide culturally competent and congruent care.

Many Navajo start the day with prayer, meditation, corn pollen, and running in the direction of the sun. Prayers ask for harmony with nature and for health and invite blessings to help the person exist in harmony with the earth and sky. Along with certain ceremonies, prayer helps the Navajo to attain fulfillment and inner peace with themselves and their environment.

MEANING OF LIFE AND INDIVIDUAL SOURCES OF STRENGTH

Spirituality for most American Indians is based on harmony with nature. The meaning of life for the Navajo is derived from being in harmony with nature. The individual's source of strength comes from the inner self and also depends on being in harmony with one's surrounding.

Many tribes are concerned about outsiders from New Age movements attempting to participate in native medicine practices without an appropriate background, knowledge, and true inner source of peace. These individuals often seek to be spiritual healers using traditional Indian medicines.

SPIRITUAL BELIEFS AND HEALTH-CARE PRACTICES

Spirituality cannot be separated from the healing process in ceremonies that are holistic in nature. Illness results from not being in harmony with nature, the spirits of evil persons such as a witch, or violation of taboos. Healing ceremonies restore an individual's balance mentally, physically, and spiritually. The following are core concepts to traditional Indian medicine:

- Indians believe in a Supreme Creator.
- Each person is a three-fold being composed of mind, body, and spirit.
- All physical things, living and nonliving, are a part of the spiritual world.
- The spirit existed before it came into the body and it will exist after it leaves the body.
- Illness affects the mind and the spirit as well as the body.
- Wellness is harmony.
- Natural unwellness is caused by violation of a taboo.
- Unnatural wellness is caused by witchcraft.
- Each of us is responsible for our own health.

Health-Care Practices

HEALTH-SEEKING BELIEFS AND BEHAVIORS

Traditional American Indian beliefs influence biomedical health-care decisions. For example, for many elderly people, the germ theory is nearly impossible to comprehend. In addition, asking clients questions to make a diagnosis fosters mistrust. This approach is in conflict with the practice of traditional medicine men, who tell people what is wrong without their having to say anything.

RESPONSIBILITY FOR HEALTH CARE

Through existing treaties, the federal government assumes responsibility for the health-care needs of American Indians. Government services respect a blending of both worlds. Some tribes have contracted for money to operate their own health-care systems. Few

American Indians on reservations have traditional health insurance, and recent efforts at health-care reform have caused many tribes to fear that the government will not continue to honor its obligations under existing treaties.

The **IHS**, a federal agency providing health services to American Indians, has shifted its focus over the last 20 years from acute care to programs directed at health promotion, disease prevention, and chronic health conditions. The tribes and the **IHS** have specific mandates to meet certain health goals and objectives for a healthy population by the year 2010. While health promotion and disease prevention is a major focus of the **IHS**, these programs are often in conflict with American Indian values. Projects promoting community involvement and culturally sensitive client education are effective strategies for implementing these goals and objectives. In the last 20 years, an increase has occurred in wellness promotion activities and a return to past traditions such as running for health, avoiding alcohol, and using purification ceremonies. Mental health programs are not well funded within the **IHS** and are thus traditionally understaffed.

The focus of acute care is curative and is based on promoting harmony with Mother Earth. Before the U.S. government assumed responsibility for health care to American Indians, health care was provided by medicine men and other traditional healers.

The use of traditional healing practices is explained to physicians practicing on the reservations, but if clients perceive reluctance to accept these practices, they do not reveal their use. This is especially true among the elderly who seek hospital or clinic treatments only when their conditions become life-threatening. Younger generations seek treatment sooner and use the health-care system more readily than do elderly people. However, if their parents are traditional, they may combine native traditional medicine with Western medicine.

Self-medication with over-the-counter drugs does not present a major health concern because there are no pharmacies on the Navajo reservation. Medications are available at **IHS** facilities at no cost.

FOLK PRACTICES

The Navajo believe wellness is a state of harmony with one's surrounding. When people are ill or out of harmony, the medicine man or, in some cases, a diagnostician tells them what they have done to disrupt their harmony. They are returned to harmony through the use of a healing ceremony. The medicine man is expected to diagnose the illness and prescribe necessary treatments for regaining health. In Western health care, the practitioner asks the client what he or she thinks is wrong and then prescribes a treatment. This practice is sometimes interpreted by the American Indian as ignorance on the part of the white healer.

BARRIERS TO HEALTH CARE

On the Navajo reservation, great distances must be traveled to reach a hospital or health-care facility. Many families do not have adequate transportation and must wait for others to transport them into town. Some urban dwellers have a car but live in an area where access to an **IHS** facility is limited. Even when a car is available, many do not have the money for gasoline. There has been a recent increase in the number of urban facilities, and some tribes have established outreach clinics that help to cope with health problems.

Immunizations may be missed because parents do not have transportation. Close attention should be paid to the immunization status of clients on arrival to the emergency department or clinic. If the client is not current with immunizations, scheduling an appointment may be a waste of time because they may not be able to return until a ride is found. Health-care providers might have better success by taking the time to administer the immunization on the spot or by making a referral to the public health nursing office.

CULTURAL RESPONSES TO HEALTH AND ILLNESS

Obtaining adequate pain control is of concern for American Indians who receive care within the context of Western medicine. Frequently, pain control is ineffective because the actual intensity of their pain is not obvious to the health-care provider and because clients do not request pain medication. The Navajo views pain as something that is to be endured, and thus, they do not ask for analgesics and may not understand that pain medication is available. Other times, herbal medicines are preferred and used without the knowledge of the health-care provider. Not sharing the use of herbal medicine is a carryover from times when individuals were not allowed to practice their native medicine.

Mental illness is perceived as resulting from witches or witching (placing a curse) on a person. In these instances, a healer who deals with dreams or a crystal gazer is consulted. Individuals may wear turquoise to ward off evil; however, a person who wears too much turquoise is sometimes thought to be an evil person and, thus, someone to avoid. In some tribes, mental illness may mean that the affected person has special powers.

The concept of rehabilitation is relatively new to American Indians because in years past they did not survive to an age where chronic diseases became an issue. Because life expectancy is increasing, an additional stress is placed on families who are expected to care for elderly relatives. Many families do not have the resources to assume this responsibility. Home health care is occasionally available, but this is a recent development that tribes are just beginning to accept. Federal public health nursing is also available to assist with home care. Those with physical or mental handicaps are not seen as different; rather, the limitation is accepted and a role is found for them within the society.

Cultural perceptions of the sick role for the American Indian are based on the ideal of maintaining harmony with nature and with others. Ill people have obviously done something to place themselves out of harmony or have had a curse placed on them. In either case, support of the sick role is not generally accepted, but rather support is directed at assisting the person with regaining harmony. Elderly people frequently work even when seriously ill and often must be encouraged to rest.

BLOOD TRANSFUSIONS AND ORGAN DONATION

Autopsy and organ donation are unacceptable practices to traditional American Indians. The concepts of organ transplant and organ donation may result in a major cultural dilemma. For example, in one case, a woman needing a kidney transplant consulted a medicine man who advised against having the transplant performed. She elected to have the transplant done against the medicine man's advice, which created a cultural dilemma for her family. As more American Indians accept biomedical care from Western medical practitioners, medicine men and traditional healing practices may be lost. Increasing use of Western medical practices on reservations must be accompanied by attempting to incorporate culturally congruent traditional care into Western practices.

Health-Care Practitioners

TRADITIONAL VERSUS BIOMEDICAL PRACTITIONERS

Native healers are divided primarily into three categories: those working with the power of good, the power of evil, or both. Generally, they are divinely chosen and promote activities that encourage self-discipline and self-control and that involve acute body awareness.

Within these three categories are several types of practitioners. Some practitioners are endowed with supernatural powers, whereas others only have knowledge of herbs and specific manipulations. The first type are people who can only use their power for good, can transform themselves into other forms of life, and can maintain cultural integration in times of stress. The second group can use their powers for both evil and good and are expected to do evil against someone's enemies. People in this group know witchcraft, poisons, and ceremonies designed to afflict the enemy. The third type is the diviner diagnostician, such as a **crystal gazer**, who can see what caused the problem, but not implement a treatment. Another example of this type is a **hand trembler**. These people, instead of using crystals, practice hand trembling over the sick person to determine the cause of an illness. A fourth group are the specialist medicine people. They treat the disease after it has been diagnosed and specialize in the use of herbs, massage, or midwifery. A fifth group are those who care for the soul and send guardian spirits to restore a lost soul. A sixth group are singers, who are considered to be the most special. They cure through the power of their song. These healers are involved in the laying on of hands and usually remove objects or draw disease-causing objects from the body while singing.

Navajo tribal practitioners divide their knowledge into preventive measures, treatment regimens, and health maintenance. An example of a preventive measure is carrying an object or a pouch filled with objects, prescribed by a medicine man, that wards off the evil of a witch. Health-care providers must not remove these objects or pouches from clients. These objects contribute

to clients' mental well-being, and their removal creates undue stress. Treatment regimens prescribed by a medicine man not only cure the body but also restore the mind. An example of a health maintenance practice among the Navajo is the Blessingway ceremony, in which prayers and songs are offered. Individuals who live off reservations frequently return to participate in this ceremony, which returns them to harmony and restores a sense of well-being.

Acceptance of Western medicine is variable with a blending of traditional health-care beliefs. Experienced **IHS** providers understand the concepts of holistic health for American Indians, and a few are beginning to make referrals to the medicine man. Few physicians possess this level of cultural experience, and there are even fewer American Indian physicians. This is also true of the nursing profession. Most registered nurses in the **IHS** are not American Indians. American Indians who seek careers in the health field often go against traditional beliefs.

Male health-care providers are generally limited in the care they provide to women, especially during their menses. Women are generally modest and wear several layers of slips. This practice is very common among elderly women.

STATUS OF HEALTH-CARE PROVIDERS

It is frequently said that if an American Indian becomes a physician, the physician must not be traditional. Therefore, many Navajo are suspicious of American Indian physicians. The factors that influence acceptance of American Indian health-care providers have not been adequately researched, but the lack of respect by some Western health-care providers for Indian beliefs has contributed to the Navajo's inability to trust them. Many health concerns of American Indians can be treated by both traditional and Western healers in a culturally competent manner when these practitioners are willing to work together and respect each other's differences.

Western practitioners, traditional medicine men, and herbal healers receive respect on the reservation. However, not all American Indians accord equal respect to these groups, and many prefer one group to the other or use all three.

CASE STUDY Mr. Begay, age 78, lives with his wife in a traditional Navajo hogan. He has lived in the same area all his life and has worked as a uranium miner until the government closed the mines. His hogan has neither electricity nor running water. Heat is provided by a fire, which is also used for cooking. Lighting is obtained from propane lanterns. Water is hauled from a windmill site 20 miles away and is stored in 50-gallon steel drums. Because the windmill freezes and the roads are often too muddy to travel in the winter, sometimes he must travel an additional 10 miles to the trading post to obtain water. Because Mr. Begay does not own a car, he must depend on transportation from extended family members who live in the same vicinity.

Mr. Begay has continually experienced shortness of breath and it is getting worse. He has been hospitalized with pneumonia several times as a result of the uranium poisoning. He had a cholecystectomy at age 62. His diet is traditional and is supplemented by canned foods, which are obtained at the trading post.

All health care is obtained at the Public Health Service Hospital in Shiprock. Neither Mr. Begay nor his wife obtain routine preventive health care. He was admitted from the clinic to the hospital with a diagnosis of pneumonia.

Mr. Begay shows clinical improvement after initial intravenous antibiotic therapy. However, his mental status continues to decline. His family feels that he should see a traditional medicine man and discusses this with his physician. The physician agrees and allows Mr. Begay to go to see the medicine man. Several members of the nursing staff disagree with the physician's decision and have requested a patient care conference with the physician. The physician agrees to the conference.

STUDY QUESTIONS

1 | Identify three physical barriers Mr. Begay must overcome to obtain health care.

2 | Discuss the benefits of Mr. Begay seeing the traditional medicine man.

3 | Identify some potential negative outcomes of Mr. Begay seeing the traditional medicine man.

4 | Identify interventions to reduce the potential for the reoccurrence of pneumonia.

5 | Identify at least two major health risks that face the Begays based on their current lifestyle.

6 | Discuss potential outcomes for negotiation during the conference.

7 | Mr. Begay's diet is described as traditional Navajo. What foods are included in this diet?

8 | What services do you anticipate for Mr. Begay when he returns home as the result of his continued need for oxygen?

9 | What might the nurse do to encourage preventive health measures for the Begay family?

10 | Identify at least three types of traditional Navajo healers.

11 | Identify contextual speech patterns of the Navajo Indians.

12 | Distinguish differences in gender roles among Navajo Indians.

13 | Identify two culturally congruent teaching methods for the Navajo client.

14 | Discuss the meaning of the First Laugh Ceremony for the Navajo.

15 | Identify two culturally congruent approaches for discussing a fatal illness with a Navajo client.

16 | Identify traditional practices used by the Navajo to start their day in regard to spirituality.

REFERENCES

Arthur, B. J. (1976). *Traditional Navajo childbearing practices: A survey of the traditional childbearing practices among elderly Navajo parents.* Unpublished master's thesis, University of Utah, Salt Lake City.

Burke, S., Kisilevsky, B., & Maloney, R. (1989). Time orientations of Indian mothers and white nurses. *Canadian Journal of Nursing Research, 21*(4), 14–20.

Carter, J. S., Pugh, J. A., & Monterrosa, A. (1996). Non-insulin-dependent diabetes mellitus in minorities in the United States. *Annals of Internal Medicine, 125*(3), 221–232.

Chisholm, J. S. (1983). *Navajo infancy: An ethnological study of child development.* New York: Aldine.

Discharry, E. K. (1986). Delivering home health care to the elderly in Zuni Pueblo. *Journal of Gerontological Nursing, 12*(7), 25–29.

Hodgins, D., & Still, O. (1989). *Lidocaine reactions in the American Indian population: quality assurance study.* Unpublished research, Tuba City Indian Health Center, Tuba City, AZ.

Indian Health Service. (2000). Overview of the context of GPRA in the Indian Health Service (2000), Rockville, MD.

Preito, D. O. (1989). American Indians in medicine: The need for Indian healers. *Academic Medicine, 64,* 388.

Social Issues Research Center. (2002). Social and cultural aspects of drinking. Retrieved May 24, 2002, from http://www.sirc.org/publink/drinking5.html.

U.S. Department of Health and Human Services. (1998). *Trends in Indian Health.* Public Health Service: Indian Health Services, Office of Planning and Evaluation. Rockville, MD.

World Health Organization Scientific Group. (1986). Primary immunodeficiency diseases. In M. M. Eibl & F. S. Rosen (Eds.), *Primary immunodeficiency diseases* (pp. 341–375). Amsterdam: Exerpta Medica.

Wilson, U. (1983). Nursing care of the American Indian patient. In M. S. Orque, B. Block, & L. S. A. Monrroy (Eds.), *Ethnic nursing care: A multicultural approach.* St. Louis, MO: Mosby.

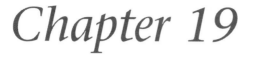

Chapter 19

People of Polish Heritage

MARTHA A. FROM

Overview, Inhabited Localities, and Topography

OVERVIEW

Over 9.4 million people in the United States and 273,000 people in Canada identify their ancestry as Polish (Statistics Canada: Ethnic Origin, 1999). Poland, whose capital city is Warsaw, is located in north central Europe. With almost 121,000 square miles, Poland is approximately the size of New Mexico, has a population of 38.6 million, and a literacy rate of 98 percent. The countries surrounding Poland are Russia, Ukraine, Belarus, and Lithuania to the east; the Czech and Slovak Republics to the south; and Germany to the west. Most of the country is a plain with no natural boundaries except the Carpathian Mountains in the south and the Oder and Neisse rivers in the west.

Between the years 1795 and 1919, Poland was divided among the countries of Prussia, Russia, and Austria and ceased to exist as a country (Davies, 1982). Through tenacity, determination, and the Catholic Church, the Poles maintained their language, culture, and heritage. Between 1920 and 1939, Poland again became a separate self-governing country after World War I. After World War II, Poland was once again reconfigured, but the country was still a separate entity. The discussion of what to do with Poland, known as the **Polish Question**, was undertaken by Stalin, Churchill, and Roosevelt at the Malta and Potsdam Conferences. In the reconfiguration, Poland lost 10,000 sq mi to the east and 50,000 sq mi to the west; a move that was "considered the most disruptive in postwar Europe" (Szulc, 1988: 85).

Polish immigrants and their descendants who have been in America for generations maintain their ethnic heritage by promoting Polish culture through attending Polish parades, eating ethnic foods, actively maintaining the Polish language, and promoting Polish interest through economic and political channels. For newer immigrant Poles, maintaining ethnic heritage means learning English and getting a good job (Erdmans, 1998). Newer immigrants are not as much concerned with raising consciousness over Polish American issues as helping families left behind in Poland and raising concerns over the political climate in Poland.

HERITAGE AND RESIDENCE

The first substantive Polish settlement in America, Panna Maria, Texas, was led by Father Leopold Moczygemba in 1864. Even though most Poles preferred living in agrarian communities, they gravitated to cities where work for laborers was plentiful. Between 1820 and 1940, more than 400,000 Polish immigrants came to America. Between 1940 and 1960, 17,500 arrived; between 1960 and 1970, 53,500; between 1970 and 1980, 37,000; between 1980 and 1990, more than 97,000; and in 1993 alone, 27,800 immigrated to the United States. Thus, the Polish immigration to America continues. Today, more than 9.4 million people of Polish descent live in America (U.S. Census, 2000).

The predominant residence for Polish immigrants in America is north of Ohio and east of the Mississippi River. At the peak of Polish migration, Chicago was considered the most well-developed Polish community in America. The city of Chicago and its suburbs has more Polish immigrants and their extended families than any other city outside Poland. Almost 2 million native and foreign-born Polish people live in New York state (Lopata, 1994). Currently, Polish communities with retirees and new immigrants are growing in Florida, Texas, and California.

Polonia was the name of Polish communities found in northeastern and midwestern cities. Members of these communities helped keep Polish nationalism alive by speaking Polish, preserving Polish customs, and attending the local Polish Catholic Church run by Polish clergy and the Felician Order of Sisters. Since Poland as a country did not exist until 1919, Poles coming to America during the 1800s and early 1900s tenaciously made sure that Polish culture continued to exist. Early Polish neighborhoods were very well organized, with religious and voluntary organizations dedicated to the support of schools, organized trade, banks, and political activities. Many of these Polish organizations are still active today. Monuments, statues, and historical sites dedicated to Polish Americans and Polish nationals can be found in towns and cities settled by Polish immigrants.

Poles as an immigrant group were slow to assimilate into multicultural America. Despite their slow assimilation, Polish Americans are not a homogeneous group. Much of the variation within this ethnic group is due to the primary and secondary characteristics of culture (see Chapter 1).

Polish Americans were well represented as part of the World War II war effort. Over 30,000 Poles were killed defending America. Even with that sense of duty and honor, however, Polish Americans were discriminated against when they were passed over for jobs because their names were difficult to pronounce. As a result, name changes became common for upwardly mobile Polish Americans who hoped to decrease discrimination and attain higher level jobs. A difficult experience for many Polish Americans is discrimination and ridicule through ethnic Polish jokes, which are similar in scope to those about Irish and Italian Americans. However, the **Solidarity** movement in the 1970s and 1980s and the election of a Polish Pope decreased the incidence of Polish jokes and made Americans realize the intellectual and political sophistication of Poles in Poland and in America. Pope John Paul II is the first Polish pope and is the first non-Italian pope since 1523.

REASONS FOR MIGRATION AND ASSOCIATED ECONOMIC FACTORS

Polish immigration to the United States occurred in three major waves. The first wave of immigrants, arriving in the mid-1800s through 1914, were considered *a chlebam*, or "bread" immigrants (Erdmans, 1998) because they came to America for economic and religious reasons. These immigrants took low-paying jobs and lived in crowded dwellings just to make a meager living.

The second wave of immigration occurred after World War II. During the war, Poland lost proportionally more people than any other country. Over 6 million of its 35 million people were killed (Brogan, 1990). "The devastation upon Poland wrought by the war staggers the human imagination" (Frydman, 1983: 617). Living conditions in Poland after World War II were very restrictive. Individuals in this second wave were primarily political prisoners, dissidents, and intellectuals from refugee camps all over Europe. Many in this group, who were educated and committed to assimilating into American culture, separated from Polonia and aligned themselves with other middle-class and professional groups in America. The upwardly mobile and middle-class aspirations of this group differed from the working-class orientation of the first- and second-generation descendants of the first wave.

The current third wave of immigrants started arriving in 1980. These immigrants reflect the ideologies from the first two waves of immigrants; that is, they come to work and are able to speak freely about political and intellectual issues. Many in this wave come to America to work with no initial interest in permanently relocating; they enter on a visitor's visa and leave their families behind in Poland. These immigrants frequently live in low-income housing, share rooms with other immigrants, and work hard to send money to their families in Poland. They quickly take any job available, particularly as laborers, domestics, and unskilled farm workers. These newer immigrants tend to save money on food by eating nutritionally inadequate diets and do not seek health care until a problem becomes serious. Networking with other Poles is their primary source of job contacts. Because many of these new immigrants have been used by unscrupulous Poles and others, they are terrified of strangers and bureaucrats who may have them deported if they are found working (No Jokes, Less solidarity, 1991). If immigrants are deported they must wait at least 7 years before they can apply for another visa to return to America.

The remaining Polish immigrants of the third wave have chosen America for political and economic reasons. This group typically consists of well-educated professionals and small business owners. They bring their families because they have consciously decided to leave Poland forever. This group epitomizes the Polish characteristics of hard work and determination. They actively seek to learn English and assimilate into their new country. Many in this group are underemployed, recognizing that this may be a necessary first step into assimilation.

Many Polish Americans from the second and third wave avoid **Polonia** communities because the ethnic **Polonias** of America are different from the Polish communities they left behind. The concerns and issues of political representation and discrimination of third- and fourth-generation first-wave immigrants living in America do not seem relevant to second- and third-wave immigrant Poles. Many **Polonia** communities are located in changing neighborhoods where other minorities have moved in. Upwardly mobile Polish Americans are leaving cities for the suburbs.

EDUCATIONAL STATUS AND OCCUPATIONS

Educational differences and assimilation into American culture vary widely among Polish immigrants. The range of socioeconomic levels and cultural philosophies often depends on when the families emigrated from Poland. Until the 1950s and 1960s, many Polish families were slow to recognize the value of education for their children. Before World War II, most Polish children went to Polish Catholic schools where they learned Polish culture, language, and Catholicism. After World War II, parents felt an acute responsibility to have their children learn English. After this, the Polish language was taught in only a few schools and the Polish language was no longer freely spoken at home.

For first- and second-generation first-wave immigrants, work was considered more important than education. Hard work and the need for material goods were things that Poles could understand. Illiterate first-wave Poles initially had difficulty with unionized labor; however, once they understood what was at stake, they became staunch union supporters. As a consequence, until the late 1950s many children followed in their fathers' footsteps by working in union jobs. They entered meat packing houses in Chicago, steel mills in Indiana, assembly lines in Detroit, and coal mines in Pennsylvania. Because young Poles continued to follow in their parents' occupational footsteps more frequently than other immigrant children, upward mobility was slower for Poles than for some other ethnic minorities (Lopata, 1994).

The second wave of Polish immigrants placed a high value on education and culture. Educated, cultured Poles were expected to read widely and speak several languages. Cultured Poles have great pride and respect for Poland's most famous people, such as Chopin, Marie Curie, Joseph Conrad, Copernicus, and Karol Wojtyla, better known as Pope John Paul II. Poles are known for epic works in prose and poetry. Major themes in Polish literature are nationality, freedom, exile, and oppression.

In the 1950s, the Polish communities in America had a renewed interest in scholarly and cultured endeavors. The Polish Institute of Arts and Sciences began publishing *The Polish Review*, a scholarly journal devoted to the works of Polish scholars, and the Kosciusko Foundation encourages cultural exchanges between Poland and America and provides scholarships to Polish American students. Once the Polish community recognized the value of education for their children, Poles became one of the highest represented ethnic groups in institutions of higher learning. "The proportion of young people who finished college was more than double that of older Polish Americans, and the proportion of young people who attended college was at least triple" (Lopata, 1994: 149).

After World War II, many Polish Catholics were blue-collar workers who valued hard work as honorable. Many feared that education and mobility were a threat to their religious and community life. For women, education was seen as even less necessary because a high value was placed on their staying at home and raising the children. Television helped change the character of ethnic communities forever because it brought the outside world into the community and into the home. This generation of first-wave descendants who did go to college valued obedience and self-control and respected authority and determination (Bukowczyk, 1987).

Communication

DOMINANT LANGUAGE AND DIALECTS

The dominant language of people living in Poland is Polish, with some regional dialects and differences. Generally, most Polish-speaking people can communicate with each other. Recently, a resurgence of interest has occurred among Poles in America in learning to speak the Polish language. Both adults and children are learning Polish in Polish churches, cultural centers, and colleges. Polish radio stations help keep an ongoing interest in the Polish language, music, and culture.

The Polish language was influenced by the countries surrounding Poland and by the Latin of 11th and 12th century kings. Depending on the regional and cultural background of the speaker, Polish may sound German, Russian, or French. The Polish language has a lyrical quality that is pleasant to the ear, even if one cannot understand the words. Poles are an animated group and facial expressions generally convey the tone of the conversation.

CULTURAL COMMUNICATION PATTERNS

Poles, as a group, tend to share thoughts and ideas freely, particularly as part of their hospitality. A guest in a Polish home is warmly welcomed and may be overwhelmed by the outpouring of generosity. Americans talk of baseball while Poles speak of their personal life, their jobs, families, spouse, and misfortunes.

To Poles, love is expressed through covert actions and displayed easily in the form of tenderness to children. However, loving phrases are not common among adult Polish Americans. Poles praise each others' deeds and good work, but they may be reluctant to acknowledge how they feel about each other. This behavior may or may not have persevered through generations of assimilated Poles.

Acknowledging the hostess is important when Poles visit each other's homes; flowers or candy are always in good taste. Normally, guests are not expected to assist the hostess in the kitchen or with cleanup after meals. Poles value thank-you letters and greeting cards.

Poles use touch as a form of personal expression of caring. Touch is common among family members and friends, but Poles may be quite formal with strangers and health-care providers. Handshaking is considered polite. In fact, not shaking hands with everyone present may be considered rude. Most Poles feel comfortable with close personal space, but personal space and distancing increases from friends to strangers.

First-generation Poles and other people from eastern European countries commonly kiss "Polish style," that is, once on each cheek and then once again. For Poles, kissing the hand is considered appropriate if the woman extends it. Two women may walk together arm in arm, or two men may greet each other with an embrace, a hug, and a kiss on both cheeks.

When interacting with others, Poles consider age, gender, and title. For example, when a group is walking through a door, an unspoken hierarchy requires the person of lower standing to hold the door for a woman or for those of a higher title. To many Americans, this behavior may seem excessive, but for Poles, it shows respect and courtesy. Polish Americans also use direct eye contact when interacting with others. Many Americans may feel uncomfortable with this sustained eye contact and may feel it is quite close to staring, but to Poles it is considered ordinary.

Most Poles enjoy a robust conversation and have a keen sense of humor. Polish humor sometimes has an openness and bawdiness that may be unnerving to those who are unaccustomed to it. Cultural nuances may make it difficult to understand the underlying meaning of some transactions. Because Poles in Poland have been censored for centuries, they have raised satire and political savvy to an art form.

TEMPORAL RELATIONSHIPS

Polish Americans are both past and future oriented. The past is very much a part of Polish culture, with the memory of World War II haunting most Poles in some way. A strong work ethic encourages Poles to plan for the future. Polish parents very much want their children to have a better life than the one they have experienced.

Punctuality is important to Polish Americans. To be late is a sign of bad manners. Depending on the status of the person for whom they are waiting, Poles may be intolerant of lateness in others. Even in social situations, people are expected to arrive on time and stay late.

FORMAT FOR NAMES

Many Polish Americans consider the use of second-person familiarity rude. Polish people speak in the third person. For example, they might ask, "would Sue like some coffee?" rather than "would you like some coffee?" Although the first expression might sound awkward, the latter expression may be considered impolite and too informal, especially if the person is older. A health-care provider is *Pani Doktor*, literally translated as "Lady Doctor," not plain "Doctor." Many Polish names are difficult to pronounce. Even though a name may be mispronounced, a high value is placed on the attempt to pronounce it correctly.

Family Roles and Organization

HEAD OF HOUSEHOLD AND GENDER ROLES

In most Polish families, the father is perceived as the head of the household. Depending on the degree of assimilation, the father may rule with absolute authority in first-, second-, and even third-generation Polish American families. Depending on circumstances, only the church may have greater authority than the father. For example, if a child wants to leave home and go to college, the priest may help in convincing the family that it is an appropriate thing to do. However, among some third- and fourth-generation Polish Americans and second- and third-wave immigrants, more egalitarian gender roles are becoming the norm.

PRESCRIPTIVE, RESTRICTIVE, AND TABOO BEHAVIORS FOR CHILDREN AND ADOLESCENTS

The most valued behavior among Polish American children is obedience. Taboo child behaviors include anything that undermines parental authority. Parents are quite demonstrative with young children, but they may not show much affection toward them once they are older than toddler age. This is the parents' way of teaching children to be strong and resilient. Many parents praise children for self-control and completing chores. Little sympathy is wasted on failure, but doing well is openly praised. Children are disciplined not to feel helpless, fragile, or dependent.

Boyd et al. (1994) conducted a study of the internalization of personality characteristics and "not-just" behaviors between Polish and Polish American mother-daughter dyads. The Polish mother-daughter dyads had a greater degree of congruence when compared with Polish American mother-daughter dyads. These results suggest that cultural and ethnic differences exist. In America, the emphasis on individualism and living independently of one's parents may contribute to these differences.

FAMILY GOALS AND PRIORITIES

Traditional family values and loyalty are strong in most Polish households. Children are very valued in the Polish American family. For many first-wave immigrants, marriage is an institution of respect and economic solidarity, and does not necessarily include romance. In the past, husbands owed their wives loyalty, fidelity, and financial support; wives owed their husbands fidelity and obedience. Children owed their parents emotional and financial support before and after marriage. An important family priority for many is to maintain the honor of the family to the larger society, have a good job, and be a good Catholic.

The elderly are highly respected in most Polish families. They attend church regularly and carry on Polish traditions. The Polish ethic of contributing to the family and enhancing family status extends to the aged as well. The elderly play an active role in helping grandchildren learn Polish customs and in helping adult children in their daily routine with families. For some families, one of the worst disgraces as seen through the eyes of the Polish community is to put an aged family member in a nursing home. Third- and fourth-generation Polish Americans may consider an extended-care facility because of work schedules and demands of care, but first-generation immigrants rarely see this as an option.

Kahana and associates (1993) studied the acceptance of nursing homes by eastern European elderly Jews and Poles living in the greater Detroit area. According to their study, Polish Americans have the most difficulty assimilating into institutional life. The Polish Americans in this sample had lived their lives in **Polonia**, were uneducated, and their main wish was to leave the institution. They felt abandoned by their children, and they were not able to find confidants in their setting. Even though these Poles were institutionalized in predominantly

Catholic nursing homes, the setting did not emphasize Polish culture or background. If Polish people are to assimilate into a nursing home, the use of the Polish language and rituals may be crucial; thus, health-care providers should assist clients in organizing these types of events for their family members or should help them select nursing homes that offer these services.

The quality of life for elderly immigrants is becoming an excellent area for research (Berdes & Zych, 2000). Immigrants who arrived before age 21 adjusted to aging much better than their elderly counterparts who arrived in America well into maturity. If the elderly Pole moved to America and was actively embraced by family and friends, adjusting to old age in America was not too difficult; however, if it was a forced choice to move to America, the elderly Pole's adjustment to living longer was difficult.

Extended family, consisting of aunts, uncles, and godparents, is very important to Poles. Longtime friends become aunts or uncles to Polish children. Numerous family rituals around holidays and family gatherings such as births, marriages, and name dates (calendar date of the patron saint for whom one is named) are times to socialize and cement relationships.

The goals of the family are to work, make economic contributions, and strive toward enhancing the position of the family in the community. The family unit bands together to help deter behaviors that might cause them shame or lower prestige in the eyes of the community. As Poles assimilate into the American culture, the American value of success may prevail. Most Poles expect their children to have an education, a well-paying job, and provide for them in their old age.

ALTERNATIVE LIFESTYLES

Alternative lifestyles are seen as part of assimilation into the blended American culture. Same-sex couples are frowned upon and may even be ostracized, depending on the level of assimilation. Older second- and third-generation Poles have one of the lowest divorce rates of white ethnic groups (Lopata, 1994), but patterns are changing with succeeding generations as they assimilate into the American lifestyle. This is not to say that marital problems do not exist but rather that the Polish value for family solidarity is strong, and divorce is truly seen as a last resort. When divorce does result, single heads of households are accepted in the Polish American community.

Workforce Issues

CULTURE IN THE WORKPLACE

Most Polish Americans are more segregated than other ethnic groups even in second-generation groups. In the past, many Poles never rose above the level of foreman. Polish American immigrants of the 1800s maintained group solidarity and could always be counted on to help their families. Because men were semiliterate and had low-level skills, they gravitated to cities like Chicago where they could work long hours as laborers and earn overtime pay. Because Poles were active in trade unions and maintained a sense of loyalty to the group, they were stronger union supporters than many other American-born workers of the 1930s and 1940s.

Polish Americans have an extensive social network, and their strong work ethic enables them to gain employment and assimilate easily into the workforce. It is still possible to spend one's entire life inside the boundaries of **Polonia**. While this may have helped immigrants in the past, it now acts as a deterrent to assimilation. Many newer immigrants move beyond the **Polonia** neighborhoods, and some even avoid them to obtain employment that will help them achieve future work goals.

ISSUES RELATED TO AUTONOMY

Some second- and third-wave Poles entering America are underemployed and may have difficulty working with authority figures that are not as well educated as they are. Poles quietly comment that they are not respected for their educational background and that they must endure decreased status to stay in America (Lopata, 1994). Poles are usually quick learners and work hard to do a job well. The Polish characteristic of praising people for their work makes Poles strong managers, but some lack sensitivity in their quest to complete tasks and please their own authority figures.

Even though nursing in Poland is considered a profession, newer immigrants may be unprepared for the level of sophistication and autonomy of American nurses. It has only been since the 1980s that nursing has entered the university setting in Poland. Most of Polish nursing education is still completed in 1- to 2-year post-high school education programs. Like many other professionals coming to America, if the Polish nurse is willing to complete the extra courses to become a registered or practical nurse, then the nurse's employment can be continued. A problem for many foreign nurses is that they may not get credit for their work experiences from their home country. So a nurse with 10 years of nursing experience may have to start with the salary and status of a new graduate.

Because Poles learn deference to authority at home, in the church, and in parochial schools, some may be less well suited for the rigors of a highly individualistic competitive market. For Poles living under the Communist political system, the American work culture may be very difficult for them to understand. Polish Americans are considered excellent workers. The strong Polish work ethic, exhibited as volunteering for overtime, being punctual, and rarely taking sick days, is valued by employers.

Native-born Polish Americans do not have difficulty with the English language. Foreign-born Poles frequently have some difficulty understanding the subtle nuances of humor. Less educated Poles tend to seek jobs as domestics or choose to perform manual labor because they do not have to rely as heavily on their language and communication skills in these occupations. New third-wave Poles, who have been working under a communist bureaucratic hierarchy, may have some difficulty with the structure and nuances of the American workforce culture. New wave Poles may be very naïve in acclimating to the American work culture and, therefore, may become frustrated in what is considered an acceptable work ethic.

Biocultural Ecology

SKIN COLOR AND OTHER BIOLOGICAL VARIATIONS

Most Poles are of medium height with a medium-to-large bone structure. As a result of foreign invasions over the centuries, Polish people may be dark and Mongol looking or fair and delicate with blue eyes and blond hair. Those with fair complexions are predisposed to skin cancer and illnesses related to exposure to environmental elements. Health-care providers must be aware of these conditions when assessing Polish clients and providing health teaching.

DISEASES AND HEALTH CONDITIONS

Risk factors for newer Polish immigrants are connected with their employment in industries, the climate of Poland, which is similar to that of the northeastern region of the United States, with short summers and long harsh winters, and the level of modern healthcare practices. This similarity encouraged Poles to settle in these areas of the United States.

Common health problems are obesity, smoking, and low leisure-time physical activity, all of which contribute to an increased incidence of heart disease. In Poland, many of the steel plants constructed after World War II were built without filtering systems and were located near major cities, thereby contributing to excessive pollution. As a result, Poland has an increased incidence of respiratory disease and cancer. Miners and workers in heavy industry are at risk for the development of pulmonary diseases. In the late 20th century, the Chernobyl incident in Russia created a new concern—that of radiation filtration into the land and water systems of eastern Poland. Time will tell the impact of this disaster on the incidence of cancer in Poland and for Poles emigrating to other parts of the world. For a long time iodine was not added to salt, so the incidence of thyroid disease was very high.

Health-care providers should carefully screen Polish immigrants for diseases common in their home country, such as dental and cardiac diseases, alcoholism, respiratory conditions, thyroid disorders, and cancer, particularly leukemia. Endemic diseases of Poland are similar to endemic diseases found in the United States. These diseases increased in Poland because of poor sanitary conditions, outdated hospitals, lack of money for preventive services, lack of access to medicines, and limited numbers of physicians, psychiatrists, physical therapists, dentists, nurses, and social workers. Culturally congruent health teaching strategies associated with risk factors for these diseases must be implemented when working with this population.

In a longitudinal study between the United States and Poland over a 10-year period, Rywik et al. (1989) compared cardiovascular diseases in male and female native Poles and Polish Americans living in rural and urban settings. The study reports that native Poles have a greater risk for cardiovascular disease than Polish Americans. This may be because Polish Americans have access to medications, so cardiovascular disease may not be as threatening to Poles in America.

VARIATIONS IN DRUG METABOLISM

Documentation on the pharmacodynamics of drug metabolism in Polish individuals is limited. The medical literature does not report any pharmacological studies specific to people of Polish descent.

High-Risk Behaviors

Alcohol abuse (Rywik et al., 1989), with its subsequent physiological and sociological effects, continues to be an ongoing concern among Polish Americans. In Poland, a high rate of alcoholic psychosis, cirrhosis of the liver, and acute alcohol poisoning exists. Other related illnesses include cancer of the gastrointestinal tract, peptic ulcer, accidents, and suicide. Alcohol abuse is an important part of the history of Poland. For many people of the first wave, alcohol was a way of relieving boredom and the severe hardships of peasant life. For many second- and third-wave immigrants, alcohol was a way of mitigating the pain of World War II and reducing depression and the symptoms of posttraumatic stress syndrome. For many second- and third-generation Poles, alcohol may still influence family patterns of behavior.

Because Poles place a high value on hospitality in both Poland and America, drinking among Poles is an accepted part of the culture. Part of being a good hostess is to have enough alcohol for every guest. For newer immigrants and older Polish Americans, vodka (or other spirits) is the alcohol of choice. Upper socioeconomic groups drink wine, and beer is consumed by all socioeconomic levels. In a study on drinking patterns of American and Polish college students, Polish students drank more than their American counterparts (Eng, Slawinska, & Hanson, 1991). Wine was the preferred drink of Polish students and beer the preferred drink of American students.

Illicit drug use is not part of the culture of Poland, but with the changing society this behavior might change. Polish Americans have a higher rate of smoking than other European Americans, but this trend may be decreasing with younger generations. Research suggests that Polish descendants start experimenting with cigarettes at the age of 14 or 15 (Wijatkowski et al., 1990).

Because alcohol use and cigarette smoking are prevalent among many Poles, it is essential for health-care providers to assess individual clients for abuse and provide counseling and referral for those who express an interest. Children of immigrants should especially be targeted for counseling regarding the health effects of smoking and alcohol consumption.

HEALTH-CARE PRACTICES

In Poland, the urban intellectual group is very interested in preventive health behaviors and exercise, with hiking and mountain climbing being important physical activities. The working class has a strong commitment to obeying laws, and seatbelt and traffic regulations are generally followed. Many Poles continue these healthy activities upon emigration. The health-care provider needs to encourage these positive health-seeking behaviors among newer immigrants.

Nutrition

MEANING OF FOOD

Food is a very important symbol of sustenance and hospitality. Most Poles extend the sharing of food and drink to people entering their homes; guests are expected to eat. Three important considerations influence Poles regarding food. First, Poland is primarily a land-based country with short summers and very cold winters. Thus, root vegetables and cabbage survive the best in this climate. Fish is limited, and game meat and pork are staples, depending on economics and availability. Second, the cold weather encourages consumption of stews, soups, and foods that have high satiety. Third, the strong Catholic influence is evidenced in many festivals and rituals, each requiring a special fast or feast. Many Poles continue these dietary practices after emigrating. Health-care providers need to assess Polish clients' dietary habits and provide nutritional information that is congruent with personal dietary choices.

COMMON FOODS AND FOOD RITUALS

Polish foods and cooking are similar to German, Russian, and Jewish practices. Staples of the diet are millet, barley, potatoes, onions, radishes, turnips, beets, beans, cabbage, cucumbers, tomatoes, apples, and wild mushrooms. Common meats are chicken, beef, and pork,

including pigs' knuckles and organ meats such as liver, tripe, and tongue. *Kapusta* (sauerkraut), *golabki* (stuffed cabbage), *babka* (coffee cake), *pierogi* (dumplings), and *chrusciki* (bowtie pastries) are common ethnic foods. Hot soups and stews are favored during bitter cold winters, and cold soups are preferred during the summer.

The meal plan for many Poles consists of a hearty breakfast of coffee, bread, cheese, sausage, and eggs. A midmorning snack consists of a sandwich and tea or coffee. The main meal in midafternoon includes soup, meat, potatoes, a hot vegetable, and dessert. In the evening, cold cuts, eggs, sour cream, bread, and grains are common. This diet is modified depending on economics and availability. Dill and paprika are the most commonly used herbs. Food is rarely eaten raw and may be pickled, which increases the sodium content.

DIETARY PRACTICES FOR HEALTH PROMOTION

The Polish American diet is frequently high in saturated fat from frying food in butter or bacon fat. The basic diet includes sour cream, butter, and fatty processed meats such as *kielbasa* and Polish ham. Clients with increased cholesterol levels, cardiovascular disease, and diabetes will require dietary counseling.

NUTRITIONAL DEFICIENCIES AND FOOD LIMITATIONS

There are no major enzyme deficiencies among Polish Americans. Native food practices may not change much when emigrating if there is a general availability of their major food groups and most ingredients are easily accessible. Often the Polish diet is deficient in fruits and vegetables. Meats and vegetables are cooked for a very long time resulting in the destruction of B vitamins and other vitamins. Because newer immigrants may live in crowded conditions and may try to save money from food purchases, they may benefit from additional education that addresses how to purchase less expensive foods and still maintain a healthy diet. Table 19–1 lists a variety of foods commonly eaten by Polish and Polish American people.

Table 19–1 Polish Foods

Common Name	Description	Ingredients
Babka	Coffeecake	Yeast bread
Barszcz	Beet soup	Served plain or with sour cream
Bigos	Hunter's stew	Stew with game, sausage, sauerkraut
Chrusciki	Polish bowties	Fried egg dough
Golabki	Cabbage rolls	Cooked cabbage stuffed with chopped meat and rice in tomato sauce
Kielbasa	Sausage	Sausage
Ogorki smietanie	Sour cream cucumbers	Sour cream, cucumbers
Pierogi	Boiled dumplings	Dumplings filled with potatoes, cheese, or sauerkraut
Sledzie	Herring	Pickled fish

Pregnancy and Childbearing Practices

FERTILITY PRACTICES AND VIEWS TOWARD PREGNANCY

Because family is very important, most Poles want children. In an agrarian society, and for early immigrants, children were considered important because they brought status to the family and were an economic necessity. However, in difficult economic times and during the years of poverty and war, abortion and child spacing were considered a necessity. In Poland, the Catholic Church strongly opposes abortion, which is the prevailing attitude of many second- and third-wave Poles in America. In Poland, women receive fully paid maternity leave for 90 days, and longer with partial payment, but many women do not take the entire leave because of trying economic circumstances. Fertility practices are balanced between the needs of the family and the laws of the Church.

PRESCRIPTIVE, RESTRICTIVE, AND TABOO PRACTICES IN THE CHILDBEARING FAMILY

Pregnant Polish Americans are expected to seek preventive health care, eat well, and get adequate rest to ensure a healthy pregnancy and baby. Immigrants who remember the war and famine, when infant mortality rates were high, pay attention to prenatal care. The emphasis on food and "eating for two" is a common philosophy. Health-care providers must pay special attention to ensure that pregnant Polish American women do not gain excess weight during pregnancy.

Because the process of childbirth was poorly understood by the early peasant society, magicoreligious and taboo beliefs continue to surround childbirth depending on the age of the Polish American. Many consider it bad luck to have a "baby shower" and even now, many Polish grandmothers may be reluctant to give gifts until after the baby is born. Birthing is typically done in the hospital. Midwives may be used if there is a community feeling that they are "just as good as the doctor."

Pregnant women usually follow the physician's orders carefully. In America, Polish women seek prenatal clinics when they cannot afford private fees. The birthing process is considered the domain of women. Newer Poles immigrating to America may not feel comfortable with men in the birthing area or with family-centered care.

Women are expected to rest for the first few weeks after delivery. To many immigrants and women who are descendants from second- and third-wave Polish Americans, breast-feeding is important. Health-care providers may need to provide active counseling and education about breast-feeding to Polish American women. They may also need to teach the proper techniques to those who choose to breast-feed and to help them to balance rest with exercise after delivery.

Death Rituals

DEATH RITUALS AND EXPECTATIONS

Most Poles have a stoic acceptance of death as part of the life process and a strong sense of loyalty and respect for their loved ones. Family and friends stay with the dying person so the dying do not feel abandoned. The Polish ethic of showing care by doing means bringing food to share, caring for children, and assisting with household chores for close family members.

Most Polish women are quick to help with the physical needs of the dying. Hospice care at home is acceptable to most Poles. Health-care providers may encounter difficulty in convincing the family that the dying member may choose not to eat as a result of the illness rather than because of stubbornness or a slur against the caretaker's cooking. Polish women may tend to hover, so health-care providers also need to help families understand that it is important for the dying person to conserve energy.

RESPONSES TO DEATH AND GRIEF

Because of the absence of embalming practices in early Poland, individuals were buried within 24 hours of their deaths. Poles of the early 20th century continued this practice by burying the deceased from the home and having home burial ceremonies, which included a wake or vigil in which family members prayed and repeated the rosary over the dead person. Late 20th century Polish American family members follow a funeral custom of having a wake for 1 to 3 days, followed by a Mass and religious burial. Most Poles honor their dead by attending Mass and making special offerings to the Church on All Souls Day, November 1. Families may continue tending the gravesite for years by pulling weeds, planting flowers, and leaving wreaths for their loved ones.

Spirituality

DOMINANT RELIGION AND USE OF PRAYER

The Catholic Church, with its required attendance at Mass on Sundays and holy days, is an integral part of the lives of most Polish people. There are holidays for every month of the year plus the rituals of baptism, confirmation, marriage, sacrament of the sick, and burial. Christmas and Easter are the two biggest feasts requiring special foods and rituals. On Christmas Eve, depending on the affluence of the family, up to 13 meatless dishes are served with the **oplatek** (wafer) that everyone at the table shares. On Christmas Day, the main meal consists of goose or turkey. The Easter holiday may begin with women bringing food to the church Easter Saturday to be blessed by the priest. On Easter Sunday, lamb or *kielbasa* and boiled eggs are served, and as a table ornament, a lamb made of salt or butter is displayed. Like many Americans of various ethnic backgrounds, Polish Americans have had a renewed interest in their ethnic roots. For example, since the 1970s, the attendance of

Polish Americans at Catholic churches in Polish neighborhoods has been on the rise.

Poles are very much concerned that churches continue to act as a vehicle of Polish culture. A group of Polish Catholics created the Polish National Church because they believed that the American Catholic Church was not meeting the needs of Polish American Catholics. Several of these churches are still in existence today in some areas of **Polonia**. Birthdays and name days are important events for Poles. One very popular song is **Sto Lat**, which means that the celebrant should live 100 years.

Religious ceremonies are a very important part of maintaining Polish culture. Polish weddings are legendary as times when family and friends get together and two families unite. One folk practice is to bring bread and salt as a symbol that there will always be plenty of food in the home. Guests always receive plenty of food and drink, and music for singing and dancing. In America, Polish weddings may only last 1 day, but plenty of food and drink are considered essential to the joyous occasion.

Primary spiritual sources are God and Jesus Christ, with first- and second-generation Polish immigrants praying to the Virgin Mary, saints, and angels to ward off evil and danger. Honor and special attention is paid to the Black Madonna or Our Lady of Czestachowa (Fig. 19–1). In Czestachowa, a town in central Poland, there is a picture of the Virgin Mary with a darkened face and two scratch marks on her face. Every year, many Poles join a pilgrimage on foot to see the Madonna. The United States has several settings honoring the Black Madonna. At times of illness and family concerns, one might hear a Pole praying or saying **Matka Boska**, which literally means "mother of God," Poland's patroness, to help in times of need.

Many older Polish people believe in the special properties of prayer books, rosary beads, medals, and consecrated objects. Early immigrants and first-generation Polish Americans commonly exhibit devotions to God in their homes, such as crucifixes and pictures of the Virgin Mary, the Black Madonna, and the Polish Pope John Paul II.

MEANING OF LIFE AND INDIVIDUAL SOURCES OF STRENGTH

Most Polish Americans have a strong work ethic and pride themselves on being fastidious and punctual. They are loyal to friends and family, have a strong sense of Catholic ideals, are self-disciplined, and are concerned about honor. Most Poles enjoy music and dancing, including the jovial Polish polka, the waltz or polonaise, and the works of Chopin and other classical composers. Liturgical music may be important to older and more religious Poles.

After years of being under Communist censorship, newer immigrants value freedom, independence, being respected for their work, and having status in the community. Most Polish Americans find meaning in family loyalty and show great generosity to friends and extended family. They want to be respected for their contribution to the world around them.

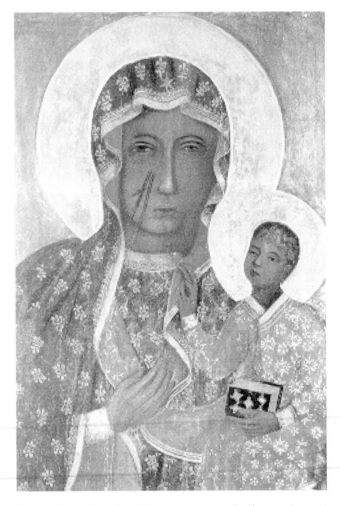

FIGURE 19–1 The Black Madonna or Our Lady of Czestachowa is an object of devotion to millions of native and immigrant Polish people. Source: The Marian Library/International Marian Research Institute, Dayton, Ohio. *http://www.udayton.edu/mary/resources/blackm/blackm03.html.*

SPIRITUAL BELIEFS AND HEALTH-CARE PRACTICES

Among the early peasants, religion had a folk tradition and formal Catholic element. Most peasants believed in mythological beings, water spirits, and house ghosts. Killing and useless slaughter of animals did not exist. All life had meaning, and if an experience could not be explained, superstition and religion filled in the gaps. This view of life is not commonly found in educated urban Poles, particularly young adults, but some immigrants from rural areas still hold to their early beliefs (Tobacyk & Tobacyk, 1992).

Health-Care Practices

HEALTH-SEEKING BELIEFS AND BEHAVIORS

Most Poles put a high value on stoicism and doing what needs to be done. Many only go to health-care providers when symptoms interfere with function, and then they may consider their advice carefully before complying. Describing anxiety and expecting nurturance is not a characteristic of most Polish adults and children. Many Poles do not discuss their treatment options and concerns with physicians and just accept the plan as outlined. Many have a strong fear of becoming dependent and "not carrying their own weight." This may also include paying medical bills. If Poles believe they cannot pay the medical bill, they may veto treatment unless the condition is life threatening. Older Poles and newer immigrants may have difficulty with the concept of Medicare, Medicaid, and managed care. Anything that lowers their status in their community is generally not acceptable. The health-care provider must describe these financial programs carefully or Poles may interpret them as charity and not follow through on prescriptions and health counseling.

Poles usually look for a physical basis of disease before considering a mental disorder. If mental health problems exist, home visits are preferred to clinic visits, and talk therapy without suitable psychosocial strategies is not maintained unless interventions are action oriented. In addition, Poles look to other family members and the community to assess the appropriateness of treatments. Polish Americans often seek self-help groups such as Alcoholics Anonymous before seeing a health-care provider. Assimilated Poles respect the health-care system and tend to seek specialists when necessary.

In Poland, health care is subsidized by the state, so cost is not an issue. The problem is that access to health care is difficult, and many people in Poland who can afford to pay higher fees to see a private physician do not have access to one. Some third-wave Poles return to Poland to have medical or surgical procedures performed because it is more affordable in their homeland.

RESPONSIBILITY FOR HEALTH CARE

Given the continuation of limited access to care in Poland and the strong work ethic of this cultural group, health promotion practices are often not valued by older Polish Americans and newer immigrants. In fact, older Polish Americans and newer immigrants commonly smoke and drink, get limited physical exercise outside of work, and have poor dental care. Partial and complete dentures are common in older Poles as one might expect in older Americans. A number of secondary teeth are often found missing in Polish American immigrant children. This often surprises school nurses who may be unaware of the limited number of dentists in Poland.

Attention to health promotion practices among women may be complicated by Polish American women's sense of modesty and religious background. Breast self-examination and pap tests are poorly understood by many older women, and practices vary depending on the woman's assimilation into American culture.

The Polish ethic of stoicism does not encourage the use of over-the-counter medications unless a symptom persists. Most Poles do not take time from work to see a health-care provider until self-help measures are no longer effective. Few Poles use vitamins unless they are suggested by a physician or a trusted family member;

even then, their extrinsic value is considered over the cost.

FOLK PRACTICES

When an older Pole is asked to undress for a physical examination, the health-care provider should pay special attention to any medals pinned to the patient's undergarments. Most of these medals have special religious significance to the wearer and should not be removed. Older Polish Americans and newer immigrants may use certain remedies to cure an illness such as tea with honey and spirits to "sweat out" a cold. Herbs and rubbing compounds also may be used for problems associated with aches, pains, and inflammation from overworked joints and muscles. Because of individual differences, every client must be assessed personally and asked specifically about use of home remedies and over-the-counter medications.

BARRIERS TO HEALTH CARE

Being unable to speak and understand English along with understanding the American health system are the greatest barriers to health care for newer Polish immigrants. In addition to overcoming the language barrier, Polish clients need health-care providers who understand Polish family values. Health-care providers also must consider that Poles often filter information through the extended family and neighborhood before accepting appropriate health-care action. Health-care providers may need to employ primary care or case management and help obtain a cultural broker from the Polish American community to help decrease the number of barriers to health care for newer immigrants.

Poles who have learned English as a second language may have some difficulty with the nuances of health-care jargon and terminology in America. The health-care provider should ask clients to restate what has been said in a discussion. If an interpreter is needed, the Polish community can usually help provide someone through an informal network. Poles are polite to authority figures and would not want to offend a health-care worker by not being agreeable; thus, they may not ask for clarification on questionable issues. Additionally, many Poles are concerned more with how a disease affects daily functioning rather than its survival rates.

CULTURAL RESPONSES TO HEALTH AND ILLNESS

Because of their strong sense of stoicism and fear of being dependent on others, many Polish Americans use inadequate pain medication and choose distraction as a means of coping with pain. When asked, many Poles either deny or diminish their pain. Poles with chronic illnesses may have similar attitudes; thus, persevering with pain is a common behavior among Poles. The health-care provider should use a visual analog scale to assess pain, assist clients with distraction techniques, and help Poles to accept pain medication as needed.

Even though Poles of the second and third wave talk

of suffering and their experiences during World War II, few turn to psychiatrists or mental health providers for help; those who do seek help, do so as a last resort. Many individuals choose their priest or a Polish volunteer-run agency over a health professional for psychiatric help.

Studies of first-time admissions to a psychiatric hospital in England (Hitch & Rack, 1980) and Australia (Krupinski, 1967) reported that eastern European refugees have a higher rate of admissions than those who are native born, and female admissions greatly outnumber male admissions. The primary diagnoses were schizophrenia and paranoia. These studies imply that people are able to overcome the initial shock of moving to a foreign country, but they do not have adequate coping skills to get through the stressors of middle age. Some of the reasons given are that people stay in **Polonia** where basic services such as grocery shopping and banking are provided. Children become the go-betweens for their parents and the larger community. As children leave their parents to start their own families, they leave their parents behind. Thus, their lack of assimilation, even 25 years later, creates stressors leading to poor coping behaviors.

Aroian (1992) describes three types of social support needed by Polish immigrants. During the first 3 years, immigrants need help finding housing and jobs, and information about getting through the system; that is, learning English, buying groceries, and learning American customs. During the next 3 to 10 years, help is required to secure credit, obtain loans, and assimilate into American life. Finally, immigrants in America for more than 10 years need support in honoring their Polish heritages through Polish networks and maintaining an American support system. After immigrants are comfortable with resettlement, feelings of grief and loss begin to be acknowledged. "The psychological adaptation to migration and resettlement requires the dual task of mastering resettlement demands and grieving, and removing the losses left in the homeland" (Aroian, 1990: 8).

Suicide rates in Poland and the United States are similar, 11.7 per 100,000 inhabitants (Kolankiewicz & Lewis, 1988). For Poland, this statistic shows improvement over previous rates, which were much higher.

Handicapped members of Polish families are usually cared for at home. The Polish characteristics of loyalty to family and the historical lack of health-care facilities in Poland make this a family duty. This same belief necessitates caring for elderly family members at home rather than placing them in a nursing home or residential care facility.

Many Poles do not assume the sick role easily and underplay their symptoms to continue functioning. If a client has an acute episode of an illness, such as the flu, the community helps to informally decide when it is time for the person to return to work. As in many other cultures, women are expected to continue their roles as wife and homemaker. When a woman is sick, other women usually help the family; men do not usually assume these roles. This practice may be different for third and fourth generations as Poles assimilate into the American culture.

BLOOD TRANSFUSIONS AND ORGAN DONATION

Given the ethic of being useful, independent, and a good Catholic, using extraordinary means to keep people alive is not commonly practiced. The individual or family determines what means are considered extraordinary. Third- and fourth-generation assimilated Polish Americans may view this issue differently. There is no taboo about receiving blood transfusions or undergoing organ transplantation. However, it is important for a family to know the extent to which a patient will be able to function following an organ transplantation. Cost is an important consideration. Most Poles do not want to be a burden on their families' physical or financial resources. On the other hand, Poles consider it their duty to care for a sick member at home.

Health-Care Practitioners

TRADITIONAL VERSUS BIOMEDICAL PRACTITIONERS

Immigrant Poles often assess health-care providers by the warmth of their manner. Newer Polish American immigrants may seek health advice from chiropractors and local pharmacists as well as neighbors and extended family. Generally, they seek biomedical advice when a symptom persists and interferes with function.

Newer immigrants coming out of a communist bureaucratic structure may not realize that patients leave the hospital early before they have healed and are fully recuperated. Newer immigrants may believe this has to do with charity care or not having enough money as opposed to the American health-care system.

STATUS OF HEALTH-CARE PROVIDERS

Physicians are held in high regard in Polish communities. Poles typically follow medical orders carefully. Poles may switch physicians if they believe they are not getting better or if a second opinion is needed. In Poland, Poles with more education are more willing than are Poles with less education to follow medical orders and continue with prescribed treatment, especially as it is related to chronic illnesses such as cardiovascular disease or diabetes. Less-educated Poles tend to change physicians if the disease does not subside fast enough. Poles respect physicians, but they want to understand the purpose of the medical treatment.

In Rempusheski's (1988) study of elderly Poles, the caring nurse was described as the nurse who knew what the patient was feeling without being told by the patient, had a quiet gentle approach, was efficient with treatments, administered medication on time, looked neat and clean, and enjoyed the work of nursing. Immigrant Poles may not realize that American nurses are expected to know about and be involved in the patients' care. Many Poles may still want the physician for the most important concerns regarding their care.

It is also important to consider how modest and self-conscious older Polish women and immigrant women may be. Polish women may actively refuse health care because they do not want to undress in front of a male provider. It may be critical to have a female provider for Polish women.

CASE STUDY Thomas Wyzinski came to America as a young boy in the 1930s, and has lived in the same Polish neighborhood his entire life. He married his neighborhood girlfriend, Zosia, and has two children. He is proud of his ethnic heritage and the fact that his wife is a "healthy looking woman and a good Polish cook." He openly boasts about how proud he is of his wife and children, but he does not like the idea that his children moved to the suburbs 15 years ago. He states, "They act so stuck up sometimes."

Mr. Wyzinski has always prided himself on working hard and earning his seniority at the electronics factory. When Thomas was younger, he was a heavy drinker, and he smoked one pack of cigarettes daily for 30 years. He gave up smoking 10 years ago and drinking about 5 years ago. He stopped smoking because he felt "winded" and stopped drinking because "I just couldn't hold it like I used to. I guess I'm just getting old."

Mr. Wyzinski has been feeling sick for the past month. Finally, his wife told him he had to go to the doctor because he was drinking so much water and was going to the bathroom all the time. Mr. Wyzinski was concerned that he could not hold his urine getting to the bathroom.

At the physician's office, his blood glucose level was 450 mg %. Thomas was told he had to go to the hospital. Protesting loudly, he called his wife and went to the hospital.

A complete physical examination revealed that his legs were swollen and that he was having trouble breathing. Thomas was prescribed furosemide (Lasix) 20 mg daily and Novolin 70/30 insulin 25 units in the morning and 10 units in the evening. He was a model patient and was discharged 3 days later.

The visiting nurse came every day for a week to teach Mr. Wyzinski diabetic care and assist him with giving himself insulin. Mr. Wyzinski was a quick learner, but he did not like the food restrictions and thought the cost of needles and insulin was too expensive. The nurse said she would call in 1 week to see how he was doing.

Mr. Wyzinski took sick days from his job for the first time in 10 years. He still felt tired but insisted on returning to work.

Mrs. Wyzinski is a full-time secretary. When the nurse called a week later, Mrs. Wyzinski told the nurse that when her husband picks her up from work she has noticed chocolate on his shirt. He denies having any desserts. She is also concerned that he may have started drinking again, and he reuses needles three times as he feels it's a waste of money to use them once and throw them out.

After 3 weeks, the swelling in his legs is still present, and Mr. Wyzinski tells his wife there is nothing to worry about. Mr. Wyzinski gets angry when his wife tells him he should call the nurse.

STUDY QUESTIONS

1 | For health teaching strategies and interventions to be successful, what is the overriding theme in working with Mr. Wyzinski?

2 | What must the health-care provider keep in mind when providing nutritional counseling to the Wyzinski family?

3 | How can meals be modified to meet the family's nutritional needs?

4 | State two short-term goals for the Wyzinski family.

5 | For the health-care provider "to be present" for this family, what personal qualities must be considered?

6 | What role might the extended family play in this situation?

7 | Prepare a flexible medication and meal schedule that would allow Mr. Wyzinski to manage his illness at work.

8 | Will Mr. Wyzinski wear a "Medical Alert" bracelet?

9 | What managed care plan might be better for the Wyzinski family than the one developed by the visiting nurse?

10 | What health promotion activities should the nurse encourage for this family?

11 | What might the health-care provider do to assist the new Polish American immigrant obtain access to health-care services?

12 | Describe the living conditions of newer Polish American immigrants in America.

13 | Identify health risks that Polish immigrants may bring with them to the United States.

14 | Describe postpartum practices for Polish American clients.

15 | Identify rituals related to terminal care for Polish Americans.

16 | Identify the primary religious practice and the use of prayer for Polish Americans.

REFERENCES

Aroian, K. J. (1990). A model of psychological adaptation to migration and resettlement. *Nursing Research, 39*(1), 5–10.
Aroian, K. J. (1992). Sources of social support and conflict for Polish immigrants. *Qualitative Health Research, 2*(2), 178–207.

Berdes, C., & Zych, A. A. (2000). Subjective quality of life of Polish, Polish-Immigrant and Polish American elderly. *International Journal of Aging and Human Development, 50*(4), 385–395.

Boyd, C. J. et al. (1994). Mother-daughter identification: Polish and Polish American mothers and their adult daughters. *Health Care For Women International, 15,* 181–195.

Brogan, P. (1990). *The captive nations of Eastern Europe: 1945–1990.* New York: Avon Books.

Bukowczyk, J. J. (1987). *And my children did not know me.* Bloomington: Indiana University Press.

Davies, N. (1982). *God's playground: A history of Poland.* New York: Columbia University Press.

Eng, R., Slawinska, J. B., & Hanson, D. J. (1991). The drinking patterns of American and Polish university students: A cross national study. *Drug and Alcohol Dependence, 27,* 167–174.

Erdmans, M. P. (1998). *Opposite Poles.* University Park: Pennsylvania State University Press.

Frydman, L. (1983). Psychiatric hospitalization in Poland. *Social Science and Medicine, 17*(10), 617–623.

Hitch, P. J., & Rack, P. H. (1980). Mental illness among Polish and Russian refugees in Bradford. *British Journal of Psychiatry, 137,* 206–211.

Kahana, E. et al. (1993). Adaptation to institutional life among Polish, Jewish, and western European elderly. In C. M. Barresi & D. E. Stull (Eds.), *Ethnic elderly and long-term care* (pp. 144–158). New York: Springer.

Kolankiewicz, G., & Lewis, P. G. (1988). *Poland.* New York: Pinter.

Krupinski, J. (1967). Sociological aspects of mental ill health in migrants. *Social Science and Medicine, 1,* 267–281.

Lopata, H. Z. (1994) *Polish Americans* (ed. 2). New Brunswick, NJ: Transaction.

No jokes, less solidarity. (1991, October 5). *Economist,* p. 33.

Rempusheski, V. (1988). Caring for self and others: Second generation Polish American elders in an ethnic club. *Journal of Cross-Cultural Gerontology, 3,* 223–271.

Rywik, S. et al. (1989). Poland and U.S. collaborative study on cardiovascular epidemiology. *Journal of Epidemiology, 130*(3), 431–445.

Statistics Canada: Ethnic origin. (1999). Ottawa, Canada: Minister of Industry Science, and Technology.

Szulc, T. (1988, January). Poland: The hope that never dies. *National Geographic,* pp. 80–117.

Tobacyk, J., & Tobacyk, Z. S. (1992). Comparisons of belief-based personality constructs on Polish and American university students. *Journal of Cross-Cultural Psychology, 23*(3), 311–325.

Wijatkowski, S. et al. (1990). Smoking behavior and personality characteristics in Polish adolescents. *The International Journal of Addictions, 25*(4), 363–373.

Chapter 20

People of Puerto Rican Heritage

TERESA C. JUARBE

Overview, Inhabited Localities, and Topography

OVERVIEW

Puerto Ricans are the third largest Hispanic cultural subgroup with a population of approximately 3 million living in the continental United States compared to 3.8 million residents in Puerto Rico (U.S. Bureau of the Census, 2000). During the last 2 decades, the composition and regions of residence for Puerto Ricans have had minor but significant changes. Sixty-one percent of Puerto Ricans live in central cities of metropolitan areas in the northeastern United States. States such as Connecticut, Florida, Illinois, and New York continue to have the largest concentration of Puerto Ricans, with many families relocating to the northwestern states.

Puerto Ricans have a unique pride in their country, culture, and music. They self-identify as *Puertorriqueños* or **Boricuans** (Taíno Indian word for Puerto Rican), or **Niuyoricans** for those born in New York. Most Puerto Ricans are between the ages of 18 and 40, with a median age of 27 years. Thirty-four percent of Puerto Ricans are age 18 and younger, and only 6 percent are age 65 and older (U.S. Bureau of the Census, 2000). During the 1990s, Puerto Rican families manifested modest health and socioeconomic improvements, but they continue to

have poor health and living conditions in the United States. In 2000, 25.8 percent of Puerto Rican families were living below the poverty level and, in 1999, 60.9 percent of full-time year-round workers had annual earnings of less than $30,000. A summary of selected sociodemographic characteristics of Puerto Ricans compared to European Americans and other Hispanic subgroups is presented in Table 20–1.

HERITAGE AND RESIDENCE

The Taíno Indians inhabited Puerto Rico until it became a Spanish colony. Puerto Ricans evolved from interracial marriages among indigenous Indians, Spaniards, and African slaves. During the Spanish-American War (1898), Puerto Rico became a colony of the United States. In 1917, Puerto Ricans were granted U.S. citizenship through the Jones Act, and in 1952 Puerto Rico became a Commonwealth. This Commonwealth "status question" is a sensitive topic for most Puerto Ricans. From the **jíbaros** (peasants) to educated political leaders, the perception of many is that the Americanos (European Americans), their culture, and politics are a potential threat to the Puerto Rican culture, language, and political future.

REASONS FOR IMMIGRATION AND ASSOCIATED ECONOMIC FACTORS

Puerto Ricans have been migrating to the United States for decades to seek employment, education, and a better quality of life. Initially, the Puerto Rican migration was fostered by a need for manual labor in the United States. By 1940, 70,000 Puerto Ricans had come to the United States. More recently, Puerto Ricans such as physi-

The author gratefully acknowledges the support and assistance of Mrs. Elizabeth Rolòn. Her Puerto Rican cultural knowledge and experiences were an inspiration for this chapter.

Table 20–1 *Selected Sociodemographic Characteristics of Puerto Ricans Compared with Whites and Other Hispanic Subgroups*

Race/ Ethnicity	Hispanic Subgroup Population (percent)	Racial and Ethnic Population in Millions	Families Living Below the Poverty Level (percent)	Unemployment Rates for Civilian Labor Force Age 16 and Older (percent)	Households with Five or More People (percent)	Population with High School Education (percent)
Whites	75.1	211.5	7.7	3.4	11.8	88.4
Hispanics	12	32.8	22.8	6.8	30.6	57
Central and South Americans	14.5	4.7	16.7	5.1	27.9	64.3
Cubans	4	1.3	17.3	5.8	14	73
Mexicans	66.1	21.7	24.1	7	35.5	51
Puerto Ricans	9	3	25.8	8.1	18.1	64.3

Source: Data were obtained from Grieco (2001), Therrien and Ramirez (2001), and the U.S. Bureau of the Census (2000).

cians, lawyers, and other professionals have migrated to enhance their educational status, social mobility, and employment opportunities. The increased number of Puerto Ricans moving to and residing in California is a reflection of this economic and social mobility.

Puerto Ricans select geographic areas where they can preserve their cultural, social, and familial wealth; enhance their assimilation into the U.S. culture; and increase their opportunities for employment and social support. For Puerto Ricans, citizenship status has created a controversial *"Va y Ven"* (go and come) circular migration (Lemann, 1991) in which individuals and families are often caught in a reverse cycle of immigration, alternatively living a few months or years in the United States and then returning to Puerto Rico.

EDUCATIONAL STATUS AND OCCUPATIONS

Education is greatly respected among Puerto Ricans. Children are praised and encouraged to become educated to improve their opportunities for the future. The educational system in Puerto Rico is similar to the system in the United States for all educational levels. Nevertheless, when children migrate from Puerto Rico to the United States, many educational organizations place them one grade below their previous academic year, as a result of language barriers.

The literacy level in Puerto Rico is 90 percent, and more than 56 percent of Puerto Ricans in the mainland have at least 1 year of college (U.S. Department of Labor, 1999). Puerto Rico boasts five well-developed and sophisticated public and private universities, plus three medical schools accredited locally and by the United States. However, in the United States, Puerto Ricans have high secondary school dropout rates (National Center for Education Statistics, 2000). Health-care providers may assess clients' literacy levels by asking how many years of education they have completed. Historically, many Puerto Ricans have valued private rather than public education. Many parents make great financial sacrifices to enable their children to attend private educational organizations, which most often are Catholic schools. Private schools are often referred to as *colegios* (colleges),

creating confusion with the American English translation of undergraduate institutions and the Central American term for college education. Instead of "college," the term *universidad* (university) is most commonly used to refer to 4-year college institutions in Puerto Rico. Bachelors and masters degrees equate to those in the United States.

Many Puerto Ricans who migrated before the 1970s had less than a fifth-grade education. Most were farmers who worked on rice, sugar cane, and coffee plantations and in the garment and manufacturing industries in northeastern and midwestern cities. However, during the past 3 decades, this pattern has begun to change as more educated Puerto Ricans migrate to the United States. After 1970, thousands of Puerto Ricans lost their jobs, suddenly finding themselves without the necessary education or training to find employment. Unemployment resulted in an increase in alcoholism, drug abuse, street crime, and family disruption and conflict.

Today, only a small percent of Puerto Ricans work in farming, forestry, or fishing, the original "catch" for U.S. migration. The overall educational attainment of Puerto Ricans age 25 and older is better than the other subgroups of Hispanics. In 1999, the percent of Puerto Ricans with less than a ninth grade education was 17.5 percent compared to 32 percent among Mexicans, 22.3 percent for Central Americans, and 18.1 percent of Cubans. Even though many Puerto Ricans value education, less than 20 percent are college educated and less than 7 percent hold an advanced degree.

Modest advances have been made in the educational status of Puerto Ricans but the unemployment status remains a challenge. Among Hispanics, Puerto Ricans have the highest unemployment rates (8.1 percent). Over the years, the most striking unemployment improvements have been those of Puerto Rican women with a 20 percent decrease in unemployment from the 1970s to the late 1990s. Puerto Rican women are more likely than men to work in managerial and professional positions. Men are more likely to work in technical, sales, administrative support, and services (U.S. Bureau of the Census, 2000).

Communication

DOMINANT LANGUAGE AND DIALECTS

Until recently, Puerto Rico was the only Spanish-speaking Latin American country in which children, beginning in kindergarten, learned to read and write English and Spanish. The issue of two official languages, English and Spanish, is a sensitive one for some Puerto Ricans who, after the U.S. occupation in 1898, were forced to learn English. At that time, many could not read and write in Spanish. This sensitivity results from the fear that speaking English would eventually replace speaking Spanish and affect Puerto Rican culture, traditions, and practices. For Puerto Ricans, language is a political issue. With each government change during the past 2 decades, the official prevailing language has been disputed and changed. Spanish is spoken at home, in schools, businesses, and the media. However, people from the metropolitan cities are more likely to read, write, and speak some English. In the United States, Puerto Ricans age 16 and over have slightly higher English literacy scores than the three other Hispanic subgroups (National Center for Education Statistics, 2000).

Puerto Ricans use the standard form of Spanish, speaking with no dialects or indigenous languages. Puerto Ricans frequently use the phrase *¡Ay bendito!* to express astonishment, surprise, lament, or pain. Some contextual differences occur, mainly in pronunciation by people from rural areas. Rural dwellers may substitute the sound of *e* for *i* and may drop the last letters of words. For example, *después* (after) may be pronounced as *dispu*, and *para donde vas* (where are you going?) may be pronounced as *pa'onde vas*. Additionally, most Puerto Ricans exchange the letter *r* for the letter *l*; for example, *animar* (encouragement) may be pronounced as *animal*, sounding like "animal." Some use a rolling *r*, a pharyngeal pronunciation that uses double *r,* such as *arroz* (rice) and *perro* (dog). Puerto Ricans speak with a melodic, high-pitched fast rhythm that may leave non–Puerto Rican health-care providers confused. This pitch and these inflections are maintained when speaking English. Because some Puerto Ricans feel uncomfortable or even insulted if people comment on their accent, the health-care provider should avoid making comments about accent, use caution when interpreting voice pitch, and seek clarification when in doubt about the content and nature of a conversation that may seem confrontational.

CULTURAL COMMUNICATION PATTERNS

Puerto Ricans are known for their hospitality and the value placed on interpersonal interaction such as *simpatía*, a cultural script where an individual is perceived as likeable, attractive, and fun loving. Puerto Ricans enjoy conversing with friends and sharing information about their families, heritage, thoughts, and feelings. They often expect the health-care provider to exchange personal information when beginning a professional relationship. The health-care provider may wish to set boundaries with discretion and *personalismo*, emphasizing personal rather than impersonal and bureaucratic relationships.

Most Puerto Ricans readily express their physical ailments and discomforts to health-care providers, with the exception of taboo issues such as sexuality. If *confianza* (trust) is established, health-care providers can establish open communication channels with individuals and family.

Spatial distancing among Puerto Ricans in the United States varies with age, gender, generation, and acculturation. Personal space may be a significant issue for some older women, particularly those from rural areas of Puerto Rico who may prefer to maintain a greater distance from men. However, Puerto Ricans born in the United States may be less self-conscious about personal space. Young Puerto Rican women may take offence to verbal and nonverbal communications that portray women as nonassertive and passive. Thus, health-care providers must carefully assess each individual's perception of distance and space.

Most Puerto Ricans are very expressive, using many body movements to convey their messages. During conversations, hand, leg, head, and body gestures are commonly used to augment messages expressed by words. Puerto Ricans express feelings and emotions through touch and are *cariñosos* (loving and caring) in verbal and nonverbal ways. Greeting Puerto Ricans with a friendly handshake is acceptable. Once trust is established, these clients might greet the health-care provider with a friendly hug. During conversations, they are likely to touch with love and affection, including a gentle hand stroke on the shoulder. Puerto Rican women greet each other with a strong familiar hug, and if among family or close friends, a kiss is included. Men may greet other men with a strong right handshake and a left hand stroking the greeter's shoulder.

Nonverbal communication plays a vital role in acquiring informed consent for health-care and research procedures, and when providing health education and discharge planning. Nonverbal communications among Puerto Ricans may include an affirmative nod with an "aha" response, but this does not necessarily mean agreement or understanding related to the conversation. Using a respectful and friendly approach, health-care providers should seek clarification of the information provided, ask for language preference in verbal and written information, and allow time for the exchange of information with questions and answers when critical decisions need to be made. Many Puerto Rican clients may prefer to read or share sensitive information, options, and decisions with close family members. Some obtain verbal approval from extended family or community members who are knowledgeable in health matters. When consent is needed from a woman, the health-care provider should ask if verbal approval or consent from the partner should be obtained first.

Traditional cultural norms discourage an overt sexual being image for women, but with family assimilation to the United States many of these traditional values disappear, in particular for young Puerto Rican men and women. When topics such as sex, sexually transmitted diseases, or other infectious diseases are discussed, an environment built on **confianza** and **personalismo** must be established if these sensitive issues are to be effectively addressed. Voice volume and tone, the degree of eye contact, spatial distancing, and time are variables that can have an impact on discussions of sensitive topics with Puerto Ricans.

The meaning and cultural value placed on direct eye contact has changed over time. Among younger Puerto Ricans and those born in the United States, eye contact is maintained and is often encouraged among those who believe in a nonsubmissive and assertive portrayal. However, among more traditional Puerto Ricans born and raised in rural areas of Puerto Rico, limited eye contact is preferred as a sign of respect, especially with the elderly who are seen as figures of respect and great wisdom.

TEMPORAL RELATIONSHIPS

Most Puerto Ricans are present oriented, having a relativistic and serene view and way of life. This relaxed attitude often frustrates business people and health-care providers. Those unaware of this cultural nuance may misinterpret this view as fatalistic. Health-care providers should respect this view and assist in identifying options, choices, and opportunities to empower individuals to change health-risk behaviors.

Most Puerto Ricans have a relativistic view of time, which may interfere with being on time for appointments. This flexible time orientation and relaxed attitude may extend to health-care appointments and interfere with the ability to provide health services within the time limited, cost-containment standard, and resources available in health-care organizations. Health-care providers should carefully explain time limits at the beginning of an interview.

FORMAT FOR NAMES

Respect for adults, parents, and the elderly is highly valued among Puerto Ricans. Respect is reflected in the way children talk, look, and refer to adults and the elderly. Rather than *Señora* (Mrs.) and *Señor* (Mr.), children and adults are expected to use the term *Doña* (Mrs.) and *Don* (Mr.) for most adults. Aunts and uncles have their name preceded by *tití* or *tío* (auntie/uncle) and *madrina* or *padrino* (godmother or godfather). These prefixes are symbols of respect and position in the family. In health-care settings, individuals expect to be addressed as *Sr.*, *Sra.*, *Don*, and *Doña*. Health-care providers should maintain their respect by using this format for names and by avoiding calling Puerto Rican clients by their first names or terms such as "honey" or "sweetheart."

Similar to other people of Hispanic heritage, Puerto Ricans have a complex system for addressing individuals, specifically women. Single women prefer to use their father and mother's surname in that order. For example, a single woman may use her name as follows: Sonia López Mendoza with López being her father's surname and Mendoza her mother's. When she is married, the husband's last name, Pérez, is added with the word *de* to

reflect that she is married. This woman's married name would be Sonia López de Pérez; the mother's surname is eliminated. In business and health-care organizations, Señora López de Pérez is the correct formal title to use when promoting conversation or building a relationship. Younger or more acculturated women may change their last names to that of their husbands. The importance and respect given to the above prescriptive name formalities are perpetuated when friendly verbal and nonverbal gestures accompany the greeting.

Family Roles and Organization

HEAD OF HOUSEHOLD AND GENDER ROLES

Despite many socioeconomic changes and changes in the position and role of Puerto Rican women, many traditional patriarchal values still define women in terms of their reproductive roles. Gender role expectations are strikingly different among more acculturated families. Traditional and newly migrated families may have expectations and view women as lenient, submissive, and always wanting to please men. Men demand respect and obedience from women and the family. Nevertheless, women play a central role in the family and the community, and the Puerto Rican family is moving toward more egalitarian relationships. Moreover, in Puerto Rico, women are making significant contributions to society by participating in politics and traditional male-oriented roles.

The classical literature of Puerto Rican women in the United States argues that Puerto Rican women "have played a paramount role in the development of the Puerto Rican community" (Comas-Díaz, 1977:1). Many of these changes in family and gender roles result from the acculturation process and the increased participation of Puerto Rican women in the workforce in the United States. Currently, more than 55 percent of Puerto Rican women in the United States are part of the civilian labor force compared to 34 percent in the early 1970s. Puerto Ricans have the largest number of female-headed households (36 percent) compared to Mexicans (21 percent), Central and South Americans (25 percent), and Cubans (18 percent). However, they continue to experience many cultural and gender roles inequalities in mean annual income when compared to non-Hispanic white women and Puerto Rican men employed in the same kind of jobs.

Through historical, social, and personal conditions, a new identity is emerging and Puerto Rican feminist voices are calling for changes in family structure, values, power, and authority. More Puerto Rican families are sharing the economic and social responsibilities of the household. However, machismo and gender roles continue to be the source of confrontations. Many Puerto Rican women are negotiating for power to equalize the dynamics of sexual relationships with Puerto Rican men, who believe women must be submissive and obedient to men in all matters. When assessing health risks and relationships, health-care providers must consider these issues and assess families for their unique patterns of relating to identify appropriate interventions.

PRESCRIPTIVE, RESTRICTIVE, AND TABOO BEHAVIORS FOR CHILDREN AND ADOLESCENTS

Children are the center of Puerto Rican family life. From childhood through adolescence, children are socialized to have respect for adults, especially the elderly. Great significance is given to the concept of **familism**, and any behavior that shifts from this ideal is discouraged and may be perceived as a disgrace to the family. Families who expect children not to contradict, argue, or disagree with their parents may have difficulties when adolescents raised in the Americanized Puerto Rican culture seek independence and struggle between traditional and contemporary family values. Many of these cultural expectations may become a serious threat to the health and educational future of young Puerto Rican adolescents. Among others, teen pregnancy, substance abuse, delinquent behaviors, and depression have been associated with these issues (National Coalition of Hispanic Health and Human Services Organizations, 1999). Mental health-care providers addressing family conflict must work within the context of the family to resolve adolescents' mental health issues rather than using individual approaches.

Several prescriptive cultural values surround health and weight. Many families believe that a healthy child is one who is *gordita* or *llenito* (diminutive for fat or overweight) and has red cheeks. Massara's (1989) early work on weight, body image perceptions, and health argues that an oversized body image may be perceived as a mirror of physical and financial wealth, even among adult women. Young mothers are often encouraged to add cereal, eggs, and *viandas* (see Nutrition) to their infant's milk bottles. Nurses are in an excellent position to educate mothers about these practices and the health risks for children who are overweight.

Many families socialize male children to be powerful and strong. This macho behavior encourages dominance over women; values obtaining social privileges; and emphasizes the pursuit of high-paying careers for their financial advantage. Although many families wish for the education of their children, a few still want educated housewives, not necessarily educated professional working women. Female children are socialized with a focus on home economics, family dynamics, and motherhood, which places women in a powerful social status. Consequently, the value placed on motherhood may be a precursor to teenage pregnancy among Puerto Rican adolescents who are seeking power, support, and cultural recognition (Orshan, 1996).

Some families abide by cultural prescriptions that encourage the initiation of sexual behaviors before marriage, extramarital sexual activity, and control over sexual relationships by men. Girls are socialized to be modest, sexually ingenuous, respectful, and subservient to men, a cultural script related to *marianismo* (Orshan, 1996; Peragallo & Alba, 1996). Discussions about sexual-

ity are considered taboo for many families, who use the term *tener relaciones* (to have relations) rather than the word "sex." Modesty is highly valued and issues such as menstruation, birth control, impotence, sexually transmitted diseases, and infertility are rarely discussed.

Less-educated families and those from rural areas may have great difficulty educating young women about sexuality and reproductive issues. Thus, many Puerto Rican adolescents depend on educational organizations to learn about menstruation and the reproductive system. The author is often asked by Puerto Rican and other Hispanic caretakers to young women about subjects such as menstruation and contraception because these topics are too embarrassing for the family to discuss openly. However, this is often not the case for preadolescents or adolescents who are exposed to information through the media, schools, and peers. Cultural respect for the role of health-care providers as educators places them in an excellent position to educate the family about sexuality issues. This respect gains them entrance into a familiar and trusted family environment that must be valued for its cultural traditions and practices.

Most families expect their children to stay home until they get married or pursue a college education. Families want to care for their young and provide them with emotional and financial support to the extent that it is feasible. Children are expected to follow family traditions and rules. The mother is expected to assume an active role disciplining, guiding, and advising children. Most fathers expect to be consulted, but they mainly see themselves as financial providers. Puerto Rican families are often very rigorous with their children's discipline. Traditional punishments include making the child who has told a lie kneel on rice until the truth is told, washing the mouth vigorously with soap for using profanity, and spanking the buttocks or lower extremities with a belt. Puerto Rican mothers tend to be very protective of their children and may use physical punishment. Many Puerto Rican mothers use threats of punishment, guilt, and discipline, which can create stress and difficulties for adolescents as they struggle with the more permissive cultural patterns of the United States, such as dating. Health-care providers should assess families for these patterns and provide counseling that promotes stability. The cultural definition of physical abuse is challenging, and health-care providers must assess each situation before determining child abuse.

FAMILY GOALS AND PRIORITIES

Family roles and priorities among Puerto Ricans are based on the concept of familism. Puerto Ricans value the unity of the family. *La familia* is the nucleus of the community and the society. The family structure may be nuclear or extended. Family members include grandparents, great-grandparents, married children, aunts, uncles, cousins, and even divorced children with their children. Two families may live in the same household.

After marriage, children live away from their parents but are expected to maintain very close ties with their families, especially the women. Most Puerto Rican families want a daughter because traditionally daughters are caretakers when parents reach advanced ages. Additionally, women continue family traditions. Male children, who are usually more independent, are valued because they continue the family name.

Because children are the center of the family, close and extended family members are expected to participate in the care of children, give support, and encourage the maintenance of cultural and religious traditions. Grandparents assume an active role in rearing grandchildren, supporting the family, babysitting, teaching traditions, disciplining, and enforcing educational activities. If the woman works outside the home, family goals and priorities may change, which often results in social and emotional burdens for women. Health-care providers can use and encourage older Puerto Ricans to introduce health promotion and disease-prevention education within their families.

As women become older, they gain status for their wisdom. Often older women have a covert power over spouses, children, and the family. Dependent elders are expected to live with their children and be cared for emotionally and financially. Informal and formal support systems are considered critical factors in promoting the health of elderly Puerto Ricans in the United States, particularly elderly women. All members of the family provide support for financial and manpower efforts needed to keep the elderly at home. Those who have higher financial liquidity may take financial responsibility in exchange for the manpower and physical efforts of those who cannot provide financially. Placements in nursing homes and extended-care facilities may be seen as inconsiderate to the elderly, and family members who must use these organizations may feel guilty and experience depression and distress. Thus, health-care providers must be sensitive to these issues by exploring alternatives for elder care and by providing information to all family members involved in this decision-making process. Discharge planning, hospice care, and other situations can be addressed in a "conference-style" approach to develop strategies for providing emotional support and assistance to family members.

Friends, neighbors, and close and distant family members are expected to visit a person during times of illness, support the family, and take an active role in family decisions and activities. A family member is expected to be at the bedside of the sick person. Health-care providers should ask the name of the family spokesperson and document it in the client's chart. Nurses may need to set boundaries about visitation, personal space, and privacy matters with clients' families.

ALTERNATIVE LIFESTYLES

During the past 2 decades, Puerto Rican families have experienced an increased incidence of pregnancy among teenagers and unmarried women. This trend is thought to be the result of the increased number of women in the labor force, high divorce rates, poverty, and the increased number of households headed by women. For health-care services to be effective in identifying appropriate interventions, health-care providers must assess social support factors and the socioeconomic status of individuals.

Homosexuality continues to be a taboo topic that carries a great stigma among Puerto Ricans. Homosexual behavior is often undisclosed to avoid family rejection and preserve family links and support. Unfortunately, the literature does not include information about these families and their lifestyles. When caring for gays and lesbians, health-care providers must inquire about their "disclosed or undisclosed status" and act according to client preferences and support resources.

Workforce Issues

CULTURE IN THE WORKPLACE

More than 67 percent of the Puerto Rican population in the United States is part of the civilian labor force, and thousands have continued to actively participate in the U.S. armed forces since World War I. Because Puerto Ricans are American citizens, they may enter the U.S. labor force without the legal implications experienced by other Hispanic subgroups who are not citizens and are undocumented. In general, men and women readily assimilate into the U.S. work environment, which is similar to their native work environment in Puerto Rico.

Nurses are among the latest group of Puerto Rican professionals who have come to the United States seeking better employment and educational opportunities. They often seek employment opportunities at federal health facilities such as the Army, Navy, Air Force, and the Veterans Administration Affairs.

Despite stereotypical views of Puerto Ricans as people who do not work and depend solely on the U.S. welfare system, most Puerto Ricans are hardworking, like to be competitive, and often make extended efforts to please their employers. Many Puerto Ricans in the labor force place a high value on their occupations, positions, and businesses. They strive for high performance even in the face of oppression; they offer little resistance and maintain the ability to be happy even when confronting oppressive situations.

Several cultural differences among Puerto Ricans, such as education, the value for honesty, integrity, personal relationships, and relativistic views of time, may have an influence in the workplace. The educational system in Puerto Rico emphasizes theoretical and practical content as well as neatness. Consequently, while most migrant Puerto Ricans are task oriented and meticulous about the presentation of their work, some have a relativistic view of time and may not value regular attendance and punctuality in the workforce. Most Puerto Ricans are cheerful, have a positive attitude, and value personal relationships at work. Work is perceived as a place for social and cultural interactions, which may include listening to background music while performing job activities. This practice can lead to loud, cheerful, and noisy conversations that may require the employer's attention.

For many women, family responsibilities, pregnancy, and the health of their children and other family members is a priority over work. For others, access to the welfare system becomes more convenient than the pride of having a secure job. In Puerto Rico, women are given a lengthy maternity leave because of the emphasis and value placed on the well-being of working women and their infants. In the U.S. labor force, many working Puerto Rican women resent the limited maternity leave supported by the American culture.

Employers may need to negotiate more flexible work responsibilities among Puerto Ricans during religious holiday celebrations such as Easter and Christmas. In Puerto Rico, schools are closed and the community celebrates a spiritual and religious recess from day-to-day activities and work responsibilities. The great solemnity and religious commitment among all religious groups bring Puerto Rican families to a societal halt for almost 6 weeks. Schools recess from early December to the middle of January, waiting for the Epiphany, *Los Tres Reyes Magos*, on January 6, and the *Octavitas*, a post-Epiphany traditional musical and cultural celebration that extends the Christmas celebration 8 more days. Many Puerto Ricans in the United States wish to use vacation and unpaid leave to spend time with their families in Puerto Rico. Traditional music, food, and folk activities during these celebrations are used to uphold ethnic pride. Holiday seasons may challenge employers who need to manage absenteeism, increased consumption of alcohol, requests for vacation, leave without pay, and decreased productivity.

With the transition of industrial to computer-related roles, musculoskeletal and cumulative trauma disorders related to ergonomics have increased. Health-care professionals should become aware of the existing controversies and health risks posed by these occupational positions to prevent repetitive injury disorders. Musculoskeletal health problems may appear earlier in this population because of workstation designs and anthropometric differences between Puerto Ricans and European Americans (Toro-Ramos & Henrich Saavedra, 1997).

ISSUES RELATED TO AUTONOMY

Puerto Rican families have traditionally socialized men into aggressive, domineering, and outspoken roles. Thus, many men display confidence at work and assume leadership positions with autonomy. However, more recent male immigrants who are less educated and have language difficulties may be reluctant to assume leadership roles, may be shy and not as outspoken, and may hesitate to challenge authority and workplace norms. Changing the conduct of these recent male immigrants in the workforce is related to the passivity and docile behaviors learned in the United States and Puerto Rican educational systems. These immigrants are more likely to conform to the behavioral norms of the workplace and avoid personal conflict or confrontations in an effort to maintain positive relationships.

Women from rural areas and traditional families are more likely to come from a submissive and noncompetitive environment. Thus they may be perceived as less determined, less confident, and less outspoken than other American women in managerial and supervisory capacities. Some women find themselves in conflict with traditional values when in a competitive, assertive work environment. Their ability to succeed in the U.S. workforce may depend on their employers' support of assertiveness and on-the-job training. In addition, women who wish to climb the career ladder may benefit from an environment that provides information, promotes confidence, fosters positive interpersonal relationships, and teaches strategies for resolving conflict.

Although most Puerto Ricans are bilingual, some may speak broken English, street English, or Puerto Rican **Spanglish** such as "I must pay billes (bills) and find dinero (money)." Younger and urban Puerto Ricans are usually more fluent in English, a skill that facilitates integration into the labor market. Older adults and people who come from a rural background may have less education, lower literacy levels, decreased English proficiency, and increased difficulty assimilating into the labor force.

Biocultural Ecology

SKIN COLOR AND BIOLOGICAL VARIATIONS

Given the heritage of Puerto Ricans who are a mixture of Native Indian, African, and Spanish heritage, some may have dark skin, thick kinky hair, and a wide flat nose; others are white skinned with straight auburn hair and hazel or black eyes. Certain traits such as skin coloring require health-care providers to vary techniques (see Chapter 2) when assessing individual Puerto Ricans for anemia and jaundice.

Limited information is available about the biocultural variations among Puerto Ricans. Although no scientific evidence exists, some posit that diseases such as hypertension and diabetes mellitus, major illnesses among Puerto Ricans in Puerto Rico and the United States, are the result of indigenous Indian and African heritage. Consequently, health-care providers should assess each person as a unique individual with awareness that standards developed for the dominant American population do not necessarily apply to the Puerto Rican population.

DISEASE AND HEALTH CONDITIONS

The health conditions of Puerto Ricans in the United States and Puerto Rico are similar with heart disease, malignant neoplasm, diabetes mellitus, unintentional injuries, and AIDS being the leading causes of death (Puerto Rico Department of Health, 1998; U.S. Department of Health and Human Services, 1999). Life expectancy among Puerto Ricans in Puerto Rico is 62 years, and 75 years among Puerto Ricans in the United States. The aging population is growing in both countries, together with an alarming increase in chronic conditions such as hypertension, diabetes, asthma, and cardiovascular disease (Puerto Rico Department of Health, 1998; U.S. Department of Health and Human Services, 1999). In the United States, Puerto Ricans have decreased mortality rates for lung, breast, and ovarian cancers, and an increased incidence of stomach, prostate, esophageal, pancreatic, and cervical cancers. In Puerto Rico, prostate, colon, and breast cancer, in that order, are the leading causes of cancer-related deaths, followed by tracheal and lung cancers (Puerto Rico Department of Health, 2000). Although the overall cancer mortality rate among Puerto Ricans is lower than for other groups, health-care providers should continue to educate Puerto Rican families about cancer prevention. Smoked, pickled, and spiced foods should be discouraged, while traditional family meals, fruits, and vegetables should be encouraged.

Puerto Ricans in the United States face a high incidence of chronic conditions such as mental illness among younger adults and cardiopulmonary and osteomuscular diseases among the elderly. Acute conditions among Puerto Ricans include a disproportionate number of acute respiratory illnesses, injuries, infectious and parasitic diseases, and diseases of the digestive system. In the Hispanic Health Assessment and Nutrition Examination Survey (HHANES), Puerto Rican children had a 6.2 percent prevalence of chronic medical conditions compared to 4 percent for Mexican American children and 3 percent for Cuban American children. Of the Puerto Rican children in this study, 62 percent had respiratory disorders; of these children, 98 percent had asthma (Martínez et al., 1991). Given these high-risk factors related to lung disorders, health-care providers need to screen Puerto Ricans for asthma and other respiratory diseases.

Puerto Rican women in the United States have a high incidence of being overweight, ranging from 38 to 41 percent; in particular this prevalence increases among the aging and women from lower socioeconomic levels (Bermudez and Tucker, 2001). Obesity and centralized body fat among these women increase the incidence of, and mortality from, diabetes, the third leading cause of death for Puerto Rican women in the mainland. Men have a lower incidence of obesity than women, and men from rural areas have lower rates of diabetes than men from urban areas. Health-care providers need to develop interventions that are appropriate to gender, age, and socioeconomic status, while giving consideration to their rural or urban living arrangements.

Dengue, a mosquito-transmitted disease caused by any of the four viral serotypes of the *Aedes aegypti* mosquito, is an endemic disease that migrants may bring to the United States. Health-care providers need to advise Puerto Rican clients and families traveling to Puerto Rico to avoid exposure to endemic areas and to use mosquito repellent and protective clothing at all times. Health-care providers should become familiar with the signs, symptoms, and current treatment recommendations for dengue fever.

Puerto Rico has a higher HIV infection rate than any state in the United States. In the United States, Puerto Ricans have the highest incidence of HIV when compared to other ethnic groups. In some states, AIDS is the leading cause of death for Puerto Rican women aged 25 to 44 (Centers for Disease Control, 1995). Puerto Rican women become HIV-positive mostly through heterosexual contact and/or intravenous drug use (Andia et al., 2001; Puerto Rico Department of Health, 1998).

VARIATIONS IN DRUG METABOLISM

Literature searches reveal no information regarding differences in drug metabolism among Puerto Ricans. Health-care providers must be aware that pharmaceutical studies conducted with European Americans may not yield the same results with Puerto Ricans; thus, individual assessments with accurate documentation of observations are imperative. Because of the African heritage of many Puerto Ricans, drug absorption, metabolism, and excretion differences experienced by African Americans and Native Americans may hold true for black Puerto Ricans. Given that some Puerto Ricans are short in stature and have higher subscapular and triceps skin folds, long trunks, and short legs, therapeutic dosages calculated for the European American population may not be appropriate for Puerto Ricans with differing physical traits.

High-Risk Behaviors

Puerto Ricans are at high risk for illnesses with increased mortality and morbidity rates related to alcoholism, smoking, illicit drug use, physical inactivity, poor dietary practices, sex-related behaviors, and underutilization of preventive health-care services. Alcoholism is the precursor of increased unintentional injuries, family disruption, spousal abuse, and mental illness among Puerto Rican families. According to the HHANES, 80 percent of Puerto Rican men and 33 percent of Puerto Rican women have high rates of alcohol consumption. Although the prevalence of alcohol consumption among Puerto Rican women is less than among Puerto Rican men and European American men and women, they drink more than Mexican, Cuban, and Central American women. This increasing pattern of alcohol consumption is attributed, in part, to acculturation into the mainstream U.S. culture and to psychosocial factors (Torres & Villaruel, 1996).

The HHANES reported that 42 percent of Puerto Rican men and 33 percent of Puerto Rican women smoke (Marks, Garcia, & Solis, 1990). However, the prevalence of smoking among Puerto Ricans is lower than that of European Americans, but higher than that for other Hispanic subgroups. Puerto Rican women have a higher prevalence of smoking than Cuban and Mexican American women, and when age is adjusted, Puerto Rican women younger than age 40 have the highest prevalence of smoking among all women in the United States. Health-care providers should consider gender and acculturation issues and build on previous successful intervention programs to develop specific programs for decreasing smoking among Puerto Rican populations. Providers must be aware that Puerto Rican adolescents, in particular women, are at higher risk of starting and continuing to smoke than other Hispanic and ethnic subgroups including African Americans and Asians (Epstein, Botvin, & Diaz, 1998).

Drug use is a significant public health problem for many Puerto Ricans whose rate of marijuana and cocaine use is often higher than that of the European American population. The last research decade clearly indicates that issues related to acculturation, peer factors, individual, family, parental, and gender-role issues are the most important risk factors in need of early health-care professional interventions to decrease susceptibility to drug addiction and delinquency (Brook, et al., 1998). Acculturation, as measured by language use, is significantly associated with marijuana and cocaine use. Many studies have shown that the longer one lives in the United States and the more acculturated one becomes, the higher the use of marijuana, smoking, and cocaine. English-speaking Puerto Ricans are five times more likely to use marijuana and two times more likely to use cocaine than Spanish-speaking Puerto Ricans (Amaro et al., 1990). Puerto Rican men use more cocaine and marijuana than women, and at least 50 percent of the men interviewed in the HHANES admitted to using marijuana at least once in their lives (Amaro et al., 1990). Among Puerto Rican men, social barriers, family demoralization, and other life problems are significant precursors for illicit drug use. However, acculturation, family factors, peer domains, language, and place of birth do not explain these patterns of illicit drug use in adolescents or men as well as they do for Puerto Rican women (Brook et al., 1997; Torres & Villaruel, 1996).

Puerto Rican women have greater drug abuse problems and a higher lifetime use of marijuana and cocaine than Mexican and Cuban American women (Amaro et al., 1990). Issues such as acculturation, self-esteem, self-concept, depression, hopelessness, and maladaptive coping behaviors are significant factors influencing the pattern and prevalence of their drug use (del Rosario Valdez, 2001). Health-care providers should develop programs that promote early interventions for the use of illicit drugs. Interventions should focus on individual psychological differences, gender issues, and other contributing factors.

Because many Puerto Ricans support machismo and submission of women, these roles foster high-risk behaviors that impede the prevention and increase the transmission of HIV. In traditional Puerto Rican culture, most men are given free will over sexual practices, including the approval and initiation of sex before marriage and extramarital affairs with other women. Some men may perceive that sexual intercourse with men is a sign of virility and sexual power rather than a homosexual behavior. Puerto Rican women are often found in a paradoxical position, as they have to deal with cultural beliefs and health-protective practices (del Rosario Valdez, 2001). Knowledge about HIV, beliefs about health and illness, and beliefs and practices related to condom use are common difficulties encountered by health-care providers in the prevention and transmission of HIV. More recently, community advocates are advocating for the improvement of housing conditions because residential status has been found to have a significant relationship with high-risk behaviors related to HIV and AIDS (Andia et al., 2000)

Lack of condom use is perhaps one of the most significant risk behaviors that need immediate attention and intervention from health-care providers. Issues such as embarrassment, cost, gender or power struggles, and abuse are among some of the barriers encountered by Puerto Rican women. Some men fear that if they use condoms they portray a less macho image, have decreased sexual satisfaction, or portray that they have a sexually transmitted disease or HIV. Additionally, the Catholic Church's opposition to the use of condoms, lower educational levels, lower socioeconomic status, and acculturation are significant variables related to the high rates of AIDS and HIV among Puerto Ricans and other Hispanics (Peragallo and Alba, 1996). Health-care providers must be aware of these barriers, assess individual perceptions of high-risk behaviors, and intervene with programs designed to meet the particular needs of clients who are at high risk for HIV infection or other sexually transmitted diseases.

Nutrition

MEANING OF FOOD

Puerto Ricans celebrate, mourn, and socialize around food. Food is used (1) to honor and recognize visitors, friends, family members, and health-care providers; (2) as an escape from everyday pressures, problems, and challenges; and (3) to prevent and treat illnesses. Puerto Rican clients may bring homemade goods to health-care providers as an expression of appreciation, respect, and gratitude for services rendered. Refusing these offerings may be interpreted as a personal rejection.

Some Puerto Ricans believe that being overweight is a sign of health and wealth. Some eat to excess believing that if they eat more their health will be better, while others pay no attention to weight control or dietary practices. Many Puerto Ricans perceive that European Americans are more preoccupied with how they look than how healthy they are. Efforts by American health-care providers directed at weight control may be seen as Americans' excessive preoccupation with a thin body image.

COMMON FOODS AND FOOD RITUALS

Traditional Puerto Rican families emphasize having a complete breakfast that begins with a cup of strong coffee or *café con leche* (coffee with milk). Some drink strong coffees such as espresso with lots of sugar; others boil fresh milk (or use condensed milk) and then add the coffee. Many families introduce children to coffee as early as 5 or 6 years of age. A traditional Puerto Rican breakfast includes hot cereal such as oatmeal; corn meal; or rice and wheat cereal cooked with vanilla, cinnamon, sugar, salt, and milk. Although less common, traditional Puerto Ricans may eat corn pancakes or fritters for breakfast.

Lunch is served by noon, followed by dinner at around 5 or 6 o'clock in the evening. It is customary to have a cup of espresso-like coffee at 10:00 A.M. and 3:00 P.M. Rice and stew *habichuelas* (beans) are the main dishes among Puerto Rican families. Rice may be served plain or cooked and served with as many as 12 side dishes. Rice cooked with vegetables or meat is considered a complete meal. *Arroz guisado* (rice stew) is seasoned with *sofrito*, a blend of spices such as cilantro, *recao* (a type of cilantro), onions, green peppers, and other nonspicy ingredients. Rice is cooked with chicken, pork, sausages, codfish, calamari, or shrimp. It is also cooked with corn, several types of beans, and *gandules* (green pigeon peas), a Puerto Rican bean that is rich in iron and protein. Rice with *gandules* is a traditional Christmas holiday dish that is accompanied by *pernil asado* (roasted pork) and *pasteles*, made with root vegetables, green plantain, bananas, or condiments and then filled with meat and wrapped with plantain leaves. Fritters are also common foods.

Puerto Ricans eat a great variety of pastas, breads, crackers, vegetables, and fruits. *Tostones*, fried green or ripe plantains, are a favorite side dish served with almost every meal. Puerto Rican families eat a variety of roots called *viandas*, vegetables rich in vitamins and starch. The most common *viandas* are celery roots, sweet potatoes, dasheens, yams, breadfruit, breadnut, green and ripe plantains, green bananas, tanniers, cassava, and chayote squash or christophines. A list of common Puerto Rican meals is presented in Table 20–2. Because Puerto Rican meals are flavorful, clients in the health-care setting may find more traditional American meals to be flavorless and unattractive. However, more acculturated Puerto Ricans are changing their traditional food practices and often follow mainland U.S. dietary practices. Health-care providers who work with traditional Puerto Rican clients should become familiar with these foods and their nutritional content to assist families with dietary practices that integrate their traditional or preferred food selections.

Table 20–2 *Common Puerto Rican Meals and Fritters*

Puerto Rican Meal	English Translation
Alcapurrias	Green plantain fritters filled with meat or crab
Arepas de maíz y queso	Corn meal and cheese fritters
Arroz con pollo	Rice with chicken
Arroz con gandules	Rice with pigeon peas
Arroz blanco (con aceite)	Plain rice (with oil)
Arroz guisado básico	Plain stewed rice
Asopao de pollo	Soupy rice with chicken
Bacalaitos	Codfish fritters
Bocadillo	Grilled sandwich
Mondongo	Tripe stew
Paella de mariscos	Seafood paella
Pastelillos de carne, queso, o pasta de guayaba	Turnovers filled with meat, cheese, or guava paste
Pollo en fricase con papas	Stewed chicken with potatoes
Relleno de papa	Potato ball filled with meat
Sancocho	*Viandas* and meats stew
Sofrito	Condiment
Surullo de queso	Corn meal fritters filled with cheese

DIETARY PRACTICES FOR HEALTH PROMOTION

Many Puerto Ricans ascribe to the hot-cold classifications of foods for nutritional balance and dietary practices during menstruation, pregnancy, the postpartum period, infant feeding, lactation, and aging. Some of the hot-cold classifications are presented in Table 20–3. Health-care providers should become familiar with these food practices when planning culturally congruent dietary alternatives.

Understanding that iron is considered a "hot" food that is not usually taken during pregnancy can assist health-care providers to negotiate approval and educate Puerto Rican women about the importance of maintaining adherence to daily iron recommendations even during pregnancy and lactation. An additional summary of Puerto Rican cultural food habits, reasons for practices, and recommendations for health-care providers during such developmental stages is presented in Table 20–4.

With the advent of alternatives to hormonal replacement therapy (HRT) (Taylor, 1999), many Puerto Rican women are using a variety of herbal and botanical remedies. Many are using relaxation, massage, acupuncture, guided imagery, chelation, biofeedback, and therapeutic touch in addition to or as an alternative to HRT. Black cohosh, evening primrose, St. John's wort, gingko, ginseng, valerian root, sarsaparilla, chamomiles, red clover, and passion flower are the most common herbs and botanical alternatives used by Puerto Rican women. Health-care professionals should understand and be able to discuss the safety and efficacy of the most frequently used alternatives. The use of HRT alternatives should be included in routine health assessment among women in this stage.

An infant is believed to be healthy if it is *gordito* (a little fat) and has red cheeks. Consequently, many mothers add ground root vegetables, eggs, hot cereals, rice, canned baby foods, and fruits and vegetables to the infant's bottle at an early age. Traditionally, when children are introduced to soft foods and vegetables, parents boil and grind root vegetables for the infant. For some, these dietary practices have changed with the availability of canned baby food. Many mothers tend to feed whole cow's milk or canned milk (Carnation) earlier than recommended in Western practice, believing that canned milk produces healthier babies. Health-care providers must educate families regarding the nutritional content of canned milk versus fresh milk, breastfeeding, and formula.

For elderly Puerto Ricans, a good diet includes meats, traditional meals, and vitamin supplements. Beverages such as fresh-squeezed orange juice, grape juice, and *ponches* (punches) are used as additional nutritional support, particularly for those who are immunosuppressed or chronically or terminally ill. If the elderly individual is believed to have low blood pressure and is weak or tired, a small daily portion of brandy may be added to black coffee to enhance the work of "an old heart." If the health-care provider criticizes these practices, it may deter the client from seeking follow-up care and decrease trust and confidence in health-care providers. Health-

Table 20–3 Puerto Rican Hot-Cold Classification of Selected Foods, Medications, Herbs, and Health-Illness Status

Hot-Cold Classification	Health-Illnesses Status	Western Medications	Traditional Herbs	Foods
Hot	GI Illnesses (constipation, diarrhea, Crohn's colitis, ulcer, bleeding) Gynecologic Issues (pregnancy, menopause) Skin Disorders (rashes, acne) Neurological Disorders (headache) Heart Disease Urologic Illnesses	Syrups Dark-colored pills Aspirin Anti-inflammatory agents Prednisone Antihypertensives Castor oil Cinnamon Vitamins (iron) Antibiotics	Teas: Cinnamon Dark-leaf teas	Cocoa products Alcoholic beverages Caffeine products Hot cereals (wheat, corn) Salt Spices and condiments Beans Nuts and seeds
Cold	Osteomuscular Illnesses (arthritis, rheumatoid arthritis, multiple sclerosis) Menstruation Respiratory illnesses	Diuretics Bicarbonate of soda Antacids Milk of magnesia	Teas: Orange-lemon chamomile Linden Mint Anise	Rice Rice and barley water Milk Sugar and sugar products Root vegetables Avocado Fruits Vegetables White meat Honey Onions

care providers must inquire about these practices and should incorporate harmless or nonconflicting practices into the diet.

During illness, Puerto Ricans pay close attention to dietary practices. Chicken soups and *caldos* (broth) are used as a hot meal to provide essential nutrients. A mixture of equal amounts of honey, lemon, and rum are used as an expectorant and antitussive. A malt drink, *malta* (grape juice), or milk is often added to an egg yolk mixed with plenty of sugar to increase the hemoglobin level and provide strength. Ulcers, acid indigestion, and stomach illnesses are treated with warm

Table 20–4 Puerto Rican Cultural Nutrition and Health Beliefs and Practices During Particular Stages

Behavioral Period	Dietary and Health Practices	Cultural Justification	Recommendation for Health-Care Professionals
Menstruation	Food Taboos: Avoid spices, cold beverages, acid-citric fruits and substances, chocolate, and coffee. Foods Encouraged: Plenty of hot fluids, such as cinnamon tea, milk with cinnamon and sugar. Teas such as chamomile, anise seed, linden tea, mint leaves. Health Practices: Avoid exercise and practice good hygiene. Do not walk barefoot. Avoid wind and rain. Stay as warm as possible.	May induce cramps, hemorrhage, clots, and physical imbalance. May produce acne during menstruation. Fluids encourage body cleaning of impurities. Hot beverages encourage circulation and reduce abdominal colic, cramps, and pain. Teas are soothing to all body systems. Exercise may increase pain and bleeding. Good hygiene is important for health. Walking barefoot during menstruation may cause rheumatoid arthritis and other inflammatory diseases. Warm temperatures promote circulation and the health of the reproductive system as well as prevent cramps.	Assess individual beliefs and acknowledge them. Incorporate traditional beliefs in treatments as required in nonsteroidal anti-inflammatories for dysmenorrhea. Encourage passive exercise. information about the role of exercise in the reduction of menstrual. Support other practices.

(Continued on following page)

Table 20–4 Puerto Rican Cultural Nutrition and Health Beliefs and Practices During Particular Stages (Continued)

Behavioral Period	Dietary and Health Practices	Cultural Justification	Recommendation for Health-Care Professionals
Pregnancy	Food Taboos: Hot food, sauces, condiments, chocolate products, coffee, beans, pork, fritters, oily foods, and citrus products.	May cause excess flatus, acid indigestion, bulging, and constipation. Chocolate and coffee may cause darker skin in fetus. Some believe citrus products may be abortive.	Encourage healthy food habits. Provide information about chocolate and coffee myths. Encourage fruits.
	Food Encouraged: Milk, beef, chicken, vegetables, fruits, *ponches*.	Considered healthy and nutritious. Increases hemoglobin, strengthens, and promotes good labor.	Discourage the use of raw eggs in beverages because of possibility of *Salmonella* poisoning.
	Health Practices: Rest and get plenty of sleep. Eat plenty of food. Follow diet cautiously. Many avoid sexual intercourse early in pregnancy. Practice good hygiene and take warm showers.	Enhances health and prevents problems during birth. Sex may cause problems with baby or preterm labor.	Encourage use of food recommended for pregnancy. Provide information about sexual activity. Encourage a balanced plan of exercise with emphasis on weight control and health of the baby.
Lactation	Food Taboos: Avoid beans, cabbages, lettuce, seeds, nuts, pork, chocolate, coffee, and hot food items at all times.	These foods cause stomach illnesses for infant and mother, including baby colic, diarrhea, and flatus.	Include a dietary plan that is balanced with substitute food items. Clarify any myths about infant diarrhea, colic, and flatus.
	Food Encouraged: Milk, water, *ponches*, chicken soup, chicken, beef, pastas, hot cereals.	Improve health and increase hemoglobin and essential vitamins. Protect mother and infant from illnesses. Fluids and ponches increase milk supply. Red meats reduce cravings.	As above with raw eggs.
	Health Practices: Avoid cold temperatures and wind. A few may avoid showering for several days during the *cuarentena* after birth. Great attention is paid to health of the mother.	Cold temperatures and winds are believed to cause stroke and facial paralysis in a new mother. Showering may cause respiratory diseases. Mother is believed to be at risk and fragile.	Provide information about reasons for stroke and facial paralysis. Provide time to ask questions and reduce anxiety during winter season deliveries.
Infant Feeding	Food Taboo: Beans, too much rice, and uncooked vegetables.	Believed to cause stomach colic, flatus, and distended abdomen. Too much rice causes constipation.	Provide information about appropriate dietary patterns for infant.
	Food Encouraged: Hot cereals, *ponches*, chicken broth or *caldos*. Fresh fruits, cooked vegetables, *viandas*. Raw eggs, cereals, baby foods in milk bottle. Fresh fruit juices. Mint, chamomile, and anise tea. Sugar and honey used for hiccups.	Believed to be nutritious, healthy, and to decrease hunger. *Caldos* are fortifying and prevent illness. Cooked vegetables are healthy and prevent constipation. Bottle food fills the baby. Fresh juices and fruits refresh the stomach. Teas help baby sleep and cure flatus. Sugar and honey have curing properties.	Instruct about infant diet and timely introduction of food items to diet. Explain consequences of excessive weight in infants. Discourage food in bottle to prevent choking.
	Health Practices: Keep baby warm while feeding.	Warm babies eat, chew, and digest food better, and choking is decreased.	Discourage raw eggs because of the risk of *Salmonella* and egg allergies and the use of honey because of the risk of botulism. Teas are harmless and provide additional fluid when used in moderation without sugar.
			Provide information about babies and choking.

milk, with or without sugar. Herbal teas are used to treat illnesses and to promote health. Most herbal teas do not interfere with medical prescriptions. Incorporating their use with traditional Western medicine may enhance compliance.

NUTRITIONAL DEFICIENCIES AND FOOD LIMITATIONS

Most Puerto Ricans moving to the United States locate in areas with Puerto Rican or Hispanic communities and where preferred foods are readily available. Traditional cooking and food practices do not necessarily change. Instead, European American foods are quickly integrated into the dietary practices, thereby increasing food diversity. Fresh fruits and juices are consumed in large quantities.

Few studies have shown significant data about nutritional deficiencies among Puerto Ricans. Studies that include small samples of Puerto Ricans show that Puerto Rican children have nutritional statuses similar to Mexican and African American children in terms of malnutrition, obesity, and short stature. Low-income Puerto Rican children and adolescents have been found to have anemia and tooth decay related to less than the recommended daily allowances of iron, folacin, thiamin, niacin, and vitamin C. In studies conducted during the late 1970s and early 1980s, such as the CDC Nutrition Surveillance Program, the Ten State Nutrition Survey, and the HHANES (Pilch, 1987), many Puerto Rican children had a high incidence of anemia, lactose malabsorption, and low levels of blood plasma vitamin A. In those studies, a large number of pregnant and lactating women were found to be anemic but not at a greater risk of impaired iron levels. Nutrition education should be a priority to improve the health of Puerto Rican families, especially children, pregnant women, and lactating mothers.

Menstruation is viewed as a time when women must care for themselves and adhere to certain dietary practices to promote health. From the onset of menstruation, young girls are encouraged to avoid foods believed to produce flatus, abdominal cramps, and colic. Hot drinks are encouraged to increase circulation and promote the elimination of metabolic waste.

Pregnancy and Childbearing Practices

FERTILITY PRACTICES AND VIEWS TOWARD PREGNANCY

Marital status, knowledge, attitudes, beliefs about the reproductive system, the role of motherhood, sexuality, and contraceptive use are factors that need to be considered when assessing and implementing culturally congruent maternal-infant interventions and educational programs. In the United States, prenatal care is a major health issue among Puerto Rican women, with many women beginning prenatal care later in their pregnancies (U.S. Department of Health and Human Services, 2000). Health-care professionals should be aware that social support has been found as one of the most significant factors related to perinatal outcomes among Puerto Rican women. Among others, social support has been found to have significant implications for stress, health behaviors, and infant health (Landale & Oropesa, 2001). Among adolescents, culturally imposed male behaviors and lack of parental guidance or supervision have been listed as predictors of teenage pregnancy (COSSMHO, 1999).

Puerto Rican women do not commonly use birth control methods such as foams, creams, and diaphragms because the Catholic Church, which only condones the rhythm method and sexual abstinence, sees them as immoral. One study showed that 40 percent of women in Puerto Rico practiced contraception through sterilization (Herold et al., 1986). According to the HHANES study, in the United States, fertility control methods used by Puerto Rican women were tubal ligation, called *La Operación* (the surgery) (23 percent); followed by oral contraceptives (8.7 percent); hysterectomies (3.5 percent); and oophorectomies (3.2 percent) (Stroup-Benham & Treviño, 1991).

Sterilization practices among Puerto Rican women came under assault following encouragement of sterilization as a method of birth control by Puerto Rican and U.S. physicians between 1965 and 1985. Sterilization choices were not made out of Puerto Rican women's free will, but in response to the social and political ideologies that view sterilization as the only lasting and effective method of birth control. According to the earlier and classical work of López (1993), sterilization became for Puerto Rican women an "element of resistance in their attempt to forge out a social space for themselves on a personal level...and an element of resistance against constraints of patriarchy/female subordination" (p. 301).

Traditionally, abortion has never been accepted except in cases in which the life of the mother was in danger. Nevertheless, this view is changing and many women now ascribe to this practice. Despite sterilization practices and the religious pressures of the Catholic Church, Puerto Rican women have fertility rates, teenage and unmarried pregnancy rates, and live-birth rates that are greater than any other Hispanic group in the United States (Orshan, 1996).

PRESCRIPTIVE, RESTRICTIVE, AND TABOO PRACTICES IN THE CHILDBEARING FAMILY

Hygiene is highly valued during pregnancy, labor, and the postpartum period. Pregnancy is a time of indulgence for Puerto Rican women. Favors and wishes are granted to women for their well-being and that of their babies. Men are socialized to be tolerant, understanding, and patient regarding pregnant women and their preferences. Pregnant Puerto Rican women are encouraged to rest, consume large quantities of food, and carefully watch what they eat. Many young Puerto Rican families prefer to attend birthing classes. Some expect women to "get fat" and place little emphasis on weight control. Strenuous physical activity and exercise are discouraged and lifting heavy objects is prohibited. Women are strongly discouraged from consuming aspirin, Alka-Seltzer, and malt beverages because these substances are believed to cause abortion.

Many women refrain from *tener relaciones*, sexual intercourse, after the first trimester to avoid hurting the fetus or causing preterm labor. Some men view this time as an opportunity for extramarital sexual affairs. Health-care providers should inquire in a nonconfrontational manner about this possibility and educate men regarding the dangers of sexually transmitted diseases and HIV.

Women prefer the bed position for labor, wish to have

their bodies covered, and prefer a limited number of internal examinations. They welcome their husbands, mothers, or sisters to assist during labor. Men are expected to be supportive. During labor, women may be loud and verbally expressive, a culturally accepted and an encouraged method for coping with pain and discomfort. Pain medications are welcomed. Health-care workers should respect these wishes and explain the necessity of invasive interventions during labor. Most women oppose having a cesarean section because it portrays a "weak woman." The health-care practitioner should discuss the possibility of a cesarean section early in the pregnancy.

Postpartum women receive care from their family and friends. Their first postpartum meal should be homemade chicken soup to provide energy and strength. Women are encouraged to avoid exposure to wind and cold temperatures, not to lift heavy objects, and not to do housework for 40 days after delivery (the *cuarentena*). Some traditional women do not wash their hair during this time. Because the mother is believed to be susceptible to emotional and physical distress during the postpartum period, family members try not to contribute to stress or to give bad news to the new mother. Fathers may be reluctant to tell the new mother about a problem with the newborn. However, most Puerto Rican women want to be told immediately about a problem with the newborn. This is a critical issue during the postpartum period, especially with premature babies, given the belief that a healthy baby is a "symbol of father's virility and a time for the woman to demonstrate her fertility, strength, and success during and after birth" (Crouch-Ruiz, 1996:26).

Some mothers might ask to talk to the pediatrician, rather than to a nurse, about infant problems. Because of the value placed on family and children, women who need to return to work early may experience great distress when they do not follow some of these cultural values or norms. Health-care providers should assess for individual perceptions and dissatisfaction with the working role and birth recuperation. Mothers who breast-feed are encouraged to drink lots of fluids such as milk and chicken soup; and if feeling weak or tired, to drink *ponches*, beverages consisting of milk or fresh juices mixed with a raw egg yolk and sugar. Hot foods such as chocolate, beans, lentils, and coffee are discouraged because they are believed to cause stomach irritability, flatus, and colic for the mother and infant.

Early studies on breast-feeding and Puerto Rican women show that only 10 to 11 percent of Puerto Rican women breast-feed (Stroup-Benham & Treviño, 1991). However, traditional Puerto Rican mothers and those from rural areas may prefer to breast-feed their babies for the first year. Mothers who work outside the home may select breast-feeding, formula, or both. However, with the introduction of formula through U.S. food stamp programs, two generations of Puerto Rican mothers have been inclined to relinquish breast-feeding and adopt formula as the primary source of infant nutrition. Because some Puerto Rican women believe that breast-feeding increases their weight, disfigures the breast, and makes them less sexually attractive, they undervalue the benefits of breast-feeding. Health-care providers need to provide information about these beliefs and educate women about breast-feeding myths and misconceptions. Because maternal grandmothers have a great influence on practices related to breast-feeding, they should be included along with significant others in educational programs that encourage breast-feeding.

Death Rituals

DEATH RITUALS AND EXPECTATIONS

Death is perceived as a time of crisis in Puerto Rican families. The body is considered sacred and guarded with great respect. Death rituals are shaped by religious beliefs and practices and family members are careful to complete the death rituals. News about the deceased should be given first to the head of the family, usually the oldest daughter or son. Because of cultural, physical, and emotional responses to grief, health-care providers should use a private room to communicate such news and have a clergy or minister present when the news is disclosed. Family privacy at this time is highly valued. Providers should allow time for family to view, touch, and stay with the body before it is removed. Traditionally, some Puerto Rican families keep the body in their home before burial. Cultural traditions and financial limitations influence this decision. Consequently, some older adults may wish to follow these death rituals in the United States. For some, funeral homes are viewed as impersonal, financially unnecessary, and detrimental to the mourning process because they detract from family intimacy.

Although the family may prefer to have all death rituals finished within a reasonable time frame, it is important to extend burial rituals until all close family members can be present. The head of the family is expected to coordinate the arrival of family members, usually creating a delay in death rituals, burial time, and an emotional burden and stress on family members. Health-care providers should ensure that members of the family are provided with support, resources, and information regarding differences in U.S. legal requirements. These requirements are often confusing and are considered insensitive, particularly with a stillbirth or when an autopsy is necessary. Authorization from several family members might be essential. Because of the spiritual and religious importance of burial traditions and rituals during these events, cremation is rarely practiced among Puerto Ricans. Among Catholics, the head of the family or other close family member is expected to organize the religious ceremonies, such as the praying of the rosary, the wake (**velorio**), and the novenas, the 9 days of rosary following the death of the family member. Family may meet at the deceased's home for several days, sometimes weeks, to support the family and talk about the deceased. Food is served throughout the day as a symbol of gratitude for those who come to pay their respects.

RESPONSES TO DEATH AND GRIEF

It is culturally acceptable for the family of the deceased to freely express themselves through loud crying and verbal expressions of grief. Some may talk in a thunderous way to God. Others may express their grief through a sensitive but continuous crying or sobbing. Some believe that not expressing their feelings could mean a lack of love and respect for the deceased. Similar to other crisis events, some may develop psychosomatic symptoms, and others may experience nausea, vomiting, or fainting spells as a result of a nervousness attack—*ataque de nervios*. Health-care providers should be nonjudgmental with clients' psychosomatic or other expressions of grief by providing a private environment and helping to minimize interruptions during that period.

Spirituality

DOMINANT RELIGION AND USE OF PRAYER

Religious beliefs among Puerto Ricans influence their approach to health and illness. Most Puerto Ricans on the mainland are Catholic (85 percent); however, over the past 4 decades, Protestant Evangelical religious movements have converted 35 percent of the Puerto Rican population in the United States. A few practice *espiritismo*, a blend of Native Indian, African, and Catholic beliefs that deal with rituals related to spiritual communications with spirits and evil forces. *Espiritistas,* individuals capable of communicating with spirits, may be consulted to promote spiritual wellness and treat mental illnesses.

In the United States, most non-Catholic Puerto Ricans are Pentecostal, and less than 7 percent are members of a Baptist denomination. The Pentecostal movement has been a strong spiritual instrument for decreasing substance abuse among Puerto Ricans by using prayer and fasting as a means for spiritual power and healing from God. Because the elderly may see illness as a result of sins, a cure should be sought through prayer or by the "laying of hands."

Upon immigration, many Puerto Ricans may feel out of place and need support resources. Many join Evangelical churches because they offer a more personal spiritual approach. These religious groups provide social support and promote harmony and spiritual–physical well-being. Health-care providers should reinforce these spiritual practices, while incorporating prescribed medications, health activities, and the prevention of risk behaviors. *Espiritistas* treat clients with mental health conditions and are often consulted to determine folk remedies compatible with Western medical treatments. Health-care providers should be aware that the elderly, those who have limited access to health care, and those who are dissatisfied with or distrust the Western medical system commonly use spiritual healers.

Among Catholics, candles, rosary beads, or a special patron or figurine might accompany the client to the health-care facility and be used during prayer rituals. To provide timely and appropriate interventions to Catholic families, health-care practitioners should inquire about the family's wishes regarding the Sacrament of the Sick. Special prayers and readings are believed to be necessary at the moment of death, and families expect to be present to recite these prayers.

MEANING OF LIFE AND INDIVIDUAL SOURCES OF STRENGTH

Puerto Ricans consider life sacred, something that individuals should preserve. Many see the quality of life as a harmonious balance among the mind, body, and spirit. Spirituality helps Puerto Ricans gain strength to deal with illness, death, and grief and ultimately promotes well-being. Most Puerto Ricans are very religious and when confronted with situations related to health, illness, work, death, or the prognosis of a terminal illness, they maintain their trust in spiritual forces. Spiritual forces assist in controlling and managing social and economic constraints. Their own personal actions are perceived as inconsequential or trivial without the trust and confidence in God's will, *Si Dios quiere* (if God wants). Rather than a fatalistic approach to life during illness, death, or health promotion, Puerto Ricans use coping mechanisms such as religious practices that are instrumental in providing control in their lives. For example, the role of religion in the lives of Puerto Ricans with chronic illnesses or with disabled children have been described as a critical source of support and a mechanism that allows for appropriate interpretation of health and illness (Skinner et al., 2001). God, who is their highest source of strength, guides life. For some, scripture readings, praise, and prayer bring inner spiritual power to the soul, *el alma*.

SPIRITUAL BELIEFS AND HEALTH-CARE PRACTICES

Spiritual practices influenced by religious groups have a great impact on the health status of Puerto Ricans in the United States. For example, Seventh Day Adventist and Pentecostal churches have had a great influence on the health of individuals by discouraging high-risk behaviors and promoting health. Through prayer, church attendance, and worship, many Puerto Ricans discover spiritual courage and inner strength to avoid high-risk behaviors such as smoking and substance abuse. Clergy and ministers are a resource for spiritual wisdom and help with a host of spiritual needs.

Although amulets have lost their popularity, some still use them. An *azabache* (small black fist) or a rabbit's foot might be used for good luck, to drive away bad spirits, and to protect a child's health. Rosary beads and patron saint figures may be placed at the head or side of the bed or on the client to protect him or her from outside evil sources. Health-care providers should ask permission before removing, cleaning, or moving these objects. A benediction may be requested before removing amulets or religious objects, giving the Sacrament of the Sick, or providing spiritual support. These objects are often used as a means of dealing with a crisis or as an expression of hope. The health-care provider should assess individual and family religious preferences and support spiritual resources according to the client or family's request.

Health-Care Practices

HEALTH-SEEKING BELIEFS AND BEHAVIORS

Most Puerto Ricans have a curative view of health. They tend to underuse health promotion and preventive services such as regular dental or physical examinations and pap smears (Marks, Garcia, & Solis, 1990). Many use emergency health-care services for acute problems rather than preventive health-care services. Acculturation, age, access to health care, education, and income influence health-seeking beliefs and behaviors. Health-care providers must develop mechanisms to integrate individual, family, and community resources to encourage a focus on health promotion and enhance early health screening and disease prevention. In particular, a great deal of attention must be provided to improve interpersonal processes of care among providers and Puerto Rican clients. In a recent study with Puerto Rican women, Davis and Flannery (2001) reported that women experienced negative interactions with providers who were perceived as the "least helpful resource." Health-care providers that offer weekend, evening, and late-night health-care services in community-based settings may increase the use of preventive services.

Good hygiene is a basic concept for health promotion among Puerto Ricans. Daily showers are essential for good health and for personal appearance. Exceptions are made during illnesses such as colds, flu, or viral infections. After surgery, some prefer to bathe using a basin of water instead of taking a shower or tub bath. Most prefer to shower and wash their hair daily; however, some women may avoid doing these activities during menstruation. During hospitalization, some refrain from having a bowel movement if they have to use a bedside commode or bedpan. Nurses are in a unique position to respectfully explore those beliefs and practices and to provide a private, nonintrusive environment for the client.

RESPONSIBILITY FOR HEALTH CARE

Most Puerto Ricans believe in "family-care," rather than self-care. Women are seen as the main caregivers and promoters of family health and are the source of spiritual and physical strength. Health-care providers should incorporate the participation of the family in the care of the ill.

Natural herbs, teas, and over-the-counter medications are often used as initial interventions for symptoms of illness. Many consult family and friends before consulting a health-care provider. Moreover, pharmacists play a vital role in symptom management. Although Puerto Rico is subject to U.S. drug administration regulations and practices, many Puerto Ricans are able to obtain controlled prescriptions from their local pharmacist in Puerto Rico. When they are in the United States, they try to obtain the same kind of services from local pharma-

cists, creating distress and frustration for both the client and the pharmacist.

Over-the-counter medications and folk remedies are often used by Puerto Ricans to treat mental health symptoms, acute illnesses, and chronic diseases. Early studies tend to show that Puerto Rican women extensively use prescription and over-the-counter medications for a variety of symptoms and discomforts (National Institute of Drug Abuse, 1987). There are no recent studies on these or other related issues for this ethnic group. Health-care providers should inquire about those practices and encourage clients to bring their medications to every visit. Engaging in a friendly conversation encourages clients to reveal their use of folk treatments, over-the-counter medications, and concurrent use of folk healers. During the past 2 decades, Puerto Ricans have become accustomed to the use of extended-care facilities and nursing homes for the elderly. However, they prefer to keep chronically or terminally ill family members at home.

FOLK PRACTICES

Espiritismo and **santería** are magicoreligious and folk-healing practices used by some Puerto Ricans. *Espiritistas* solve problems by communicating with spirits. The **Santería** focuses on health promotion and personal growth and development. Clients who use these folk practices visit **bótanicas**, folk religious stores, and use natural herbs, aromatic incenses, special bathing herbs, prayer books, prayers, and figurines for treating illness and promoting good health. Providers must examine their own views about traditional practices and healers, and refrain from making prejudicial comments that may inhibit collaboration with folk healers.

Puerto Ricans may use folk practices for shortness of breath, nausea, and vomiting. Asphyxia or shortness of breath is believed to be caused by lack of air in the body. Fanning the face or blowing into the client is believed to provide oxygen and relieve dyspnea. Some may use tea from an alligator's tail, snails, or *savila* (plant leaves) for illnesses such as asthma and congestive heart failure.

Nausea and vomiting may be embarrassing and cause alarm to many Puerto Rican clients. Many believe that smelling or rubbing isopropyl alcohol (*alcolado*) may help alleviate these symptoms. Some place a damp cloth on the forehead to refresh the "hot" inside the body and relieve nausea. Some put the head between the legs to stop vomiting. Mint, orange, or lemon tree leaves are boiled and used as tea to relieve nausea and vomiting. Rectal suppositories are believed to induce diarrhea. Health-care practitioners should provide clear information about suppositories and the etiologic cause of symptoms.

BARRIERS TO HEALTH CARE

The medically indigent in Puerto Rico receive free health-care services through the Department of Health. In the United States, accessing health-care services is a complex issue for many Puerto Ricans. A recent analysis of insurance coverage and use of health services showed that 22 percent of Puerto Ricans are uninsured, and those who are insured are likely to receive services through public health insurance coverage (Treviño et al., 1991). Lack of access to health care limits the use of preventive health-care services such as routine dental and physical examinations, prenatal care, postpartum care, and the prevention and treatment of chronic illnesses such as hypertension, diabetes, and cancer. Additional barriers to using health-care services include poor English language skills, low acculturation, poor socioeconomic status, and lack of transportation and childcare.

CULTURAL RESPONSES TO HEALTH AND ILLNESS

When a family member is ill, other family members and friends become a source of support and care. Puerto Ricans may be loud and outspoken in expressing pain. Health-care providers should not censure this expression of pain or judge it as an exaggeration. This expressive behavior is a socially learned mechanism to cope with pain. *Ay!* is a common verbal moaning expression for pain (*dolor*). Because rural elderly individuals might have difficulty interpreting and quantifying pain, the use of numerical pain-identifying scales may be inappropriate. Most people prefer oral or intravenous medications for pain relief rather than intramuscular injections or rectal medications. Additionally, herbal teas, heat, and prayer are used to manage pain.

Because mental illness carries a stigma, obtaining information or talking about mental illness with Puerto Rican families may be difficult. Some might not disclose the presence or history of mental illnesses even in a trusting environment. Additionally, Puerto Ricans may have a different cultural perception about the etiology, meaning, and treatment of mental illnesses. A mental illness may result from a terrible experience, a crisis, or the action of evil forces or spirits. Some perceive that symptoms of mental illness result from *nervios* (nerves), having done something wrong, or failing God's commandments. When someone is anxious or overcome with emotions or problems, he or she is just *nervioso*. Similarly, someone who is experiencing despair, anorexia, bulimia, melancholy, anxiety, or lack of sleep may be *nervioso(a)*, or suffering from *ataque de nervios* (an attack of nerves) rather than being clinically depressed, manic-depressive, or mentally ill. These conditions may be used to camouflage mental illness. Given the high incidence of depression (Munet-Vilaro, Folkman & Gregorich, 1999; Oquendo et al., 2001), this is a critical mental health issue for Puerto Ricans. Providers must acknowledge the confidentiality of information when obtaining a history. If trust is developed, practitioners may get a more accurate response to their questions.

Health-care providers must become familiar with the vocabulary used to describe signs and symptoms of mental illnesses among this group. Families must be provided with clear and relevant information about the diagnosis, treatment, and etiology of mental illnesses to enhance adherence to treatment and follow-up care. In addition, health-care providers should be aware of traditional healing practices and be sensitive to mental health

services for Puerto Rican families. Community-based settings such as churches, schools, and childcare centers are excellent environments for promoting the physical and mental health among Puerto Ricans.

Genetic or physical defects among Puerto Ricans may be seen as a result of heredity, suffering, or lack of care during pregnancy. Less educated individuals may place guilt and blame on the mother or father. Caregivers must provide information about the causes of genetic defects and reduce stress and guilt for parents. For decades, some Puerto Rican families cared for impaired family members in a covert environment, away from the eyes of the community. Presently, families are more open about these family members and care for the physically and mentally challenged at home, which is preferred over acute or long-term care facilities. The role of familism is of particular importance for Puerto Ricans as they provide caregiving in an interdependent network of extended family members that provide social support, solidarity, *cariño*, and resources for the family (Magaña, 1999). Sociocultural differences exist in parental beliefs and attitudes when caring for children with disabilities. Puerto Rican parents develop a sense of interdependence and overprotection that is expressed through extreme nurturing behaviors and positive caring behaviors. As a result, conventional test scores for family functioning may not be appropriate to interpret child development and family adaptation. Health-care providers should be aware of these differences and act with caution when interpreting these results (Gannotti et al., 2001). Caregivers' stress should be a key component of the health assessment of these families. Health-care providers should supply information about community resources, support groups, and culturally appropriate mental health services.

BLOOD TRANSFUSIONS AND ORGAN DONATION

For many Puerto Ricans, organ donation is seen as an act of goodwill and a gift of life. However, autopsy may be seen as a violation of the body. When discussions regarding autopsies and organ donations are necessary, the health-care provider must proceed with patience and provide precise and simple information. A clergy or minister may be helpful and may be expected to be present at the time of death. Although there are no proscriptions against blood donation and blood transfusion, many Puerto Ricans may be reluctant to engage in these procedures for fear of contracting HIV. Health-care providers need to carefully explore these beliefs and dispel myths.

Health-Care Providers

TRADITIONAL VERSUS BIOMEDICAL PRACTITIONERS

Many Puerto Ricans use traditional and folk healers such as **espiritistas** and **santeros** along with Western health-care providers. Some *espiritismo* practices are used to deal with the power of good and evil spirits in the physical and emotional development of the individual. **Santeros**, individuals prepared to practice *santería*, are consulted in matters related to the belief of object intrusion, diseases caused by evil spirits, the loss of the soul, the insertion of a spirit, or the anger of God.

Modesty is a highly valued quality. An intimate and unobtrusive environment is preferred for disclosing health-related concerns. Individuals expect a respectful environment, a soft tone of voice, and time to be heard, explain concerns, and ask questions when discussing health matters. Rooms without doors are considered disrespectful and conspicuous, particularly if the visit requires the removal of clothing. Some Puerto Ricans may have a gender or age bias against health-care providers. Men prefer male physicians for care and may feel embarrassed and uncomfortable with a female physician. A few individuals discount the academic and intellectual competencies of female physicians and may distrust their judgment and treatment. Some Puerto Rican women feel uncomfortable with a male physician, while a few prefer a male doctor. Elderly Puerto Ricans may prefer older health-care providers because they are seen as wise and mature in matters related to health, life experiences, and the use of folk practices and remedies. To build the client's confidence, younger and female health-care providers must demonstrate an overall concern for the client and develop respect and understanding by acknowledging and incorporating traditional healing practices into treatment regimens.

STATUS OF HEALTH-CARE PROVIDERS

Puerto Ricans hold health-care providers in high regard; that is, they are seen as wise figures of authority. Distrust may develop if the health-care provider (1) lacks respect for issues related to traditional health practices, (2) ignores personalism in the relationship, (3) does not use advanced technological assessment tools, and (4) has a physical or personal image that differs from the traditional "well-groomed white attire" image. Overall, however, Puerto Ricans are well-educated health consumers and expect high-quality care blended with traditional practices and reliable technological approaches (Pérez-Montijo et al., 1996).

CASE STUDY   Mr. López, age 62, lives with his second wife Mirna, age 51, his parents-in-law, his 4-year-old grandson, and his 3 children; Carmen (age 21), Daniel (age 17), and Consuelo (age 16). He owns a small car shop in Denver, Colorado. They came from Puerto Rico after experiencing financial hardships. Mirna used to work as a teacher, but since they had children she has devoted her time to being a housewife and, more recently, to being a caregiver for her parents and grandchild, Paquito. They are both devout Catholics and are active members of the local Spanish-speaking parish.

The López family has health insurance and both of Mirna's parents are covered through Medicare. Mirna is the administrator for her parent's finances (social security pension) and her own home. They live in a four-bedroom home in the back of Mr. Lopez's car shop. Carmen is a single mom that works full-time in a shoe store. She takes care of her financial needs and those of her 4-year-old son. She sleeps in the same room with her sister and her son and contributes to the financial needs of the family.

Mirna's mother, age 66, has been in the hospital three times during the last year for the management of diabetes. Her father, age 67, had a myocardial infarction 6 months ago and is in cardiac rehabilitation. Paquito has asthma and was in the emergency room twice during the last 3 months. Mrs. López has been feeling tired, with headaches, irregular menses, bleeding, and abdominal pain. She experienced a fainting episode during her father's hospitalization and she was found to have anemia. She was given instructions for follow-up care, but she cancelled her appointment twice to accommodate her parents and Paquito's medical care appointments. Both Mr. López and Mirna's parents believe that as a result of all of these problems, Mirna is having *ataques de nervios.*

During the last 7 months, there have been several family arguments about home rules, family values, and responsibilities. The last discussion took place 3 weeks ago. The discussion emerged when Consuelo got home at 11 P.M. and her parents confronted her. She has been skipping classes and dating an older man. When her brother became part of the discussion, she told the family of his gay "friends," and he angrily disclosed and responded: "Yes, I am gay and so what." Carmen has decided to move out with her son and is advising her mother to place her grandparents in a senior housing facility.

Mr. López came with his wife to her first primary health-care appointment in 5 years. His last visit to a primary care provider was 12 years ago, before he got the family life insurance. Both look tired and overwhelmed. Mr. López is quietly listening to the health-care encounter and Mrs. López has been crying through most of the appointment.

STUDY QUESTIONS

1   List the two most significant primary care needs for Mrs. López.

2   Identify primary care interventions for Mrs. López.

3   Discuss a culturally relevant approach to schedule Mr. López for a primary care appointment.

4   Identify potential barriers and their solutions for the continuation of care for Mrs. López.

5   What are the high-risk physical, mental, and spiritual behaviors exhibited by this family?

6   Identify health-care utilization barriers for all family members.

7   List potential medical and mental health diagnoses for each member of this family.

8 Discuss gender and family roles in the context of the traditional Puerto Rican culture.

9 Identify potential factors that may affect the physical and mental health well-being of Consuelo, Daniel, and Paquito.

10 Identify Puerto Rican spiritual practices appropriate for this family.

11 If the family decides to make changes in their living arrangements, what would be the most appropriate approach? Why?

12 What interpersonal processes of care may enhance or hinder the health-care encounter with the members of this family?

13 Identify culturally congruent interventions to facilitate the health care of Mr. and Mrs. López.

14 Discuss the importance of *respeto* and **familism** in the López family.

15 Identify culturally congruent interventions for the management of adolescent-related health such as sexuality, family roles, delinquency, and substance abuse.

16 Identify health promotion and disease prevention strategies for each member of this family. Consider issues related to aging, pediatric and child care, and women's health.

17 What interactions may lead to foster *simpatía* and *personalismo* in the health-care encounter?

REFERENCES

Amaro, H. et al. (1990). Acculturation and marijuana and cocaine use: Findings from the HHANES 1982–1984. *American Journal of Public Health, 80,* (Suppl.), 54–60.

Andia, J. F. et al. (2001). Residential status and HIV risk behaviors among Puerto Rican drug injectors in New York, and Puerto Rico. *American Journal of Drug and Alcohol Abuse, 27*(4), 719–735.

Bermudez, O. I., and Tucker, K. L. (2001). Total and central obesity among elderly Hispanics and the association with Type 2 diabetes. *Obesity Research, 9*(8), 443–451.

Brook, J. S. et al. (1997) African-American and Puerto Rican Drug Use: A longitudinal study. *Journal of the American Academy of Child Adolescent Psychiatry, 36*(9), 1260–1268.

Brook, J. S. et al. (1998) Similar and different precursors to drug use and delinquency among African Americans and Puerto Ricans. *Journal of Genetic Psychology, 159*(1), 13–29.

Centers for Disease Control. (1995, February 10). Update: AIDS among women in the United States 1994. *MMWR, 44,* 81–83.

Comas-Díaz, L. (1977) Mental health needs of Puerto Rican women in the United States. In R. Sánchez and R. Martínez-Cruz, R. (eds.): *Essays on la mujer* (pp. 1–10). Anthology No. 1. Los Angeles: Chicano Studies Center for Publications.

Crouch-Ruiz, E. (1996). The birth of a premature infant in a Puerto Rican family. In S. Torres (Ed.): *Hispanic voices: Hispanic health educators speak out* (pp. 26–28). New York: National League for Nursing.

Davis, R. E., & Flannery, D. D. (2001). Designing health information delivery systems for Puerto Rican women. *Health Education and Behavior, 28*(6), 680–695.

del Rosario Valdez, M. (2001). A metaphor for HIV-positive Mexican and Puerto Rican women. *Western Journal of Nursing Research, 23*(5), 517–535.

Epstein, J. A., Botvin, G. J., & Diaz, T. (1998). Ethnic and gender differences in smoking prevalence among a longitudinal sample of inner-city adolescents. *Journal of Adolescent Health, 23,* 160–166.

Gannotti, M. E. et al. (2001). Sociocultural influences on disability status in Puerto Rican children. *Physical Therapy, 81*(9), 1512–1523.

Grieco, E. (2001). *The White Population: 2000: Census 2000 Brief.* U.S. Department of Commerce. Economics and Statistics Administration. U.S. Census Bureau. Washington, DC: U.S. Government Printing Office.

Herold, J. M. et al. (1986). Contraceptive use and the need for family planning in Puerto Rico. *Family Planning Perspectives, 18,* 190–192.

Landale, N. S., & Oropesa, R. S. (2001). Migration, social support and perinatal health: An origin-destination analysis of Puerto Rican women. *Journal of Health and Social Behaviors, 42*(2), 166–183.

Lemann, N. (1991, December 1). The other underclass. *Atlantic Monthly, 268,* 96–110.

López, I. (1993). Agency and constraint: Sterilization and reproductive freedom among Puerto Rican women in New York City. *Urban Anthropology, 22,* 299–323.

López, L. M., & Másse, B. R. (1993). Income, body fatness, and fat patterns in Hispanic women from the Hispanic Health and Nutrition Examination Survey. *Health Care for Women International, 14,* 117–128.

Magaña, S. M. (1999). Puerto Rican families caring for an adult with mental retardation: Role of familism. *Journal of Mental Retardation, 104*(5), 466–482.

Marks, G., Garcia, M., & Solis, J. (1990). Health risk behaviors of Hispanics in the United States: Results from the HHANES 1982–1984. *American Journal of Public Health, 80* (Suppl.) 20–26.

Martínez, F. S. et al. (1991). Selected measures of health status for Mexican-American, mainland Puerto Rican, and Cuban-American children. *Journal of the American Medical Association, 265,* 227–232.

Massara, E. B. (1989). *!Que gordita!: A study of overweight among Puerto Rican women.* New York: AMS Press.

Munet-Vilaro, F., Folkman, S., & Gregorich, S. (1999). Depressive symptomatology in three Latino groups. *Journal of Nursing Research, 21*(2) 209–224.

National Center for Education Statistics. (2000). *Digest of Education Statistics by Selected Characteristics: Outcomes of Education.* Washington, DC: Author.

National Coalition of Hispanic Health and Human Services Organizations (COSSMHO). (1999). *The State of Hispanic Girls.* Washington, DC: COSSMHO Press.

National Institute of Drug Abuse. (1987). *1985 National household survey on drug abuse: Population estimates* (DHHS Publication No. ADM 87–1539). Rockville, MD: U.S. Government Printing Office.

Oquendo, M. A. et al. (2001). Ethnic and sex differences in suicide rates relative to major depression in the United States. *American Journal of Psychiatry, 158*(10), 1652–1658.

Orshan, S. A. (1996). Acculturation, perceived social support, and self-esteem in primigravida Puerto Rican teenagers. *Western Journal of Nursing Research, 18,* 460–473.

Peragallo, N. P. & Alba, M. L. (1996). HIV/AIDS: Risk factors, incidence, and interventions among Latinos in the United States. In S. Torres (Ed.): *Hispanic voices: Hispanic health educators speak out* (pp. 126–142). New York: National League for Nursing.

Pérez-Montijo et al. (1996). The health of Puerto Ricans. In S. Torres (Ed.): *Hispanic voices: Hispanic health educators speak out* (pp. 49–84). New York: National League for Nursing.

Pilch, S. M. (1987). Analysis of vitamin A from the Health and Nutrition Examination Surveys. *Journal of Nutrition, 117,* 636–640.

Puerto Rico Department of Health. (1998). *AIDS Surveillance Program.* Río Piedras, PR: Central Office for AIDS and Communicable Disease.

Puerto Rico Department of Health. (1998). *Annual Vital Statistics Report for 1998: Mortality.* Volume II. Auxiliary Secretary for Planning, Evaluation, Statistics and Information Systems. San Juan, Puerto Rico: Puerto Rico Health Department, Statistics Division.

Puerto Rico Department of Health. (2000). *Annual Vital Statistics Report for 1998: Natality.* Volume II. Auxiliary Secretary for Planning, Evaluation, Statistics and Information Systems. San Juan, Puerto Rico: Puerto Rico Health Department, Statistics Division.

Skinner, D. G. et al. (2001). Role of religion in the lives of Latino families with young children with developmental delays. *American Journal of Mental Retardation, 106*(4), 297–213.

Stroup-Benham, C. A., and Treviño, F. M. (1991). Reproductive characteristics of Mexican-American, Puerto Rican and Cuban-American women. *Journal of the American Medical Association, 265,* 222–226.

Taylor, M. (1999). Alternatives to conventional hormonal replacement therapy. *Contemporary OB/GYN, 12*(3), 23–54.

Therrien, M., & Ramirez, R. (2001). *The Hispanic population in the United*

States: Population Characteristics. U. S Department of Commerce. Economics and Statistics Administration. U.S. Census Bureau. Washington, DC: U.S. Government Printing Office.

Toro-Ramos, Z. R., & Henrich Saavedra, M. A. (1997). Anthropometric table for the Puerto Rican industrial population. *Computers and Industrial Engineers, 33*, 213–216.

Torres, S., & Villaruel, A. (1996). Health risk behaviors for Hispanic women. *Annual Review of Nursing Research, 5*, 293–319.

Treviño, F. M. et al. (1991). Health insurance coverage and utilization by Mexican-Americans, Mainland Puerto Ricans, and Cuban Americans. *Journal of the American Medical Association, 265*, 233–237.

U.S. Bureau of the Census. (2000). *U.S. Hispanic Population: 2000*. Current Population Survey, March 2000, PG-4. U. S Department of Commerce.

Economics and Statistics Administration. U.S. Census Bureau. Washington, DC: U.S. Government Printing Office.

U.S. Department of Health and Human Services. (2000). *Healthy people 2010: National health promotion and disease prevention objectives*. Retrieved May 24, 2002, from http://odphp.osophs.dhhs.gov/pubs/hp2000/21cps2.htm.

U.S. Department of Health and Human Services. (1999). *Health U.S. 1995*. Leading causes of death and number of deaths, according to sex, detailed race and Hispanic origin: U.S. 1980 and 1993. Public Health Service, National Vital Statistics.

U.S. Department of Labor. (1999). *Puerto Rico Fact Sheet*. Department of Education, Puerto Rico Government. San Juan, P. R.: Department of Labor.

Chapter 21

People of Vietnamese Heritage

THU T. NOWAK

Overview, Inhabited Localities, And Topography

OVERVIEW

Vietnam is located at the extreme southeastern corner of the Asian mainland along the South China Sea. Bordered by China on the north and Laos and Cambodia (Kampuchea) on the west, it has a landmass of 127,330 sq mi, which is about the size of New Mexico. Although relatively narrow in width, its north-south length equals the distance from Minneapolis to New Orleans. The population is approximately 78.8 million, and it is the 14th most populous country in the world. Vietnam consists largely of a remarkable blend of rugged mountains and the broad, flat Mekong and Red River deltas, which mainly produce rice. Other features are a long, narrow coastal plain and other riverine lowlands, where most ethnic Vietnamese live. Much of the rest of the country is covered with tropical forests.

HERITAGE AND RESIDENCE

The Vietnamese, a Mongolian racial group closely related to the Chinese, make up approximately 85 percent of the population of Vietnam. The terms *Southeast Asian refugee*, **Indochinese**, and *Vietnamese* are not synonymous. Indochina is a supranational region that includes Vietnam, Laos, and Cambodia. Muecke (1983a) distinguished 11 different **Indochinese** groups based on ethnicity, habitat, and differences in language and religion. Included among these are Laotian, Cambodian,

Thai, and Hmong and Tai Dam mountain people in Laos and in northern Vietnam. One factor in providing proper health care to Vietnamese in America is understanding that they differ substantially between and among themselves, depending on the primary and secondary characteristics of culture (see Chapter 1). Clear differences exist among Vietnamese, Cambodians, and Laotians with respect to premigration experiences, influencing subsequent manifestations of psychological distress.

Approximately 1.2 million Vietnamese live in the United States, the vast majority having arrived only since 1975. California has the largest number, followed by Texas. The influx of Vietnamese and other Southeast Asians is perhaps the most complex and unusual phase of immigration ever experienced by the United States. Although the movement of refugees from Cuba to the United States is comparable in scope, Vietnamese immigrants confronted a unique set of problems, including dissimilarity of culture, no family or relatives here to offer initial support, and a negative identification with the unpopular Vietnam War. Many Vietnamese are involuntary immigrants. Their expatriation was unexpected and unplanned, and their departures were often precipitous and tragic. Escape attempts were long, harrowing and, for many, fatal. Survivors were often placed in squalid refugee camps for years.

The first wave of Vietnamese immigration began in April 1975 when South Vietnam fell into the communist control of North Vietnam and the Viet Cong. At that time, many South Vietnamese businessmen, military officers, professionals, and others closely involved with America feared persecution by the new regime and sought to escape. American ships and aircraft rescued some. The 130,000 Vietnamese refugees who arrived in the United States in 1975 came mainly from urban areas, especially Saigon, and consequently had some prior orientation to Western culture. Many spoke English or soon learned English in relocation centers. More than half were Christian. Sixty-two percent consisted of family units of at least five people, and nearly half were female. They were dispersed over much of the United States, often in the care of sponsoring American families. One year after arrival, 90 percent were employed, and by the mid-1980s their average income matched that of the overall American population. These first-wave immigrants adjusted well in comparison to the subsequent wave of refugees.

Over the next few years, many Vietnamese grew disenchanted with communism and their decreased living standard. Great numbers had been forced into labor in new countryside settlements and young men were often fearful of being called to fight against China or in the new war with Cambodia. More than 100,000 Vietnamese left their homeland in 1978 and more than 150,000 left in 1979. Some left by land across Cambodia or Laos, commonly joining refugees from those countries in an effort to reach Thailand. For more than a decade, many others, known as the "boat people," departed Vietnam in small, often unseaworthy and overcrowded vessels in hopes of reaching Malaysia, Hong Kong, the Philippines, or another noncommunist port. Half died during their journey. Many were forcibly repatriated to Vietnam or eventually returned voluntarily; others continue to languish in camps.

Most of the second-wave refugees represented lower socioeconomic groups and had less education and little exposure to Western cultures. Most did not speak English. This wave of Vietnamese included far more young men than women, children, or older people, which disrupted intact families and normal gender ratios. Many spent months or years in refugee camps under deplorable and regimented conditions. When they finally arrived in the United States and Canada, many did not fit into American communities, did not learn English effectively, and remained unemployed or obtained menial jobs. These hardships contributed to physical problems, psychological stress, and depression. Some exceptions were found among the ethnic Chinese refugees, who often came from the established business community and could afford to keep extended families together.

A third wave of immigration started in 1979 with creation of the Orderly Departure Program, which provided safe and legal exit for Vietnamese seeking to reunite with family members already in America. Initially small in scope, this program eventually supported the annual air travel of tens of thousand of ethnic Vietnamese and Chinese Vietnamese to the United States.

In 1987, a fourth wave of immigration began with passage of the Amerasian Homecoming Act, which provided for the entry of former South Vietnamese military officers, other political detainees, children of American servicemen and Vietnamese women, and their close relatives.

REASONS FOR MIGRATION AND ASSOCIATED ECONOMIC FACTORS

Vietnamese, whether as immigrants or sojourners, have fled their country to escape war, persecution, or possible loss of life. Better-educated first-wave immigrants from urban areas had professional, technical, or managerial backgrounds. Less-educated second-wave immigrants from more rural areas were fishermen, farmers, and soldiers and had only minimal exposure to Western culture. Factors influencing the ability of displaced Vietnamese to obtain employment include higher education and the ability to speak English on arrival. Thus, the second-wave immigrants are significantly more disadvantaged.

Because most refugee heads of households worked, families were not totally dependent on welfare for financial assistance. Many worked for comparatively low wages, and their families often required some supplemental aid. However, "like other Indochinese groups, the Vietnamese are becoming independent of the welfare system at a relatively fast rate. Pride, a tradition of hard work, and the pooling together of family resources account for their aversion to relying on outside assistance" (Calhoun, 1986:16).

EDUCATIONAL STATUS AND OCCUPATIONS

Vietnamese place a high value on education and accord scholars an honored place in society. The teacher is highly respected as a symbol of learning and culture. In contrast to American schools' emphasis on experimentation and critical thinking, Vietnamese schools emphasize observation, memorization, and repetitive learning. Most Vietnamese men and women in America are very educationally oriented, and take full advantage of educational opportunities when possible.

Gold (1992) reported that 78 percent of the refugees who arrived between 1975 and 1977 had been in white-collar occupations in Vietnam, compared with 49 percent of those coming since 1978. The latter group experienced greater difficulty in adapting economically and suffered higher levels of unemployment and welfare dependency (64 percent). Professionals, mostly men, and unskilled laborers are often unable to find work in their former fields, with the recent reduction in professional, technical, and managerial positions in the United States and an increased concentration of craft, operative, and service employment. Some Vietnamese fishermen on the Gulf Coast of Texas have been able to maintain their traditional occupation, but experience hostility from American fishermen who consider them competitors.

Communication

DOMINANT LANGUAGE AND DIALECTS

Ethnic Vietnamese speak a single distinctive language, with northern, central, and southern dialects, all of which can be understood by anyone speaking any one of these dialects. The language differs from those spoken in the neighboring countries of Laos and Cambodia and from those spoken by highland tribal groups of Southeast Asia. The Vietnamese language resembles Chinese and contains many borrowed words, but someone speaking one of these languages cannot necessarily understand the other. All words in Vietnamese consist of a single syllable, although two words are commonly joined with a hyphen to form a new word. Contextually, the Vietnamese language is musical and flowing. It is polytonal, with each tone of a vowel conveying a different meaning to the word. The language is spoken softly and its monosyllabic structure lends itself to rapidity, but spoken pace varies according to the situation. Whereas grammar is mostly simple, pronunciation can be difficult for westerners, mainly because each vowel can be spoken in five or six tones that may completely change the meaning of the word. Vietnamese is the only language of the Asian mainland that, like English, is regularly written in the Roman alphabet. Although the letters are the same, pronunciation of vowels may vary radically depending on associated marks indicating tone and accent, and certain consonant combinations take on unusual sounds.

Even if someone learns how to pronounce and translate Vietnamese, problems may remain with respect to intended meaning of various words. One minor but perennial stumbling point with potential medical connotations is that the word for "blue" and "green" is the same. More important, the word for "yes," rather than expressing a positive answer or agreement, may simply reflect an avoidance of confrontation or a desire to please the other person. The terms *hot* and *cold,* rather than expressing physical feelings associated with fever and chills, may actually relate to other conditions associated with perceived bodily imbalances. Various medical problems might be described differently from what a westerner might expect; for example, a "weak heart" may refer to palpitations or dizziness, a "weak kidney" to sexual dysfunction, a "weak nervous system" to headaches, and a "weak stomach or liver" to indigestion (Muecke, 1983b).

Most Vietnamese refugees, even those who have been in the United States for many years, do not feel competent in English. Although many refugees eventually learn English, their skills may not be sufficient to communicate in psychiatric interviews, which are usually carried out at a highly abstract level.

Health-care providers may need to watch clients for behavioral cues, use simple sentences, paraphrase words with multiple meanings, avoid metaphors and idiomatic expressions, ask for correction of understanding, and explain all points carefully. Approaching Vietnamese clients in a quiet, unhurried manner, opening discussions with small talk, and directing the initial conversation to the oldest member of the group facilitates communication.

CULTURAL COMMUNICATION PATTERNS

Traditional Vietnamese religious beliefs transmitted through generations produce an attitude toward life that may be perceived as passive. For example, whenever confronted with a direct but delicate question, many Vietnamese cannot easily give a blunt "no" as an answer because they feel that such an answer may create disharmony. Self-control, another traditional value, encourages keeping to oneself, whereas expressions of disagreement that may irritate or offend another person are avoided. Individuals may be in pain, distraught, or unhappy, yet rarely complain except perhaps to friends or relatives. Expression of emotions is considered a weakness and interferes with self-control. Vietnamese are unaccustomed to discussing their personal feelings openly with others. Instead, at times of distress or loss, they often complain of physical discomforts, such as headaches, backaches, or insomnia.

The strong influence of the Confucian code of ethics means that proper form and appearance are important to Vietnamese people and form the foundation for nonverbal communication patterns. For example, the head is a sacred part of the body and should not be touched. Similarly, the feet are the lowest part of the body, and to place one's feet on a desk is considered offensive to a Vietnamese person. To signal for someone to come by using an upturned finger is a provocation, usually done to a dog; waving the hand is considered more proper.

Hugging and kissing are not seen outside the privacy of the home. Men greet each other with a handshake but do not shake hands with a woman unless she offers her hand first. Women do not usually shake hands. It is acceptable practice for two men or two women to walk hand in hand and does not carry sexual connotations. However, for a man to touch a woman in the presence of others is insulting.

Looking another person directly in the eyes may be deemed disrespectful. Women may be reluctant to discuss sex, childbearing, or contraception when men are present and demonstrate this unwillingness by giggling, shrugging their shoulders, or averting their eyes. Negative emotions and expressions may be conveyed by silence or a reluctant smile. A smile may express joy, convey stoicism in the face of difficulty, indicate an apology for a minor social offense, or be a response to a scolding to show sincere acknowledgment for the wrongdoing or to convey the absence of ill feelings. Vietnamese prefer more distance during personal and social relationships than other cultures, but extended Vietnamese families of many individuals live comfortably together in close quarters.

TEMPORAL RELATIONSHIPS

Vietnamese religion and tradition place emphasis on continuity, cycles, and worship of ancestors. Traditional Vietnamese may be less concerned about the present and precise schedules than are European Americans. To cope with their changed situation, many Southeast Asian refugees concentrate on the present and to some extent on the future.

Asians frequently arrive late for appointments. Noncompliance in keeping appointments may relate to not understanding oral or written instructions, or not knowing how to use the telephone. On the other hand, many Vietnamese Americans fully understand the significance of punctuality.

One other aspect of time involves the treatment of age. Vietnamese people pay much less attention to people's precise ages than Americans. Actual dates of birth may pass unnoticed, with everyone celebrating their birthdays together during the Lunar New Year (**Tet**) in January or February. In addition, a person's age is calculated roughly from the time of conception; most children are considered to already be a year old at birth and gain a year each **Tet**. A child born just before **Tet** could be regarded as 2 years old when only a few days old by American standards. Because the practice of determining age is so different in Vietnam, many immigrants may have difficulty determining their exact birth date and are often given January 1 as a date of birth for official records.

FORMAT FOR NAMES

Most Vietnamese names consist of a family name, a middle name, and a given name of one or two words, always written in that order. There are relatively few family names, with Nguyen (pronounced "nwin") and Tran accounting for more than half of all Vietnamese names. Other common family names are Cao, Dinh, Hoang, Le, Ly, Ngo, Phan, and Pho. There are relatively few middle names, with Van being used regularly for men and Thi (pronounced "tee") for women. Given names frequently have a direct meaning, such as a season of year or object of admiration. Family members often refer to offspring by a numerical nickname indicating their order of birth.

This practice may increase the difficulty of modern recordkeeping and identification of specific individuals. It is therefore advantageous to use the family name in combination with the given name. Indeed, Vietnamese refer to each other by given name both in formal and informal situations. For example, a typical woman's name is Tran Thi Thu. That is how she would write or give her name if requested. She would expect to be called simply "Thu" or sometimes "*Chi* (sister) Thu" by friends and family. In other situations she would expect to be addressed as *Cô* (Miss) or *Ba* (Mrs.) Thu. If married to a man named Nguyen Van Kha, the proper way to address her would be as Mrs. Kha, but she would retain her full three-part maiden name for formal purposes. The man would always be known as Kha or *Ong* (Mr.) Kha. Some Vietnamese American women have adopted their husband's family name. Children always take the father's family name.

Family Roles and Organization

HEAD OF HOUSEHOLD AND GENDER ROLES

The traditional Vietnamese family is strictly patriarchal and is almost always an extended family structure, with the man having the duty of carrying on the family name through his progeny. Some families who are not accustomed to female authority figures may have diffi-

culty relating to women as professional health-care providers. With the move into Western society, the father may no longer be the undisputed head of the household, and the parents' authority may be undermined. Immigrant Vietnamese families frequently experience role reversals, with wives or children adapting more easily than men to the Western workplace, becoming the primary providers, and thus gaining increased authority. Some families adapt well to this situation, whereas others experience resentment and hostility, which may erupt into child or wife abuse, depression, and alcoholism (Gold, 1992).

A Vietnamese woman lives with her husband's family after marriage but retains her own identity. Within the family, the division of labor is gender related: the husband deals with matters outside the home, and the wife is responsible for the actual care of the home. Although her role in family affairs increases with time, a Vietnamese wife is expected to be dutiful and respectful toward her husband and his parents throughout the marriage. Vietnamese women often make family health-care decisions.

Vietnamese refugees of all subgroups have various degrees of reversal of the provider and recipient roles that existed among family members in Vietnam. "Women's jobs," such as hotel maid, sewing machine operator, and food service worker, are more readily available than male-oriented unskilled occupations. Role reversals between parents and children are also common because children often learn the English language and American customs more rapidly than their parents and may be able to find employment more quickly than their parents.

Vietnamese families in the United States experience a tendency toward nuclearization, a growth in spousal interaction and interdependency, more egalitarian spousal relations, and shared decision making.

PRESCRIPTIVE, RESTRICTIVE, AND TABOO BEHAVIORS FOR CHILDREN AND ADOLESCENTS

Traditionally, children are expected to be obedient and devoted to their parents, their identity being an extension of the parents. Children are obliged to do everything possible to please their parents while they are alive and to worship their memory after death. The eldest son is usually responsible for rituals honoring the memory and invoking the blessings of departed ancestors. This pattern may be ingrained from early childhood.

Vietnamese children are prized and valued because they carry the family lineage. For the first 2 years, their mothers primarily care for them; thereafter, their grandmothers and others take on much of the responsibility. Parents usually do not discipline or place extensive limits on their children at a young age. Generally, Vietnamese do not use corporal punishment such as spanking; rather, they speak to the children in a quiet, controlled manner.

Young people are expected to continue to respect their elders and to avoid behavior that might dishonor the family. As a result of the effects of their exposure to Western cultures, a disproportionate share of young people in the refugee population, which has a median age of 18, have difficulty adapting to this expectation. A conflict often develops between the traditional notion of filial piety, with its requisite subordination of self and unquestioning obedience to parental authority, and the pressures and needs associated with adaptation to American life. Ironically, successful relationships with Americans at school have placed Vietnamese adolescents at risk for conflicts with their parents. Conversely, failure to form such relationships has sometimes appeared to be a precursor of emotional distress. Parents do, however, show relative approval for adolescent freedom of choice regarding dating, marriage, and career choices.

The extreme bipolarities of the adaptation of Vietnamese youth is sometimes overemphasized. One group, usually the children of the first-wave refugees, are often portrayed as academic superstars. At the other end of the social spectrum are the criminal and gang elements, who often direct their activities against other Asian immigrants. Most Vietnamese adolescents, however, fall between these two extremes and have the same pressures and concerns as other youths.

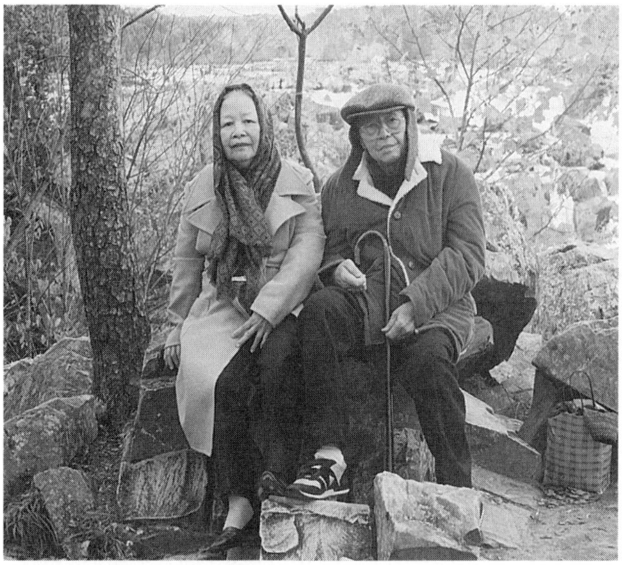

FAMILY GOALS AND PRIORITIES

The traditional Vietnamese family is perhaps the most basic, enduring, and self-consciously acknowledged form of national culture among refugees, providing life-long protection and guidance to the individual. It is customarily a large, patriarchal, and extended family unit, including minor children, married sons, daughters-in-law, unmarried grown daughters, and grandchildren under the same roof. Other close relatives may be included within the extended family structure. The family is explicitly structured with assigned priorities, identifying parental ties as paramount. A son's obligations and duties to his parents may assume a higher value than those to his wife, children, or siblings. Sibling relationships are considered permanent. Vietnamese self is defined more along the lines of family roles and responsibilities and less along individual lines. These mutual family tasks provide a framework for individual behavior, promoting a sense of interdependence, belonging, and support. The traditional family has been altered as a consequence of Western influence, urbanization, and the war-induced absence of men. Nevertheless, many Vietnamese continue to uphold this social form as the preferable basis of social organization in the United States. As mentioned in the previous section, exposure of the younger generation to American culture can become a source of conflict with considerable family strain as adolescents are influenced by the perceived American values of individuality, independence, self-assertion, and egalitarian relationships.

Traditionally, elders are honored and have a key role in most family activities for transmitting guidelines related to social behavior, preparing younger people for handling stressful life events, and serving as sources of support in coping with life crises. Elders are usually consulted for important decisions. Addressing a client in the presence of an elder, whether they speak English or not, may be interpreted as disrespectful to the family.

Homesickness and bewilderment are especially acute

FIGURE 21–1 Elders are honored in traditional Vietnamese culture, but the effects of American culture on immigrant families may sometimes be troubling to elderly Vietnamese Americans.

in older refugees when confronted with the strange Western culture and despair about the future (Fig. 21–1). Accustomed to considerable respect and esteem in their homeland, they may feel increasingly alienated and alone as the younger generations adopt new values and ignore the counsel and values of the elders. Living within the family unit facilitates the social adjustment of elderly refugees into American society. However, those who live in overcrowded households and in households with children under the age of 16 experience a poorer adjustment.

Traditional Vietnamese are class conscious and rarely associate with individuals at different levels of society. Traditional respect is accorded to people in authoritative positions who are well educated or otherwise successful, or who have professional titles. However, class distinctions are sometimes blurred in the turmoil of war and resettlement. Two concepts govern the gain and loss of prestige and power, thereby maintaining face: **mien**, based on wealth and power, and **lien**, based on demonstration of control over and responsibility for moral character. For example, to smile in the face of adversity is to maintain **lien** and is considered of great importance.

ALTERNATIVE LIFESTYLES

The complex extended Vietnamese family in America is extremely vulnerable to change. Many young people, frequently unmarried couples, seek their own living accommodations away from the control of older generations. Unattached male refugees may join **pseudofamilies**, households made up of close and distant relatives and friends that share accommodations, finances, and companionship. These families form an important source of social support in the refugee communities. Because of the high regard for chastity placed on Vietnamese adolescents, the number of single-parent households is low.

Workforce Issues

CULTURE IN THE WORKPLACE

First-wave immigrants adjusted well to the American workplace, and within a decade, their average income equaled that of the general U.S. population. Many later immigrants, who had less education and did not know English, ended up working in lower-paying jobs. However, some learned English and opened their own businesses and prospered.

Traditionally, priority is given to the concerns of the family, rather than to those of the employer. However, this emphasis is not a detriment to productivity in work habits, because a good work record and steady pay brings honor and prosperity to the family. The Vietnamese are highly adaptable and adjust their work habits to meet requirements for successful employment.

Most Vietnamese respect authority figures with impressive titles, achievement, education, and a harmonious work environment. They may be less concerned about such factors as punctuality, adherence to deadlines, and competition. Other traditions include a willingness to work hard, sacrificing current comforts, and saving for the future to ensure that they assimilate well into the workforce. Many seek the same material, financial, and status rewards that beckon native-born Americans.

ISSUES RELATED TO AUTONOMY

Confucianism and its stress on the maintenance of formal hierarchies within governmental, religious, and educational institutions; commercial establishments; and families have heavily influenced the Vietnamese outlook. This cultural background results in conformity and reluctance to undertake independent action. At the same time, the cultural outlook of company and family values superseding personal values creates a cohesive work group.

Vietnamese quickly learn vocabulary for pragmatic communication but may have difficulty with complex verbal skills. Values related to their own culture discourage disclosure of inner thoughts and feelings. These barriers adversely affect employment opportunities and limit their ability to communicate needs relative to social, psychological, and economic matters. Despite extensive English instruction programs, many Vietnamese may still lack transcultural communication skills. Employers may need to allow extra time, provide visually oriented instructions, and provide programs that enhance communications to promote increased harmony in the workplace.

Biocultural Ecology

SKIN COLOR AND OTHER BIOLOGICAL VARIATIONS

Vietnamese are members of the Mongolian or Asian race. Although their skin is often referred to as "yellow," it varies considerably in color, ranging from pale ivory to dark brown. Mongolian spots, bluish discolorations on the lower back of a newborn child, are normal hyperpigmented areas in many Asians.

To assess for oxygenation and cyanosis in dark-skinned Vietnamese, the health-care provider must examine the sclera, conjunctiva, buccal mucosa, tongue, lips, nailbeds, palms of the hands, and soles of the feet. These same areas should be observed for signs of reactions during blood transfusions, giving special attention to diaphoresis on the forehead, upper lip, and palms, which may signify impending shock.

One of the first signs of iron deficiency anemia is pallor, which varies with skin tones. Dark skin loses the normal underlying red tones so that Vietnamese clients with brown skin will appear yellow-brown. Petechiae and rashes may be hidden in dark-skinned individuals as well, but they can be detected by observing for patches of melanin in the buccal mucosa and on the conjunctiva. Jaundice can be observed in dark-skinned Vietnamese by a yellow discoloration of the conjunctiva. Because many dark-skinned individuals have carotene deposits in the subconjunctival fat and sclera, the hard palate should also be assessed.

The Vietnamese are usually small in physical stature and light in build relative to most European Americans. Adult women average 5 feet tall and weigh 80 to 100 lbs. Men average a few inches taller and weigh 110 to 130 lbs. Although Roberts and associates (1985) reported no significant difference in birth weight between refugee babies and those of other parents, Vietnamese children are small by American standards, not fitting the published growth curves. Barry and associates (1983) found that 47 percent of the refugee children are below the fifth percentile in height for age, and 22 percent are below the fifth percentile in weight for age on standard American growth curves. However, no clinical evidence shows that such development is the result of disease or malnutrition. According to Pickwell (1982), 72 percent of refugee children examined fall below the 10th percentile for weight, stature, or both in relation to age. However, when these are plotted on the weight-for-stature graphs, they fall within the normal range. Thus, growth charts commonly used in America cannot provide adequate assessments for evaluating the physical development of Vietnamese children. Other parameters, such as parental height and weight, apparent state of health, the energy level of the child, and progressive development over time need to be considered. The development of standing, walking, and language skills begin at a slightly later age in Vietnamese children, but they rapidly catch up with American norms by the age of 1.5 to 2 years (Sokoloff, Carlin, & Pham, 1984).

Typical physical features of the Vietnamese include inner eye folds that make the eyes look almond shaped, sparse body hair, and coarse head hair. Vietnamese also have dry earwax, which is gray and brittle. People with dry earwax have few apocrine glands, especially in the underarm area and thus produce less sweat and associated body odor. Asians generally have larger teeth than European Americans, creating a normal tendency toward a prognathic profile, the mouth area coming out farther than the upper part of the face. In addition, there may be a torus, bony protuberance, on the midline of the palate or on the inner side of the mandible near the second premolar. Mandibular tori occur in about 40 percent of Asians as compared with only 7 percent of Americans (Overfield, 1977).

Betel nut pigmentation may be found in some Vietnamese adults, resulting from the practice of chewing betel leaves (*chau*). This practice is common among older women and has a narcotic effect on diseased gums. Some elderly women lacquer their teeth, believing that it strengthens the teeth and symbolizes beauty and wealth.

DISEASES AND HEALTH CONDITIONS

Vietnamese women have the highest rate of cervical cancer of any female population in the United States that has been surveyed, approximately 43 per 100,000 or 6 times the national average (Wright, 2000). The prevalence of the disease is the result of lack of education, reluctance to seek early treatment, fear that nothing can be done, low utilization of annual Pap smears, and failure to follow up on abnormal Pap smears. Some evidence also implicates human papilloma virus (HPV), a sexually transmitted etiological factor in the pathogenesis of cervical cancer. It may be that the enormous and lengthy military activity and social disruption in Vietnam led to extensive utilization of multiple sexual partners by men and hence a spread of sexually transmitted problems, including HPV, to women. Cancer and other problems common to Vietnamese people may also be associated with the widespread application of chemical agents during the Vietnam War.

Mental health research has indicated that Vietnamese refugees have disturbingly high rates of depression, generalized anxiety disorders, and post-traumatic stress associated with military combat, political imprisonment, harrowing events during escapes by sea, and brutal pirate attacks. Chronic personal and emotional problems often stem from post-traumatic stress experiences in this population.

Of immediate concern to health-care providers working with Vietnamese refugees is the treatment of infectious conditions that jeopardize both the refugee and the resident population. Some refugees suffer from malaria, parasites, and other problems associated with the tropics. Catanzaro and Moser (1982) reported that Vietnamese have a lower incidence of intestinal parasites, anemia, and hepatitis B antigenemia than other refugee groups. However, 69 percent of tuberculin tests return positive in the Vietnamese, and this high rate of positive results correlates with their origins from crowded, poorly ventilated cities. Screening of second-wave refugees reveals a higher incidence of tuberculosis, intestinal parasitism, anemia, malaria, and hepatitis B. Sutter and Haefliger (1990) reported an estimated annual risk for tuberculosis of 2.2 percent in Vietnamese people, and also noted that the disease was most likely present before arrival in refugee camps. Hepatitis B virus is hyperendemic in Indochina, with most people being infected during childhood and spreading the infection to others. HBV vaccination is recommended for all newborn refugee children.

Other endemic diseases include leprosy (a rate of about 20 to 30 cases per 1000 population as compared with a U.S. rate of fewer than 0.25 per 1000 population); high levels of parasitism, particularly the intestinal nematodes *Ascaris* (roundworm) and *Trichuris* (whipworm), which are associated with contaminated or poorly cooked foods, and the liver fluke *Clonorchis*, which is introduced in raw, pickled, or dried fish (Dao, Gregory, & McKee, 1984), *Necator* (hookworm), and malaria with the arrival of refugees.

To determine the presence of parasites, health-care providers must assess for symptoms of anemia, lassitude, failure to thrive, abdominal pain, weight loss, and skin rashes. In the first two waves of refugees, major health problems also included skin infections caused by fungus, impetigo, scabies, and lice (7 to 15 percent); infections of the upper respiratory tract and otitis media (20 percent); anemia including parasitic iron deficiency (16 to 40 percent), with a higher occurrence in young children; hemoglobin disorders (30 percent); chronic diseases (10 percent); and malnutrition and poor immunization status (Ross, 1982).

Two clinical illnesses that may mimic tuberculosis, melioidosis and paragonimiasis, are also reported among refugees. Sutherland and associates (1983) reported that 14 percent of the Vietnamese refugees in their Mayo Clinic study exhibited microcytosis, which can lead to an incorrect diagnosis of iron deficiency and inappropriate treatment with iron. Erythrocytic microcytosis in Southeast Asians is most likely a reflection of the presence of thalassemia or of hemoglobin E trait, conditions which are usually harmless and need no treatment. These disorders should be suspected in people with findings consistent with tuberculosis but with a negative purified protein derivative response (Ross, 1982).

Screening immigrants for syphilis shows an incidence as low as 1 to 5 percent. Sporadic cases and limited outbreaks of cholera, measles, diphtheria, epidemic conjunctivitis, and typhoid fever fail to show notable secondary spread (Ross, 1982). Observations at the Mayo Clinic (Sutherland et al., 1983) reported that refugee populations are young and generally healthy, despite a prevalence rate of 82 percent for intestinal parasites. Additionally, moderate to severe dental problems may occur in newer immigrants, especially children.

VARIATIONS IN DRUG METABOLISM

Little pertinent drug research exists specifically on the Vietnamese. Clinical studies comparing other Asians with European Americans provide some idea of what might be expected. For example, the Chinese are twice as sensitive to the effects of propranolol on blood pressure and heart rate; experience a greater increase in heart rate from atropine; require lower doses of benzodiazepines, diazepam, and alprazolam because of their increased sensitivity to the sedative effects of these drugs; require lower doses of imipramine, desipramine, amitriptyline, and clomipramine; and are less sensitive to cardiovascular and respiratory side effects of analgesics (for example, morphine) but more sensitive to their gastrointestinal side effects. Asians require lower doses of neuroleptics (for example, haloperidol) (Levy, 1993).

Lin and Shen (1991) expressed concern about the lack of research on pharmacotherapy specifically related to major depressive and post-traumatic stress disorders in Southeast Asian refugees. They suggested that drug metabolism is comparable to that of other Asian groups with important common traits such as genetic, cultural, and environmental influences. Asian diets, for example, are similar in carbohydrate-to-protein ratio, which significantly influences the metabolism of some commonly prescribed drugs. Also, because most Asians come from areas with similar degrees of socioeconomic development, exposure to various enzyme-inducing agents, such as drugs and industrial toxins, is likely to be similar. On the other hand, the exposure of the refugees to war, trauma, starvation, and other adverse conditions could have an effect on the enzyme systems governing psychotropic medications. One precaution involves the continued extensive use of traditional herbal medicines by the refugees. Some of these herbal drugs have active pharmacologic properties that may interact with psychotropic drugs. For example, some may cause atropine psychosis when ingested concomitantly with tricyclic antidepressants or low-potency neuroleptics.

Significantly lower dosages of psychotropic medications are prescribed in Asian countries than are common in Western countries (Rosenblat & Tang, 1987). Low doses of antidepressant medications are often effective. Weight standards for neuroleptic dose ranges are significantly lower in Asians than in White Americans (Lin & Finder, 1983). Because Vietnamese are considerably smaller than most white Americans, medication dosages may need to be reduced. Vietnamese generally consider American medicines more concentrated than Asian medicines; thus, they may take only half of the dosage prescribed. Additionally, many Asian people are slow metabolizers of alcohol. Thus, Asians are more sensitive than European Americans to the adverse effects of alcohol as expressed by facial flushing, palpitation, and tachycardia.

High-Risk Behaviors

Alcohol and tobacco use by Vietnamese has been reported to be relatively low. However, some adolescents have turned to alcohol, often drinking alone and claiming it helps them forget what they experienced in their homeland (Felice, 1986). Fitzpatrick and associates (1987) cautioned that peer pressure to drink and experiment with drugs might be greater than previously realized for Indochinese teenagers. Yu (1991) reported a substantial increase in smoking among Asian American women in general. Jenkins and colleagues (1992) found the incidence of smoking among men in California was higher in Vietnamese than in Chinese or Hispanics.

Data suggest a possible high mortality from cancer at certain sites among Vietnamese (Jenkins et al., 1990). Cigarette smoking, excessive dietary intake of fat, low dietary intake of fiber, and consumption of alcohol have been linked epidemiologically to an increased risk of cancer. In a survey of Vietnamese adults in the San Francisco area, 13 percent had never heard of cancer,

27 percent did not know that cigarette smoking can cause cancer, and 28 percent believed that cancer is contagious. Although hepatitis B–related liver cancer is endemic among Vietnamese, 48 percent had never heard of hepatitis B. Among men, 56 percent are smokers versus 32 percent in the general population. Of those, 88 percent report smoking high-tar, high-nicotine brands. Most wanted to quit and said that their physicians had advised them to quit or reduce smoking. Cigarette smoking in men is strongly associated with incomes below the poverty level, residence in the United States of 9 years or less, not knowing that smoking causes cancer, and limited English proficiency. Only 9 percent of Vietnamese women are smokers versus 27 percent of women in general.

The prevalence of alcohol consumption is 67 percent among Vietnamese men and only 18 percent among women, versus 66 percent and 47 percent, respectively, in the general population. Binge drinking is reported by 35 percent of men.

Among women, 89 percent say they had never heard of the Pap test; after this procedure is explained, 32 percent say they never had one (versus 9 percent of American women). In addition, 28 percent of women never had a breast examination and 83 percent never had a mammogram.

Lung cancer is 18 percent higher among Southeast Asian men than among European American men, and the incidence of liver cancer is more than 12 times higher among Southeast Asian men and women. The high rate of liver cancer is associated with the prevalence of hepatitis B in Southeast Asian immigrants. High rates of gastrointestinal cancer may be due to asbestos in some parts of the world that is used in the process of "polishing" rice. Thus, imported rice should always be washed.

Asians may be less aware of hypertension than are people of other races. In one study, 85 percent of Southeast Asians did not know what to do to prevent heart disease (Chen et al., 1991).

Young Asians are less sexually active than other groups and have a lower risk of acquired immunodeficiency syndrome (AIDS). Vietnamese also have a lower incidence of AIDS than the Japanese (Cochran, Mays, & Leung, 1991). Indochinese teenagers may have a high rate of certain hemoglobinopathies, and their pairing poses an increased risk of passing these conditions to their offspring (Fitzpatrick et al., 1987).

Trichinosis risk is 25 times greater in Southeast Asian refugees than in the general population. This increased risk is related to undercooking pork and purchasing pigs directly from farms.

Depression is the greatest threat to refugee health. At least half of Vietnamese clients are diagnosed with depression, anxiety, or both. The risk of developing depression is moderated by social support from the established ethnic community and by having an intact marriage. However, sponsorship by groups with a different religion than that of the refugees can act as an additional source of stress (Beiser, Turner, & Ganesan, 1989).

Possibly related to psychological pressures on refugees is the occurrence of sudden unexplained death syndrome (SUDS), a phenomenon reported mainly for the Hmong, but also affecting Vietnamese and other Asian groups. Nearly all deaths involve physically healthy, young adult men who die at night or during sleep (Baron et al., 1983). The Centers for Disease Control (1990) reported 117 cases from 1981 to 1988 and suggested that a structural abnormality of the cardiac conduction system and stress may be risk factors for SUDS. The exact cause of the deaths remains unknown. These deaths may be a form of unconscious suicide associated with nightmares brought on by intensive feelings of depression and survivor guilt (Tobin & Friedman, 1983).

Health-Care Practices

The Vietnamese approach to health care is one of ambivalence. Many Vietnamese immigrants are accustomed to dependence on the family unit and traditional means of providing for health needs. They may be distrustful of outsiders and Western methods. Most are familiar with immunizations and diagnostic tests. They want to avoid health problems and are anxious to follow reasonable procedures. Newly arrived refugees are less likely to seek Western health care, but Vietnamese are the most likely of the Southeast Asians to seek care and to do so earlier (Strand & Jones, 1983). Most Southeast Asian refugees want to go to a physician for an illness, but they rarely seek care when they are asymptomatic and few are familiar with the appointment system. Some regard the most convenient physician as the closest one not requiring an appointment and accepting medical coupons, which usually translates into a hospital emergency room (Muecke, 1983a).

The Vietnamese family may not seek outside assistance for illness until it has exhausted its own resources. The family may try various home remedies, allowing the condition to become serious before seeking professional assistance. Once a physician or nurse has been consulted, the Vietnamese are usually quite cooperative and respect the wisdom and experience of health-care professionals. Hospitalization is viewed as a last resort and is acceptable only in case of emergency when everything else has failed. With respect to mental health, Vietnamese do not easily trust authority figures, including treatment staff, because of their refugee experiences.

Nutrition

MEANING OF FOOD

Meals are an important time to the Vietnamese, allowing the entire family to come together and share a common activity. Preparation is precise and may occupy much of the day. Celebrations and holidays involve elaborately prepared meals.

COMMON FOODS AND FOOD RITUALS

Because of their size, the normal daily caloric intake of the Vietnamese is approximately two-thirds that of average Americans. Rice is the main staple in the diet, providing up to 80 percent of daily calories. Other common foods are fish (including shellfish), pork, chicken, soybean curd (tofu), noodles, various soups, and green vegetables. Preferred fruits are bananas, mangoes, papayas, oranges, coconuts, pineapples, and grapefruits. Soy sauce, garlic, onions, ginger root, lemon, and chili peppers are used as seasoning.

The Vietnamese eat almost exclusively white or polished rice, disdaining the more nutritious brown or unpolished variety. Rice and other foods are commonly served with *nuoc mam*, a salty, marinated fish sauce. A meal typically consists of rice, *nuoc mam* and a variety of other seasonings, green vegetables, and sometimes meat cut into slivers. Chicken and duck eggs may be used. The Vietnamese prefer white bread, particularly French loaves and rolls, and pastry. A regular dish is *pho*, a soup containing rice noodles, thinly sliced beef or chicken, and scallions.

Other Vietnamese dishes resemble Chinese foods commonly seen in the United States. Some of these include *com chien* (fried rice) and *thit bo xau ca chua* (beef fried with tomatoes). Perhaps the favorite of Americans is *cha gio* (pronounced "cha-yuh"), a combination of finely chopped vegetables, mushrooms, meat or bean curd, rolled into delicate rice paper and deep fried. It is served as part of elaborate meals or during celebrations; proper preparation may require many hours.

Vietnamese eat three meals a day: a light breakfast, a large lunch, and dinner with optional snacks. Meals are served communal style, with food being placed in the center of the table or passed around with everyone taking what they wish. Children wait for their elders to pass each dish. Chopsticks and sometimes spoons are used for eating. Knives are seldom necessary at the table, since meat and vegetables are usually cut into small pieces before serving. Stir frying, steaming, roasting, and boiling are the preferred methods of cooking. Hot tea is the usual beverage.

DIETARY PRACTICES FOR HEALTH PROMOTION

A predominant aspect of the traditional Asian system of health maintenance is the principle of balance between two opposing natural forces, known as **am** and **duong** in Vietnamese. These forces are represented by foods that are considered hot (**duong**) or cold (**am**). The terms have nothing to do with temperature and are only partly associated with seasoning. Rice, flour, potatoes, most fruits and vegetables, fish, duck, and other things that grow in water are considered cold. Most other meats, fish sauce, eggs, spices, peppers, onions, candies, and sweets are hot. Tea is cold, coffee is hot, water is cold, and ice is hot.

Illness or trauma may require therapeutic adjustment of hot-cold balance to restore equilibrium. Hot foods and beverages, used to replace and strengthen the blood, are preferred after surgery or childbirth. During illness, certain foods are consumed in greater quantity, such as a light rice gruel (*chao*) mixed with sugar or sweetened condensed milk, and a few pieces of salty pork cooked with fish sauce. Fresh fruits and vegetables are usually avoided, being considered too cold. Water, juices, and other cold drinks are restricted. Nutritional counseling should take into consideration these factors and other aspects of the usual Vietnamese diet, because advice to simply eat certain kinds of American foods may be ignored.

NUTRITIONAL DEFICIENCIES AND FOOD LIMITATIONS

The traditional Vietnamese diet is basically nutritious, comparing favorably with U.S. federal guidelines for a diet low in fat and sugar, high in complex carbohydrates, and moderate in fiber. However, the prevalence of anemia in children may be associated with an iron deficiency (Goldenring, Davis, & McChesney, 1982). The Vietnamese diet may also be deficient in calcium and zinc, but exceedingly high in sodium, with implications relevant to hypertension.

Most Vietnamese adults and many children have lactose intolerance, which may cause problems in schools, other institutional settings, and adoptive families. Health-care providers may need to encourage the use of substitute milk products that use soybeans.

Before 1975, immigrants encountered difficulty in preparing traditional dishes, especially in areas with no established Vietnamese community. Even then, the determined housewife could assemble most necessary ingredients through judicious selections at ethnic American, Chinese, Korean, and Indian groceries. Today, nearly all common Vietnamese foods are available at reasonable costs in the United States, except perhaps for certain native fruits and vegetables. In addition, Vietnamese Americans have changed their diet to a degree, often increasing their fat intake.

Pregnancy and Childbearing Practices

FERTILITY PRACTICES AND VIEWS TOWARD PREGNANCY

Indochinese women have children over a longer period of life than European Americans, evidenced by females aged 40 to 44 having a birth rate nearly 14 times as great as their European American counterparts (Hopkins & Clarke, 1983). Their fertility rate is about three times that of American women but, in general, they know little about contraception. Abortions are commonly performed in their homeland because pregnancy outside of marriage is considered a disgrace to the family.

After arriving in the United States, women often desire information on contraception but are afraid to ask. The problem stems in part from their cultural background and emphasis on premarital modesty and virginity. However, when contraception was addressed and information made available at the Mayo Clinic, 80 percent of Vietnamese women chose some method of contraception. Practitioners should avoid forceful family planning indoctrination on the first encounter, but such information is usually well received on subsequent visits.

Women over age 40 have an average of six pregnancies and four births, representing losses due to sponta-

neous and induced abortions and stillbirths. With a correction for a 6 percent reported rate of induced abortions, fetal death rates appear to be as high as 44 per 1000 live births, whereas in California the death rate is 8 per 1000. The neonatal death rate reported by one group was 184 per 1000 live births, in contrast to the California rate of 14 per 1000 (Minkler, Korenbrot & Brindis, 1988).

PRESCRIPTIVE, RESTRICTIVE, AND TABOO PRACTICES IN THE CHILDBEARING FAMILY

Prescriptive food practices for a healthy pregnancy include noodles, sweets, sour foods, and fruit but avoidance of fish, salty foods, and rice. After birth, to restore equilibrium and provide adequate warmth to the breast milk, women consume soups with chili peppers, salty fish and meat dishes, and wine steeped with herbs. In addition to hot and cold, foods are classified as tonic and **wind**. Tonic foods include animal protein, fat, sugar, and carbohydrates; they are usually also hot and sweet. Sour and sometimes raw and cold foods are classified as antitonic. **Wind** foods, often classified as cold, include leafy vegetables, fruit, beef, mutton, fowl, fish, and glutinous rice. It is considered critical to increase or decrease foods in various categories to restore bodily balances upset by unusual or stressful conditions such as pregnancy. While the balance of foods may be followed, the terminology is not consistently used.

During the first trimester, the expectant mother is considered to be in a weak, cold, and antitonic state. Therefore she should correct the imbalance by eating hot foods, such as ripe mangoes, grapes, ginger, peppers, alcohol, and coffee. To provide energy and food for the fetus, she is prescribed tonic foods, including a basic diet of steamed rice and pork. Cold foods, including mung beans, green coconut, spinach, and melon, and antitonic foods, such as vinegar, pineapple, and lemon, are avoided during the first trimester.

In the second trimester, the pregnant woman is considered to be in a neutral state. Cold foods are introduced and the tonic diet is continued.

During the third trimester, when the woman may feel hot and suffer from indigestion and constipation, cold foods are prescribed and hot foods are avoided or strictly limited. Tonic foods, which are believed to increase birth weight, are restricted to reduce the chances of a large baby, which would make birthing difficult. **Wind** foods are generally avoided throughout pregnancy, as they are associated with convulsions, allergic reactions, asthma, and other problems. This regimen may appear more complex and restrictive than it actually is in practice. Most women use it only as a general guide, commonly restricting, rather than totally abstaining from, the proscribed foods. A great variety of food, including rice, many kinds of vegetables and fruits, various seasonings, and certain meats and fish are generally permissible throughout pregnancy.

Intensive prenatal care is not the norm in Southeast Asia. Many women do not seek medical attention until the third trimester because of cost, fear, or lack of perceived need. Vietnamese women who are generally better educated seek early prenatal care more than other

Southeast Asians (Hopkins & Clarke, 1983). Of the Vietnamese American women interviewed by Calhoun (1985), 75 percent thought that monthly examinations were important; however, for obstetric and gynecologic matters, they tended to feel more comfortable with a female physician or midwife.

Traditionally, Vietnamese women maintain physical activity to keep the fetus moving and to prevent edema, miscarriage, or premature delivery. Prolonged labor may result from idleness, and an undesirable large baby may result from afternoon napping. Additional restrictive beliefs include avoiding heavy lifting and strenuous work, raising the arms above the head, which pulls on the placenta causing it to break, and sexual relations late in pregnancy, which may cause respiratory stress in the infant. In Vietnam, many consider it taboo for pregnant women to attend weddings or funerals. However, they often look at pictures of happy families and healthy children, believing that it helps give birth to healthy babies.

In Vietnam, most children are delivered in a screened-off portion of the home or in a special birth house by certified midwives, although some are born in hospitals with Western-trained physicians in attendance. Southeast Asians generally dislike invasive procedures, such as episiotomies, cesarean sections, circumcisions, nasal oxygen, and intravenous fluids. However, unlike some women of other ethnic groups, Vietnamese women may ask for anesthesia during labor and delivery. Otherwise, once in labor the Vietnamese woman tries to maintain self-control and may even smile continuously. Her period of labor is usually short, and there may be no warning of impending delivery. Although a special bed may be available, the mother may prefer walking around during labor and squatting during the birth process. This position is less traumatic than others, both for mother and baby and results in fewer and less serious lacerations.

Because the head is considered sacred, neither that of the mother nor of the infant should be touched or stroked. Removal of vernix from the infant's head can cause distress. The American practice of inserting intravenous devices into infants' scalps can be particularly stressful to Vietnamese families. Health-care providers need to stress the importance and necessity of this invasive procedure and select other venous routes if possible.

Customary practices include clearing the neonate's throat using the finger, cutting the umbilical cord with a nonmetal instrument, quickly burying the placenta to protect the infant's health, and ritual cleansing for the mother that does not involve actual bathing with water. In the United States, Vietnamese husbands may be present during the birthing process, although they may not assist.

Because body heat is lost during delivery, Vietnamese women avoid cold foods and beverages and increase consumption of hot foods to replace and strengthen their blood. Ice water and other cold drinks are usually not welcome, and most raw vegetables, fruits, and sour items are taken in lesser amounts. Prescriptive foods include steamed rice, fish sauce, pork, chicken, eggs, soups with chili or black peppers, other highly seasoned and salty items, wine, and sweets.

Because water is cold, women traditionally do not fully bathe, shower, or wash their hair for a month after delivery. Some Vietnamese women have complained that they were adversely affected by showering shortly after delivery in American hospitals. Others, however, have welcomed the opportunity to shower and seem willing to give up other traditional practices. Postpartum women also avoid drafts and strenuous activity; wear warm clothing; stay in bed, indoors, or both for about a month; and avoid sexual intercourse for months. In the past, postpartum women remained in a special bed above a slow-burning fire. This practice still continues with the use of hot water bottles or electric blankets.

Other women in the family assume responsibility for the baby's care. The mother's inactivity and dependence on others may be incorrectly interpreted by health-care workers as apathy or depression. A newborn is often dressed in old clothes, it is considered taboo to praise the child lest jealous spirits steal the infant. The mother may be reluctant to cut the child's hair or nails for fear that this might cause illness. The infant is generally maintained on a diet of milk for the first year, with the introduction of rice gruel at around 6 months. There is little formal toilet training; the child usually learns by imitating an older child.

Breast-feeding is customary in Vietnam, but since resettlement some variations on this practice have been instituted. Some Southeast Asian women discard colostrum and feed the baby rice paste or boiled sugar water for several days. This does not indicate a decision against breast-feeding. After the milk comes in, both mother and young benefit from the hot foods consumed by the mother for the first month. Then, however, a conflict arises: the mother believes that hot foods benefit her health but that cold foods ensure healthy breast milk. Having the mother change from breast-feeding to formula can easily solve this dilemma. However, if the mother cannot afford formula, she may use fresh milk or rice boiled with water, which may result in anemia and growth retardation. Some health-care professionals, concerned about these developments and their impact on the infant's health, have recommended programs that might restore conditions conducive to traditional breast-feeding.

Death Rituals

DEATH RITUALS AND EXPECTATIONS

Vietnamese accept death as a normal part of the life process. The traditional stoicism of the Vietnamese, the influence of Buddhism with its emphasis on cyclic continuity and reincarnation, and the pervading association of current activities with ancestral spirits and burial places contribute to attitudes toward death.

Most Vietnamese have an aversion to hospitals and prefer to die at home. Some believe that a person who dies outside the home becomes a wandering soul with no place to rest. Family members think that they can provide more comfort to the dying person at home. Sixty percent of women in one survey said that if someone in their family were dying, they would not want that person told; 95 percent said that they would want a priest or minister with them when they died, and 95 percent indicated a belief in life after death (Calhoun, 1985, 1986). Ancestors are commonly honored and worshipped and are believed to bestow protection on the living.

Southeast Asians tend not to want to artificially prolong life and suffering, but it may still be difficult for relatives to consent to terminating active intervention, which might be viewed as contributing to the death of an ancestor who would shape the fates of the living (Muecke, 1983a).

Few Vietnamese families consent to autopsy unless they know and agree with the reasons for it. Older Vietnamese, on realizing the inevitability of death, sometimes purchase coffins in advance, display them beneath the household altar, and choose burial sites with a favorable position. Although Vietnamese custom is associated with proper burial practices and maintenance of ancestral tombs, cremation is an acceptable practice to some families.

RESPONSES TO DEATH AND GRIEF

Vietnamese families may wish to gather around the body of a recently deceased relative and express great emotion. Traditional mourning practices include the wearing of white clothes for 14 days, the subsequent wearing of black armbands by men and white headbands by women, and the yearly celebration of the anniversary of a person's death. Such observances, together with ritual cleaning and worship at ancestral graves, help reinforce family ties and are deeply woven into Vietnamese culture. Departure from Vietnam has greatly curtailed the observance of these practices, leaving a painful void for many refugees.

Priests and monks should only be called at the request of the client or family. Clergy visitation is usually associated with last rites by the Vietnamese; especially those influenced by Catholicism, and can actually be upsetting to hospitalized clients. Sending flowers may be startling, as flowers usually are reserved for the rites of the dead.

Spirituality

DOMINANT RELIGION AND USE OF PRAYER

The major religions practiced by the Vietnamese are Buddhism, Confucianism, and Taoism; a few Vietnamese are Christians, most of whom are Catholic. There are a number of other religions, and these are basically offshoots and combinations of the major faiths. Animism is found mainly among the highland tribes. Many Vietnamese believe that deities and spirits control the universe and that the spirits of dead relatives continue to dwell in the home.

Most Vietnamese are Buddhists but some almost never visit temples or perform rituals. Others, both Buddhist and Christian, may maintain a religious altar in the home and conduct regular religious observances. In cases of severe illness, prayers and offerings may be made at a temple.

MEANING OF LIFE AND INDIVIDUAL SOURCES OF STRENGTH

While the wish to bring honor and prosperity to the family remains a dominant force for most Vietnamese, many find meaning in life from the practice of Buddhism or other religions. Some are driven by the desire to learn, to relieve suffering, to produce beauty, to assist the progress of civilization, and to gain strength from participating in ethnic community activities.

"The family is the main reference point for the individual throughout his life, superseding obligations to country, religion, and self. The family is responsible for all decisions and individual actions" (Calhoun, 1986:15). The family is the fundamental social unit and the primary source of cohesion and continuity.

SPIRITUAL BELIEFS AND HEALTH PRACTICES

Vietnamese religious practices are influenced by the Eastern philosophies of Buddhism, Confucianism, and Taoism. Central to Buddhism is the concept of following the correct path of life, thus eliminating suffering that is caused by desire. Another tenet is that the world is a cycle of ordeals: to be born, grow old, fall ill, and die. In addition, people's present lives predetermine their own and their dependents' future lives.

Confucianism stresses harmony through maintenance of the proper order of social hierarchies, ethics, worship of ancestors, and the virtues of chastity and faithfulness. Taoism teaches harmony, allowing events to follow a natural course that one should not attempt to change. These beliefs have contributed to an attitude, which may be perceived as passive by westerners, characterized by maintenance of self-control, acceptance of one's destiny, and fatalism toward illness and death.

Health-Care Practices

HEALTH-SEEKING BELIEFS AND BEHAVIORS

One dominant theory influencing health-care practices among the Vietnamese is a metaphysical explanation that views health as only one facet of a comprehensive scheme of life. Good health is achieved by having harmony and balance with the two basic opposing forces, **am** (cold, dark, female) and **duong** (hot, light, male). An excess of either force may lead to discomfort or illness.

Naturalistic explanations for poor health include eating spoiled food and exposure to inclement weather. The natural element known as **cao gio** is associated with bad weather and cold drafts and causes problems such as the common cold, mild fever, and headache. Countermeasures involve dietary, herbal, hygienic, and simple medical practices. Collectively, these measures are categorized as *thuoc nam*, the traditional southern medicine of Vietnam, and *thuoc bac*, the more formal northern or Chinese medicine. One final explanation for illness places blame on supernaturalistic causes, such as gods, spirits, or demons. Illness may be seen as a punishment for offending such an entity or violating some religious or moral code.

The belief that life is predetermined is a deterrent to seeking health care. For many Vietnamese, diagnostic tests are baffling, inconvenient, and often unnecessary. Procedures such as circumcision or tonsillectomy, which biomedicine considers simple, are generally unknown to the Vietnamese. Invasive procedures are frightening. The prospect of surgery can be terrifying. A great fear of mutilation stems from widespread beliefs among non-Christians that souls are attached to different parts of the body and can leave the body, causing illness or death. Loss of blood from any route is feared, and the Vietnamese may refuse to have blood drawn for laboratory tests. The client may complain, though not to the health-care worker, of feeling weak for months. A Vietnamese client in America may feel that any body tissue or fluid removed cannot be replaced, and the body suffers the loss in this life as well as into the next life.

The concept of long-term medication for chronic illnesses and acceptance of unpleasant side effects and increased autonomic symptoms, which are standard components of modern Western medicine, are not congruent with traditional notions of safe and effective treatment of illnesses.

RESPONSIBILITY FOR HEALTH CARE

In Vietnam, the family is the primary provider of health care, even in hospitals. This practice survives because of tradition and a shortage of professional personnel. Their own families attend hospitalized clients day and night. The importance of including family members in all major treatment decisions regarding physical and mental health must be stressed, including elder family members or clan leaders.

Health care in Vietnam is crisis oriented, with symptom relief as the goal. Vietnamese typically deal with illness by means of self-care, self-medication, and the use of herbal medicines. Facsimiles of Western prescription drugs are sold over the counter throughout Southeast Asia, which may explain the increasing resistance of bacteria to several readily available antibiotics.

Many Vietnamese believe that Western medicine is very powerful and cures quickly, but few understand the risks of overdosages or underdosages. Some believe that Asians have a different physical constitution than European Americans, so that Western drugs and drug dosages that are appropriate for European Americans may not be appropriate for Asians. Consequently, they may politely accept the prescription, but not fill it. If they have filled it, they may not take the medicine or they may adjust the dosage without telling the health-care provider to avoid hurting or embarrassing anyone. Clients being treated for depression who fail to take their antidepressants evidence improvement after receiving instructions for taking their medication (Lin & Shen, 1991). Vietnamese clients may not follow prescribed schedules of medication for the treatment and prevention of tuberculosis. Extensive education, repetition of instructions, and home visitations are necessary.

It has been found, unfortunately, that most Vietnamese women who have abnormal Pap smears fail to return for follow-up care, thereby contributing to the shockingly high incidence of cervical cancer in the population (Wright, 2000). That problem has been associated with lack of organized language services and, thus, a failure by the women to comprehend the severity of the situation and the potential for recovery if regular treatment begins early enough. To increase follow-up visits and care, it may be necessary to carefully explain the problems that may result if there is no action relative to an abnormal Pap smear. Women should understand that lack of symptoms or pain may be only temporary and that experiences of acquaintances may not apply to them. Persistent reminding, as part of an overall effort to improve communication and information dissemination, has been suggested as the best way to encourage Vietnamese women to undergo regular cancer screening and follow-up treatment.

FOLK PRACTICES

The forces of **am** (cold) and **duong** (hot) are pervasive forces in the practice of traditional Vietnamese medicine. **Am** represents factors that are considered negative, feminine, dark, and empty, whereas **duong** represents those that are positive, masculine, light, and full. These terms are applied to various parts, organs, and processes of the body. For example, the inside of the body is **am**, and the surface is **duong**. The front part of the body is **am**, and the back is **duong**. The liver, heart, spleen, lungs, and kidneys are **am**, and the gallbladder, stomach, intestines, bladder, and lymph system are **duong**. **Am** stores strength, and care must be taken not to use it up too quickly. **Duong** protects the body from outside forces and, if not cared for, the organs are thrown into disorder. Proper balance of these two life forces ensures the correct circulation of blood and good health. If the balance is not proper, life is short.

Diseases and other debilitating conditions result from either cold or hot influences. For example, diarrhea and some febrile diseases are due to an excess of cold, whereas pimples and other skin problems result from an excess of hot. Countermeasures involve using foods, medications, and treatments that have properties opposite those of the problem, and avoiding foods that would intensify the problem. Asian herbs are cold and Western medicines are hot. A widely held belief among Vietnamese refugees is that Asian medicine relieves symptoms of a disease more quickly than Western medicine, but that Western medications can actually cure the illness. Many prefer Asian methods for children. Reliance on traditional folk medicine is declining in the United States, partly because of the unavailability of suitable shamans and traditional herbs.

The following are common treatments practiced in Vietnam and continued to some degree in the United States:

Cao gio, literally meaning "rubbing out the wind" is used for treating colds, sore throats, flu, sinusitis, and similar ailments. An ointment or hot balm oil is spread across the back, chest, or shoulders and rubbed with the edge of a coin (preferably silver) in short, firm strokes. This technique brings blood under the skin, resulting in dark ecchymotic stripes, so the offending wind can escape. Health-care professionals must be careful not to interpret these ecchymotic areas as evidence of child abuse. However, dermabrasion may provide a portal for infection.

Be bao or ***bar gio***, skin pinching, is a treatment for headache or sore throat. The skin of the affected area is repeatedly squeezed between the thumb and forefinger of both hands, as the hands converge toward the center of the face. The objective is to produce ecchymoses or petechiae.

Giac, cup suctioning, another dermabrasive procedure, is used to relieve stress, headaches, and joint and muscle pain. A small cup is heated and placed on the skin with the open side down. As the cup cools, it contracts the skin and draws unwanted hot energy into the cup. This treatment leaves marks that may appear as large bruises.

Xong, an herbal preparation, relieves motion sickness or cold-related problems. Herbs or an agent such as Vicks Vaporub is put into boiling water and the vapor is inhaled. Small containers of aromatic oils or liniments are sometimes carried and inhaled directly.

Moxibustion is used to counter conditions associated with excess cold, including labor and delivery. Pulverized wormwood or incense is heated and placed directly on the skin at certain meridians. (See Fig. 21–2.)

Acupuncture, acupressure, and acumassage relieve symptomatic stress and pain (see Glossary).

Balms and oils, such as Red Tiger balm, available in Asian shops, are applied to affected areas for relief of bone and muscle ailments.

Herbal teas, soups, and other concoctions are taken for various problems, generally in the sense of using cold measures to overcome hot illnesses.

Eating organ meats such as liver, kidneys, testes, brains, and bones of an animal is said to increase the strength of the corresponding human part.

Two additional practices in Vietnam are consuming gelatinized tiger bones to gain strength and taking powdered rhinoceros horn to reduce fever. At least 430 folk medicines used by Vietnamese contain ingredients from endangered, threatened, or protected species (Gaski & Johnson, 1994).

BARRIERS TO HEALTH CARE

Barriers to adequate health care for Vietnamese people include:

1 Subjective beliefs and the cost of health care

2 Lack of a primary provider

3 Differences between Western and Asian health-care practices

4 Caregivers' judgment of Vietnamese as deviant and unmotivated because of noncompliance with medication schedules, diagnostic tests, follow-up care, and their failure to keep appointments

5 Inability to communicate effectively in the English language with recent immigrants who lack

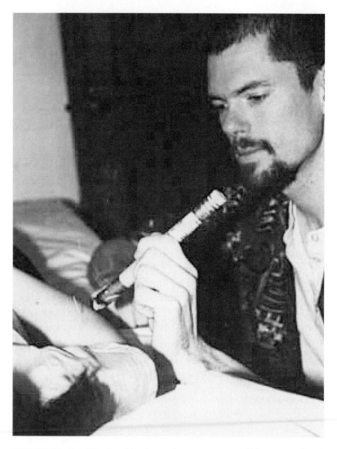

FIGURE 21–2 **Moxibustion** is used to counter conditions associated with excess cold, including labor and delivery. Pulverized wormwood or incense is heated and placed directly on the skin at certain meridians. (From Ancient Way Acupuncture and Herbs. Klamath Falls, Oregon. *www.AncientWay.com.*)

confidence in their ability to communicate their needs; failure of providers to communicate

6 Avoidance of Western practitioners out of fear that traditional methods will be criticized

7 Fear of conflicts and ridicule resulting in loss of face

8 Lack of knowledge of the availability of resources

Additional barriers exist for Vietnamese people when seeking mental health care. These include fear of stigmatization, difficulty locating agencies that can provide assistance without distorted professional and cultural communication, and unwillingness to express inner feelings.

CULTURAL RESPONSES TO HEALTH AND ILLNESS

Fatalistic attitudes and the belief that problems are punishment may reduce the degree of complaining and expression of pain among the Vietnamese, who view endurance as an indicator of strong character. One accepts pain as part of life and attempts to maintain self-control as a means of relief. A deep cultural restraint against showing weakness limits the use of pain medication. However, the sick person is allowed to depend on family and receives a great deal of attention and care.

Many Vietnamese believe that mental illness results from offending a deity and that it brings disgrace to the family and, therefore, must be concealed. A shaman may be enlisted to help, and additional therapy is sought only with the greatest discretion and often after a dangerous delay. Emotional disturbance is usually attributed to possession by malicious spirits, the bad luck of familial inheritance, or for Buddhists, to bad karma accumulated by misdeeds in past lives. The term *psychiatrist* has no direct translation in Vietnamese and may be interpreted to mean nerve physician or specialist who treats crazy people. The nervous system sometimes is seen as the source of mental problems, neurosis being thought of as "weakness of the nerves" and psychosis as "turmoil of the nerves."

To overcome these problems, Kinzie and associates (1982) and Buchwald and colleagues (1993) developed a Vietnamese depression scale, which uses terms that allow an English-speaking practitioner to make a cross-cultural assessment of the clinical characteristics of depressed Vietnamese clients. Health-care providers working with Vietnamese clients may find this scale useful when providing mental health services.

Physically disabled people are common and readily seen in Vietnam. To the extent that resources allow, they are treated well and cared for by their families and the government. In contrast, a mentally disabled person may be stigmatized by the family and society and can jeopardize the ability of relatives to find marriage partners. The mentally disabled are usually harbored within their families unless they become destructive; then they may be admitted to a hospital.

BLOOD TRANSFUSIONS AND ORGAN DONATION

Because many Vietnamese believe that the body must be kept intact even after death, they are averse to blood transfusions and organ donation. Many Vietnamese, even those whose families have long been Christian, may object to removal of body parts or organ donation. However, some staff in a rural hospital in Vietnam donated blood after learning that the body replenished its blood supply. The smaller size of Vietnamese adults makes many of them ineligible to donate a full unit of blood. Other Vietnamese people, who may prefer cremation, will donate body parts under certain circumstances.

Health-Care Practitioners

TRADITIONAL VERSUS BIOMEDICAL PRACTITIONERS

Four kinds of traditional and folk practitioners exist in Vietnam. The first group includes Asian physicians who are learned individuals and employ herbal medication and acupuncture. The second group consists of more informal folk healers who use special herbs and diets as cures based on natural or pragmatic approaches. The secrets of folk medicine are passed down through the generations. The third group comprises various forms of spiritual healers, some with a specific religious outlook

and others with powers to drive away malevolent spirits. The fourth group is made up of magicians or sorcerers who have magical curative powers, but no communication with the spirits. Many Vietnamese consult one or more of these healers in an attempt to find a cure.

While many Vietnamese have great respect for professional, well-educated people, they may be distrustful of outside authority figures. Most Vietnamese have come to America to escape oppressive authority. Refugees generally expect health-care professionals to be experts. A common suspicion is that divulging personal information for a medical history could jeopardize their legal rights. Respect and mistrust are not mutually exclusive concepts for Vietnamese seeking care from Western practitioners.

Acknowledgment and support of traditional belief systems are important in building a trusting relationship. Traditional healers often provide the Vietnamese with necessary social support.

Traditional Asian male practitioners do not usually touch the bodies of female clients and sometimes use a doll to point out the nature of a problem. While most Vietnamese might no longer insist on the use of this practice, adults, particularly young and unmarried women, are more comfortable with health-care providers of the same gender. Pelvic examinations on unmarried women should not be made on the first visit or without careful advanced explanation and preparation. When such an examination is necessary, the woman may want her husband present. If possible, the practitioner and an interpreter should both be female. Women may not want to even discuss sexual problems, reproductive matters, and birth control techniques until after an initial visit and confidence has been established in the practitioner.

STATUS OF HEALTH-CARE PROVIDERS

Because of the shortage of physicians in Vietnam, medical assistants, nurses, village health-care workers, self-trained individuals, and injectionists practice Western medicine. Paralleling these approaches are the traditional systems of Asian and folk medicine. All are respected and have high status and may be used concurrently or separately, according to the illness and varying beliefs of each individual.

CASE STUDY Cao Thi Xuan, age 48, arrived in Arlington, Virginia, about 5 years ago directly from Vietnam under the Orderly Departure Program. Her husband, Nguyen Van Minh, now a cook at a restaurant owned by his brother, had come several years earlier with their son, Danh, now age 19, and daughter, Tuyet, 23. Xuan's departure had been delayed several times through a combination of clearance problems and a commitment to remaining to care for an elderly father, who now has died. Although she had a high school education in Vietnam and studied some English, she is not fluent and finds paperwork and communication with Americans difficult, if not impossible. She is now usually at home or visiting

Vietnamese friends, but also works part time at the restaurant.

While pleased with some aspects of life in the United States, Xuan is somewhat upset by the radical differences from the traditional Vietnamese lifestyle, notably the role of young people. Her daughter, "Tilly," as she is known to American friends, has adapted well to the United States, speaks English fluently, has completed college, and holds a good job as a computer programmer, but spends a great deal of time away from the family. Her son, often called "Danny," drifts back and forth, has dropped out of school, has no steady employment, and often accompanies members of a local Vietnamese gang. When he does return home, he is subjected to criticism from other family members, especially his father, though Xuan tends to be somewhat protective.

Xuan considers herself in good health and is not aware of any problems, other than worry and tiredness. She had not been to any Western doctor or clinic since her examination before immigration. However, after persuasion by Tilly and a number of female acquaintances, she agreed to go to a clinic for a general examination, including mammogram and Pap smear. The results were mostly favorable but the Pap smear showed some abnormalities and she was asked to return for follow-up testing.

Confused and troubled, Xuan has not complied with the clinic's instructions. She told Tilly and others that she feels fine and has noticed no pain or symptoms. Moreover, she already had been seeing an elderly local Vietnamese woman reputed to be a traditional "healer" and has been given various herbal concoctions. That has been comforting to her and she feels it is sufficient. She was upset by her experience at the clinic, especially the invasive tests by a male doctor, and by her inability to communicate effectively.

STUDY QUESTIONS

1 What is the preferred form of address for Xuan, Minh, and Tilly, and how should their names be recorded?

2 Identify the most critical cultural factors affecting Vietnamese people after immigration, and how might they apply in the case of Xuan's family, especially Tilly and Danny?

3 What information can be provided to Xuan and her family to help improve compliance with clinical instructions and other aspects of physical health?

4 What should Xuan know about dangers and treatment of cervical cancer, especially with respect to Vietnamese women?

5 How might Xuan's clinical experience be improved, particularly with respect to communication, presence of others, and designation of the examiner?

6 What questions should be asked regarding Xuan's traditional treatments?

7 Explain some of the major religious factors influencing the Vietnamese outlook toward health care.

8 Distinguish ethnic Vietnamese from other Southeast Asian groups.

9 What are generally considered the most serious health problems for Vietnamese refugees?

10 What is the role of the family in Vietnamese health care?

11 Explain the connotations of "hot" and "cold" in traditional Vietnamese health care.

12 Discuss some of the customary practices in a Western hospital that might be upsetting to a pregnant or postpartum Vietnamese woman.

13 Name three traditional Vietnamese treatments and their connotations to Western professionals.

REFERENCES

Baron, R. C. et al. (1983). Sudden death among Southeast Asian refugees. *Journal of the American Medical Association, 250*(21), 2947–2951.

Barry, M. et al. (1993). Clinical findings in Southeast Asian refugees. *Journal of the American Medical Association, 249*(23), 3200–3203.

Beiser, M., Turner, R., & Ganesan, S. (1989). Catastrophic stress and factors affecting its consequences among Southeast Asian refugees. *Social Science Medicine, 28*(3), 183–195.

Buchwald, D. et al. (1993). Prevalence of depressive symptoms among established Vietnamese refugees in the United States. *Journal of General Internal Medicine, 8*(2), 76–81.

Calhoun, M. A. (1985). The Vietnamese woman: Health/illness attitudes and behaviors. *Health Care for Women International, 6*(1–3), 61–72.

Calhoun, M. A. (1986). Providing health care to Vietnamese in America: What practitioners need to know. *Home Health-care Nurse, 4*(5), 14–22.

Catanzaro, A., & Moser, R. J. (1982). Health status of refugees from Vietnam, Laos, and Cambodia. *Journal of the American Medical Association, 247*(9), 1303–1308.

Centers for Disease Control (1990). Update: Sudden unexplained death syndrome among Southeast Asian refugees—United States. *Journal of the American Medical Association, 260*(14) 2033.

Chen, M. S. et al. (1991). Providing heart health for Southeast Asians: A database for planning interventions. *Public Health Reports, 106*(3), 304–309.

Cochran, S. D., Mays, V. M. & Leung, L. (1991). Sexual practices of heterosexual Asian-American young adults: Implications for risk of HIV infection. *Archives of Sexual Behavior 20*(4), 381–391.

Dao, A. H., Gregory, D. W., & McKee, C. (1984). Specific health problems of Southeast Asian refugees in middle Tennessee. *Southern Medical Journal, 77*(8), 995–997.

Felice, M. E. (1986). Reflections on caring for Indochinese children and youths. *Developmental and Behavioral Pediatrics, 7*(2), 124–130.

Fitzpatrick, S. et al (1987). Health care needs of Indochinese refugee teenagers. *Pediatrics, 79*(1), 118–124.

Gaski, A. L., & Johnson, K. A. (1994). *Prescription for extinction: Endangered species and patented Oriental medicines in trade.* Washington, DC: Traffic USA.

Gold, S. J. (1992). Mental health and illness in Vietnamese refugees. *Western Journal of Medicine, 157*(3), 290–294.

Goldenring, J. M., Davis, J., & McChesney, M. (1982). Pediatric screening of Southeast Asian immigrants. *Clinical Pediatrics, 21*(10), 613–616.

Hopkins, D. D., & Clarke, N. G. (1983). Indochinese refugee fertility rates and pregnancy risk factors: Oregon. *American Journal of Public Health, 73*(11), 1307–1309.

Jenkins, C. N. H. et al. (1990). Cancer risks and prevention practices among Vietnamese refugees. *Western Journal of Medicine, 153*(1), 34–39.

Jenkins, C. N. H. et al. (1992). Cigarette smoking among Chinese, Vietnamese, and Hispanics: California 1989–1991. *Morbidity and Mortality Weekly Report, 41*(20), 362–367.

Kinzie, J. D. et al. (1982). Development and validation of a Vietnamese-language depression rating scale. *American Journal of Psychiatry, 139*(10), 1276–1281.

Levy, R. A. (1993). Ethnic and racial differences in response to medicines: Preserving individualized therapy in managed pharmaceutical programmes. *Pharmaceutical Medicine, 7,* 139–165.

Lin, K., & Finder, E. (1983). Neuroleptic dosage for Asians. *American Journal of Psychiatry, 140*(4), 490–491.

Lin, K., & Shen, W. W. (1991). Pharmacotherapy for Southeast Asian psychiatric patients. *Journal of Nervous and Mental Disease, 179*(6), 346–350.

Minkler, D. H., Korenbrot, C., & Brindis, C. (1988). Family planning among Southeast Asian refugees. *Health Care Delivery, 148*(3), 349–354.

Muecke, M. A. (1983a). Caring for Southeast Asian refugee patients in the USA. *American Journal of Public Health, 73*(4), 431–438.

Muecke, M. A. (1983b). In search of healers: Southeast Asian refugees in the American health care system. *Western Journal of Medicine, 139*(6), 835–840.

Overfield, T. (1977). Biological variation. *Nursing Clinics of North America, 12*(1) 19–27.

Pickwell, S. M. (1982). Primary health care for Indochinese refugee children. *Pediatric Nursing, 8*(2), 104–107.

Roberts, N. S. et al. (1985). Intestinal parasites and other infections during pregnancy in Southeast Asian refugees. *Journal of Reproductive Medicine, 30*(10), 720–725.

Rosenblat, R., & Tang, S. W. (1987). Do Oriental psychiatric patients receive different dosages of psychotropic medication when compared with Occidentals? *Canadian Journal of Psychiatry, 32,* 270–273.

Ross, T. F. (1982). Health care problems of Southeast Asian refugees. *Western Journal of Medicine, 136*(1), 35–43.

Sokoloff, B., Carlin, J., & Pham, H. (1984). Five-year follow-up of Vietnamese refugee children in the United States. *Clinical Pediatrics, 23*(10), 565–570.

Strand, P. J., & Jones, W. (1983). Health service utilization by Indochinese refugees. *Medical Care, 21*(11), 1089–1098.

Sutherland, J. E. et al. (1983). Indochinese refugee health assessment and treatment. *Journal of Family Practice, 16*(1), 61–67.

Sutter, R. W., & Haefliger, E. (1990). Tuberculosis morbidity and infection in Vietnamese in Southeast Asian refugee camps. *American Review of Respiratory Disease, 141*(6), 1483–1486.

Tobin, J. J., & Friedman, J. (1983). Spirits, shamans, and nightmare death: Survivor stress in a Hmong refugee. *American Journal of Orthopsychiatry, 53*(3), 439–448.

Wright, J. B. (2000). 2000 Assembly on Cervical Cancer Among Vietnamese-American Women. National Asian Women's Health Organization, Annandale, VA.

Yu, E. S. H. (1991). The health risks of Asian Americans. *American Journal of Public Health, 81*(11), 1391–1393.

Appendix

Cultural and Racial Diseases and Illnesses

Causes are grouped into three categories, genetic, lifestyle, and environment.

Lifestyle causes include cultural practices and behaviors that can generally be controlled: for example, smoking, diet, and stress.

Environment causes refer to the external environment (e.g., air and water pollution) and situations over which the individual has little or no control over (e.g., presence of malarial mosquitos, exposure to chemicals and pesticides, access to care, and associated diseases).

Cultural/Racial Group	Diseases/Disorders	Causes
Black populations	Sickle cell disease	Genetic, environment
	Hypertension	Genetic, lifestyle
	Systemic lupus erythematosus	Genetic with an environmental trigger
	Diabetes mellitus	Genetic, lifestyle
	Glaucoma	Genetic
	Cardiovascular disease	Genetic, environment, lifestyle
	Prostate cancer	Genetic, environment
	Hemoglobin C disease	Genetic
	Hereditary persistence of hemoglobin F	Genetic
	Glucose-6-phosphate dehydrogenase deficiency	Genetic
	β-Thalassemia	Genetic
	Haitian	
	Malaria	Environment
	Tuberculosis	Lifestyle, environment
	Diabetes mellitus	Genetic, environment, lifestyle
	Hypertension	Genetic, lifestyle
	Kenyan	
	Nasopharyngeal cancer	Lifestyle
	Esophageal cancer	Lifestyle, environment?
	Zairian & Ugandan	
	Stomach cancer	Lifestyle
	Duodenal ulcers	Unknown
	Rhodesian	
	Stomach cancer	Lifestyle

Cultural/Racial Group	Diseases/Disorders	Causes
	Sub-Saharan African	
	Liver cancer	Environment
	100 degrees north and south of the equator	
	Burkitt lymphoma	Environment
Hispanics	Lactase deficiency	Genetic
	Diabetes mellitus	Genetic, lifestyle, environment
	Cleft lip/palate	Lifestyle
	Dental caries	Lifestyle, environment
	Cardiovascular disease	Genetic, environment, lifestyle
	Tuberculosis	Environment, lifestyle
	Hypertension	Genetic, environment, lifestyle
	Costa Rican	
	Malignant osteoporosis	Environment? Genetic?
	Puerto Rican	
	Cardiovascular disease	Genetic, environment, lifestyle
	Hypertension	Genetic, environment, lifestyle
	Dengue fever	Environment
	Breast cancer	Genetic, lifestyle
	Prostate cancer	Genetic, environment, lifestyle
Arabs/Middle Easterners	Familial Mediterranean fever	Genetic
	Familial paroxysmal polyserositis	Genetic
	Tuberculosis	Environment, lifestyle
	Malaria	Genetic, environment
	Trachoma	Environment, lifestyle
	Typhoid fever	Environment
	Glucose-6-phosphate dehydrogenase deficiency	Genetic
	Sickle cell disease	Genetic, environment
	Thalassemia	Genetic
	Hepatitis A and B	Environment, lifestyle
	Iranian	
	Dubin-Johnson syndrome	Genetic
	Epilepsy	Genetic
	Iraqi	
	Ichthyosis vulgaris	Genetic
	Yemeni	
	Phenylketonuria	Genetic
	Glucose-6-phosphate dehydrogenase deficiency	Genetic
	Lebanese	
	Dyggve-Melchior-Clausen syndrome	Genetic
	Familial hypercholesterolemia	Genetic
	Egyptians	
	Schistosomiasis	Lifestyle, environment
	Trachoma	Environment, lifestyle
	Typhoid fever	Environment
	Tuberculosis	Lifestyle, Environment
	β-Thalassemia	Genetic

Cultural/Racial Group	Diseases/Disorders	Causes
	Saudi Arabians	
	Metachromatic leukodystrophy	Genetic
Asian/Pacific Islanders	**Chinese**	
	α-Thalassemia	Genetic
	Glucose-6-phosphate dehydrogenase deficiency	Genetic
	Lactase deficiency	Genetic
	Nasopharyngeal cancer	Environment, lifestyle
	Liver cancer	Environment, lifestyle
	Stomach cancer	Unknown, lifestyle and/or environment
	Cardiovascular disease	Genetic, lifestyle, environment
	Hepatitis B	Genetic, lifestyle, environment,
	Tuberculosis	Environment, lifestyle
	Diabetes mellitus	Genetic, lifestyle, environment
	Japanese	
	Vogt-Koyanagi-Harada syndrome	Genetic
	Cardiovascular disease	Genetic, lifestyle, environment
	Asthma	Lifestyle, environment
	Takayasu disease	Genetic
	Acatalasemia	Genetic
	Cleft lip/palate	Lifestyle, genetic
	Oguchi disease	Genetic
	Lactase deficiency	Environment, lifestyle
	Stomach cancer	Genetic, lifestyle, environment
	Hypertension	Genetic, lifestyle, environment
	Asian Indian	
	Cancer of the cheek	Lifestyle
	Ichthyosis vulgaris	Genetic
	Tuberculosis	Lifestyle, environment
	Malaria	Environment
	Rheumatic heart disease	Environment
	Cardiovascular disease	Genetic, lifestyle, environment
	Sickle cell disease	Genetic
	Filipino	
	Diabetes mellitus	Genetic, environment, lifestyle
	Hyperuricemia	Lifestyle
	Cardiovascular disease	Genetic, lifestyle, environment
	Hypertension	Genetic, lifestyle, environment
	Thalassemia	Genetic
	Glucose-6-phosphate dehydrogenase deficiency	Genetic
	Lactase deficiency	Genetic
	Vietnamese	
	Nasopharyngeal cancer	Lifestyle, environment
	Lactase deficiency	Genetic
	Posttraumatic stress disorder	Environment
	Tuberculosis	Lifestyle, environment
	Malaria	Environment
	Hepatitis B	Environment, lifestyle
	Melioidosis	Environment, lifestyle
	Paragonimiasis	Environment, lifestyle
	Leprosy	Genetic

Cultural/Racial Group	Diseases/Disorders	Causes
	Hmong and Laotian	
	Nasopharyngeal cancer	Lifestyle, environment
	Lactase deficiency	Genetic
	Tuberculosis	Environment, lifestyle
	Hepatitis B	Genetic, environment, lifestyle
	Korean	
	Stomach cancer	Lifestyle
	Liver cancer	Genetic, environment
	Hypertension	Genetic, lifestyle, environment
	Schistosomiasis	Environment, lifestyle
	Hepatitis A and B	Environment, lifestyle
	Lactase deficiency	Genetic
	Osteoporosis	Genetic, lifestyle
	Peptic ulcer disease	Lifestyle, environment
	Insulin autoimmune deficiency disease	Genetic
	Renal failure	Lifestyle
European American ethnic white populations	Skin cancer	Environment, lifestyle
	Appendicitis	Unknown
	Diverticular disease	Diet, genetic?
	Colon cancer	Diet, genetic?
	Hemorrhoids	Lifestyle, unknown
	Cardiovascular disease	Genetic, diet, lifestyle, environment
	Varicose veins	Genetic
	Diabetes mellitus	Genetic, diet
	Multiple sclerosis	Environment
	Obesity	Lifestyle
	English	
	Cystic fibrosis	Genetic
	Hereditary amyloidosis, type III	Genetic
	Rosacea	Genetic
	French Canadian	
	Sickle cell disease	Genetic, environment
	Osteoporosis	Lifestyle, genetic
	Osteoarthritis	Genetic
	Cardiovascular disease	Genetic, lifestyle, environment
	Lung cancer	Environment, lifestyle
	Breast cancer	Genetic, lifestyle
	Cystic fibrosis	Genetic
	Phenylketonuria	Genetic
	Tyrosinemia	Genetic
	Morquio syndrome	Genetic
	Hypercholesterolemia	Genetic, lifestyle
	Greek	
	Tay-Sachs disease	Genetic
	Cardiovascular disease	Genetic, environment, lifestyle
	Malaria	Environment
	Tuberculosis	Environment, lifestyle
	Glucose-6-phosphate dehydrogenase deficiency	Genetic
	Hepatitis A and B	Environment, lifestyle
	Finns	
	Stomach cancer	Diet
	Congenital nephrosis	Genetic
	Generalized amyloidosis, type V	Genetic
	Polycystic liver disease	Genetic

Cultural/Racial Group	Diseases/Disorders	Causes
	Retinoschisis	Genetic
	Aspartylglycosaminuria	Genetic
	Diastrophic dwarfism	Genetic
	Retinoschisis	Genetic
	Choroideremia	Genetic
Italian		
	Vogt-Koyanagi-Harada syndrome	Genetic
	β-Thalassemia	Genetic
	Recurrent polyserositis	Genetic
	Hypertension	Lifestyle, genetic
	Nasopharyngeal cancer	Lifestyle
	Stomach cancer	Lifestyle
	Liver cancer	Lifestyle
	Familial Mediterranean fever	Genetic
	Glucose-6-phosphate dehydrogenase deficiency	Genetic
Jewish		
	Lactase deficiency	Genetic
	Werdnig-Hoffmann disease	Genetic
	Mucolipidosis IV	Genetic
	Phenylketonuria	Genetic
	Kaposi sarcoma	Genetic
	Gaucher disease	Genetic
	Niemann-Pick disease	Genetic
	Tay-Sachs disease	Genetic
	Riley-Day syndrome	Genetic
	Torsion dystonia	Genetic
	Factor XI (PTA) deficiency	Genetic
	Cystinuria	Genetic
	Ataxia-telangiectasia	Genetic
	Familial Mediterranean fever	Genetic
	Metachromatic leukodystrophy	Genetic, unknown
	Bloom syndrome	Genetic, diet
	Myopia	Genetic, lifestyle
	Polycythemia vera	Genetic, lifestyle
	Hypercholesterolemia	Genetic
	Breast cancer	Environment, lifestyle
	Diabetes mellitus	Genetic, lifestyle, environment
Polish		
	Phenylketonuria	Environment
	Respiratory diseases	Environment, lifestyle
	Cardiovascular diseases	Diet
Appalachian		
	Black lung	Environment, lifestyle
	Emphysema	Unknown
	Tuberculosis	Genetic, lifestyle, environment
	Hypochromic anemia	Environment, lifestyle
	Cardiovascular disease	Genetic, lifestyle
	Sudden infant death syndrome	Genetic
	Diabetes mellitus	Genetic
	Otitis media	Lifestyle
Scandinavians		
	Cholelethiasis	Genetic, lifestyle
	Sjögren-Larsson syndrome	Genetic
	Krabbe disease	Genetic, environment, lifestyle
	Phenylketonuria	Genetic

Cultural/Racial Group	Diseases/Disorders	Causes
	Irish	
	Phenylketonuria	Genetic
	Neural tube defects	Genetic
	Cardiovascular disease	Genetic
	Alcoholism	Genetic
	Skin cancer	Genetic
	Amish	
	Limb-girdle muscular dystrophy	Genetic
	Ellis-van Creveld syndrome	Genetic
	Dwarfism	Genetic, unknown
	Polydactylism	Genetic
	Cartilage hair hypoplasia	Genetic
	Phenylketonuria	Genetic
	Glutaric aciduria	Genetic
	Manic-depressive disorder	Genetic
	Pyruvate kinase deficiency	Genetic
	Hemophilia B	Genetic
Native American/ Alaskan natives	Diabetes mellitus	Genetic, lifestyle, environment
	Cholelithiasis	Lifestyle
	Lactase deficiency	Genetic
	Liver disease	Environment, lifestyle
	Hepatitis B	Environment, lifestyle
	Nasopharyngeal cancer	Environment, lifestyle
	Tuberculosis	Environment, lifestyle
	Alcoholism	Lifestyle, genetic
	Navajo	
	Ear anomalies	Genetic
	Arthritis	Genetic
	Severe combined immunodeficiency syndrome	Genetic
	Navajo neuropathy	Genetic
	Albinism	Genetic
	Tuberculosis	Environment, lifestyle
	Hopi	
	Tyrosinase-positive albinism	Genetic
	Trachoma	Environment, lifestyle
	Pueblo	
	Albinism	Genetic
	Zuni	
	Tyrosinase-positive albinism	Genetic
	Eskimo	
	Hereditary amyloidosis	Genetic
	Congenital adrenal hyperplasia	Genetic
	Methemoglobinemia	Genetic
	Lactase deficiency	Genetic
	Pseudocholinesterase deficiency	Genetic
	Haemophilus influenza type B	Genetic?

Glossary

A

aagwachse: An Amish folk illness referred to in English as *livergrown*, with symptoms of abdominal distress thought to be caused by too much jostling, especially for infants during buggy rides.

abnemme: An Amish folk illness characterized by "wasting away," usually affecting infants or young children who seem to be too lean and not active.

abwaarde: Amish term for ministering to someone by being present and serving when someone is sick in bed.

Acadia: Part of the Canadian Maritime provinces.

Acadian: Early French settler of Acadia; a French dialect spoken by people in Acadia.

acculturate: To modify the culture of a group or individual as a result of contact with another group or individual.

adab: Egyptian word for politeness.

Ainu: Indigenous people of uncertain origin in northern Japan.

Allah: The greatest and most inclusive of the names of God. An Arabic word used to describe the God worshipped by Muslims, Christians, and Jews.

am: A pervasive force in Vietnamese traditional medicine which is associated with cold conditions and things that are dark, negative, feminine, and empty.

amal: Egyptian voodoo-like action done to bring bad luck or illness to an unloved person.

Americanos: Hispanic name given to people from the European American culture.

amor propio: Filipino term for saving face.

Anabaptist: Adherent of radical wing of the Protestant Reformation who espouses baptism of adult believers.

andarun: Iranian term meaning inner self.

antyesti: Hindu equivalent of last rites.

Appalachian Regional Commission: Federal Commission established in the 1960s to improve economic conditions in Appalachia. This includes appropriations for improving and building roads, establishing loans for small businesses, and attracting industry to the area.

Arabic: The Semitic language of the Arabs.

arwah: Egyptian word for the spirits.

asafetida bag: Odorous combination of roots and herbs, usually made into a poultice, enclosed in a bag, and worn around the neck or some other part of the body for the purpose of warding off contagious illnesses.

Ashkenazi: Descended from Eastern Europe and Russia.

assimilate: To gradually adopt and incorporate the characteristics of the prevailing culture.

atma: Eternal soul in Hindu.

atary: An Iranian herb shop.

attitude: A state of mind or feeling with regard to some matter of a culture.

augmented families: A term used in African American culture to refer to children who are raised in households in which they are not related to the head of that household.

¡ay bendito!: A frequently used Puerto Rican expression that expresses astonishment, surprise, lament, or pain.

Ayurveda: Traditional Asian Indian medicine.

B

bahala na: Filipino term meaning it is up to God.

baklava: Turkish pudding.

Baltics dainas: Latvian songs.

barrenillos: Spanish word for obsessions.

baten: Iranian term for inner self.

be bao or bat gio: Vietnamese folk practice where the skin is pinched with the objective of producing ecchymosis and petechiae. This is practiced to relieve sore throats and headaches.

Bedouins: Egyptian desert inhabitants.

Behçet's disease: Endemic disease in Turkey characterized by chronic inflammatory disorders of the blood vessels with recurrent ulcerations of the oral and pharyngeal mucous membranes and the genitalia, skin lesions, severe uveitis, retinal vasculitis, and optic atrophy.

being: The essence of existence in an unqualified state and conceived as an essential of nature where one does not need to be actively engaged in an activity.

belief: Something accepted as true, especially as a tenet or a body of tenets accepted by people in an ethno-cultural group.

bisprechung: German term for formal conversation and discourse.

African Americans: A term used to describe Americans of African descent.

Black bourgeoisie: African American families who achieve middle- and upper-class status.

Black English: A dialect used by African Americans.

boat people: Haitian or Cuban entrants who arrive in small boats. They are usually of undocumented status.

Boricua: Puerto Rican term used with great pride. Name given to Puerto Rico by the Taino Indians.

botanica: Traditional Cuban or other Spanish store selling a variety of herbs, ointments, oils, powders, incenses, and religious figurines used in Santería.

brauche: Folk healing art common among Pennsylvania Germans.

braucher: Amish practitioner of *brauche,* a folk healer.

Briefe zum Himmel: German for the tooth fairy.

bris or brit milah: Ritual circumcision of a male Jewish child.

bruderschaft-trinken: When German friends formally shift to the more intimate form of address, they hook arms and sip from a glass. Then they shake hands and announce their first names.

Burakumin: Japanese term for Korean descendants or descendants of the ***burakumin***, the "untouchable" caste who cared for the dead and tanned leather in feudal times.

Bureau of Indian Affairs: Federal agency responsible for ensuring services to Native Americans, Alaskan Indians, and Eskimo tribes.

C

caida de la mollera: A condition of fallen fontanelle that is thought to occur because the infant was withdrawn too harshly from the nipple; common among some Spanish-speaking populations.

cao gio: Vietnamese practice of placing ointments or hot balm oil across the chest, back, or shoulders and rubbing with a coin. Used to treat colds, sore throats, flu, and sinusitis.

cariñoso(a): Hispanic term denoting caring in both verbal and nonverbal communications.

catimbozeiros: Portuguese word for sorcerer. Can be a folk practitioner.

Celtic: Belonging to a group of Indo-European languages: Irish, Welsh, or Breton.

chesm-i-bad: Iranian term meaning evil eye.

Chicano(a): A Mexican American.

choteo: Cuban term for a lighthearted attitude, involving teasing, bantering, and exaggeration.

Chondo Kyo: Korean naturalistic religion which combines Confucianism, Buddhism, and Daoism.

clan: A division of a tribe tracing descent from a common ancestor.

collectivist culture: A group of people who place a higher value on the family than on the individual.

Colored: A term once used to describe African Americans.

comadre: Portuguese word for godmother.

community: A group or class of people having a common interest or identity living in a specified locality.

compadre: Portuguese term for godfather.

compadrazgo: Spanish for a system of personal relationships in which friends or relatives are considered part of the family whether or not there is a blood relationship.

confianza: Hispanic term for trust developed between individuals, which is essential for effective communication and interpersonal interactions in health-care settings.

conformity: concept with an emphasis on familialism rather than individualism within the Arab culture, conformity to adult rules is favored. Correspondingly, child-rearing methods are oriented toward accommodation and cooperation.

conservative: Jewish term meaning between Reform and Orthodox in terms of religious practice.

contadini: Italian word for peasants.

Copts: Christian Egyptians.

cornicelli: Italian red horns: a symbol of good luck.

cosmology: A branch of philosophy that deals with the origin, processes, and structure of the universe.

Creole: Rich and expressive language derived from two other languages, such as French and Fon, an African tongue.

cross-cultural: Making comparisons between or among cultural groups.

crystal gazer: A Navajo folk healer that interprets dreams.

cultural awareness: Having more to do with an appreciation of the external signs of diversity such as the arts, music, dress, and physical characteristics.

cultural competence: Having an awareness of one's own existence, sensations, thoughts, and environment without letting them have an undue influence on those from other backgrounds. (See Chapter 1 for a more extensive definition.)

cultural diversity: Representing a variety of different cultures.

cultural imperialism: The practice of extending the policies and practices of one organization (usually the dominant one) to disenfranchised and minority groups.

cultural imposition: The intrusive application of the majority cultural view upon individuals and families.

cultural relativism: The belief that the behaviors and practices of people should be judged only from the context of their cultural system.

cultural sensitivity: Having to do with personal attitudes and not saying things that may be offensive to someone from a cultural or ethnic background different from the health-care provider's background.

culturally conscious: Having an awareness of one's own existence, sensations, thoughts, and environment and not letting them have an undue influence over the cultural characteristics of another individual, family, group, or community.

culture: The totality of socially transmitted behavior patterns, arts, beliefs, values, customs, lifeways, and all other products of human work and thought characteristics of a population of people that guides their worldview and decision making. These patterns may be explicit or implicit, are primarily learned and transmitted within the family, and are shared by the majority of the culture.

curandeiro: Portuguese folk practitioner whose healing powers are divinely given.

curandero: A traditional folk practitioner common in Spanish-speaking communities. Treats traditional illness not caused by witchcraft.

D

daadihaus: Amish grandparents' cottage adjacent to farmhouse.

dainos ruta: Lithuanian term for songs.

dan wei: Functional unit of Chinese society. The work unit or the neighborhood unit that is responsible to and for the Chinese people's way of life.

dao: The balance between *yin* and *yang*.

decaimientos: Cuban condition related to tired blood.

decensos: Spanish term for fainting spells.

demut: German for humility, a priority value for the Amish. The effects of which may be seen in details such as the height of the crown of an Amish man's hat, as well as in very general features such as the modest and unassuming bearing and demeanor usually shown by Amish in public. This behavior is reinforced by frequent verbal warnings against its opposite, *hochmut,* pride or arrogance, which is to be avoided.

Diet: The Japanese parliament.

Deitsch: Pennsylvania German, sometimes incorrectly anglicized as Pennsylvania Dutch, an American dialect derived from several uplands and Alemanic German dialects, with an admixture of American English vocabulary.

doing: A state of being actively engaged in an activity for the purpose of accomplishing something.

doog: Yogurt soda (Iranian term).

dozens: A joking relationship between two African Americans in which it is permitted to make fun of each other without taking offense.

dulse: Iodine rich edible seaweed used in clarifying beer and wine and as a suspension medium in some medicines. Also known as Irish moss.

duong: Vietnamese force used in traditional health practice which is associated with things positive, masculine, light, and full.

E

ebo: The sacrificial offering made to establish communication between the spirits and human beings in the Santería religion.

Eid: Iranian term for celebration of a feast; e.g., *Eid Gorgan* (day/feast ending pilgrimage to Mecca; *Eid Fetr* (last day of the month of Ramadan.

Eire: Gaelic name for Ireland.

el ataque/ataque de nervios: A hyperkinetic spasmodic activity common in Spanish-speaking groups. The purpose is to release strong feelings or emotions. The person requires no treatment, and the condition subsides spontaneously. Is an expression of deep anger or depression.

empacho: A condition common among some Spanish speaking populations and is believed to be caused by a bolus of food stuck in the gastrointestinal tract. Massage of the abdomen is thought to relieve the condition.

endropi: Greek word for shame.

escondido: Portuguese term that means hidden and refers to undocumented aliens who remain hidden.

espiritualista (espirituista): Spanish or Portuguese folk practitioners who receive their talent from "God"; they treat conditions thought to be caused by witchcraft.

ethnic group: A group of people who have had different experiences from the dominant culture by status, background, residence, religion, education, or other factors that functionally unify the group and act collectively on each other. Pertaining to a religious, racial, national, or cultural group.

ethnic identity: A subjective sense of social boundary (social emphasis) or a self-definition which answers the question "Who am I?"

ethic of neutrality: Avoiding aggression and assertiveness, not interfering with others' lives unless asked to do so, avoiding dominance over others, and avoiding arguments and seeking agreement.

ethnocentrism: The tendency for human beings to think that our own ways of thinking, acting, and believing are the only right, proper, and natural ones and to believe that those who differ greatly are strange, bizarre, or unenlightened.

ethnocultural: A group of people who have had different experiences from the dominant culture by status, ethnic background, residence, religion, education, or other factors that functionally unify the group and act collectively on each other.

evli: Turkish word for marriage.

F

falling out: A sudden collapse, paralysis, and inability to see or speak. This behavior is noted among African Americans during a funeral or other tragic experiences.

familism: A social pattern where family solidarity and tradition assume a superior position over individual rights and interests.

family: Two or more people who are emotionally involved with each other. They may, but not necessarily, live in close proximity to each other.

fatalism: The acceptance that occurrences in life are predetermined by fate and cannot be changed by human beings.

fatback: A term for salt pork.

fayots: Canadian pea soup in Acadia.

Filipino: Preferred term for someone from the Philippines. Same as Pilipino.

Francophone: People living in Canada using French as their first language.

Frau: German title for a married woman; equivalent to "Mrs." in English.

Fraulein: German title for an unmarried woman; equivalent to "Miss" in English.

freindschaft: Amish three-generational extended family network of relationships.

Freundschaftkarten: German for Groundhog Day.

G

galang: Filipino term for respect.

garm: Iranian term meaning hot.

garmie: Iranian digestive problem caused from eating too much hot food.

gelassenheit: Amish term for submission, yielding, surrender of self and ego to the higher will of the group or deity.

generalization: Reducing numerous characteristics of an individual or group of people to a general form that renders them indistinguishable.

gesprach: German term used for casual conversation.

geophagia: The eating of nonfood substances such as clay, cornstarch, or charcoal during pregnancy.

ghalbam gerefth: Iranian term for distress of the heart.

giac: Vietnamese dermabrasive procedure with cup suctioning.

giagia: Greek word for grandma.

giri: Japanese term for the sense of obligation that exists between people who are socially interconnected.

global society: Seeing the world as one large community of multicultural people.

gohan: Japanese term for rice, particularly the sticky rice that is preferred by Japanese.

gol-i-gov zabon: Iranian term for foxgloves.

Great Eid: Islamic feast of four days.

great potato famine: Time in Ireland (1848–1850s) when the main crop, potatoes, failed; millions of Irish emigrated to escape starvation.

guanxi: Chinese term where relatives are expected to help each other through connections, which are used by Chinese society in a manner similar to the use of money in other cultures.

Gullah: A creole language spoken by African Americans who reside on or near the sea islands off Georgia (e.g., Hilton Head, Myrtle Beach).

H

hadith: The oral tradition of the Prophet Muhammad; collection of words and deeds that form the basis of Muslim law.

Haitians: People from the Caribbean island of Haiti.

Halakha: Jewish laws or commandments.

halal: The lawful: that which is permitted by Allah; also, the term used to describe ritual slaughter of meat.

Han: Largest ethnic group of Chinese

hand trembler: A Navajo traditional healer.

hanyak: Korean traditional herbal medicine used to create harmony between oneself and the larger cosmology and is a healing method for body and soul.

haram: The unlawful: that which is prohibited by Allah; anyone who engages in what is prohibited is liable to incur punishment in the hereafter (as well as legal punishment in countries which incorporate Islamic law into legal codes).

Hasidic: Jewish ultra-Orthodox sect.

health: A state of wellness which is defined by the people within their ethnocultural group and generally includes physical, mental, and spiritual states as they interact with the family, community, and global society.

Hebrew: The language of Israel and Jewish prayer.

hegab: Egyptian amulet kept close to the body to protect against evil eye and bad spirits.

hejab: Iranian term for any behavior that expresses modesty in public; e.g. in women, modest attire (loose dress or head scarf) or shy, self-limiting behavior in relating to the other gender.

Herr: German title equivalent to "Mr." in English.

hijab: Modest covering of a Muslim woman; concealing the head and the body except for the hands and face with loosely fitting, nontransparent clothing.

high blood: Too much blood in circulation in the body or pressure that is too high. Term commonly used by African Americans and Appalachians.

hilot: Filipino folk healer and massage therapist.

hindi ibang tao: Filipino term for insider.

Hinduism: Predominant religion of Asia Indians.

Hispanic: An American of Spanish or Latin American origin.

hiya: Filipino word for shame.

hogan: An earth covered Navajo dwelling.

home: In the Appalachian context, a connectedness to the land more than a physical dwelling.

honor: Spanish term for goodness or virtue, which can be diminished or lost by an immoral or unworthy act.

hot-and-cold theory: Hispanic concept that illness is caused when the body is exposed to an imbalance of hot and cold. Foods are also classified as hot or cold.

humanism: asserts that all human beings are fundamentally equal in worth, that they have common resources, and that they are alike in fundamental ways.

hwangap: At the age of 60 a person starts the calendar cycle over again. This becomes a significant celebration in Korean society.

hwa-byung: Korean traditional illness that occurs from repressing anger or other strong emotions.

I

igang tao: Filipino term for outsider.

individualistic culture: A group of people who place a higher value on the individual than on the family or other group unit.

intercultural: Within a cultural group.

il mal occhio: Italian word for evil eye.

Imam: Muslim leader of the prayer; usually the most learned member of the local Islamic community.

Indian Health Service: Federal agency that has the responsibility for providing health services to Native Americans.

Indochinese: Individuals originating from Viet Nam, Cambodia, or Laos.

insallah: Arabic phrase meaning "if God wills."

insider: Someone who is known to and accepted by the group; usually has special knowledge regarding the values and beliefs of the group.

Islam: A monotheistic religion in which the supreme deity is Allah; according to Muslim belief, God imparted his final revelations—the Holy Qur'an—

through his last prophet, Mohammed, thereby completing Judaism and Christianity.

issei: A first-generation Japanese immigrant.

itami: Japanese term for pain.

itheram: Egyptian word for respect.

J

jenn: Egyptian world for the devil.

jerbero: A Spanish folk practitioner who specializes in treating health conditions through the use of herbal therapy.

jibaro: Puerto Rican word for peasant.

jing: Chinese term for passages throughout the body that are interrelated and connected; includes the 14 meridians called the *jing luo*.

jing luo: Chinese term for organ system.

jing ye: Chinese term for body fluids, including the *jing*, the clear, thin fluids which moisturize the skin and warm the muscles, and the *ye*, the thicker and heavier fluids which moisten the joints.

jinn: In Iran, spirits created by God from smokeless fire; they inhabit a world parallel to that of humans; some are righteous and others are evil.

Joual: French dialect incorporating English words into a syntax and grammar that is essentially French.

K

kaddish: Jewish prayer said for the dead.

kaffeeklatsch: German term for "gossip session."

kampo: Japanese term for East Asian or Chinese medical practices and botanical therapies.

kango-san/kango-fu: Japanese term for registered nurse.

karma: Hindu term for actions performed in the present life and the accumulated affects from past lives.

kashrut or kashrus: Jewish laws that dictate which foods are permissible under religious law.

ki: Japanese term for the energy that flows through living creatures.

kibun: Korean term related to mood, current feelings, and state of mind.

Koran: *See* Qur'an.

kosher: Kashrut laws in the Jewish religion.

koumbari: Greek word for coparents.

L

lace curtain Irish: Name given to Irish in America who left inner city enclaves and moved to the suburbs.

la gente de la raza: A phrase that denotes a genetic determination to which all Spanish speaking people belong, regardless of class differences or place of birth.

Ladino(a): Originally, a person with Jewish and Spanish background.

Latino(a): A person from Latin America.

lavash: Iranian flat thin bread made with wheat.

laying on of hands: A spiritual practice of placing one's hands on an individual for the purpose of healing.

lien: Vietnamese concept that represents control over and responsibility for moral character.

limerick: An Irish humorous poem receiving its name from the County of Limerick in Ireland.

low blood: Too little blood, too low blood count, or too thin blood. Term is commonly used by African Americans and Appalachians.

M

maalesh: Arabic term meaning "never mind, it doesn't matter"; substantial efforts are directed at maintaining pleasant relationships and preserving dignity and honor; hostility in response to perceived wrongdoing is warded off by an attitude of *maalesh*.

machismo: A sense of masculinity that stresses virility, courage, and domination of women. Includes the need to display physical strength, bravery, and virility.

madichon: Haitian term used to indicate that a child's future will be marred by misfortune because he or she has disrespected his or her elders.

magissa: Greek folk healer.

mai: One of the elements of traditional Chinese medicine that encompasses the Chinese pulses and vessels.

mal ojo: Spanish for the "evil eye," a hex condition with unspecific signs and symptoms thought to be caused by an older person admiring a younger person. The condition can be reversed if the person doing the admiring touches the person being admired.

masallah: Turkish word meaning may "God bless and protect."

marielitos: Cuban immigrants who arrived in 1980 on a massive boatlift from Muriel Harbor to Key West, Florida.

matiasma: Greek work for the evil eye.

Matka Boska: Poland's patroness to help in time of need. Literally means "mother of God."

Métis: People of mixed Native American and European, especially French Canadian, heritage.

mezaj: Iranian term for a person's humoral temperament.

mezuzah: A container with Biblical writings; placed on the doorpost of homes or hung around the neck on a necklace.

mestizo(a): A person of mixed Spanish and Native American heritage.

Mezzogiorno: Southern Italy.

mien: Vietnamese concept that is based on wealth and power.

mikveh: Jewish term for a ritual bath, after a woman's menstrual period is over.

minyan: Ten adults needed for prayer in the Jewish faith.

Mohel: Ritual circumciser in the Jewish faith.

moreno: Portuguese individual who has black or brown hair and dark eyes.

morita therapy: An indigenous Japanese school of psychotherapy.

mosque: Muslim place of worship.

Moslem: *See* Muslim

moxibustion: Vietnamese health-care practice where pulverized wormwood is heated and placed directly on the skin at specified meridians to counter conditions associated with excess cold.

mukrah: Arabic term meaning undesirable but not forbidden.

mulatto: Person of mixed European and African heritage.

mundang: Korean folk healer who has special abilities for communicating with the spirits and in treating illnesses after all other means of treatment are exhausted.

muska: Turkish tradition of writing a prayer on a piece of paper, wrapping it in fabric, and hidden in the home or worn by a person seeking help for emotional problems.

Muslim: Person who follows the Islamic faith, the second largest world religion.

Mohammed: Prophet of God and founder of Islam.

N

nabat: Iranian concentrated sugar used for treating stomach upsets.

naharati: Iranian term meaning generalized distress.

Navajo neuropathy: A neurological condition confined to Navajo Indians; characterized by a complete absence of myelinated fibers resulting in short stature, sexual infantilism, systemic infection, hypotonia, areflexia, loss of sensation in the extremities, corneal ulcerations, acral mutilation, and painless fractures.

nazar: Turkish word for envy.

nazar boncuk: Small blue bead used among Turkish people to protect a child from the evil eye.

nevra: Greek folk illness.

nervioso(a): Hispanic term used to describe signs and symptoms of nervousness, anxiety, sadness, and grief.

Neshasteh: Wheat starch is combined with boiling water and drunk for sore throats or coughs and also used to stop diarrhea.

Nihon/Nippon: The name for Japan in Japanese.

Nihonjin: Japanese term for a native of Japan.

nisei: Japanese term for the second generation of an immigrant family.

Niuyorican: Term used to identify the cultural pride of Puerto Rican generations born and reared in New York.

noruz or norooz: Iranian New Year, non-Islamic, first day of spring.

nubians: Black Egyptians living around and south of Aswan.

O

o-bento: Japanese term for box lunch.

obi: The sash for a Japanese kimono or an abdominal binder.

o-cha: Japanese term for green tea.

office lady: A young woman who works in a Japanese office providing hospitality to visitors and performing limited clerical functions.

o-furo: The Japanese bath.

Old Order Amish: Most conservative and traditionalist group among the followers of Jacob Ammann, today simply called Amish, but technically known as Old Order Amish Mennonite, to distinguish them from other related Amish and Mennonite groups.

onore della famiglia: Italian term for family honor.

oplatek: Polish wafer that everyone shares and is served at Christmas time.

oppression: Haitian aliment related to asthma and describes a state of anxiety and hyperventilation.

ordnung: The codified rules and regulations that govern the behavior of a local Amish church district, or congregation, local consensus of faith and practice. Also the German term for order.

orishas: The gods or spirits in Santería.

orthodox: Traditional Judaism.

o-shogatsu: The Japanese New Year celebrated for several days around January 1.

outsider: Someone who is not known to members of the group and assumed that they do not have the special knowledge regarding the values and beliefs that an insider has.

P

padrone: Italian word for master, head of the family.

pabasa: Filipino term for novena.

pakikisama: Filipino term for yielding to the leader or the majority.

pakiramdam: Filipino term for shared inner feeling with another person.

pappous: Greek word for grandfather.

patrao: Portuguese term for employer.

pazienza: Italian word for patience/long suffering.

person: A human being who is constantly adapting to their environment biologically, psychologically, and socially.

personalismo: Spanish word for emphasis on intimate, personal relationships as more important than impersonal, bureaucratic relationships.

philptimo: Greek work for respect.

phylacto: Greek amulet worn to ward off envy.

Pilipino: Filipino word for Filipino.

pidgin: A simplified language used for communicating between speakers of different languages.

pogrom: Organized persecution or massacre of a minority group.

Polish question: The discussion between Stalin, Churchill, and Roosevelt at the Potsdam and Malta Conferences as to what to do with Poland after World War II.

Polonia: Communities heavily occupied by Polish immigrants and descendants of Polish Nationals.

postmodernism: holds the stance that everything is social construction, which leads to contention that context is all important.

practika: Greek herbal remedies.

primary characteristics of culture: the primary characteristics of culture are nationality, race, color, gender, age, and religious affiliation.

pseudofamilies: Vietnamese households made up of close and distant relatives and friends that share accommodations, finances, and fellowship.

Pu tong hua: The recognized language of China.

Q

Quebecer: Descendant of early French settlers, now living in Quebec Province, Canada.

qi: One of five substances or elements of Traditional Chinese Medicine encompassing the foundation of the energy of the body, environment, and universe. Includes all sources and expenditures of energy.

Qur'an: (also Koran) Muslim holy book; believed by Muslims to contain God's final revelations to mankind.

R

rabbi: Jewish religious leader.

race: having to do with genetic differences such as blood type, skin color, and other physical characteristics.

refugee: Someone who flees from their home country due to political, religious, or other type of oppression. The host country assigns refugee status.

Ramadan: The ninth month of the Islamic year during which Muslims are required to fast during daylight hours for thirty days.

reconstructionism: a mosaic of the three main branches of Judaism and is as an evolving religion of the Jewish people and seeks to adapt Jewish beliefs and practices to the needs of the contemporary world.

refakatci: Turkish word for someone who stays overnight in the hospital with a sick person.

reform: Liberal/progressive Judaism.

remedios caserios: Portuguese (Brazilian) home medicine or remedy.

remedios populares: Portuguese (Brazilian) folk medicine practitioner.

respeto: Hispanic term denoting respect; refers to the qualities developed for others such as parents, the elderly, and educated people who are expected to be honored, admired, and respected,

ruta: Plant having a special place in Lithuanian gardens.

S

Saiidis: Egyptian group living south of Cairo.

sake: Japanese rice wine, used ritually as well as socially.

salary man: Japanese term for a white male worker or company man.

sand painting: Navajo art work originally designed on the hogan floor and then destroyed and returned to the earth. Currently, sand paintings are created and sold commercially.

sansei: Japanese term for the third generation of an immigrant family.

Santería: A 300-year-old Afro-Cuban religion that syncretizes Roman Catholic elements with ancient Yoruba tribal beliefs and practices.

santero: A practitioner of Santería.

sard: Iranian term meaning cold.

sardie: Iranian digestive problem from eating too much cold food.

secondary characteristics of culture: Includes educational status, socioeconomic status, occupation, military experience, political beliefs, urban/rural residence, enclave identity, marital status, parental status, physical characteristics, sexual orientation, gender issues, and reason for migration (sojourner, immigrant, or undocumented status).

Sensei: Japanese term for "master," used to address teachers, physicians, or those in seniority in a corporate setting.

sephardic: Jewish term for being descended from Spain, Portugal, the Mediterranean, Africa, or Central and South America.

settlement: Aggregation of Amish church districts, usually the result of intentional geographical grouping.

severe combined immune deficiency syndrome: An immune deficiency syndrome (unrelated to AIDS), characterized by a failure of antibody response and cell mediated immunity.

shanty Irish: Term describing Irish who lived in urban Irish ethnic enclaves.

shen: One of five substances or elements of Traditional Chinese Medicine encompassing the spirit.

shaitsu: Japanese term for acupressure therapy.

Shinto: The indigenous religion of Japan.

sikkeenah: Egyptian word for knife.

simpatia: Spanish term for smooth interpersonal relationships, characterized by courtesy, respect, and the absence of harsh criticism or confrontation.

sit a spell: Process of engaging in nonhierarchical relaxed conversation in order to get to know the beliefs and feelings of others.

Small Eid: Islamic holy feast of three days.

sobador: A Spanish folk practitioner similar to a chiropractor who treats illnesses and conditions affecting the joints and musculoskeletal system.

sojourner: Someone who relocates with the intention of remaining only a short time and then returning home.

solidao: Portuguese word for loneliness.

solidarity: A union of interests, purposes, and sympathies promoting fellowship with Polish nationals.

soul food: Traditional diet of African Americans.

Spanglish: Sentence structure that includes both English and Spanish words.

speaking in tongues: Praying in a language that is not understood by anyone except the person reciting the prayer.

stereotyping: An oversimplified conception, opinion, or belief about some aspect of an individual or group of people.

sto lat: Polish phrase meaning that the celebrant should live a hundred years.

subculture: A group of people who have had different experiences from the dominant culture by status, ethnic background, residence, religion, education, or other factors that functionally unify the group and act collectively on each other.

susto: "Magical fright," a condition thought to be caused by witchcraft; symptoms can be quite varied and include both mental and physical concerns.

synagogue: Jewish house of worship.

T

ta'arof: Iranian ritual expressing courtesy.

tabi'at: Iranian term for a person's makeup, nature, or genetic build.

tae kyo: Korean word that literally means "fetus education," with the objective being health and well-being of fetus and mother through art, beautiful objects, and a serene environment.

tae mong: Korean term that signifies the beginning of pregnancy. The pregnant woman dreams of conception of the fetus.

Tagalog: Filipino national language.

tagdir: Iranian term for destiny, future mapped out by powers greater than oneself, beyond individual control.

Taglish: Dialect mixing English and Tagalog.

tatami: Traditional Japanese floor coverings made out of straw.

Tet: Asian Lunar New Year celebrated in January or February.

Torah: The five books of Moses. Referred to in the Jewish faith.

transcultural: making comparisons for similarities and differences between cultures.

treyf: Jewish term for forbidden or unclean.

tribe: A Native American social organization comprising several local villages, bands, districts, lineages, or other groups who share a common ancestry, language, and culture.

Tridosha: Theory that the body is made up of five elements: fire, air, space, water, and earth.

Turkiye: Turkish word for the country, Turkey.

tzedakah: Jewish term that means righteousness and sharing and is a central concept to Judaism; commonly used to indicate charity.

U

universal ethics: the belief that each culture decides what is right or wrong and what is good or bad.

utang na loob: Filipino term for gratitude.

V

values: Principles and standards that have meaning and worth to an individual, family, group, or community. Associated with what is important to a cultural or ethnic group or individual.

velorio: Spanish term for a wake; a festive occasion following the burial of a person.

vendouses: Greek practice of cupping.

verguenza: Spanish term for a consciousness of public opinion and the judgment of the entire community.

viandas: Spanish term for root vegetables.

via nuova: Italian word for new way.

via vecchia: Italian word for old way.

visiting: High frequency custom of family-to-family home visits that help to maintain kinship and church ties and the flow of information within the Amish community.

voudou/voodoo: Vibrant religion born from slavery and revolt; the word means "sacred" in the African language of Fon.

W

waham: Egyptian word for cravings during pregnancy.

wake: A watch over a deceased person before burial and is usually accompanied by a celebration, which may include feasting.

warm hands: Healing art related to therapeutic touch, regarded by Amish as a gift to be applied for the good of others in need of healing, a form of brauche.

wesel: Polish phrase for a wedding sequence.

Western ethics: The beliefs that are held by individualistic societies can be applied to all cultural groups.

wetback: A derogatory term applied to undocumented aliens of Mexican or Latin American descent.

wind: A classification for Vietnamese foods that is closely related to cold foods.

witchcraft: A belief that illness or harm can come to you via supernatural forces.

worldview: The way an individual or group of people look upon their universe to form values about their life and the world around them.

X

xue: One of five substances or elements of Traditional Chinese Medicine encompassing the blood

Y

yarmulke: Jewish head covering.

yang: In Chinese belief system, it is one of two opposing principles of the balance of life; it can be either a single phenomenon or a state of being of a phenomenon. *See also yin.*

yangban: Korean term meaning upper class.

yerbero: Same as *Jerbero.*

Yiddish: A language often spoken by elderly Jews.

yin: In Chinese belief system it is one of two opposing principles of the balance of life; it can be either a single phenomenon or a state of being of a phenomenon. *See also yang.*

Z

zaher: Iranian term for public persona.

zang fu: Chinese term for the tissues of the bones, tendons, flesh, blood vessels, and skin.

zeranghi: Iranian term for cleverness.

zar: An Egyptian trans-meditative ceremony.

zong: Vietnamese herbal preparation which relieves motion sickness or cold related problems.

Zhong guo: The principal term used to denote China; other Chinese words are added to this term to denote Chinese, Chinese language, and Chinese people.

Index

Page numbers followed by *b* indicates boxes; those followed by *f* indicate figures; and those followed by *t* indicate tables.